Evidence-based Sports Medicine

Second Edition

Evidence-based Sports Medicine

Second Edition

Edited by

Domhnall MacAuley
Visiting Professor
Faculty of Life and Health Science
University of Ulster
Belfast
United Kingdom
Specialist in Sport and Exercise Medicine

and

Thomas M. Best
Professor and Pomerene Chair in Family Medicine
Chief, Division of Sports Medicine
Ohio State University
Columbus
Ohio
USA

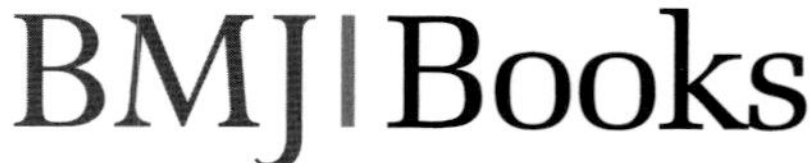

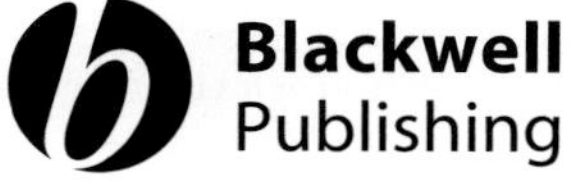

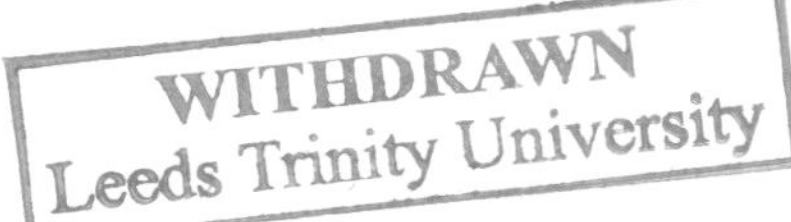

BMJ Books is an imprint of the BMJ Publishing Group Limited, used under licence

Blackwell Publishing, Inc., 350 Main Street, Malden, Massachusetts 02148-5020, USA
Blackwell Publishing Ltd, 9600 Garsington Road, Oxford OX4 2DQ, UK
Blackwell Publishing Asia Pty Ltd, 550 Swanston Street, Carlton, Victoria 3053, Australia

First published 2002
Second edition 2007

2 2008

Library of Congress Cataloging-in-Publication Data

Evidence-based sports medicine / edited by Domhnall MacAuley and Thomas M. Best.—2nd ed.
p. ; cm.
Includes bibliographical references and index.
ISBN 978-1-4051-3298-5 (hbk. : alk. paper)
1. Sports medicine. 2. Evidence-based medicine. I. MacAuley, Domhnall. II. Best, Thomas M.
[DNLM: 1. Athletic Injuries—therapy. 2. Evidence-Based Medicine. QT 261 E93 2007]
RC1210.E925 2007
617.1′027—dc22

2006025870

A catalogue record for this title is available from the British Library

Set in 9.5/12pt Minion by Graphicraft Limited, Hong Kong
Printed and bound in Singapore by Fabulous Printers Pte Ltd

Commissioning Editor: Mary Banks
Editorial Assistant: Victoria Pittman
Development Editor: Lauren Brindley
Production Controller: Rachel Edwards

For further information on Blackwell Publishing, visit our web site:
http://www.blackwellpublishing.com

The publisher's policy is to use permanent paper from mills that operate a sustainable forestry policy, and which has been manufactured from pulp processed using acid-free and elementary chlorine-free practices. Furthermore, the publisher ensures that the text paper and cover board used have met acceptable environmental accreditation standards.

Contents

Updates website: www.evidbasedsportsmedicine.com

Contributors

Roald Bahr, MD, PhD

Oslo Sports Trauma Research Center, Norwegian School of Sport Sciences, PO Box 4014, Ulleval Stadion, 0806 Oslo, Norway

Graham Bailie, FRCS (Tr & Orth), MMedSci

Specialist Registrar in Orthopaedic Surgery, Royal Victoria Hospital, Grosvenor Road, Belfast BT12 6BA, UK

Kim Bennell, BAppSci(physio), PhD

Centre for Health, Exercise and Sports Medicine, Faculty of Medicine, Dentistry and Health Sciences, University of Melbourne, Parkville, Victoria 3010, Australia

Thomas M. Best, MD, PhD, FACSM

Professor and Pomerene Chair in Family Medicine; Chief, Division of Sports Medicine; Director, Primary Care Sports Medicine Fellowship; Medical Director, The OSU Sports Medicine Center, The Ohio State University, 2050 Kenny Road, Pavilion, Suite 3100, Columbus, OH 43221, USA

Chris Bleakley, PhD, BSc, MCSP, SRP

Physiotherapist and Research Associate, University of Ulster, Shore Road, Jordanstown, Co. Antrim BT37 0QB, UK

Peter Brukner, MBBS, FRACSP

Centre for Health, Exercise and Sports Medicine, Faculty of Medicine, Dentistry and Health Sciences, University of Melbourne, Parkville, Victoria 3010, Australia

A. John Campbell

Professor of Geriatric Medicine, Department of Medical and Surgical Sciences, University of Otago Medical School, PO Box 913, Dunedin, New Zealand

Peter J. Carek, MD, MS

Director, Trident/MUSC Family Medicine Residency Program, Professor Department of Family Medicine, Medical University of South Carolina, 9298 Medical Plaza Drive, Charleston, SC 29406, USA

Jill L. Cook, BApp Sci(Phty), Phd

Associate Professer, Musculoskeletal Research Centre, La Trobe University, Bundoora, Victoria 3086, Australia

Matthew W. Cooke, PhD, FRCS(Ed), FCEM, DipIMC

Professor of Emergency Medicine, Warwick Medical School, Medical School Building, Gibbe Campus, Coventry CV4 7AL, and Heart of England NHS Foundation NHS Trust, UK

Ian Corry, MD, FRCS (Orth), Dip Sports Med

Consultant Orthopaedic Surgeon, Royal Victoria Hospital, Grosvenor Road, Belfast BT12 6BA, UK

Andrew Currie, BSc (Hons)

Graduate Medical Student, Warwick Medical School, Medical School Building, Gibbet Hill Campus, Coventry CV4 7AL, UK

Joanne Dear, BSc (Hons), MSc

Senior Research Fellow, Research Centre, The British School of Osteopathy, 275 Borough High Street, London SE1 1JE, UK

David J. Deehan

Department of Orthopaedics, Freeman Hospital, Freeman Road, High Heaton, Newcastle upon Tyne NE7 7DN, UK

William W. Dexter, MD, FACSM

Director, Sports Medicine Program, Maine Medical Center, 272 Congress Street, Portland, ME 04101, USA

William R. Donaldson, MD

Clinical Professor, Department of Orthopedics, Tufts–New England Medical Center, 750 Washington Street, Box 143, Boston, MA 02111, USA

Fredrick J. Dorey, PhD

Adjunct Professor, Department of Orthopedic Surgery, University of California, Los Angeles, CA 90095, USA

Anthony Festa, MD

Chief Resident, Department of Orthopaedic Surgery, Tufts-New England Medical Center, 750 Washington Street, Box 143, Boston MA, O2111, USA

Anastasia M. Fischer, MD

Sports Medicine Program, Maine Medical Center, 272 Congress Street, Portland, ME 04101, USA

Peter A. Fricker, OAM, MBBS, FACSP, FRACP (Hon)

Director of Medical Services, Australian Institute of Sport, Leverrier Crescent, Bruce, ACT 2617, Australia

Simon P. Frostick, MA, DM, FRCS

Professor of Orthopaedics, Department of Musculoskeletal Science, The Royal Liverpool University Hospitals, Liverpool L69 3GA, UK

Michael J. Hayton, BSc (Hons), MB.ChB, FRCS (Orth)

Consultant Orthopaedic Surgeon, Wrightington Hospital, Hall Lane, Appley Bridge, Wigan WN6 9EP, UK

Bryan Heiderscheit, PT, PhD

Assistant Professor, Department of Orthopedics and Rehabilitation, University of Wisconsin School of Medicine and Public Health, 1300 University Avenue, 4120 MSC, Madison, WI 53706-1532, USA

Stanley A. Herring, MD

Clinical Professor, Departments of Rehabilitation Medicine, Orthopaedics and Sports Medicine, and Neurological Surgery, Harborview Medical Center, University of Washington, 325 Ninth Avenue, Seattle, WA, USA

Duncan Hodge, MD

Department of Orthopedic Surgery, Northern California Permanente Medical Group, Walnut Creek Medical Center, 1425 S. Main Street, Medical Office Building, 1st Floor, Walnut Creek, CA 94596, USA

Jennifer M. Hootman, PhD, ATC, FACSM

Epidemiologist, Arthritis Program, Division of Adult and Community Health, Centers for Disease Control and Prevention, 4770 Buford Highway NE, Mailstop K-51, Atlanta, GA 30341, USA

Deiary Kader, MD, FRCS (Tr&Orth)

Consultant Orthopaedic Surgeon, Queen Elizabeth Hospital, Gateshead, Tyne and Wear, NE9 6SX, UK

Anne-Maree Keenan, BAppSc (Pod), MAppSc

Academic Unit of Musculoskeletal Medicine, University of Leeds, Chapel Allerton Hospital, Chapeltown Road, Leeds LS7 4SA, UK

Karim M. Khan, MD, PhD

Department of Family Practice, School of Human Kinetics, University of British Columbia, 211/2150 Western Parkway, Vancouver, BC V6T 1Z6, Canada

Bart Koes

Professor of General Practice, Department of General Practice, Erasmus University Medical Center, Rotterdam, PO Box 1738, 3000 DR Rotterdam, The Netherlands

Karl B. Landorf, DipAppSc (Pod), GradDipEd, PhD

Senior Lecturer and Research Coordinator, Department of Podiatry, Faculty of Health Sciences, La Trobe University, Bundoora, Victoria 3086, Australia

Jeremy Lewis, PhD, MCSP, MAPA, MMACP, MMPA

Consultant Shoulder Physiotherapist, St. George's Hospital, London, UK Visiting Reader, St. George's University of London, Research Lead, Therapy Department, Chelsea and Westminster Hospital, London, UK

Greg Lovell, MBBS, Dip, DHM, FACSP, FASMF

Sports Physician, Department of Sports Medicine, Australian Institute of Sport, Leverrier Crescent, Bruce, ACT 2617, Australia

Domhnall MacAuley, MD, FRCGP, FFPHMI, FFSEM

Visiting Professor, Faculty of Life and Health Science, University of Ulster, and Specialist in Sport and Exercise Medicine, Hillhead Family Practice, 33 Stewartstown Road, Belfast BT11 9FZ, UK

Christopher A. McGrew, MD

Department of Orthopedics and Rehabilitation, and Department of Family and Community Medicine, University of New Mexico Health Sciences Center, 2211 Lomas Boulevard NE, Albuquerque, NM 87106, USA

Paul McCrory, MBBS, PhD, FRACP, FACSP, FACSM, FASMF, GradDipEpidStats

Neurologist and Sports Physician, Centre for Health, Exercise and Sports Medicine, University of Melbourne, Parkville, Victoria 3010, Australia

Nicola Maffulli, MD, MS, PhD, FRCS(Orth)

Professor of Trauma and Orthopaedic Surgery, Department of Trauma and Orthopaedic Surgery, Keele University School of Medicine, Thornburrow Drive, Hartshill, Stoke on Trent, Staffs ST4 7QB, UK

Gladys Onambele-Pearson, BSc, MSc, PhD

Research Fellow, Department of Exercise and Sports Science, Institute for Biophysical and Clinical Research into Human Movement, Manchester Metropolitan University, Hassall Road, Alsager, Stoke on Trent ST7 2HL, UK

Joanna Picot

Medical Researcher, Wessex Institute for Health Research and Development, Mailpoint 728, University of Southampton, Bolderwood SO16 7PX, UK

Felix S.F. Ram

Senior Lecturer in Respiratory Medicine and Clinical Pharmacology, School of Health Sciences, Massey University-Auckland, Private Bag 102 904, North Shore Mail Centre, Auckland, New Zealand

John C. Richmond, MD

Chairman, Department of Orthopaedic Surgery, New England Baptist Hospital, 125 Parker Hill Avenue, Boston MA 02120, USA

M. Clare Robertson

Research Associate Fellow, Department of Medical and Surgical Sciences, University of Otago Medical School, PO Box 913, Dunedin, New Zealand

Gerald Ryan, MD

Associate Professor, Department of Family Medicine, University of Wisconsin Medical School, 777 S Mills Street, Madison, WI 53715, USA

John M. Ryan, FRCSEd (A&E), FCEM, FFSEM, DCH, DipSportsMed

Consultant in Emergency Medicine, Emergency Department, St. Vincent's University Hospital, Elm Park, Dublin 4, Ireland

Raymond A. Sachs, MD

Department of Orthopedic Surgery, Southern California Permanente Medical Group, San Diego, and Assistant Clinical Professor of Orthopedic Surgery, University of California, 350 Dickinson Street, San Diego, CA 92103, USA

Marc R. Safran, MD

Associate Professor, Department of Orthopedic Surgery, University of California at San Francisco, 500 Parnassus Avenue, Box 0728, San Francisco, CA 94143, USA

Alasdair J.A. Santini, FRCS(Glasg,Eng), FRCS(Orth)

Consultant Orthopaedic Surgeon, The Royal Liverpool and Broadgreen University Hospitals, Liverpool L69 3GA, UK

Marc Sherry, PT, LAT, CSCS

Senior Physical Therapist and Athletic Trainer, University of Wisconsin Sports Medicine Clinic, Research Park Clinic, 621 Science Drive, Madison, WI 53711, USA

Ian Shrier MD, PhD, Dip Sport Med, FACSM

Past-president, Canadian Academy of Sport Medicine, and Associate Professor McGill University, Centre for Clinical Epidemiology and Community Studies, SMBD-Jewish General Hospital, 3755 Côte Ste-Catherine Road, Montreal, Quebec H3T 1E2, Canada

Christopher J. Standaert, MD

Clinical Assistant Professor, Departments of Rehabilitation Medicine, Orthopedics and Sports Medicine, and Neurological Surgery, Harborview Medical Center, University of Washington, 325 Ninth Avenue, Seattle, WA, USA

T. Duncan Tennent, FRCS (Orth)

Consultant Orthopaedic Surgeon, St. George's Hospital, Blackshaw Road, London SW17 0QT, and Honorary Senior Lecturer, St. George's Hospital Medical School, London, UK

Martin Underwood

Professor of General Practice, Institute of Community Health Sciences, Barts and the London Medical School, Queen Mary's School of Medicine and Dentistry, Queen Mary, University of London, Abernethy Building, Mile End, London E1 2AT, UK

Daniëlle van der Windt, PhD

Department of General Practice, EMGO Instituut, Vrije Universiteit Medical Centre, van der Boechorststraat 7, 1081 BT Amsterdam, The Netherlands and Primary Care Musculoskeletal Research Centre, Keele University, Keele, Staffordshire ST5 5BG, UK

C. Niek van Dijk

Department of Orthopedic Surgery, Academic Medical Center, Meibergdreef 9, PO Box 22660, 1100 DD, Amsterdam, The Netherlands

Abel Wakai, MD, FRCSI

Specialist Registrar in Emergency Medicine, Emergency Department, St. Vincent's University Hospital, Elm Park, Dublin 4, Ireland

Weiya Zhang, BSc, MSc, PhD

Associate Professor of Musculoskeletal Epidemiology, Academic Rheumatology, University of Nottingham, Clinical Sciences Building, City Hospital, Nottingham NG5 1PB, UK

Preface

It was perhaps only a decade ago that a formal definition of evidence-based medicine (EBM) was clearly articulated.[1] Sport and exercise medicine is now taking its place as an equal with other specialties in the era of EBM. As the quality of research improves and the knowledge base widens, it is now increasingly possible to base one's clinical decisions on higher-level evidence. Evidence-based sports medicine, once a new term, is no longer such a surprising expression, and we have become much more selective in our acceptance of original research and review articles. Anecdote has given way to evidence, opinion has given ground to research, and patients expect us to help guide their decisions on the basis of the latest findings in the literature. Best practice does not mean how you have learned to practice—it means learning from the best available evidence.

Sports-medicine practitioners have begun to look more closely at their own practice and question what they do. It may not have been doctors who were first to recognize the importance of evidence-based decision-making; our physiotherapy colleagues were perhaps the pioneers. But as we began to audit our practice, we began to realize the value of data and to see the potential for measuring our performance. The growth of university departments of sport and exercise medicine and the academic development of the discipline has led to a much better understanding of the importance of research. Journals now have a much sharper focus on the quality of the papers they publish. The methodological quality of published research has paralleled the interest in evidence-based medicine in our discipline. Prospective data collection, randomization, blinding, and appropriate control groups are continuing to find their way into a greater number of studies. And along with the increasing numbers of randomized controlled trials, there is now an opportunity to synthesize these findings and bring them together in systematic reviews of the literature. The process of systematic review assists the sports-medicine practitioner in interpreting study results and in understanding the relative validity of these results in the hierarchy of evidence. Whereas in the past we might have been satisfied with a narrative review, we now look for meta-analyses and systematic reviews.

The science of the systematic review has also evolved, and through efforts of the Cochrane Collaboration we now have well-established guidelines on how to undertake systematic reviews. Similarly, our colleagues in Australia have developed the PEDro database, a truly innovative concept in sport and exercise medicine. There are now well-accepted guidelines in systematic reviews. The *British Medical Journal* recommends reporting using the guidelines of the QUORUM group. There are recognized methods of selecting appropriate evidence, and we now grade the evidence.

It is our hope that the second edition of this book has captured the evolution and maturity of evidence-based sports medicine. In clinical practice, caring for patients generates many questions about diagnosis, prognosis, and treatment that should challenge all of us to keep abreast of the current literature. Conscientiously practicing EBM is one way to ensure that clinicians keep up to date with the exponential growth in the medical literature. This should be an ongoing exercise designed to improve our skills in asking questions, finding the best evidence, critically appraising it, integrating it with our clinical expertise and our patients' unique features, and applying the results to clinical practice. The best available clinical evidence is typically derived from clinical research that is patient-centered, that evaluates the accuracy and precision of diagnostic tests and prognostic markers, and takes into account the efficacy and safety of therapeutic, rehabilitative, and preventive regimens.

All of our authors were asked to provide the latest up-to-date and highest-quality research that answered a specific question. As can be seen, we still have level 4 or level 5 evidence for many of these questions. In other cases, a number of level 1 studies are now available that provide the basis for a structured systematic review. A new feature of this second edition is a greater emphasis on the reliability and validity of the clinical examination, perhaps somewhat of a lost art in today's practice of "high-technology" medicine. Many of the pearls we were taught in our younger days have never been properly evaluated and instead were accepted as dogma because an authoritative professor, through his or her name or stature alone, convinced us this was the right way to do things. For example, we now recognize that a clinician's use of tests relies heavily on pretest clinical assessment.[2] We have also tried to maintain consistency with the first edition by asking each author to provide key summary points and questions that address critical take-home messages.

In no way does this collection of 30 chapters do complete justice to the progress made in EBM and sports medicine. Topics were selected that we felt best illustrated the growth of our field and the potential for future research—we still have a long way to go! Our hope is that both undergraduate students and busy practitioners will read this book and become more engaged in the application of EBM to sports medicine. We appreciate the time and effort made by our authors, and we wish you success in the classroom and in your practice.

Domhnall MacAuley
Thomas M. Best

References

1 Sackett DL, Rosenberg WM, Gray JA, Haynes RB, Richardson WS. Evidence based medicine: what it is and what it isn't. *BMJ* 1996; **312**:71–72.

2 Straus SE, Sackett DL. Using research findings in clinical practice. *BMJ* 1998; **317**:339–342.

SECTION 1
Prevention

CHAPTER 1

Is it possible to prevent sports and recreation injuries? A systematic review of randomized controlled trials, with recommendations for future work

Jennifer M. Hootman

Introduction

To determine whether the prevention of sports injuries merits the attention of the public health authorities and clinical institutions, we need to know whether sports and recreation injuries are a substantial problem, and if so, whether there are factors that can be changed in order to remedy the problem. Figure 1.1 illustrates a sports injury prevention model, the "sequence of prevention," first proposed by van Mechelen and colleagues[1] and used by others to illustrate the process and to promote the critical need for advances in sports injury prevention.[2–7] Some advances have already been seen, including the First World Congress on Sports Injury Prevention (convened in Oslo, Norway in June 2005), special journal supplements focusing on sports injury prevention, and multiple reviews on the topic.[2,5,6] In this chapter, I will review and update the scientific evidence on the topic of sports injury prevention, attempting to answer the question: "Is it possible to prevent sports injuries?"

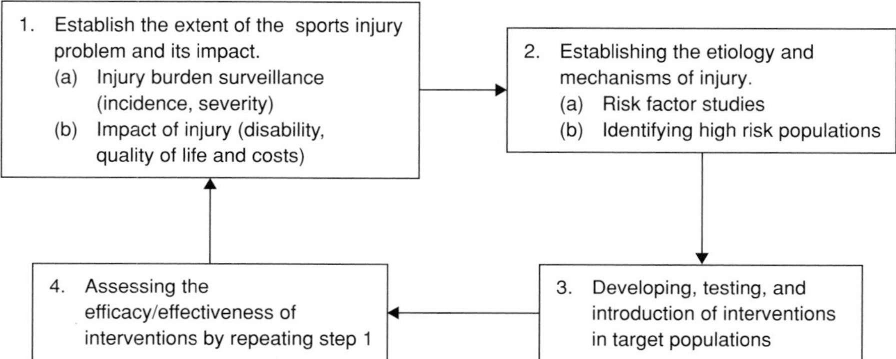

Figure 1.1 A modified version of the "sequence of prevention," an injury prevention model proposed by van Mechelen and colleagues (adapted with permission from ref. 1).

Methods

Inclusion/exclusion criteria

The following inclusion and exclusion criteria were developed and used for computerized bibliographic database searches and to define the final studies to be included in the review.

Inclusion criteria

- *Age range:* all.
- *Publications:* English-language, 1980–July 2005.
- *Interventions:* clinical or community-based, randomized controlled trials.
- *Outcomes:* injury frequency or rates, incidence of injury, hazard ratios; with or without exposure time data.
- *Sport:* sports and recreation activities, including school (interscholastic, intercollegiate, and intramural), community-based activities (Little League, soccer leagues, etc.), recreational individual sports (tennis, skiing, etc.), or team sports (volleyball, soccer, rugby, etc.).

Exclusion criteria

- Fall-related hip fractures.
- Military populations—specifically, recruits in basic or advanced training. Studies including students at U.S. military academies who participate in intramural or intercollegiate athletes were eligible.
- Bicycling (recreational and competitive) and other wheeled activities (skateboarding, scooters, rollerblading, etc.).

Retrieval of published studies

A comprehensive computer bibliographic database search was conducted using MEDLINE, EMBASE and the Cumulative Index to Nursing and Allied Health Literature (CINAHL) for the dates 1980 through July 2005. The search terms used included: 1, "injury" OR "trauma" AND 2, "sports" OR "exercise" OR "athletic" OR "athlete," AND 3, "prevention," and were combined with the Cochrane highly sensitive search strategy for randomized controlled trials (RCTs).[8] The final search results were limited to English-language publications. Figure 1.2 illustrates the subsequent flow of the study selection process. All abstracts identified in the bibliographic search (n = 172) were read and evaluated according to the *a priori* inclusion/exclusion criteria. Any study not explicitly meeting the stated exclusion criteria at this stage was kept for further review. Complete copies of the 27 studies selected at this stage were requested through interlibrary loan. Hand searching of the reference lists of the 27 papers received, as well as the reference lists of select review papers[3,9–12] yielded another 22 potentially relevant papers. Of the 49 total papers identified, one was immediately excluded because it was a duplicate publication from the same study. The remaining 48 papers were evaluated a final time using a checklist of the inclusion/exclusion criteria stated above. This stage excluded 21 papers, leaving 27 RCTs for inclusion in this review.

Quality assessment

Each study meeting the inclusion criteria was evaluated using the methodological quality scoring scale developed by Jadad *et al.*,[13] with slight modifications. The three-item Jadad scale is an easy-to-use scale, with established psychometric properties, that assesses each study with regard to randomization, double-blinding, and reporting of withdrawals

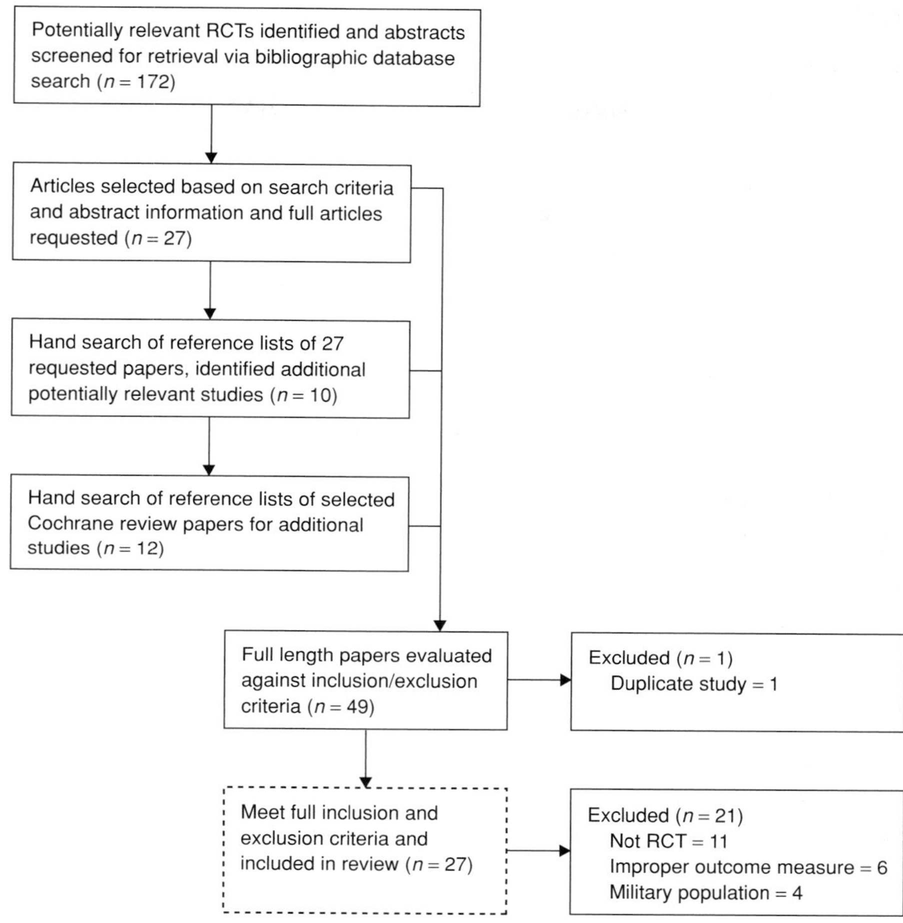

Figure 1.2 Flow chart of study selection for randomized controlled trials (RCTs) included in the review.

or participants lost to follow-up. The total score ranges from a minimum of 0 to a maximum of 5.

Since it is impossible to blind participants to select types of interventions used in sports medicine (e.g., exercise, braces, etc.), the second criterion regarding double-blinding was modified for this study. Studies received one point if the methods stated that the person or persons doing the assessments were blinded to the intervention assignment. An additional point was awarded if the process of blinding the assessors was described and appropriate. Since all studies had to be randomized controlled trials according to the inclusion criteria (assigned one point for the first criterion), the range of possible scores on the Jadad scale for this review was 1 to 5.

Data abstraction/statistical analysis

Information on the intervention type, publication year, subjects, country of origin, sport, primary and secondary outcome measures and quality scores were abstracted from each study and entered into a spreadsheet. Average quality scores were computed for each of the four intervention types.

RCTs were grouped according to the type of intervention: 1, neuromuscular, functional, or proprioceptive exercise programs (n = 12); 2, protective or prophylactic equipment (n = 10); 3, educational programs (n = 2); and 4, other programs (one warm-up/cool-down/stretching program and one multiple-component program). Several individual studies could be included in more than one category or had more than one comparison, since these reports included multiple interventions in the same study. For example, Stasinopoulos[14] compared three intervention groups: a technical sport-specific skill training group, an ankle disk proprioception exercise group, and an ankle orthosis group. Three separate outcome comparisons were presented for this study: technical skill versus orthosis, ankle disk exercise versus orthosis, and orthosis versus technical skill. For each of the four intervention types, a level of evidence rating was assigned using the Oxford Centre for Evidence-based Medicine criteria.[15]

For pooling of the 27 included studies, the data that were abstracted and entered into an analysis database included the author, year, quality score, effect (primary injury outcome), number injured (intervention and control), and number not injured (intervention and control) for each study. Mantel–Haenszel odds ratios (OR), 95% confidence intervals (CI) and Forrest plots were created, and summary effectiveness estimates were calculated using Comprehensive Meta-Analysis software (BioStat, Inc., Englewood, New Jersey, USA). Both fixed and random-effects models are presented, but since interventions were combined across sports, populations, and countries of origin (with possible heterogeneity), an *a priori* decision was taken to use the random-effects estimate and 95% confidence interval as the primary measure of effectiveness. The *Q*-statistic to test for homogeneity was also used to confirm heterogeneity.[16]

Results

Description of interventions

Neuromuscular, functional or proprioceptive exercise programs. The 12 studies classified in this category basically consisted of: 1, sport-specific or skill-specific functional exercise training (i.e., acceleration/deceleration activities, technical skills for landings and take-offs, plyometric and agility tasks, and power, strengthening and stabilization exercises, n = 5;[17–21] 2, balance or proprioception training programs, mostly using ankle disks/balance boards (n = 4);[22–25] and 3, a combination of both (n = 3).[14,26,27] The length of the interventions ranged from 7 weeks to the entire sport season. In general, details regarding the frequency per week, session duration, and length of the intervention were poorly reported.

Protective or prophylactic equipment. Of the 11 studies in this category, five investigated the effectiveness of ankle or knee braces/orthoses,[14,23,28–30] two studied custom mouth guards,[31,32] two studied wrist protectors,[33,34] and one each studied break-away bases in softball and baseball[35] and different shoe styles (high versus low top)[36] in basketball.

Educational programs. The two studies investigating educational approaches to injury prevention both used video formats to present information to subjects. One study[37] showed a 45-minute video on skiing injury prevention and proper equipment use during a bus ride to a ski resort. The other study[38] used a 2-hour workshop format to present a video analysis of injury mechanisms in soccer, followed by a group discussion.

Other interventions. One study[39] described a seven-component global soccer injury prevention program that included correction of training errors, provision of safety equipment, prophylactic ankle taping, controlled rehabilitation of injuries, exclusion of players with knee instability, education, and on-field medical supervision. The other study[7] consisted of a warm-up/cool-down and stretching program for runners.

Qualitative summary

Table 1.1 summarizes the studies by the four categories of intervention type and by individual studies. For neuromuscular, functional, or proprioception exercise programs, the majority (92%) of the studies reported significant reductions in injury outcomes and on average scored 2.4 in terms of methodological quality. Sixty-four percent of protective equipment interventions reported significant reductions in injury outcomes and had an average quality score of 2.7. Only half (50%) of the educational and other intervention types reported reduced injury outcomes and scored relatively low in terms of quality (educational = 1.5 and other = 1.0). Of the 27 studies, most (n = 16) originated from Scandinavian or European countries, six from the United States, and five from other countries.

Rating the evidence

On the basis of the Oxford Centre for Evidence-based Medicine levels of evidence, the studies included in both the neuromuscular, functional, or proprioception exercise and the protective or prophylactic equipment categories meet the 1A level of evidence, in which evidence is based on reports from large RCTs or systematic reviews. The educational program studies were graded A4 (evidence from at least one RCT) and the "Other" intervention group was graded A3 (evidence from at least one moderate-sized RCT or systematic review) (Table 1.1).

Quantitative summary

Pooled summary estimates are presented in Fig. 1.3 for the two intervention types that included more than two studies. Pooled estimates for the two educational program interventions were not significant (random-effects model OR 0.87; 95% CI, 0.34–2.21; $P = 0.77$) and are therefore not included in Fig. 1.3. Pooled estimates could not be calculated for the "Other" intervention types due to a lack of sufficient information in the printed manuscripts and the obvious heterogeneity between the two studies included in this category. All 12 of the neuromuscular, functional, or proprioception exercise studies reported data that could be pooled. However, one study in the protective equipment group[31] did not report sufficient raw data for summary estimates to be calculated, and therefore only nine studies were included in this analysis.

Neuromuscular, functional and proprioception exercise interventions. The Q-statistic to test for homogeneity indicated significant heterogeneity (Q-value 32.3, $P < 0.001$). Pooled effect estimates for the random-effects model suggest that neuromuscular, functional, or proprioception exercise interventions can reduce sports injuries by 65% (OR 0.35; 95% CI, 0.23–0.52; $P < 0.0001$).

Table 1.1 Summary of evidence for the effectiveness of interventions to prevent sports injuries, arranged by intervention type and individual studies

Evidence summary by intervention type

Intervention type (n*)	Components of interventions	Those favoring intervention† % (n)	Average quality score‡	Level of evidence§
Neuromuscular, functional, and/or proprioception exercise programs (n = 12)	Neuromuscular training programs, stability, power and strength exercises, balance and proprioception activities, sport- and skill-specific training	92% (11)	2.4	A1
Protective or prophylactic equipment interventions (n = 11)	Mouth guards, ankle braces and stirrup orthoses, lateral knee braces, break-away bases, wrist protectors, shoe styles	64%	2.7	A1
Educational programs (n = 2)	Video and video + group discussion	50% (1)	1.5	A4
Other (n = 2)	Warm-up/cool down and stretching program and multiple-component program	50% (1)	1.0	A3

Evidence summary for individual studies by intervention type

Neuromuscular, functional, and/or proprioception exercise programs

First author	Year	Country	Sport or activity	Intervention	Primary findings +/–†	Quality score‡
Tropp[23] (ankle disk vs. control)	1985	Sweden	Soccer	Ankle disk training	+	2
Wester[25]	1996	Denmark	Recreational athletes	Ankle disk training	+	2
Holme[19]	1999	Denmark	Recreational athletes	Strength and balance exercise	+	2
Wedderkopp[26]	1999	Denmark	Handball	Ankle disk + functional exercise training	+	1
Heidt[18]	2000	United States	Soccer	Frappier Acceleration Training Program	+	3

Soderman[22]	2000	Sweden	Soccer	Ankle disk training	–	2
Wedderkopp[27]	2003	Denmark	Handball	Ankle disk + functional exercise training	+	1
Sherry[21]	2004	United States	Recreational athletes	Progressive agility and trunk stabilization exercises	+	3
Stasinopoulos[14]	2004	Greece	Volleyball		+	2
Ankle disk vs. orthosis				Ankle disk training		
Skill vs. orthosis				Technical sport-specific skill training		
Verhagen[24]	2004	Denmark	Volleyball	Ankle disk training	+	3
Emery[17]	2005	Canada	PE students	Home-based balance training exercises	+	3
Olsen[20]	2005	Sweden	Handball	Strength, power, balance and technical skill program	+	5

Protective or prophylactic equipment interventions

First author	Year	Country	Sport or activity	Intervention	Primary findings +/–†	Quality score‡
Tropp[23] (orthosis vs. control)	1985	Sweden	Soccer	Ankle stirrup orthosis	+	2
Janda[35]	1988	United States	Baseball/softball	Break-away bases	+	4
Sitler[29]	1990	United States	Football	Lateral knee braces	+	2
Barrett[36]	1993	United States	Basketball		–	3
High top vs. low top				High-top basketball shoes		
High top + stirrup vs. low top				High top + air stirrup basketball shoes		
Sitler[28]	1994	United States	Basketball	Semi-rigid ankle stabilizing brace	+	1
Surve[30]	1994	South Africa	Soccer	Ankle stirrup orthosis	+	1
Ronning[34]	2001	Norway	Snowboarding	Wrist brace	+	5
Machold[14]	2002	Austria	Snowboarding	Wrist brace	+	3
Stasinopoulos[14] (orthosis vs. skill)	2004	Greece	Volleyball	Ankle stirrup orthosis	–	2
Barbic[31]	2005	Canada	Football/rugby	WIPSS Brain-Pad mouth guard	–	5
Finch[32]	2005	Australia	Australian football	Custom mouth guard	–	2

Continued

Table 1.1 (*Continued*)

Educational programs **First author**	**Year**	**Country**	**Sport or activity**	**Intervention**	**Primary findings +/–[†]**	**Quality score[‡]**
Jorgenson[37]	1998	Denmark	Downhill skiing	Educational video	+	1
Arnason[38]	2005	Iceland	Soccer	Educational video + group workshop	–	2

Other interventions **First author**	**Year**	**Country**	**Sport or activity**	**Intervention**	**Primary findings +/–[†]**	**Quality score[‡]**
Ekstrand[39]	1983	Sweden	Soccer	Multiple-component injury prevention program	+	1
Van Mechelen[7]	1993	Netherlands	Runners	Warm-up, stretching, cool-down	–	1

* A total of 27 studies were included in this review. Several studies had multiple intervention groups and subsequent comparisons, which are labeled separately in the lower part of the table.

† Number and percent of studies in each category reporting positive outcomes. Individual studies were graded positive (+) if significant ($P < 0.05$) reductions in injury or re-injury outcomes for their stated primary outcome measure were reported, and negative (–) if no statistical differences were reported.

‡ Quality scores ranged from 1 to 5, using a modified Jadad Scale for assessing study quality.[13]

§ Evidence levels based on the Oxford Centre for Evidence-based Medicine chart:[15]

A1, evidence comes from large randomized controlled trials (RCTs) or systematic review/meta-analysis.

A2, evidence comes from at least one high-quality cohort.

A3, evidence comes from at least one moderate-sized RCT or systematic review.

A4, evidence comes from at least one RCT.

B, evidence comes from at least one high-quality, nonrandomized study.

C, evidence based on expert opinion.

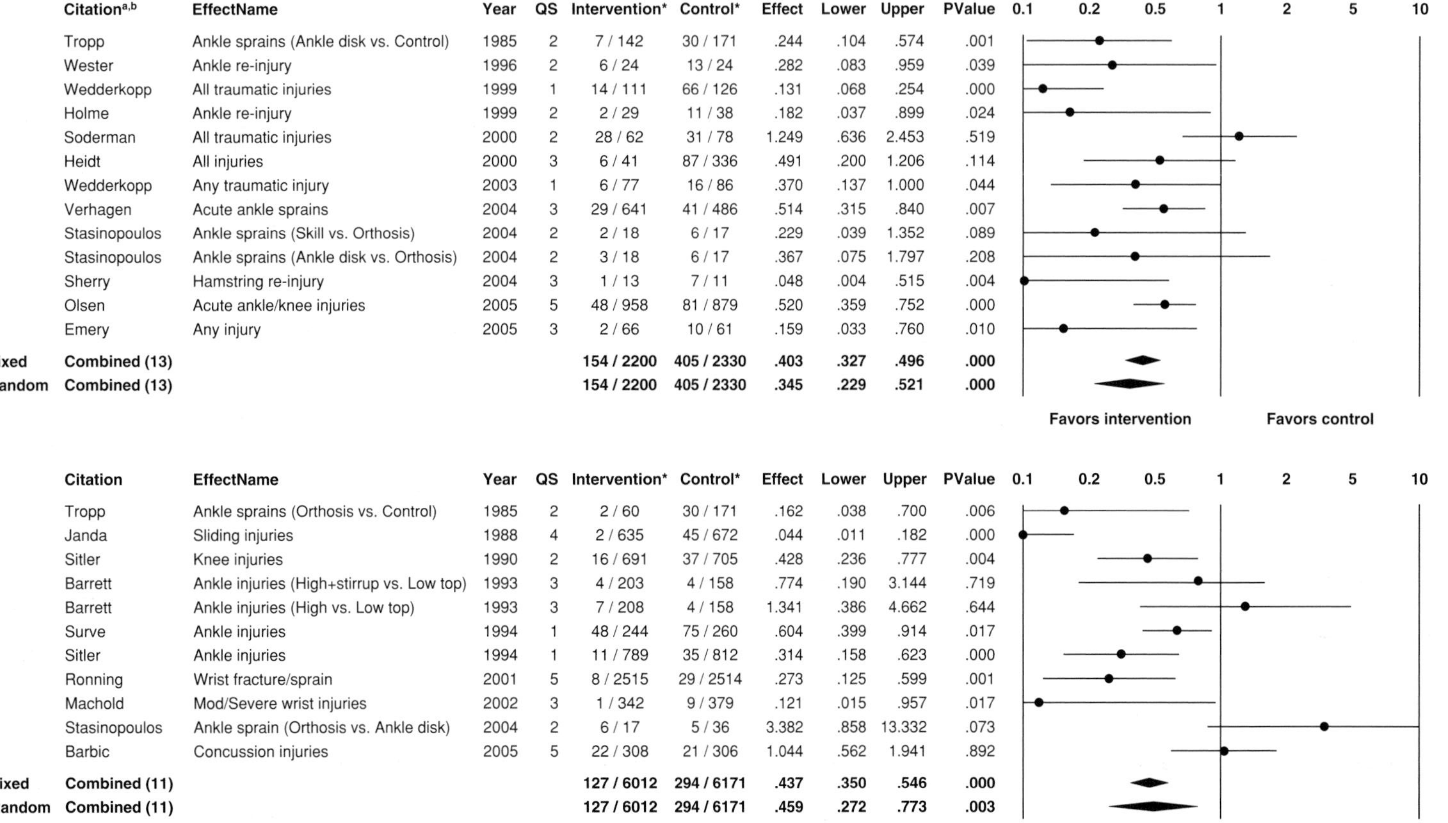

	Citation[a,b]	EffectName	Year	QS	Intervention*	Control*	Effect	Lower	Upper	PValue
	Tropp	Ankle sprains (Ankle disk vs. Control)	1985	2	7 / 142	30 / 171	.244	.104	.574	.001
	Wester	Ankle re-injury	1996	2	6 / 24	13 / 24	.282	.083	.959	.039
	Wedderkopp	All traumatic injuries	1999	1	14 / 111	66 / 126	.131	.068	.254	.000
	Holme	Ankle re-injury	1999	2	2 / 29	11 / 38	.182	.037	.899	.024
	Soderman	All traumatic injuries	2000	2	28 / 62	31 / 78	1.249	.636	2.453	.519
	Heidt	All injuries	2000	3	6 / 41	87 / 336	.491	.200	1.206	.114
	Wedderkopp	Any traumatic injury	2003	1	6 / 77	16 / 86	.370	.137	1.000	.044
	Verhagen	Acute ankle sprains	2004	3	29 / 641	41 / 486	.514	.315	.840	.007
	Stasinopoulos	Ankle sprains (Skill vs. Orthosis)	2004	2	2 / 18	6 / 17	.229	.039	1.352	.089
	Stasinopoulos	Ankle sprains (Ankle disk vs. Orthosis)	2004	2	3 / 18	6 / 17	.367	.075	1.797	.208
	Sherry	Hamstring re-injury	2004	3	1 / 13	7 / 11	.048	.004	.515	.004
	Olsen	Acute ankle/knee injuries	2005	5	48 / 958	81 / 879	.520	.359	.752	.000
	Emery	Any injury	2005	3	2 / 66	10 / 61	.159	.033	.760	.010
Fixed	**Combined (13)**				**154 / 2200**	**405 / 2330**	**.403**	**.327**	**.496**	**.000**
Random	**Combined (13)**				**154 / 2200**	**405 / 2330**	**.345**	**.229**	**.521**	**.000**

	Citation	EffectName	Year	QS	Intervention*	Control*	Effect	Lower	Upper	PValue
	Tropp	Ankle sprains (Orthosis vs. Control)	1985	2	2 / 60	30 / 171	.162	.038	.700	.006
	Janda	Sliding injuries	1988	4	2 / 635	45 / 672	.044	.011	.182	.000
	Sitler	Knee injuries	1990	2	16 / 691	37 / 705	.428	.236	.777	.004
	Barrett	Ankle injuries (High+stirrup vs. Low top)	1993	3	4 / 203	4 / 158	.774	.190	3.144	.719
	Barrett	Ankle injuries (High vs. Low top)	1993	3	7 / 208	4 / 158	1.341	.386	4.662	.644
	Surve	Ankle injuries	1994	1	48 / 244	75 / 260	.604	.399	.914	.017
	Sitler	Ankle injuries	1994	1	11 / 789	35 / 812	.314	.158	.623	.000
	Ronning	Wrist fracture/sprain	2001	5	8 / 2515	29 / 2514	.273	.125	.599	.001
	Machold	Mod/Severe wrist injuries	2002	3	1 / 342	9 / 379	.121	.015	.957	.017
	Stasinopoulos	Ankle sprain (Orthosis vs. Ankle disk)	2004	2	6 / 17	5 / 36	3.382	.858	13.332	.073
	Barbic	Concussion injuries	2005	5	22 / 308	21 / 306	1.044	.562	1.941	.892
Fixed	**Combined (11)**				**127 / 6012**	**294 / 6171**	**.437**	**.350**	**.546**	**.000**
Random	**Combined (11)**				**127 / 6012**	**294 / 6171**	**.459**	**.272**	**.773**	**.003**

Figure 1.3 Study characteristics, summary estimates, and Forrest plots for the primary injury outcomes for (**a**) neuromuscular, functional, or proprioception exercise programs, and (**b**) protective or prophylactic equipment interventions. QS, quality score; Effect, Mantel–Haenszel odds ratio; Lower, lower boundary of 95% confidence interval; Upper, upper boundary of 95% confidence interval.

Protective or prophylactic equipment interventions. The Q-statistic to test for homogeneity indicated significant heterogeneity (Q-value 37.7, $P < 0.0001$). Pooled effect estimates for the random-effects model suggest that protective or prophylactic equipment interventions can reduce sports injuries by 54% (OR 0.46; 95% CI, 0.27–0.77; $P = 0.003$).

Discussion

The answer to the question: "Is it possible to prevent sports injuries?" is essentially "yes." The results of this systematic review suggest that sports injuries can be reduced by 54–65%, depending on the type of intervention. For some interventions, effectiveness is even greater among persons with previous injuries. This review could only pool studies on the basis of two very general groupings of intervention types and suggests that there is still a critical need for well-designed sport-specific or activity-specific studies to identify risk factors for injuries, to develop and test interventions, and to document post-intervention changes in the injury burden using the "sequence of prevention" model proposed by van Mechelen *et al.*[1]

One area that warrants further inspection and discussion is the relatively enhanced effectiveness for various exercise programs and ankle-stabilizing braces (semi-rigid braces or stirrup orthoses) among those with a previous history of ankle injuries. Several studies reported subgroup analyses for individuals who had prior injuries in comparison with individuals without. In all cases, individuals with previous ankle injuries had a significant reduction in the incidence of injury even if the intervention was not effective among individuals without prior injuries. Five studies[14,17,22–24] reported that interventions were more effective for ankle disk training/balance exercises among individuals with a previous ankle injury. Four studies[23,28,31,36] found similarly enhanced intervention effectiveness for various types of ankle stabilizers (rigid stirrup orthosis, semi-rigid ankle braces, high-top basketball shoes) among those with a previous ankle injury. These subgroup findings suggest that the potential "best practice" would be to recommend prophylactic ankle bracing and ankle disk/balance exercise programs for athletes participating in jumping and twisting sports who have a history of ankle injuries.

What is interesting in the results of this review is the fact that most of the sports injury prevention work is being done in Scandinavian and European countries. There is a dearth of well-designed studies from the United States, Canada, Australia, and Africa, and none from other continents, despite the fact that sports and recreational activities are popular pastimes across the globe. In addition, there are no studies for many types of sports and activities that are very popular worldwide. Soccer has considerable worldwide participation and was the sport most often studied (six studies) in this review. However, the numbers of children and adults participating in many different sports or activities, such as football, baseball, and softball, walking and running, aerobics, swimming, and others, are high[40,41] and this suggests that attention should be paid to injury prevention in a wider variety of activities and across different age groups.

In general, the quality of the studies included was relatively poor (average score 2.4 out of 5), and only four individual studies scored above a 4. The reason for this is unclear, but it is likely to be multifactorial. One reason may be that there is a lack of training opportunities for sports-medicine researchers in the methods of RCT study design, conduct, and analysis, and only a handful of agencies funding research in this area. There is also a lack of the sport-specific and activity-specific injury risk factor information that is needed to design appropriate interventions. These data often have to come from expensive and long-term longitudinal cohort studies, which may explain the difficulty in conducting such studies. Also, in comparison with clinical settings, conducting research on the athletic field or in recreational sports settings may be fraught with "uncontrollable" factors (weather, field conditions, spectator behavior, etc.), the inability to blind subjects to some types of intervention (exercise, bracing/taping, etc.), and there may be an inherent "distrust" of researchers on the athletic fields on the part of coaches, parents, and athletes. The issue of poor study quality is not a new problem in this field; others have also discussed this limitation and called for more high-quality research.[3,9,42–44]

Another factor related to study quality is the type of instrument used to rate study methodology. A wide variety of quality rating instruments have been published in the literature, none however, specific to sports injury prevention RCT study designs. The Jadad scale[13] was chosen for its ease of use and because it has been shown to be reliable[45] and had been used previously[42] in sports injury prevention research. Three Cochrane reviews used a generic, 11-item scoring tool developed by the Cochrane Musculoskeletal Injuries Group.[10–12] A series of systematic reviews published by the U.S. Centers for Disease Control and Prevention developed a 100-point, checklist-type tool to rate study quality.[43,44,46–48] To date, there has not been any consistent use of a single quality assessment tool in the field of sports injury prevention. The field is unique in terms of factors that may bias study design and execution, and as such, a rating scale specific to the field may need to be developed and psychometrically tested. This tool would need to be very flexible to accommodate different sports, different populations, and different types of intervention.

The studies included in this review were deliberately limited to RCTs, which may be considered both a strength and a limitation. This study design is considered the "gold standard" for assessing intervention effectiveness and is often used to inform clinical decisions. An RCT, if properly conducted, can help control for various biases that cannot be assessed or controlled with other experimental or observational study designs.[49,50] Due to the difficulties in conducting RCTs in the sports setting discussed above, some may feel that limiting evidence for effectiveness to this stringent type of study design may be overly conservative.[51] Studies using quasi-experimental or observational study designs may still be informative in terms of prevention effectiveness, but were not included in this review, and this may be viewed as a limitation.[52] Even when effective interventions exist, there is still considerable difficulty in disseminating these interventions to the populations who will benefit the most from them.

A decade has passed since the publication of the landmark report *Physical Activity and Health: a Report from the Surgeon General.*[53] In the ensuing years, public health, clinical, and community-based organizations have been promoting moderate daily physical activity for all persons in order to benefit their health. Despite this, physical inactivity is still a critical problem both in the United States[54] and worldwide. The benefits of an active lifestyle are well known, but the risks associated with physical activity and exercise are less well understood. One of the most common possible adverse events associated with exercise and/or sports participation is musculoskeletal injury. To better promote safe, yet healthful, physical activity and exercise, we need evidenced-based information regarding injury mechanisms and risk factors that can be used to develop and evaluate injury prevention programs.

Recommendations

Clinical practice

• Comprehensive neuromuscular, functional exercise and/or proprioception training programs should be incorporated into all conditioning activities for soccer, volleyball, handball and other sports with a high incidence of lower-extremity injuries, especially ankle sprains.

• Participants in sports that involve jumping, twisting, and pivoting should be counseled to wear ankle-stabilizing devices such as a rigid stirrup orthosis or a semi-rigid brace. Such prophylactic ankle stabilizers should be strongly recommended to athletes with prior ankle injuries.

Future research

• Develop and implement standardized data systems for sports injury research.

• Increase training and funding opportunities for sports-medicine researchers to gain skills and experience in conducting clinical or community-based intervention studies and outcomes research.

• Recruit multidisciplinary partners, including health-care providers (physicians, nurses, etc.), allied health practitioners (Certified Athletic Trainers, physical therapists, exercise physiologists, etc.), coaches, athletic administration personnel, and parents to improve the evaluation and dissemination of effective methods of injury prevention.

• Convene an international sports injury prevention forum/network to develop a sports injury research agenda.

• Expand the reach of known effective interventions and evaluate promising interventions across activities and populations.

Summary

• Some sports and recreation-related injuries can be prevented.

• Level 1A evidence suggests that neuromuscular, functional, or proprioception exercise programs and prophylactic equipment are effective in reducing sports injuries.

• There is a critical need for high-quality randomized controlled trials of injury prevention interventions among physically active children and adults.

Key messages

• Sports injuries can be prevented.

• Neuromuscular, functional or proprioception exercise programs should be a integral part of sport training.

• A suggested "best practice" would be to recommend prophylactic ankle bracing and ankle disk/balance exercise programs for athletes participating in jumping and twisting sports who have a history of ankle injuries.

Sample examination questions

Multiple-choice questions (answers on page 602)

1 For the purposes of this review, "neuromuscular, functional, or proprioception exercise programs" consisted of all of the following except:
   A Ankle disk/balance board training

B Acceleration/deceleration activities
C Calisthenics
D Plyometrics/agility training

2 What type of interventions had the highest proportion of studies reporting significant reductions in injury outcomes?
A Neuromuscular, functional, or proprioception exercise programs
B Protective or prophylactic equipment
C Educational
D Other

3 In terms of pooled effect estimates, which interventions were effective in reducing sports injuries by more than 50%? (Choose two.)
A Neuromuscular, functional, or proprioception exercise programs
B Protective or prophylactic equipment
C Educational
D Other

Essay questions

1 Define a common sports-related injury and, using the "sequence of prevention" model, describe the burden, risk factors, and development and evaluation of a sports injury prevention program for this injury problem.
2 In terms of summarizing intervention effectiveness, why is it crucial to report the details of individual interventions in publications?
3 As judged by the quality-scoring scale used in this study, the overall quality of studies included in this review was low. Discuss factors that may contribute to poor study quality in studies of sports injury prevention and how they may be improved in future research.
4 Discuss three ways in which the reach of effective sports injury interventions can be increased.

References

1 van Mechelen W, Hlobil H, Kemper H. Incidence, severity, aetiology and prevention of sports injuries: a review of concepts. *Sports Med* 1992; **14**:82–99.
2 Chalmers D. Injury prevention in sport: not yet part of the game? *Inj Prev* 2002; **8**(Suppl IV):iv22–iv25.
3 Parkkari J, Kujala U, Kannus P. Is it possible to prevent sports injuries? Review of controlled clinical trials and recommendations for future work? *Sports Med* 2001; **31**(14):985–995.
4 Bahr R, Krosshaug T. Understanding injury mechanisms: a key component of preventing injuries in sport. *Br J Sports Med* 2005; **39**:324–329.
5 Engebretsen L, Bahr R. An ounce of prevention? *Br J Sports Med* 2005; **39**:312–313.
6 Shephard R. Towards an evidence based prevention of sports injuries. *Inj Prev* 2005; **11**:65–66.
7 van Mechelen W, Hlobil H, Kemper H, Voorn W, de Jongh H. Prevention of running injuries by warm-up, cool-down, and stretching exercises. *Am J Sports Med* 1993; **21**:711–719.
8 Higgins JPT, Green S, editors. *Cochrane Handbook for Systematic Reviews of Interventions* 4.2.5 [updated May 2005]. http://www.cochrane.org/resources/handbook/hbook.htm (accessed 22 August 2005).
9 Emery C. Risk factors for injury in child and adolescent sports: a systematic review of the literature. *Clin J Sport Med* 2003; **13**:256–268.
10 Handoll HH, Rowe BH, Quinn KM, de Bie R. Interventions for preventing ankle ligament injuries. *Cochrane Database Syst Rev* 2001; (3):CD000018.
11 Rome K, Handoll HH, Ashford R. Interventions for preventing and treating stress fractures and stress reactions of bone of the lower limbs in young adults. *Cochrane Database Syst Rev* 2005; (2):CD000450.
12 Yeung EW, Yeung SS. Interventions for preventing lower limb soft-tissue injuries in runners. *Cochrane Database Syst Rev* 2001; (3):CD001256.

13 Jadad AR, Moore RA, Carroll D, *et al.* Assessing the quality of reports of randomized clinical trials: is blinding necessary? *Control Clin Trials* 1996; **17**:1–12.
14 Stasinopoulos D. Comparison of three preventive methods in order to reduce the incidence of ankle inversion sprains among female volleyball players. *Br J Sports Med* 2004; **38**:182–185.
15 Centre for Evidence-based Medicine (Oxford, UK). Levels of Evidence (May 2001). http://www.cebm.net/levels_of_evidence.asp#levels (accessed 22 August 2006).
16 Fleiss J, Gross A. Meta-analysis in epidemiology, with special reference to studies of the association between exposure to environmental tobacco smoke and lung cancer: a critique. *J Clin Epidemiol* 2001; **44**:127–139.
17 Emery CA, Cassidy JD, Klassen TP, Rosychuk RJ, Rowe BH. Effectiveness of a home-based balance-training program in reducing sports-related injuries among healthy adolescents: a cluster randomized controlled trial. *CMAJ* 2005; **172**:749–754.
18 Heidt R, Sweeterman L, Carlonas R, Traub J, Tekulve F. Avoidance of soccer injuries with preseason training. *Am J Sports Med* 2000; **28**:659–662.
19 Holme E, Magnusson S, Becher K, Bieler T, Aagaard P, Kjaer M. The effect of supervised rehabilitation on strength, postural sway, position sense and re-injury risk after acute ankle ligament sprain. *Scand J Med Sci Sports* 1999; **9**:104–109.
20 Olsen O, Myklebust G, Engebretsen L, Holme I, Bahr R. Exercises to prevent lower limb injuries in youth sports: cluster randomized controlled trial. *BMJ* 2005; **330**:1–7.
21 Sherry MA, Best TM. A comparison of 2 rehabilitation programs in the treatment of acute hamstring strains. *J Orthop Sports Phys Ther* 2004; **34**:116–125.
22 Soderman K, Werner S, Pietila T, Engstrom B, Alfredson H. Balance board training: prevention of traumatic injuries of the lower extremities in female soccer players? A prospective randomized intervention study. *Knee Surg Sports Traumatol Arthrosc* 2000; **8**:356–363.
23 Tropp H, Askling G, Gillquist J. Prevention of ankle sprains. *Am J Sports Med* 1985; **13**:259–262.
24 Verhagen E, van der Beek A, Twisk J, Bouter L, Bahr R, van Mechelen W. The effect of a proprioceptive balance board training program for the prevention of ankle sprains: a prospective controlled trial. *Am J Sports Med* 2004; **32**:1385–1393.
25 Wester J, Jespersen S, Nielsen K, Neumann L. Wobble board training after partial sprains of the lateral ligaments of the ankle: a prospective randomized study. *J Orthop Sports Phys Ther* 1996; **23**:332–336.
26 Wedderkopp N, Kaltoft M, Lundgaard B, Rosendahl M, Froberg K. Prevention of injuries in young female players in European team handball: a prospective intervention study. *Scand J Med Sci Sports* 1999; **9**:41–47.
27 Wedderkopp N, Kaltoft M, Holm R, Froberg K. Comparison of two intervention programmes in young female players in European handball—with and without ankle disc. *Scand J Med Sci Sports* 2003; **13**:371–375.
28 Sitler M, Ryan J, Wheeler B, *et al.* The efficacy of a semirigid ankles stabilizer to reduce acute ankle injuries in basketball: a randomized clinical study at West Point. *Am J Sports Med* 1994; **22**:454–461.
29 Sitler M, Ryan J, Hopkinson W, *et al.* The efficacy of a prophylactic knee brace to reduce knee injuries in football: a prospective, randomized study at West Point. *Am J Sports Med* 1990; **18**:310–315.
30 Surve I, Schwellnus MP, Noakes T, Lombard C. A five-fold reduction in the incidence of recurrent ankle sprains in soccer players using the sport-stirrup orthosis. *Am J Sports Med* 1994; **22**:601–606.
31 Barbic D, Pater J, Brison R. Comparison of mouth guard designs and concussion prevention in contact sports: a multicenter randomized controlled trial. *Clin J Sport Med* 2005; **15**:294–298.
32 Finch C, Braham R, McIntosh A, McCrory P, Wolfe R. Should football players wear custom fitted mouthguards? Results from a group randomised controlled trial. *Inj Prev* 2005; **11**:242–246.
33 Machold W, Kwasny O, Eisenhardt P, *et al.* Reduction of severe wrist injuries in snowboarding by an optimized wrist protection device: a prospective randomized trial. *J Trauma* 2002; **52**:517–520.
34 Ronning R, Ronning I, Gerner T, Engebretsen L. The efficacy of wrist protectors in preventing snowboarding injuries. *Am J Sports Med* 2001; **29**:581–585.
35 Janda D, Wojtys E, Hankin F, Benedict M. Softball sliding injuries: a prospective study comparing standard and modified bases. *JAMA* 1988; **259**:1848–1850.
36 Barrett J, Tanji J, Drake C, Fuller D, Kawasaki R, Fenton R. High- versus low-top shoes for the prevention of ankles sprains in basketball players: a prospective randomized study. *Am J Sports Med* 1993; **21**:582–585.

37 Jorgensen U, Fredensborg T, Haraszuk J, Crone K. Reduction of injuries in downhill skiing by use of an instructional ski video: a prospective randomised intervention study. *Knee Surg Sports Traumatol Arthrosc* 1998; **6**:194–200.

38 Arnason A, Engebretsen L, Bahr R. No effect of a video-based awareness program on the rate of soccer injuries. *Am J Sports Med* 2005; **33**:77–84.

39 Ekstrand J, Gillquist J, Liljedahl S. Prevention of soccer injuries: supervision by doctor and physiotherapist. *Am J Sports Med* 1983; **1**:116–120.

40 Powell K, Heath G, Kresnow M, Sacks J, Branche C. Injury rates from walking, gardening, weightlifting, outdoor bicycling and aerobics. *Med Sci Sports Exerc* 1998; **30**:1246–1249.

41 Sporting Goods Manufacturers Association. Sports Participation in America 2006. http://www.sgma.com (accessed 22 August 2006).

42 Olsen L, Scanlan A, MacKay M, *et al.* Strategies for prevention of soccer related injuries: a systematic review. *Br J Sports Med* 2004; **38**:89–94.

43 Thacker SB, Stroup DF, Branche CM, Gilchrist J, Goodman RA, Weitman EA. The prevention of ankle sprains in sports: a systematic review of the literature. *Am J Sports Med* 1999; **27**:753–760.

44 Thacker S, Gilchrist J, Stroup D, Kimsey CD. The prevention of shin splints in sports: a systematic review of the literature. *Med Sci Sports Exerc* 2002; **34**:32–40.

45 Brouwers MC, Johnston ME, Charette ML, Hanna SE, Jadad AR, Browman GP. Evaluating the role of quality assessment of primary studies in systematic reviews of cancer patient guidelines. *BMC Med Res Methodol* 2005; **5**(1):8. Available at: http://www.biomedcentral.com/1471-2288-5-8 (accessed 22 August 2006).

46 Jones B, Thacker S, Gilchrist J, Kimsey C, Sosin D. Prevention of lower extremity stress fractures in athletes and soldiers: a systematic review. *Epidemiol Rev* 2002; **24**:228–247.

47 Thacker SB, Stroup DF, Branche CM, Gilchrist J, Goodman RA, Porter Kelling E. Prevention of knee injuries in sports: a systematic review of the literature. *J Sports Med Phys Fitness* 2003; **43**:165–179.

48 Thacker S, Gilchrist J, Stroup D, Kimsey C. The impact of stretching on sports injury risk: a systematic review of the literature. *Med Sci Sports Exerc* 2004; **36**:371–378.

49 Kestle J. Clinical trials. *World J Surg* 1999; **23**:1205–1209.

50 Sackett DL, Straus S, Richardson W, Rosenberg W, Haynes R. *Evidence-based Medicine: How to Practice and Teach EBM*, 2nd ed. Edinburgh: Churchill Livingstone, 2000.

51 Grossman J, Mackenzie F. The randomized controlled trials: gold standard, or merely standard? *Perspect Biol Med* 2005; **48**:516–534.

52 MacLehose RR, Reeves BC, Harvey IM, Sheldon TA, Russell IT, Black AM. A systematic review of comparisons of effect sizes derived from randomised and non-randomised studies *Health Technol Assess* 2000; **4**(34):1–4.

53 U.S. Department of Health and Human Services. *Physical Activity and Health: a Report of the Surgeon General.* Atlanta: National Center for Chronic Disease Prevention and Health Promotion, Centers for Disease Control and Prevention, 1996.

54 Centers for Disease Control and Prevention. Adult participation in recommended levels of physical activity: United States, 2001 and 2003. *Mort Morb Weekly Rep* 2005; **54**:1208–1212.

CHAPTER 2

Evidence-based preparticipation physical examination

Peter J. Carek

Introduction

The preparticipation physical examination (PPE) has become a requirement and represents the standard of care for athletes in many countries as they prepare for organized athletic participation. This requirement appears to have been established due to both medical and legal concerns regarding athletes who may be at increased risk for severe injury or death due to participation in athletics. While a PPE is a requirement based on the policies of sponsoring or regulatory institutions, a detailed description regarding the specific content of these examinations is usually not provided. The specific content of the PPE has been recommended and extensively reviewed by numerous authorities in sports medicine.[1–30]

Although the PPE has been adopted by many organizations, agreement on the content and usefulness of the PPE has been a topic of considerable debate.[31–34] Nevertheless, many sponsoring institutions and governing bodies continue to require the medical evaluation prior to competition in organized athletics.

Internationally, the PPE is not a universal requirement. In the United States, most states require a PPE for high school student athletes. The Italian government has required screening and medical clearance of all young athletes since 1971. In contrast, the British perspective is that while identifying people at risk is vital for effective intervention, widespread population screening is not appropriate, particularly in relation to cardiomyopathy.[31] Rather than providing a PPE, a process of profiling or ongoing monitoring of player health and performance has been introduced to elite-level athletes in Great Britain.[35] While validity has yet to be studied, profiling is intended to minimize the incidence of illness, fatigue, and overuse injuries.

Several medical organizations in the United States recommend the completion of a medical evaluation prior to participation in athletics. The American College of Sports Medicine states that it is essential for prospective athletes to complete a preparticipation evaluation.[36] In 1976, the American Medical Association's Committee on Medical Aspects of Sports developed a statement of Rights of the Athlete and included a statement that each athlete is entitled to adequate health supervisions, including a thorough preparticipation physical examination.[37]

Several years ago, the American Academy of Family Physicians, the American Academy of Pediatrics, the American Medical Society for Sports Medicine, the American Orthopedic Society for Sports Medicine, and the American Osteopathic Academy of Sports Medicine established the Preparticipation Physical Examination Task Force. The recommendations of this task force, which were recently updated, serve as a guide for the physician conducting these examinations for their local high school and collegiate athletes.[38–40] The American Heart Association (AHA) and 26th Bethesda Conference have contributed various guidelines for athletic preparticipation cardiovascular screening.[41,42] Despite being required, the preparticipation screening process used by many U.S. colleges and universities appears to have limited potential to detect cardiovascular abnormalities capable of causing sudden death in competitive student-athletes.[33]

In addition to being a requirement for athletic participation, several studies have found that many athletes utilize this examination as their only contact with a health-care provider.[43,44] Furthermore, mass preparticipation screening events may serve to provide public awareness of a physician's or medical group's interest in providing sports-medicine services.

Athletic mortality and morbidity

The mortality associated with athletic participation is most often the result of acute sudden cardiac death, a condition that occurs in about 0.5 per 100,000 high school athletes per academic year.[41,45] Screening for predisposing conditions is severely limited by several factors: the low prevalence of relevant cardiovascular lesions in the general youth population, the low risk of sudden death even among persons with an unsuspected abnormality, and the relatively large size of the competitive athletic population.[41,46] An estimated 200,000 children and adolescents would have to be screened with the current techniques available in order to detect the 500 athletes who are at risk for sudden cardiac death and the one individual who would actually experience it.[47]

At present, the common cardiac conditions that limit athletic participation are nearly never detected during the PPE. The most prevalent congenital heart diseases (ventricular septal defect, atrial septal defect, patent ductus arteriosis, pulmonic stenosis, and aortic stenosis) are generally recognized early in life and are therefore unlikely to be first detected during the preparticipation process.[48] Even when cardiac abnormalities are detected, the findings leading to disqualification are most often rhythm and conduction abnormalities, valvular abnormalities, and systemic hypertension that are not the cardiac abnormalities noted to be associated with sudden cardiac death in athletes.[49,50] In an analysis of 125,408 athletes, 3190 (2.5%) were disqualified.[51] Cardiovascular abnormalities (e.g., arrhythmias, valvular abnormalities, including mitral valve prolapse, and hypertension) lead to the disqualification in one-half of the affected individuals. Less frequent abnormalities resulting in disqualification included congenital, rheumatic, or ischemic disease, pericarditis, and cardiomyopathies.

Certain populations of athletes appear to be at higher risk for sudden cardiac death. For instance, four sports (American football, basketball, track, and soccer) are associated with a majority of the sudden deaths. Additionally, approximately 90% of athletic-field deaths have occurred in males and most of the individuals affected were high school athletes.[41,52,53]

The prevalence of underlying cardiovascular disease varies according to ethnic background and nationality. The Brugada syndrome—in which right bundle-branch block with persistent ST segment elevation in the right precordial leads is associated with susceptibility to ventricular tachyarrhythmias and sudden cardiac death—is more prevalent in those of Asian descent.[54] While hypertrophic cardiomyopathy is the most common cause

Table 2.1 Rates of clearance, clearance with a medical condition, or full restriction

Reference	Athletes (n)	Pass (%)	Pass with condition (%)	Fail (%)
Goldberg, 1980[56]	701	85.2	13.5	1.3
Linder, 1981[57]	1268	94.8	5.0	0.2
Tennant, 1981[58]	2719	89.6	9.2	1.2
Thompson, 1982[59]	2670	89.2	9.6	1.2
DuRant, 1985[60]	922	94.4	5.6	0.3
Risser, 1985[61]	2114	96.6	3.1	0.3
Magnes, 1992[62]	10540	89.4	10.2	0.4
Rifat, 1995[63]	2574	84.8	12.6	2.6
Lively, 1999[64]	596	85.9	13.9	0.2

of sudden death in athletes in the United States, arrhythmogenic right ventricular dysplasia (ARVD) is the most common cause of sudden death among Italian athletes.[55]

More frequently than mortality, athletic participation places the individual at risk for acute injury or worsening of an underlying medical condition. While a majority of athletes are cleared during the PPE without significant medical or orthopedic abnormalities being noted, the PPE often detects conditions that may predispose the athlete to injury or limit full participation in certain activities. In previous reported results of mass preparticipation screening events, approximately 5–15% of athletes require further evaluation; less than 3% fail the examination and are denied participation (Table 2.1).[56–64] These conditions are usually limited to several organ systems (i.e., musculoskeletal and cardiovascular) (Table 2.2).[39,46,63,64]

Currently, the recommended PPE includes the acquisition of specific historical information and the completion of a limited physical examination in an attempt to detect medical conditions in the athlete that may predispose them to injury or death. Additional evaluation and determination of level of participation is based on the findings in the history and physical.

Preparticipation evaluation

Medical history

A medical history should be obtained from each participant (grade of recommendation: B). A complete medical history has been shown to identify approximately 75% of problems that affect initial athletic participation and serves as the cornerstone of the PPE.[56,61] Unfortunately, these studies noted that the sensitivity of the recommended questionnaires is approximately 50%, far below the usual standard expected from a medical screening test.[30]

Most conditions requiring further evaluation or restriction have been reported to be identified during this aspect of the examination process. Rifat *et al.* noted that the history accounted for 88% of the abnormal findings and 57% of the reasons cited for activity restriction.[63] The Preparticipation Physical Evaluation Task Force has developed a history form that emphasizes the areas of greatest concern for sports participation.[38] In particular, specific questions regarding risk factors and symptoms of cardiovascular disease are asked (Table 2.3). A positive response to any of these questions should be confirmed and further

Table 2.2 Medical and orthopedic conditions found in junior/senior high school[63] and college-aged[64] athletes resulting in additional recommendations

	Rifat, 1995* n = 2574		Lively, 1999† n = 596
	Pass with follow-up and/or restriction (12.6%)	**Fail with follow-up (2.6%)**	**Follow-up or restriction (14.1%)**
Medical (% of overall total)	76.6	74.1	55.4
Cardiovascular	18.3	35.0	63.0
Dermatologic	6.8		
Endocrinologic	0.4		
Ear, nose, and throat	9.6	2.5	
Gastrointestinal	0.9		2.2
Genitourinary	9.6	12.5	8.7
Gynecologic			4.4
Infectious	0.4		6.5
Neurologic			6.5
Ophthalmologic	26.0	25.0	6.5
Psychological			2.2
Pulmonary	14.2	2.5	
Other‡	13.7	22.5	
Total medical (%)	100.0	100.0	100.0
Orthopedic (% of overall total)	23.4	25.9	44.6
Ankle/foot	14.9	7.7	2.7
Back/neck	22.4	14.3	5.4
Elbow			5.4
Hand/wrist	1.5		10.9
Knee	41.8	7.1	43.2
Leg			5.4
Shoulder			27.0
Nonspecific pain/injury	19.4	71.4	
Total orthopedic (%)	100.0	100.0	100.0

* Two individuals failed (nonspecific pain/injury).
† One individual failed (complicated pregnancy).
‡ "Other" includes abdominal pain, allergy, bruising, chest pain, chronic/recurrent illness, dizziness/syncope with exercise, surgery (recent).

evaluation conducted if necessary and warranted based on further questioning. Unfortunately, most athletes with hypertrophic cardiomyopathy do not report a history of syncope with exercise or a family history of premature sudden cardiac death due to the disease. Furthermore, a specific, effective evaluation that should be conducted either to identify a specific cause for the issue presented by a positive response or to exclude potential life-threatening conditions has not been delineated nor studied.

As musculoskeletal injury is a common cause for disqualification of an athlete, the medical history should attempt to detect any underlying condition that predisposes an athlete to injury.[56,61,63] In terms of anatomical sites, the most common injury to restrict participation is a knee injury, followed by an ankle injury.[65] The strongest independent

Table 2.3 Medical history questions regarding the presence of cardiovascular risk factors

- Have you ever passed out during or after exercise?
- Have you ever been dizzy during or after exercise?
- Have you ever had chest pain during or after exercise?
- Do you get tired more quickly than your friends do during exercise?
- Have you ever had racing of your heart or skipped heartbeats?
- Have you had high blood pressure or high cholesterol?
- Have you been told you have a heart murmur?
- Has any family member or relative died of heart problems or of sudden death before age 50?
- Have you had a severe viral infection (for example, myocarditis or mononucleosis) within the last month?
- Has a physician ever denied or restricted your participation in sports for any heart problem?

predictor of sports injuries is a previous injury (odds ratio 9.4) and exposure time (OR 6.9).[66] DuRant *et al.* found that having previously experienced a knee injury or having undergone knee surgery was significantly associated with knee injuries during the subsequent sports season when compared to individuals who did not report previous knee injury or surgery (30.6% vs. 7.2%; $P = 0.0001$).[65]

Additional historical information has been recommended for inclusion. For example, the athlete should be questioned about the presence of wheezing during exercise. Due to the high rate of recurrence and potential for long-term adverse effects, a history of previous concussions should be obtained. Other issues to be addressed should include presence of a single bilateral organ and use of performance-enhancing medication. Finally, female athletes should be questioned regarding their menstrual history and other symptoms or signs of the female athletic triad (eating disorder, amenorrhea, and osteoporosis).[67]

The recent recommendations by the PPE task force and others have included questions regarding lifestyle choices and preventive services not previously recommended for this particular examination.[38] While most athletes believe that the PPE prevents/helps to prevent injuries when there is no clear evidence to support this assumption, athletes are not consistently receptive to some preventive health screening.[44] For example, some athletes do not feel comfortable with certain issues being raised (i.e., gynecologic health, eating disorders, alcohol and nicotine use).

The information provided by athletes and their parents should always be reviewed carefully. In two separate studies, minimal agreement was found between histories obtained from athletes and parents independently.[61,68] Of particular note, unreliable information may be obtained regarding cardiovascular and musculoskeletal issues.[68] As the source that provides the most accurate history is unclear, both the parents and student athletes should be questioned and specific answers confirmed.

Physical examination

For the PPE, a limited physical examination is recommended (grade of recommendation: C).[38] The screening physical examination should include vital signs (i.e., height, weight, and blood pressure) and visual acuity testing as well as a cardiovascular, pulmonary, abdominal, skin, genitalia (for males), and musculoskeletal examination. Further examination should be based on issues elicited during the history.

Due to the recognition that a cardiac etiology is the most common cause of sudden death in the young, athletic population, the cardiovascular examination requires an additional level of detail (grade of recommendation: C). Auscultation of the heart should be performed initially with the patient in both standing and supine position. Auscultation should also occur during various maneuvers (i.e., squat-to-stand, deep inspiration, or Valsalva's maneuver) as these maneuvers can clarify the type of murmur. Any systolic murmur of grade III/VI or louder, any murmur that disrupts normal heart sounds, any diastolic murmur, or any murmur that intensifies with the previously described maneuvers should be evaluated further through diagnostic studies (e.g., electrocardiography or echocardiography) or consultation prior to participation. Sinus bradycardia and systolic murmurs are commonly found, occurring in over 50% and between 30% and 50% of athletes, respectively, and do not warrant further evaluation in the asymptomatic athlete.[69] Third and fourth heart sounds are also commonly found in asymptomatic athletes without underlying heart disease.[69,70]

Noninvasive cardiac testing (e.g., electrocardiography, echocardiography, or exercise stress testing) are not considered a routine aspect of the screening PPE (grade of recommendation: B).[38] These tests are not cost-effective in a population at relatively low risk for cardiac abnormalities and cannot consistently identify athletes at actual risk.[71–75] A high proportion of normal athletes have abnormal electrocardiograms with increased voltage (left ventricular hypertrophy, left and right atrial enlargement), repolarization changes, and Q waves as well as resting bradycardia and abnormal atrioventricular conduction.[76] The sensitivity of the electrocardiogram in identifying significant cardiovascular disease has been noted to be 50% and the positive predictive value was 7%.[75]

A benefit of an initial cardiovascular screening protocol that included family and personal history, physical examination, basal 12-lead electrocardiography, and limited exercise testing has been reported.[50] In this study, the authors reported that hypertrophic cardiomyopathy was an uncommon cause of death in young competitive athletes and suggested that the identification and disqualification of affected athletes at screening before participation in competitive sports may have prevented sudden death due to hypertrophic cardiomyopathy. The rate of sudden death among athletes compared to controls was noted to be significantly greater among the athletes in this study. Of note, over 25% of nonathletes experiencing sudden death in this study were found to have an "other" or unidentified cause (compared to 10% of athletes) making comparison between the two groups difficult.

Maron *et al.* noted in a large group of intercollegiate competitive athletes that the inclusion of electrocardiography as a primary screening test did not appear to appreciably enhance the sensitivity of an informed history and physical examination in detecting important cardiovascular disease.[77] Furthermore, electrocardiography was responsible for a large number of false positive observations. In a review of two large registries comprised of young competitive athletes who died suddenly, Basso *et al.* noted that standard testing with electrocardiography (ECG) under resting or exercise conditions would unlikely provide clinical evidence of myocardial ischemia and would not be reliable as screening tests in large athletic populations.[78]

The sensitivity of electrocardiography in detecting cardiovascular abnormalities requiring further testing before approval for participation in sports could be given was greater compared to cardiac history, auscultation/inspection, or blood pressure measurement.[73] While athletes were not approved for cardiovascular conditions such as arrhythmias/conduction abnormalities, hypertension, and severe aortic root regurgitation, hypertrophic cardiomyopathy was not identified in an athlete in this study. The 12-lead electrocardiography was found to be the most cost-effective preparticipation cardiovascular screening modality compared to a specific cardiovascular history and physical examination and two-dimensional echocardiography ($44,000 per year of life gained compared to $84,000 and $200,000, respectively).[74,79]

Echocardiography and stress testing are the most commonly recommended diagnostic tests for patients with an abnormal cardiovascular history or examination. With the assistance of clinical information, echocardiography has been previously reported to be able to distinguish the nonobstructive hypertrophic cardiomyopathy from the athletic heart syndrome.[80,81]

Unfortunately, echocardiography lacks specificity in terms of diagnosing hypertrophic cardiomyopathy and determining the patients with hypertrophic cardiomyopathy at risk for sudden cardiac death. In a study by Pelliccia *et al.*, a substantial minority of subjects (11%) were found to have a clinically significant increased ventricular wall thickness which made clinical interpretation of the echocardiographic findings difficult in individual athletes.[75] Furthermore, some patients with hypertrophic cardiomyopathy are able to tolerate particularly intense athletic training and competition for many years, and even maintain high levels of achievement without incurring symptoms, disease progression, or sudden death.[72] Echocardiography is unable to identify these athletes.

Therefore, the identification of athletes with underlying cardiovascular disease placing them at risk for sudden cardiac death is extremely difficult. In addition to the inadequacies of current screening methods, the specific characteristics of the underlying condition make successful screening challenging. In a systemic review of hypertrophic cardiomyopathy, Maron clarified and summarized the relevant clinical issues regarding this genetic cardiac disease.[82] The highest risk for sudden death in hypertrophic cardiomyopathy has been associated with any of the following: prior cardiac arrest or spontaneous sustained ventricular tachycardia; family history of premature hypertrophic cardiomyopathy-related death; syncope and some cases of near-syncope; multiple and repetitive or prolonged bursts of nonsustained ventricular tachycardia on serial ambulatory ECG recordings; hypotensive blood pressure response to exercise; and extreme left ventricular hypertrophy (LVH) with a maximum wall thickness ≥ 30 mm.[82] The hypertrophic cardiomyopathy phenotype is not a static disease manifestation; LVH can appear at virtually any age and can increase and decrease dynamically throughout life. Sudden death associated with hypertrophic cardiomyopathy most commonly occurs during mild or sedentary activities, but is not infrequently related to vigorous physical exertion.

A screening musculoskeletal history and examination in combination can be used for asymptomatic athletes with no previous injuries (Table 2.4) (grade of recommendation: A4).[83] An accurate history is able to detect over 90% of significant musculoskeletal injuries. The screening physical examination is 51% sensitive and 97% specific.[83] If the athlete has either a previous injury or other signs or symptoms (i.e., pain, tenderness, asymmetries in muscle bulk, strength, or range of motion, and any obvious deformity) detected by the general screening examination or history, the general screen should be supplemented with relevant elements of an anatomical site-specific examination.

Additional forms of musculoskeletal evaluation are often performed for athletes to determine their general state of flexibility and muscular strength. While various degrees of hyperlaxity, muscular tightness, weakness, asymmetry of strength or flexibility, poor endurance, and abnormal foot configuration may predispose an athlete to increased risk

Table 2.4 The "90-second" musculoskeletal screening examination

Instruction	Observations
Stand facing examiner	Acromioclavicular joints: general habitus
Look at ceiling, floor, over both shoulders, touch ears to shoulder	Cervical spine motion
Shrug shoulders (resistance)	Trapezius strength
Abduct shoulders to 90° (resistance at 90°)	Deltoid strength
Full external rotation of arms	Shoulder motion
Flex and extend elbows	Elbow motion
Arms at sides, elbows at 90° flexed; pronate and supinate wrists	Elbow and wrist motion
Spread fingers; make fist	Hand and finger motion, strength, and deformities
Tighten (contract) quadriceps; relax quadriceps	Symmetry and knee effusions, ankle effusion
"Duck walk" away and towards examiner	Hip, knee, and ankle motions
Back to examiner	Shoulder symmetry; scoliosis
Knees straight, touch toes	Scoliosis, hip motion, hamstring tightness
Raise up on toes, heels	Calf symmetry, leg strength

of injury during sports competition, the studies have failed to demonstrate conclusively that injuries are prevented by interventions aimed at correcting such abnormalities.[84–87] Meeuwisse and Fowler reported that new injuries were found to have no relationship to previous injury, flexibility, range of motion, strength or other factors identifiable on preseason musculoskeletal examination.[88] As noted by Garrick, little if any evidence exists regarding the premise that any level of loss of motion or strength is predictive of an increased likelihood of subsequent injury.[89] Additionally, evidence that stretching to increase range of motion prevents injury is lacking. In a systematic review to assess the evidence for the effectiveness of stretching as a tool to prevent injuries in sports, stretching was not significantly associated with a reduction in total injuries (OR 0.93, 95% CI, 0.78 to 1.11).[90] Smith and Laskowski noted that the absence of concrete recommendations concerning the findings from a preparticipation screening examination are attributable to the lack of consensus regarding the threshold for abnormality, the unavailability of data indicating the predictive value of specific physical abnormalities for injury, and the lack definitive proof that corrective interventions alter outcome.[91]

The remainder of the physical examination is limited to the following anatomical areas: General appearance, eyes/ears/nose/throat, lymph nodes, lungs, and abdomen. The genitalia in males are examined, mainly in order to identify the presence of an inguinal hernia. The effectiveness of this partial examination in identifying asymptomatic conditions that require further evaluation and potential treatment or that restrict an individual from athletic participation is unclear and not well studied.

Historically, studies have not supported the use of routine laboratory or other screening tests such tests as urinalysis, complete blood count, chemistry profile, lipid profile, ferritin level, or spirometry during the PPE (grade of recommendation: B).[92–95] In light of these recommendations, several authors have recommended screening for specific conditions, especially in specific athletic populations.

For instance, Fallon recommended screening for hematological and iron-related abnormalities in athletes entering an elite training program.[96] In support of this recommendation, previous reports have suggested that athletes in general may be prone to iron deficiency.[97–102] Clement *et al.* observed iron deficiency more frequently in exercising females compared to exercising males,[97] and Dickerson *et al.* specifically associated iron deficiency with running.[98] Adolescent athletes of both genders, gymnasts in particular, were prone to nonanemic iron deficiency.[103] Eliakim *et al.* found low ferritin levels in 13% of the Israeli National Olympic gymnastic team.[104]

Several studies have also found evidence to support the presence of non-anemia iron deficiency in the physically active population. Throughout a long-term period (6 months) of moderate exercise, previously sedentary women developed depleted iron stores (serum ferritin < 15 ng/mL).[105] In a study of 851 male athletes, physical activity of increasing duration and workload lead to decreased ferritin levels irrespective of the athlete's discipline.[106] Runners had a more pronounced effect.

In contrast to the above studies, other studies have failed to provide consistent evidence regarding the association between an increase in physical activity and a decrease in serum ferritin. Milman and Kirchhoff did not find an association between serum ferritin and physical activity.[107] Following a resistance-training program twice weekly for 12 weeks, serum ferritin concentrations decreased significantly in women but were unchanged in men.[108] Bourque *et al.* examined the effects of 12 weeks of endurance exercise training in iron status measures in previously inactive women and compared the effects of weight-bearing endurance exercise training and non-weight bearing endurance exercise on iron status measures.[109] The results indicated that participation in 12 weeks of moderate-intensity endurance exercise training (walking/running or cycling) resulted in no negative effects on selected measures of iron status in healthy, previously untrained women with normal iron stores (serum ferritin ≥ 20 μg/L).

As the prevalence of exercise induced bronchoconstriction (EIB) in athletes has been reported to range from 6–12% to nearly 21% in a group of elite athletes, screening for this condition is often recommended.[110–113] Despite this relatively high prevalence, screening for this condition is difficult. Many athletes who report symptoms of EIB do not demonstrate laboratory study results consistent with this diagnosis. Less than half (46%) of intercollegiate athletes referred for pulmonary function tests based on a medical history consistent with EIB had a positive laboratory exercise challenge test.[114] Only 76% of male college football players with symptoms suggestive of EIB had a positive methacholine challenge test.[115] In a study of elite athletes, 45% of those subjects reporting symptoms had a negative exercise challenge test.[116] Holzer *et al.* found that 28% of elite summer sort athletes reported one or more respiratory symptom but did not have a positive bronchial provocation challenge.[117]

In contrast, Rundell *et al.* found that only 61% of athletes positive to a field exercise challenge reported symptoms.[116] Holzer *et al.* observed that only 60% of elite athletes with a positive eucapnic voluntary hyperpnea challenge test reported symptoms.[117]

Therefore, the sensitivity and specificity of testing for EIB is inadequate for an effective medical screening tool. Recently, Hammerman *et al.* noted that a free running test may be a good test for identifying and assessing the athlete with EIB.[118]

In addition to medical screening tests, baseline functional status determination of the athlete in specific areas has been promoted. As majority of athletes participating in contact sports give a history of prior concussion, several authorities have recommended that a baseline neuropsychological examination, preferably using a computerized test battery, should be performed in order to guide return to play following subsequent concussive injury.[119,120] Although no published controlled studies at the present time provide an evidence-based decision in regards to baseline neuropsychological assessment, the expert consensus group from the First World Conference on Sport-Related Concussion held in Vienna in 2001 determined that all return-to-play decisions should be based on individual recovery assessment and that neuropsychological testing is the cornerstone of management strategy.[121]

The PPE is only one aspect of an overall program of risk assessment for athletic participation. In addition to the PPE, physicians should consider exploring other aspects of sports participation to assist athletes in reducing the risk of injury. Practice patterns, rules, equipment, or other factors may have a greater effect on decreasing the mortality and morbidity associated with athletic participation. A marked decrease in cervical spine injuries occurred following the rule change in football banning both deliberate "spearing" and the use of the top of the helmet as the initial point of contact in making a tackle.[122]

Determination of clearance

Occasionally, an abnormality or condition is found that may limit an athlete's participation or predispose him or her to further injury. In these cases, the examining physician should review the following questions as the overall question of participation is being debated:[38]

- Does the problem place the athlete at increased risk for injury?
- Is another participant at risk for injury because of the problem?
- Can the athlete safely participate with treatment (i.e., medication, rehabilitation, bracing, or padding)?
- Can limited participation be allowed while treatment is being completed?
- If clearance is denied only for certain sports or sport categories, in what activities can the athlete safely participate?

A specific risk-analysis providing the physician with further guidance in answering the above questions has not been developed. Furthermore, the specific threshold used in the decision is dependent on numerous factors, including the specific sport, desires of the athlete and parent, and available equipment.

The determination of clearance to participate in a particular sport should be based on previously published guidelines such as the recommendations by the American Academy of Pediatrics, the 26th Bethesda Conference and the American Heart Association (grade of recommendation: C).[41,123,124] Participation recommendations are based on the specific diagnosis, though multiple factors such as the classification of the sport and the specific health status of the athlete affect the decision.[124–126] Whether these specific guidelines for clearance effectively limit participation of athletes at risk for further injury without limiting participation for athletes with minimal or no risk is unclear and has yet to be studied. Furthermore, the effect of inappropriately excluding the individual with minimal or no risk of athletic associated injury or death is unclear.

Additional considerations

While current research demonstrates that the PPE has no effect on the overall morbidity and mortality rates in athletes, other objectives may be fulfilled by these examinations. The determination of general health, the counseling on health-related issues, and the assessment of fitness level for specific sports are several other objectives often identified as being fulfilled during the PPE. Furthermore, no harmful effects of these examinations have been reported. The PPE has also become institutionalized in the athletic and sports-medicine community. As such, physicians should base their PPE on the best available evidence using standard PPE form such as the one recommended by Matheson *et al.*[38]

In general, the current recommended PPE fails to meet many of its intended objectives, including the detection of conditions that may predispose to injury or conditions that may be life-threatening or disabling. This ineffectiveness has been studied by several authors. Glover and Maron found that the preparticipation athletic screening for cardiovascular disease in U.S. high schools may be inadequate, is implemented by a variety of health-care workers with varying levels of expertise, and may be severely limited in its power to detect potentially lethal cardiovascular abnormalities.[32] Gomez *et al.* found that 17.2% of high schools used PPE forms with all the elements of the cardiac history recommended by the consensus panel and the PPE varies among states.[127] While an effective screening tool has yet to be developed, many authorities believe the preparticipation screening process used by many U.S. colleges and universities appears to have limited potential to detect cardiovascular abnormalities capable of causing sudden death in competitive student-athletes based on the finding that untested guidelines were not being met.[33]

These observations may represent an impetus for change and improvement in the preparticipation screening process for high school athletes. Unfortunately, the standardized evaluation that has been recommended has not been shown to be better the reported inadequate forms used by some states or to no preparticipation screening. Even when completed by physicians with sports-medicine training and experience, over one-third of athletes reported having had a bad-quality preparticipation sports examination.[128] According to these athletes, medical history taking was poor and physical examination restricted to blood pressure measurement and/or chest listening and not targeted enough to past athletic injuries.

As previously noted, the PPE has become a requirement and the standard of care for athletes in many countries as they prepare for organized athletic participation. As such, several key issues regarding this examination exist.

Key messages

- The mortality associated with athletic participation is most often the result of acute sudden cardiac death and certain populations of athletes appear to be at higher risk. Furthermore, the prevalence of underlying cardiovascular disease varies according to ethnic background and nationality.
- A complete medical history has been shown to identify approximately 75% of problems that affect initial athletic participation. For the PPE, a limited physical examination is recommended. A screening musculoskeletal history and examination in combination can be used for asymptomatic athletes with no previous injuries.
- Noninvasive cardiac testing (e.g., electrocardiography, echocardiography, or exercise stress testing) and the use of routine laboratory or other screening tests such tests as urinalysis, complete blood count, chemistry profile, lipid profile, ferritin level, or spirometry during the PPE is not supported by studies currently available.
- The determination of clearance to participate in a particular sport should be based on previously published guidelines such as the recommendations by the American Academy of Pediatrics, the 26th Bethesda Conference and the American Heart Association.

Sample examination questions

Multiple-choice questions (answers on page 602)

1 A preparticipation physical examination (PPE) for athletics is a universally accepted medical screening instrument utilized in all countries.
   A True
   B False

2 While hypertrophic cardiomyopathy is the most common cause of sudden death in athletes in the United States, the following is the most common cause of sudden death among Italian athletes:
   A Brugada syndrome
   B Arrhythmogenic right ventricular dysplasia (ARVD)
   C Essential hypertension
   D Mitral valve prolapse

3 The strongest independent predictor of sports injuries is:
   A Decreased flexibility
   B Imbalance of agonist–antagonist muscle strength
   C Abnormal foot configuration
   D A previous injury

4 Studies have supported the general use of spirometry during the preparticipation physical examination (PPE) in order to screen for underlying exercise-induced bronchospasms (EIBs).
   A True
   B False

Essay questions

1 The current recommended preparticipation physical examination (PPE) fails to meet many of its intended objectives, including the detection of conditions that may predispose to injury or conditions that may be life-threatening or disabling. Furthermore, clearance criteria may inappropriately restrict individuals at low or no risk for athletic related injury. Describe the current issues that limit the effectiveness of the PPE in identifying at risk athletes as well as the potential implications of unnecessary restrictions.

2 Currently, the mortality associated with athletic participation is most often the result of acute sudden cardiac death. Describe the cardiac abnormalities and methods of diagnosis of these conditions most frequently found in athletes experiencing sudden cardiac death and the athletic population that appears to be at higher risk.

3 Occasionally, an abnormality or condition is found that may limit an athlete's participation or predispose him or her to further injury. Describe potential criteria that may be used by the physician to determine the clearance status for an athlete with such an abnormality or condition.

Case study 2.1

James, an 18-year-old high-school football player, presents for his routine preparticipation physical examination. On review, you note that he has experienced acute loss of consciousness during exercise and he has a family history of sudden cardiac death in an uncle aged 28. As team physician, you need to determine an appropriate cardiovascular evaluation.

Case study 2.2

You are the team physician for the local high school. Before the football season, a group of parents approach you regarding preparticipation physical examinations. Due to recent news reports regarding mortality associated with participation in high school sports, they would like to have an extensive medical evaluation of the high school athletes, including an electrocardiogram, spirometry, and laboratory studies. They are seeking your advice regarding appropriate screening tests for their high school athletes.

Summarizing the evidence: grades of recommendations for the preparticipation physical examination for athletics

Recommendation	Results	Level of evidence*
Medical history		C
Limited physical examination		C
Additional detail of cardiovascular examination		C
Exclusion of noninvasive cardiac testing	Numerous large studies with descriptive data†	B
Screening musculoskeletal examination	One randomized trial	A4
Exclusion of routine laboratory or other screening tests such as urinalysis, complete blood count, chemistry profile, lipid profile, ferritin level, or spirometry	Numerous large studies with contrasting descriptive data	B
Determination of clearance based on published guidelines		C

* A1: evidence from large randomized controlled trials (RCTs) or systematic review (including meta-analysis).†
A2: evidence from at least one high-quality cohort.
A3: evidence from at least one moderate-sized RCT or systematic review.†
A4: evidence from at least one RCT.
B: evidence from at least one high-quality study of nonrandomized cohorts.
C: expert opinions.
† Arbitrarily, the following cut-off points have been used: large study size: ≥ 100 patients per intervention group; moderate study size ≥ 50 patients per intervention group.

References

1 Runyan DK. The pre-participation examination of the young athlete. *Clinical Pediatrics* 1983; 22:674–679.
2 Strong WB, Steed D. Cardiovascular evaluation of the young athlete. *Primary Care* 1984; 11:61–75.
3 Rowland TW. Preparticipation sports examination of the child and adolescent athlete: changing views of an old ritual. *Pediatrician* 1986; 13:3–9.
4 Kibler WB, Chandler TJ, Uhl T, Maddux RE. A musculoskeletal approach to the preparticipation physical examination. *Am J Sports Med* 1989; 17:525–531.
5 McKeag DB. Preparticipation screening of the potential athlete. *Clin Sports Med* 1989; 8:373–397.
6 Fields KB, Delaney M. Focusing the preparticipation sports examination. *J Fam Pract* 1990; 30:304–312.
7 Garrick JG. Orthopedic preparticipation screening examination. *Ped Clin N Am* 1990; 37:1047–1056.

8 Tanji JL. The preparticipation physical examination for sports. *Am Fam Physician* 1990; **42**:397–402.

9 Ball RM. The sports preparticipation evaluation. *N J Med* 1991; **88**:629–633.

10 Smith DM, Lombardo JA, Robinson JB. The preparticipation evaluation. *Primary Care* 1991; **18**:777–807.

11 Dyment PG. The orthopedic component of the preparticipation examination. *Pediatric Annals*. 1992; **21**:159–162.

12 Henderson JM. The preparticipation screening evaluation. *J Med Assoc Georgia* 1992; **81**:277–282.

13 Hoekelman RA. The preparticipation sports physical examination [editorial]. *Pediatr Ann* 1992; **21**:145–146.

14 Overbaugh KA, Allen JG. The adolescent athlete. Part I: preseason preparation and examination. *J Pediatr Health Care* 1994; **8**:146–151.

15 Strong WB. Preparticipation physical examination: it should be required. *Arch Pediatr Adolesc Med* 1994; **148**:99–100.

16 Hergenroeder AC. The preparticipation sports examination. *Pediatr Clin North Am* 1997; **44**:1525–1540.

17 Bratton RL. Preparticipation screening of children for sports. *Sports Med* 1997; **24**:300–307.

18 Cantwell JD. Preparticipation physical evaluation: Getting to the heart of the matter. *Med Sci Sports Exerc* 1998; **10** (Suppl):S341–S344.

19 Clinkenbeard D, Wright P. The preparticipation physical examination and its current status in Oklahoma. *J Okla State Med Assoc* 1998; **91**:155–61.

20 Myers A, Sickles T. Preparticipation sports examination. *Prim Care* 1998; **25**:225–236.

21 Metzl JD. The adolescent preparticipation physical examination: is it helpful? *Clin Sports Med* 2000; **19**:577–592.

22 Lyznicki JM, Nielsen NH, Schneider JF. Cardiovascular screening of student athletes. *Am Fam Physician* 2000; **62**:765–784.

23 McKeag DB, Sallis RE. Factors at play in the athletic preparticipation examination. *Am Fam Physician* 2000; **61**:2617–2618.

24 Stickler GB. Are yearly physical examinations in adolescents necessary? *J Am Board Fam Pract* 2000; **13**:172–177.

25 Carek PJ, Hunter MH. The preparticipation physical examination for athletes: a critical review of current recommendations. *Lebanese Med J* 2001; **49**:292–297.

26 Lombardo JA, Badolato SK. The preparticipation physical examination. *Clinical Cornerstone* 2001; **3**:10–25.

27 Carek PJ, Mainous AG. A thorough yet efficient exam identifies most problems in school athletes. *J Fam Pract* 2003; **52**:127–134.

28 Seto CK. Preparticipation cardiovascular screening. *Clin Sports Med* 2003; **22**:23–35.

29 Armsey TD, Hosey RG. Medical aspects of sports: epidemiology of injuries, preparticipation physical examination, and drugs in sports. *Clin Sports Med* 2004; **23**:255–279.

30 Wingfield K, Matheson GO, Meeuwisse WH. Preparticipation evaluation: an evidence-based review. *Clin J Sport Med* 2004; **14**:109–122.

31 MacAuley D. Does the preseason screening for cardiac disease really work?: the British perspective. *Med Sci Sports Exerc* 1998; **30**:S345–S350.

32 Glover DW, Maron BJ. Profile of preparticipation cardiovascular screening for high school athletes. *JAMA* 1998; **279**:1817–1819.

33 Pfister GC, Puffer JC, Maron BJ. Preparticipation cardiovascular screening for US collegiate student-athletes. *JAMA* 2000; **283**:1597–1599.

34 Reich JD. It won't be me next time: an opinion on preparticipation sports physicals. *Am Fam Physician* 2000; **61**:2618, 2620, 2625, 2629.

35 Batt ME, Jacques R, Stone M. Preparticipation examination (screening): practical issues as determined by sport. *Clin J Sport Med* 2004; **14**:178–182.

36 American College of Sports Medicine. Sideline preparedness for the team physician: a consensus statement. Available at: http://www.acsm.org/pdf/sideprep.pdf. Accessed : May, 2005.

37 American Medical Association. Medical Evaluation of the Athlete: A Guide. Revised. Chicago, Ill: American Medical Association; 1976.

38 Matheson GO, Boyajian-O'Neill LA, Cardone D, *et al. Preparticipation Physical Examination*, 3rd ed. Minneapolis: McGraw-Hill, 2005: 1–98.

39 Smith DM, Kovan JR, Rich BSE, Tanner SM. *Preparticipation Physical Evaluation*, 2nd ed. Minneapolis: McGraw-Hill, 1997: 1–46.
40 Lombardo JA, Robinson JB, Smith DM, *et al. Preparticipation Physical Examination*, 1st ed. Kansas City, MO: American Academy of Family Physicians, American Academy of Pediatrics, American Medical Society for Sports Medicine, American Orthopedic Society for Sports Medicine, American Osteopathic Academy of Sports Medicine, 1992.
41 Maron BJ, Thompson PC, Puffer JC, *et al.* Cardiovascular preparticipation screening of competitive athletes: a statement for health professionals from the sudden death committee (clinical cardiology) and congenital cardiac defects committee (cardiovascular disease in the young), American Heart Association. AHA Medical/Scientific Statement. *Circulation* 1996; **94**:850–856.
42 Maron BJ, Araujo CG, Thompson PD, *et al.* Recommendations for preparticipation screening and the assessment of cardiovascular disease in masters athletes: an advisory for healthcare professionals from the working groups of the World Heart Federation, the International Federation of Sports Medicine, and the American Heart Association on Exercise, Cardiac Rehabilitation, and Prevention. *Circulation* 2001; **103**:327–334.
43 Krowchuk DP, Krowchuk HV, Hunter M, *et al.* Parents' knowledge of the purposes and content of preparticipation physical examinations. *Arch Pediatr Adolesc Med* 1995; **149**:653–657.
44 Carek PJ , Futrell MA. Athlete's view of the preparticipation physical examination: attitudes toward certain health screening questions. *Arch Fam Med* 1999; **8**:307–312.
45 Maron BJ, Gohman TE, Aeppli D. Prevalence of sudden cardiac death during competitive sports activities in Minnesota high school athletes. *J Am Coll Cardiol* 1998; **32**:1881–1884.
46 American Medical Association Board of Trustees, Group on Science and Technology. Athletic participation examinations for adolescents. *Arch Pediatr Adolesc Med* 1994; **148**:93–98.
47 Epstein SE, Maron BJ. Sudden death and the competitive athlete: perspectives on preparticipation screening studies. *J Am Coll Cardiol* 1986; **7**:220–30.
48 Beckerman J, Wang P, Hlatky M. Cardiovascular screening of athletes. *Clin J Sports Med* 1994; **14**:127–133.
49 Pelliccia A, Maron BJ. Preparticipation cardiovascular evaluation of the competitive athlete: perspectives from the 30-year Italian experience. *Am J Cardiol* 1995; **75**:827–829.
50 Corrado D, Basso C, Schiavon M, Thiene G. Screening for hypertrophic cardiomyopathy in young athletes. *N Engl J Med* 1998; **339**:364–369.
51 Zeppilli P. Il concetto di idoneita e non ideoneita cardiovaculare allo sport sotto il profile clinico e medico-legale. In: Zeppilli P, ed. *Cardiologia dello Sport.* Rome: Casa Editrice Scientifica Internazionale, 1990: 269–274.
52 Maron BJ, Gohman TE, Aeppli D. Prevalence of sudden cardiac death during competitive sports activities in Minnesota high school athletes. *J Am Coll Cardiol* 1998; **32**:1881–1884.
53 Cantu RC, Mueller FO. Fatalities and catastrophic injuries in high school and college sports, 1982–1997. *Phys Sportsmed* 1999; **27**:35–48.
54 Brugada P, Brugada J. Right bundle branch block, persistent ST segment elevation and sudden cardiac death: a distinct clinical and electrocardiographic syndrome. A multicenter report. *J Am Coll Cardiol* 1992; 20:1391–1396.
55 Thiene G, Nava A, Corrado D, *et al.* Right ventricular cardiomyopathy and sudden death in young people. *N Engl J Med* 1988; **318**:129–133.
56 Goldberg B, Saranti A, Witman P, *et al.* Pre-participation sports assessment: an objective evaluation. *Pediatrics* 1980; **66**:736–745.
57 Linder CW, DuRant RH, Seklecki RM, *et al.* Preparticipation health screening of young athletes: results of 1268 examinations. *Am J Sports Med* 1981; **9**:187–193.
58 Tennant FS Jr, Sorenson K, Day CM. Benefits of preparticipation sports examinations. *J Fam Pract* 1981; **13**:287–288.
59 Thompson TR, Andrish JT, Bergfield JA. A prospective study of preparticipation sports examinations of 2670 young athletes: method and results. *Cleve Clin Q* 1982; **49**:225–233.
60 DuRant R, Seymore C, Linder CW, *et al.* The preparticipation examination of athletes: comparison of single and multiple examiners. *Am J Dis Child* 1985; **139**:657–661.
61 Risser WL, Hoffman HM, Bellah GG Jr. Frequency of preparticipation sports examinations in secondary school athletes: are the University Interscholastic League guidelines appropriate? *Tex Med* 1985; **81**:35–39.

62 Magnes SA, Henderson JM, Hunter SC. What limits sports participation: experience with 10,540 athletes. *Phys Sportsmed* 1992; 20:143–160.
63 Rifat SF, Ruffin MT, Gorenflo DW. Disqualifying criteria in preparticipation sports evaluation. *J Fam Pract* 1995; **41**:42–50.
64 Lively MW. Preparticipation physical examinations: a collegiate experience. *Clin J Sport Med* 1999; **9**:3–8.
65 DuRant RH, Pendergrast RA, Seymore C, Gaillard G, Donner J. Findings from the preparticipation athletic examination and athletic injuries. *Am J Dis Child* 1992; **146**:85–91.
66 Van Mechelen W, Twisk J, Molendijk A, *et al.* Subject-related risk factors for sports injuries: a 1-yr prospective study in young adults. *Med Sci Sports Exerc* 1996; **28**:1171–1179.
67 Rumbell JS, Lebrun CM. Preparticipation physical examination: selected issues for the female athlete. *Clin J Sport Med* 2004; **14**:153–160.
68 Carek PJ, Futrell MA, Hueston WJ. The preparticipation physical examination history: who has the correct answer? *Clin J Sports Med* 1999; **9**:124–128.
69 Huston TP, Puffer JC, Rodney WM. The athletic heart syndrome. *N Engl J Med* 1985; **313**:24–32.
70 Crawford MH, O'Rourke RA. The athlete's heart. *Adv Intern Med* 1979; **24**:311–329.
71 Lewis JF, Maron BJ, Diggs JA, *et al.* Preparticipation echocardiographic screening for cardiovascular disease in a large, predominantly black population of collegiate athletes. *Am Coll Cardiol* 1989; **64**:1029–1033.
72 Maron BJ, Klues HG. Surviving competitive athletes with hypertrophic cardiomyopathy. *Am J Card* 1994; **73**:1098–1104.
73 Fuller CM, McNulty CM, Spring DA, *et al.* Prospective screening of 5,615 high school athletes for risk of sudden death. *Med Sci Sports Exer* 1997; **29**:1131–1138.
74 Fuller CM. Cost effectiveness of analysis of high school athletes for risks of sudden death. *Med Sci Sports Exer* 2000; **32**:887–890.
75 Pelliccia A, Maron BJ, Culasso F, *et al.* Clinical significance of abnormal electrocardiographic patterns in trained athletes. *Circulation* 2000; **102**:278–284.
76 Sharma S, Whyte G, Elliott P, *et al.* Electrocardiographic changes in 1000 highly trained junior elite athletes. *Br J Sports Med* 1999; **33**:319–324.
77 Maron BJ, Bodison SA, Wesley YE, Tucker E, Green KJ. Results of screening a large group of intercollegiate competitive athletes for cardiovascular disease. *J Am Coll Cardiol* 1987; **10**:1214–1221.
78 Basso C, Maron BJ, Corrado D, Thiene F. Clinical profile of congenital coronary artery anomalies with origin from the wrong aortic sinus leading to sudden death in young competitive athletes. *J Am Coll Cardiol* 2000; **35**:1493–1501.
79 Risser WL, Hoffman HM, Bellah GG Jr, Green LW. A cost–benefit analysis of preparticipation sports examination of adolescent athletes. *J School Health* 1985; **55**:270–273.
80 Pelliccia A, Maron BJ, Spataro A, Proschan MA, Spirito P. The upper limit of physiologic cardiac hypertrophy in highly trained elite athletes. *N Eng J Med* 1991; **324**:295–301.
81 Maron BJ, Pelliccia A, Spirito P. Cardiac disease in young trained athletes: insights into methods for distinguishing athlete's heart from structural heart disease with particular emphasis on hypertrophic cardiomyopathy. *Circulation* 1995; **91**:1596–1601.
82 Maron BJ. Hypertrophic cardiomyopathy: a systematic review. *JAMA* 2002; **287**:1308–1329.
83 Gomez JE, Landry GL, Bernhardt DT. Critical evaluation of the 2-minute orthopedic screening examination. *Am J Dis Child* 1993; **147**:1109–1113.
84 Abbott HG, Kress JB. Preconditioning in the prevention of knee injuries. *Arch Phys Med Rehabil* 1969; **50**:326–333.
85 Jackson DW, Jarrett H, Bailey D, *et al.* Injury prediction in the young athlete: a preliminary report. *Am J Sports Med* 1978; **6**:6–14.
86 Nicholas JA. Injuries in knee ligaments: relationship to looseness and tightness in football players. *JAMA* 1970; **212**:2236–2239.
87 Willems TM, Witvrouw E, Delbaere K, *et al.* Intrinsic risk factors for inversion ankle sprains in male subjects. *Am J Sports Med* 2005; **33**:415–423.
88 Meeuwisse WH, Fowler PJ. Frequency and predictability of sports injuries in intercollegiate athletes. *Can J Sports Sci* 1988; **13**:35–42.
89 Garrick JG. Preparticipation orthopedic screening evaluation. *Clin J Sport Med* 2004; **14**:123–6.

90 Thacker SB, Gilchrist J, Stroup DF, *et al.* The impact of stretching on sports injury risk: a systematic review of the literature. *Med Sci Sports Exerc* 2004; **36**:371–378.

91 Smith J, Laskowski E. The preparticipation physical examination: Mayo Clinic experience with 2,739 examinations. *Mayo Clin Proc* 1998; **73**:419–429.

92 Dodge WF, West EF, Smith EH, Bruce Harvey 3rd. Proteinuria and hematuria in schoolchildren: epidemiology and early natural history. *J Pediatr* 1976; **88**:327–347.

93 Peggs JF, Reinhardt RW, O'Brien JM. Proteinuria in adolescent sports physical examinations. *J Fam Pract* 1986; **22**:80–81.

94 Rupp NT, Brudno DS, Guill MF. The value of screening for risk of exercise-induced asthma in high school athletes. *Ann Allergy* 1993; **70**:339–342.

95 Feinstein RA, La Russa J, Wang-Dohlman A, *et al.* Screening adolescent athletes for exercise-induced asthma. *Clin J Sports Med* 1996; **6**:119–123.

96 Fallon KE. Utility of hematological and iron-related screening in elite athletes. *Clin J Sport Med* 2004; **14**:145–152.

97 Clement DB, Taunton JE, Poskitt K. Iron deficiency anaemia in a distance runner. *Can Fam Physician* 1982; **28**:1008–1010.

98 Dickerson DH, Wilkinson RL, Noakes TD. Effects of ultra-marathon training and racing on hematologic parameters and serum ferritin levels in well-trained athletes. *Int J Sports Med* 1982; **3**:111–117.

99 Dufaux B, Hoederath A, Streitberger I, Hollman W, Assman G. Serum ferritin, transferrin, haptoglobin and iron in middle- and long-distance runners, elite rowers and professional racing cyclists. *Int J Sports Med* 1981; **2**:43–46.

100 Ehn L, Carlmark B, Hoglund S. Iron status in athletes involved in intense physical activity. *Med Sci Sports Exerc* 1980; **12**:61–64.

101 Finch CA, Gollnick PD, Hlastala MP, *et al.* Lactic acidosis as a result of iron deficiency. *J Clin Invest* 1979; **64**:129–137.

102 Wishnitzer R, Vorst E, Berebi A. Bone marrow iron depression in competitive distance runners. *Int J Sports Med* 1983; **4**:27–30.

103 Constantini NW, Eliakim A, Zigel L, Yaaron M, Falk B. Iron status in highly active adolescents: evidence of depleted iron stores in gymnasts. *In J Sport Nutr Exerc Metab* 2000; **10**:62–70.

104 Eliakim A, Namet D, Constantini N. Screening blood tests in members of the Israeli National Olympic team. *J Sports Med Phys Fitness* 2002; **42**:250–255.

105 Rajaram S, Weaver CM, Lyle RM, *et al.* Effects of long-term moderate exercise on iron status in young women. *Med Sci Sports Exerc* 1995; **27**:1105–1110.

106 Schumacher YO, Schmid A, Grathwohl D, Bültermann D, Berg A. Hematological indices and iron status in athletes of various sports and performances. *Med Sci Sports Exerc* 2002; **43**:869–875.

107 Milman N, Kirchhoff M. Relationship between serum ferritin and risk factors for ischemic heart disease in 2235 Danes aged 30–60 years. *J Internal Med* 1999; **245**:423–433.

108 Murray-Kolb LE, Beard JL, Joseph LJ, *et al.* Resistance training affects iron status in older men and women. *In J Sport Nutr Exerc Metab* 2001; **11**:287–298.

109 Bourque SP, Pate RR, Branch JD. Twelve weeks of endurance exercise training does not affect iron status measures in women. *J Am Diet Assoc* 1997; **97**:1116–1121.

110 Corrigan B, Kazlauskas R, Medication use in athletes selected for doping control at the Sydney Olympics (2000). *Clin J Sport Med* 2003; **13**:33–40.

111 Randolph C, Randolph M, Fraser B. Exercise-induced asthma in school children. *J Allergy Clin Immunol* 1991; **87**:341.

112 Kawabori I, Pierson WE, Conquest LL, *et al.* Incidence of exercise-induced asthma in children. *J Allergy Clin Immunol* 1976; **58**:447–455.

113 Rupp NT, Guill MF, Brudno DS. Unrecognized exercise-induced bronchospasm in adolescent athletes. *Am J Dis Child* 1992; **146**:941–944.

114 Rice SG, Bierman CW, Shapiro GG, *et al.* Identification of exercise-induced asthma among intercol legiate athletes. *Ann Allergy* 1985; **55**:790–793.

115 Weiler JM, Metzger JW, Donnelly AL, *et al.* Prevalence of bronchial hyperresponsiveness in highly trained athletes. *Chest* 1986; **90**:23–28.

116 Rundell KS, Im J, Mayers LB, *et al.* Self-reported symptoms and exercise-induced asthma in the elite athlete. *Med Sci Sports Exerc* 2001; **33**:208–213.

117 Holzer K, Anderson SD, Douglass J. Exercise in elite summer athletes: challenges for diagnosis. *J Allergy Clin Immunol* 2002; **110**:374–380.

118 Hammerman SI, Becker JM, Rogers J, Quedenfeld TC, D'Alsonzo GE. Asthma screening of high school athletes: identifying the undiagnosed and poorly controlled. *Ann Allergy Asthma Immunol* 2002; **88**:380–384.

119 Johnston K, McCrory P, Mohtadi N, *et al.* Evidence based review of sport-related concussion: clinical science. *Clin J Sport Med* 2001; **11**:150–160.

120 McCrory P, Collie A, Anderson V, Davis G. Can we manage sport related concussion in children the same as in adults? *Br J Sports Med* 2004; **38**:516–519.

121 Aubry M, Cantu R, Dvorak J, *et al.* Summary and agreement statement of the first International Conference on Concussion in Sport, Vienna 2001. *Br J Sports Med* 2002; **36**:6–10.

122 Torg JS, Vegso JJ, Sennett B, Das M. The National Football Head and Neck Injury Registry: 14-year report on cervical quadriplegia, 1971 through 1984. *JAMA* 1985; **254**:3439–3443.

123 Anonymous. 26th Bethesda Conference: recommendations for determining eligibility for competition in athletes with cardiovascular abnormalities. *Med Sci Sports Exerc* 1994:**26** (10 Suppl):S223–83.

124 American Academy of Pediatrics. Medical conditions affecting sports participation. *Pediatrics* 2001; **107**:1206–1207.

125 Moeller JL. Contraindications to athletic participation: cardiac, respiratory, and central nervous system conditions. *Phys Sportsmed* 1996; **8**:47–59.

126 Moeller JL. Contraindications to athletic participation: spinal, systemic, dermatologic, paired-organ, and other issues. *Phys Sportsmed* 1996; **9**:57–78.

127 Gomez JE, Lantry BR, Saathoff KN. Current use of adequate preparticipation history forms for heart disease screening of high school athletes. *Arch Pediatr Adolesc Med* 1999; **153**:723–726.

128 Laure P. High-level athlete's impressions of their preparticipation sports examination. *J Sports Med Phys Fitness* 1996; **36**:291–292.

CHAPTER 3
Does stretching help prevent injuries?

Ian Shrier

Since the first edition of this book, several other authors have performed systematic reviews on this topic and reached the same conclusions: stretching prior to exercise does not prevent injury.[1–3] This concept is now also being promoted to a wider audience than simply sports-medicine clinicians.[4,5] However, practicing evidence-based medicine means that everything constitutes work in progress, and it is important to update the knowledge base on any question continuously. With respect to original clinical research, two recent studies are added to this review.[6,7] Two tangential studies have not been included: Malliaropoulos *et al.*[8] studied the effects of stretching once per day versus four times per day, but did not include a no-stretch control group. Sherry and Best[9] compared stretching and isolated hamstring strengthening versus progressive agility and trunk stabilization. Although these studies are valid, they did not address the question with which this chapter is concerned and are not included in the analysis.

Introduction

Over the past 30 years, sports-medicine professionals have promoted stretching as a way to decrease the risk of injury.[10–15] Two potential mechanisms are often proposed by which stretching could decrease injury: a direct decrease in muscle stiffness via changes in passive viscoelastic properties, or an indirect decrease in muscle stiffness via reflex muscle inhibition and consequent changes in viscoelastic properties due to decreased actin–myosin cross-bridges. These changes in muscle stiffness would allow for an increased ROM (ROM) around a joint (within this paper, I will use the term flexibility as a synonym for range of motion (ROM) because that is the common use of the term by clinicians even though it may have other meanings in other domains), which is believed to decrease the risk of injury. However, there are several important points the reader must consider.

First, both the muscle–tendon unit and the joint capsule may limit ROM. Flexibility is usually considered the ROM limited by muscle–tendon, and mobility is usually considered the ROM limited by capsule/ligament. These differences should be taken into account when reading the literature.

Second, stretching must be differentiated from ROM. There are many individuals who have excellent ROM but never stretch, and many individuals who stretch but continue to have limited ROM. Therefore, different injury rates in people with different ROMs may not be related to the effect of stretching, but rather to the underlying interindividual variations in tissue properties (e.g., strength), anatomy, etc. To understand the specific effect of stretching, one should limit the review to studies that directly look at the intervention of stretching.

Third, stretching immediately before exercise may have different effects than stretching at other times and should be considered as a separate intervention. Whereas there is a considerable amount of clinical data on stretching immediately before exercise, there is much less data on stretching at other times.

Fourth, some people claim that negative results in some studies are due to improper stretching technique. Because the effects of stretching are believed to occur through changes in stiffness and ROM, an "improper" technique implies that the ROM is not increased. If ROM is increased without causing an immediate injury, then by definition the stretches were done properly.

Fifth, warm-up is not synonymous with stretching. In the colloquial sense, warm-up means any activity performed before participating in sport. Used in this sense, stretching is only one component of warm-up, and if stretching is included in the pre-exercise activity, I explicitly state that stretching was used. The other component of warm-up is participating in an activity that requires active muscle contractions. This type of warm-up can be divided into general or sport-specific warm-up. In a general warm-up, the objective is to increase body temperature. As such, the muscles used are either not the muscles required in the activity (e.g., a pitcher jogs before a game), or do not reflect the type of activity in sport (e.g., jumping jacks prior to sprinting). In sport-specific warm-up, the activity is the same but performed at a lower intensity (e.g., jogging slowly before starting a running race). Whether warm-up itself prevents injury or improves performance is beyond the scope of this chapter. However, if it does, the reader should be aware that the mechanism of action (e.g., temperature, muscle fiber energetics, central programming of muscle contractions, proprioception) will dictate whether one type of warm-up is superior to another. In this chapter, I will use warm-up to mean performing an activity prior to sport and specify if it was general or sport-specific where possible.

Sixth, the term "dynamic stretching" is currently used differently by different people, but in essence it refers to the stretching of a muscle by contracting and relaxing the antagonist muscle. For example, if a subject uses the hip abductor muscles to swing the lower limb laterally until the adductor muscles are stretched and then relaxes the abductors and contracts the adductors to swing the lower limb medially, and repeats this several times, some would consider this a dynamic stretch of the adductor and abductor muscles. There is some preliminary evidence that dynamic stretching is less effective than static stretching at improving range of motion (ROM: 4.3° vs. 11.4°).[16] There is no research on injury rates with this type of stretching, and therefore all claims are conjectural. One should note that dynamic stretching includes both classical stretching and warm-up at the same time. Because dynamic stretching requires the muscles to contract, other possible mechanisms include central programming of muscle contraction/coordination and decreased fatigue through increased warm-up activity. Those who promote dynamic stretching as a method to prevent injury should provide some evidence that supports their claim. Further, if they want to demonstrate that it is the stretch that is important as opposed to the general warm-up that also occurs, then the control group intervention should include warm-up activity.

In this chapter, I will first review new findings that have changed our understanding of what stretching actually does to muscle. This will include changes at the level of the whole muscle (e.g., compliance) and at the level of the myofiber. Next, I will review the clinical evidence surrounding the protective effect of stretching both immediately before exercise, and at other times. Finally, I will review the basic science evidence to see whether it supports or contradicts the clinical evidence. The use of stretching as performance enhancement has been discussed elsewhere.[17]

Physiology of stretching

Immediate effects

Stretching is believed to increase the ROM around a joint through decreases in viscoelasticity and increases in the compliance of muscle. What are compliance and viscoelasticity? Compliance is the reciprocal of stiffness, and mathematically it is equal to the length change that occurs in a tissue divided by the force applied to achieve the change in length. A tissue that is easy to stretch is compliant because it lengthens with very little force. Viscoelasticity refers to the presence of both elastic behavior and viscous behavior. An elastic substance will exhibit a change in length for a given force, and will return to its original length immediately on release (e.g., a regular store-bought elastic). The effect is not dependent on time. However, a viscous substance exhibits flow and movement (e.g., molasses), which is dependent on time.[18] Experimentally, viscous behavior produces "creep" if the force is held constant (i.e., the length continues to increase slowly even though the applied force is constant) or "stretch relaxation" if the length is held constant (i.e., the force on the tissue decreases if the tissue is stretched and then held at a fixed length). When the force is removed, the substance slowly returns to its original length. This is different from plastic deformation, in which the material remains permanently elongated even after the force is removed (e.g., a plastic bag[18]). The reader should note that stretching affects tendons and other connective tissue in addition to muscle. However, within the context of normal stretching, the stiffness of a muscle–tendon unit is mostly related to the least stiff section (i.e., resting muscle) and is minimally affected by the stiffness of tendons.

Stretching appears to affect the viscoelastic behavior of muscle and tendon, but the duration of the effect appears short. In one study, canine gastrocnemius muscle was repeatedly stretched to a fixed length and the force was measured. The force required to produce the length change declined over 10 repetitions and was fairly stable after four stretches.[19] The authors did not measure how long the effect lasted. In humans, Magnusson originally found that increased ROM was lost by 60 min if the subjects remained at rest after stretching. Because they did not take measurements at intervals, the effect could have lasted anywhere from 1 to 60 min.[20] In a later study designed to further narrow the interval for the effect, the same group found that the increased ROM lasted less than 30 min even if the person warmed up prior to the stretch and continued to exercise.[21] More studies are needed to see exactly how long the effect does last—e.g., 1 min, 5 min, 15 min, etc.

As one observes people, it becomes clear that some are naturally flexible even though they never stretch, whereas others remain inflexible no matter what they do. The effect of stretching also appears to be specific to individuals and also muscle-specific. For instance, within every study, some individuals have large increases in ROM with stretching whereas others do not, both in animal studies[19] and human studies.[22,23] In addition, stretching appears less effective in increasing hip external rotation and abduction in comparison with hip flexion.[24] Finally, the effects of stretching for 60 s versus 30 s were found to be greater in the elderly[25] but not in younger populations.[26] If true, the optimal duration and frequency for stretching may be different for different muscle groups or individuals. This appears logical, given that different muscles have different temperatures (superficial muscles are colder than deep muscles) and different amounts of pennation (i.e., the angle of sarcomeres to the direction of force when the muscle contracts—e.g., gastrocnemius muscle), and different subjects have different baseline muscle compliances. More research is needed on which variables are responsible (and to what degree) for the variation observed in response to stretching protocols.

Stretching also appears to increase the pain threshold during a muscle stretch—i.e., it acts like an analgesic.[27–29] In these series of studies, subjects' muscles were stretched until they felt pain, and the stretch stopped. After the subjects stretched, the expected increased ROM before pain was felt was associated with both an increased length and force across the muscle. Had the increased ROM been limited to viscoelastic changes, the muscle length would have increased, but the force applied would have been less or unchanged. The only explanation for an increase in force before pain is felt is that stretching acts like an analgesic. Finally, the analgesia is at least partially due to the effects at the spinal cord or cerebral level, because during unilateral proprioceptive neuromuscular facilitatory (PNF) stretching, the ROM in the unstretched leg also increases.[30]

PNF stretching is also an interesting example of the way in which myths can be propagated within the medical literature. When they were first proposed in the early 1970s, PNF techniques were based on the basic science finding that stretching/activity of the antagonist muscle creates reciprocal inhibition of the agonist muscle.[31] When tested, PNF techniques were indeed shown to increase ROM more than static stretching. However, these initial studies did not measure muscle activity, so the reason for the increased ROM was not known. In fact, when electromyographic findings were recorded in 1979, the reciprocal inhibition theory was disproved.[30,32] Although these results have been confirmed more recently,[28,33,34] the myth of reciprocal inhibition continues to be promoted in textbooks and the medical literature. In fact, muscles are electrically silent during normal stretches until the end ROM is approached. Surprisingly, PNF techniques actually increase the electrical activity of the muscle during the stretch,[30,32,33] even though the ROM is increased.[28,32,34,35] This suggests firstly, that PNF stretching is associated with a more pronounced analgesic effect, and secondly that the muscle is actually undergoing an eccentric contraction during a "PNF stretch."

Although stretching may affect the viscoelastic properties of resting muscle, it does not affect the compliance of *active* muscle. Compliance of resting muscle is almost exclusively due to the muscle cytoskeleton,[36,37] whereas compliance of active muscle is directly dependent on the number of active actin–myosin cross-bridges.[38–41] Because injuries are believed to occur when the muscle is active (i.e., during eccentric contractions),[42] compliance during activity should be more important than compliance at rest.

In summary, stretching decreases viscoelasticity of muscle for less than 30 min, and the increased ROM is at least partially due to an analgesic effect mediated at the level of the spinal cord or higher.

Long-term effects

Although the immediate effects of a single stretching session produce a decrease in viscoelasticity and an increase in stretch tolerance, the effect of stretching over 3–4 weeks appears to affect only stretch tolerance, with no change in viscoelasticity.[35,43] In this case, a second explanation for the increased stretch tolerance besides an analgesic effect is possible; regular stretching may induce muscle hypertrophy.

Animal research has shown that muscles that are stretched for 24 h per day for several days will actually increase in cross-sectional area (or decrease in cross-sectional area less than if casted without stretch), even though they are not contracting.[44–46] This is known as stretch-induced hypertrophy. These studies all used cast-immobilization[44,46] or weights to stretch the muscle continuously 24 h/day over 3–30 days.[45] This is of course very different from human stretching programs, which involve stretching for only 30–60 s/day for any particular muscle group. In this connection, Black and Stevens[47] recently found that 2 min stretching of the mouse extensor digitorum longus muscle per day for 12 days did not reduce the force or work deficit created by an acute eccentric-induced injury. However, it must be remembered that stretch-induced hypertrophy may be affected by the presence of injury, and that the stretching period was only 12 days. Therefore, the possibility remains that some hypertrophy will occur in healthy muscle or if muscles are stretched over a longer period of time.

There is some supporting evidence for stretch-induced hypertrophy in humans. If hypertrophy occurred, one would expect force to increase with an isolated stretching program. In a recent review, I showed that stretching regularly over weeks not prior to exercise improves results on tests of maximal voluntary contraction, jumping height and possibly running speed.[17] However, there is an alternative hypothesis as well—a reduction in central neuromuscular inhibition. In most subjects, an electrically-stimulated muscle produces more force than a maximal voluntary contraction, and this means that the central nervous system is unable to fully activate the muscle.[48] If regular stretching reduced this central inhibition, a greater force would occur. Although neuromuscular adaptation is known to be the prime reason for an increase in untrained individuals, its role is thought to be minimal in the type of trained individuals participating in the studies cited in the review. The differentiation between these two theories (hypertrophy and reduction of inhibition) is theoretically simple: getting trained people to stretch regularly for several weeks and measure cross-sectional muscle area with magnetic resonance imaging and neuromuscular inhibition with twitch interpolation. This study remains to be done.

Finally, if stretch-induced hypertrophy does occur, it should be associated with an increase in stiffness, because of the increased muscle cross-sectional area. For example, the stiffness of an elastic band doubles when the cross-section of an elastic band is doubled (e.g., by folding it over itself), even though the elastic itself has not changed. Therefore, a thicker muscle should also be stiffer. However, the stiffness of human muscles does not change over time with stretching.[35,43] Therefore, if stretch-induced hypertrophy is occurring in this situation, then there must be associated changes in the viscoelastic properties of the individual muscle fibers to explain the lack of increase in whole-muscle viscoelasticity. This would only be observable through isolated fiber studies and could not be done *in vivo*.

Does stretching prevent injury?

Methods

The MEDLINE and EMBASE databases were searched for all clinical articles related to stretching and injury, using the strategy outlined in Table 3.1. All titles were scanned, and

Table 3.1 MEDLINE (PubMed search engine) and EMBASE search strategies, searching all fields, including MEDLINE Subject Headings (MeSH) and text words between 1996 and September 2003. The text-word strategy retrieves any article that includes the word in the title or abstract (if the abstract is included in MEDLINE). The symbol "*" in the search acts as a wildcard for any text

Item	Search	MEDLINE	EMBASE
1	Stretch*	30731	12795
2	Sprain OR strain OR injur*	682286	339533
3	Sport OR athlet* OR activ*	2223441	997212
4	1 AND 2 AND 3 (limited to human studies)	554	474

the abstracts of any potentially relevant articles were retrieved for review. All studies that used stretching as an intervention, included a comparison group, and had some form of injury risk as an outcome were included for this analysis. In addition, all pertinent articles from the bibliographies of these papers were also reviewed. Finally, a citation search was carried out on the key articles. Forrest plots were generated using Cochrane Review Manager version 4.2.7.

Results

Every study has limitations. This does not usually invalidate the research, but only limits the interpretation of the study. This chapter summarizes the main weaknesses of the studies and illustrates how the data can still be interpreted for clinical usefulness.

Does pre-exercise stretching prevent injuries?

Only 17 of the articles retrieved from the search strategy used a control group to analyze whether pre-exercise stretching prevents injury and all were included in this analysis. Of these, seven articles suggested it is beneficial (Table 3.2),[6,7,49–53] three articles suggested it is detrimental (Table 3.3),[54–56] and seven articles suggested no difference (Table 3.3).[57–63]

Figure 3.1 shows the relative risks or odds ratios or hazard ratios (with 95% confidence intervals) for all the prospective studies. A close examination of these studies suggests that the clinical evidence does not support the hypothesis that stretching before exercise prevents injury. Because the methodology differed greatly between the studies, an overall summary statistic is inappropriate. The values shown in the figures are for qualitative purposes only and are used to show the effect of stretching before versus not before exercise, and the inclusion/exclusion of certain studies.

Positive studies. When grouped together, four of the seven studies that showed a positive effect actually evaluated a complete program that included many co-interventions in addition to stretching prior to exercise. First, Ekstrand *et al.* found that elite soccer teams that were part of an experimental group (pre-exercise warm-up, leg guards, special shoes, taping ankles, controlled rehabilitation, education, and close supervision) had 75% fewer injuries in comparison with the control group of soccer teams.[52] However, it is impossible to determine which of the interventions might be responsible for the decrease in injury rates. Second, in a similar study completed a year earlier, Ekstrand *et al.* found less

Table 3.2 Brief summary of the clinical studies that suggest stretching immediately before exercise may prevent injury. For the relative risk (RR) or odds ratios (OR), a value above 1 means a higher rate of injury in people who stretch

Reference	Population	Study design	Results	Comments
Ekstrand *et al.*[52]	180 elite male soccer players	RCT intervention of warm-up, stretch, leg guards, prophylactic ankle taping, controlled rehabilitation, information, supervision	The group that received the combined intervention had a RR of 0.18 (0.6 injuries/month versus 2.6 injuries per month)	The multiple interventions prevent one from concluding that pre-exercise stretching is beneficial
Bixler & Jones[51]	5 high-school football teams	Pseudo-RCT intervention of half-time stretching and warm-up	Intervention group had 0.3 injuries per game vs. 0.8 injuries per game for control group	If an intervention team did not stretch at half-time, they were considered as part of the "control data." No numbers given for changes in exposure. With increased exposure and constant risk, frequency of injuries is expected to increase. Therefore, risks cannot be calculated. Also, there was a co-intervention of warm-up
Ekstrand *et al.*[64]	180 elite male soccer players	1-year prospective cohort study	"All seven quadriceps strain affected players of teams in which shooting at the goal occurred before warm-up ($P < 0.058$)" "Hamstring strains were most common in teams not using special flexibility exercises ($t = 2.1$)"	No real analysis of stretching before exercise. Multiple co-interventions

Wilber *et al.*[50]	518 recreational cyclists	Survey of overuse injuries and other related factors	Only results available are "stretching before cycling (1 vs. 2 minutes, $P < 0.007$) . . . had a significant effect on those female cyclists who sought medical treatment for groin/buttock conditions"	Response rate of 518/2500. The association between stretching and injuries to other body parts (e.g., knees, back) was not reported, even though data available. Not clear if people stretched before injury, or because of injury. Effect only in women and not in men
Cross *et al.*[49]	195 Division III college football players	Chart review, pre–post stretching intervention using historical controls. Stretching immediately before exercise	43/195 injuries pre-intervention, and 21/195 post-intervention ($P < 0.05$)	Use of historical controls is poor design. Likely to have had high rate of injuries and decided to introduce stretching. If true, results are likely by chance due to regression towards the mean
Amako *et al.*[6]	901 military recruits	Prospective, exposure decided by company commander. Intervention 4 upper extremity stretches, 7 lower extremity stretches, 7 trunk stretches. Static stretch for 30 s pre- and post-exercise	Risk of injury 11.2% in stretching group and 14.1% in control group ($P = 0.12$)	The company commander chose whether their group would be exposed to the intervention, and groups may train differently. Further, non-stretch group was not prevented from stretching. Finally, group also stretched after activity, so not purely pre-exercise stretch intervention
McKay *et al.*[7]	Elite and recreational, male and female basketball players	Observational study during competitions	OR_{adj}: 0.38 (95% CI, 0.16 to 0.92)	Note that there was a coding error in OR in the article; this is corrected here and the OR represents the odds of injury with stretching versus the odds of injury without stretching. This study examined basketball, but there was no adjustment for position or ankle taping

Table 3.3 Brief summary of the clinical studies that suggest stretching immediately before exercise does not prevent injury. For the relative risk (RR), odds ratio (OR) or hazard ratio (HR), a value above 1 means a higher rate of injury in people who stretch

Reference	Population	Study Design	Results	Comments
Pope *et al.*[62]	1538 male military recruits	12-week RCT	Univariate HR 0.95 (95% CI, 0.77 to 1.18) Multivariate HR 1.04 (95% CI, 0.82 to 1.33)	Large sample size. Military recruits do not perform same activities as elite athletes, but the activity is probably very similar to recreational athletes. Compliance and follow-up is easy in this group
Pope *et al.*[63]	1093 male military recruits	12-week RCT stretch calves	HR 0.92 (95% CI, 0.52 to 1.61)	Although stretching didn't reduce risk, there was a 5-fold increased ankle injury if ankle ROM only 34° ($P < 0.01$)
Van Mechelen *et al.*[61]	421 male recreational runners	16-week RCT matched on age and weekly running distance	RR 1.12	Intervention was warm-up and pre-exercise stretching. There was a lot of "noncompliance" in each group
Macera *et al.*[58]	583 habitual runners	1-year prospective cohort	OR for men 1.1, for women 1.6	Response rate 966/1576. Stretching data was only controlled for age. Stretching was not included in the multiple regression analysis because it was insignificant in the univariate analysis
Walter *et al.*[59]	1680 community road race runners	1-year prospective cohort	Comparison group was people who always stretch. RR: Never stretched: 1.15, 1.18; sometimes stretch: 0.56, 0.64; usually stretch: 1.05, 1.25	To be consistent with other articles, the RR was converted so that the numbers reflect the risk of people who always stretch. These numbers are controlled for running distance and frequency, type of runner, use of warm-up, injuries in past year

Howell[54]	17 elite women rowers	Cross-sectional	Stretching associated with injuries	Not clear if people stretched before injury, or because of injury
Brunet *et al.*[60]	1505 road race recreational and competitive runners	Survey of past injuries and other related factors	Similar frequencies of injuries among those who stretch and those who don't	Response rate unknown. Cross-sectional study design, but injury profile was "any injury" and not recent injury. Not clear if people stretched before injury, or because of injury
Blair *et al.*[57]	438 habitual runners	Survey of past injuries and other related factors	Only results available are "frequency of stretching . . . were not associated with running injuries"	Response rate 438/720. This article comprises three studies. Only the cross-sectional study directly looked at stretching habits. Not clear if people stretched before injury, or because of injury
Kerner[56]	540 people buying running shoes	Survey of past injuries and other Related factors	Only results available are "A comparison of subjects who warmed up prior to running (87.7%) and those who did not (66%) revealed a higher frequency of pain in the former"	Response rate 540/800. No data available to determine clinical relevance. Not clear if people stretched before injury, or because of injury
Jacobs[55]	451 10-km race participants	Survey of past injuries and related factors	~90% of injured people stretched, compared to ~80% of non-injured people	Response rate 451/550. Not clear how 550 were chosen from potential 1620. Univariate analysis only. Not clear if people stretched before injury, or because of injury

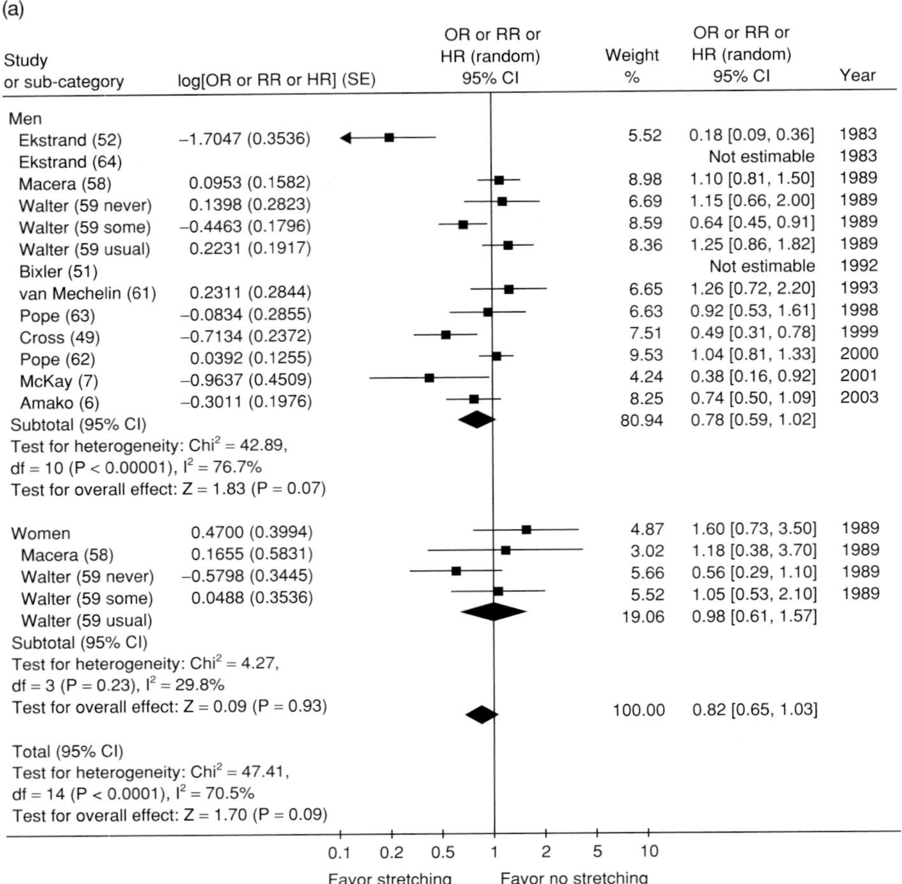

Figure 3.1 In (a), the relative risks or odds ratios or hazards ratio (±95% confidence intervals) are plotted for all randomized controlled trials and cohort studies grouped by men or women. (Note that the McKay study included both women and men in the same analysis, but is grouped with men). A value greater than 1 means an increased risk for people who stretch before exercise, and a value below 1 means a decreased risk of injury for people who stretch before exercise. There were two studies[51,64] in which there were insufficient data in the article to calculate the relative risk or odds ratio. The study by Ekstrand *et al.*[52] was calculated for strains and sprains only, and as if each person was only injured once. The study by Walter *et al.*[59] compared several groups with "Always stretched before exercise" (a relative risk above 1 means the "always" group had a higher injury rate). The test of heterogeneity suggests that the results are very heterogeneous. In this situation, sources of heterogeneity should be sought out. In (**b**), the same data are shown, but I have omitted the studies in which stretching may very well not have been the reason for the differences between groups. The more likely reasons in these studies are co-interventions[6,52] and regression to the mean.[49] The test of heterogeneity still suggests some heterogeneity (most likely due to the study by McKay on basketball injuries), but much less. Qualitatively, the overall effect of stretching before exercise suggests no clinically relevant benefit.

(b)

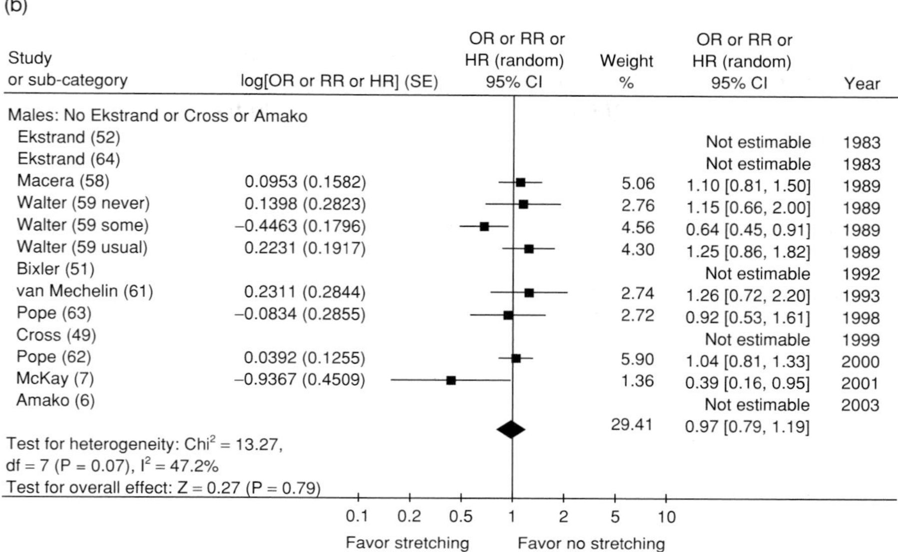

Figure 3.1 *(Continued)*

hamstring and quadriceps strains in elite soccer players who performed warm-up, skill exercises, and stretching exercises before soccer.[64] In a third study,[51] high-school football teams were pseudorandomized to either stretching or warm-up during half-time. The hypothesis was that athletes become stiff during half-time and that stretching at half-time might decrease third quarter injuries. In addition to the co-intervention, this study had problems with randomization and compliance, and did not use the recommended "intention-to-treat" analysis. Finally, the intervention in the Amako *et al.* study was stretching both before and after exercise,[6] and there is some evidence that regular stretching not prior to exercise is beneficial (see the section on "Does stretching after or outside periods of exercise prevent injuries?" below).

Of the remaining three studies, the methodology was weak in two. First, Cross *et al.* used a cohort design with historical controls and found that pre-exercise stretching decreased injuries.[49] Historical controls are only appropriate if certain assumptions are met. For instance, if there were an unusually high injury rate one year by chance, one would expect the injury rate to return to normal the following year. If the medical staff had introduced an intervention to decrease injuries after the high injury rate year, they would mistakenly attribute the decrease in injuries to their intervention. Statistically, this is called regression towards the mean. Studies using historical controls only provide strong evidence when the rates are stable over a number of years, and then fall (or rise) for a few years following the introduction of an intervention. Therefore, without knowing the rates of injury for several seasons before and after the intervention, nor the reason why the intervention was applied during that particular year, the most likely reason for the drop in injury rates in the Cross *et al.* study is regression towards the mean. Second, in a cross-sectional study, women cyclists who stretched before exercise had less groin and buttock pain, but the effect was not observed in men.[50] Because the physiological effect of stretching is similar in both groups, these results are difficult to interpret.

The remaining study examined ankle injuries in basketball players.[7] This was the only study to look at higher intensity exercise and showed a mild protective effect, but did not adjust for position of play or presence of ankle taping. With respect to the basic science evidence, strain rates (analogous to high-intensity vs. low-intensity exercise) did not affect the relationship between compliance and length/energy absorbed before failure.[65] Therefore, intensity is unlikely to modify the effect of stretching and injury, and more research is needed before stretching should be recommended in high-intensity sports.

In summary, although there are some strong studies for which pre-exercise stretching was associated with a reduction in injury rates, the presence of probable effective co-interventions or other limitations suggests that whatever evidence is in favor is weak.

Negative studies. There have been three studies (all cross-sectional) that suggested stretching before exercise may increase the risk of injury.[54–56]

In a cross-sectional study, Howell found that 13 of 13 elite rowers who stretched had back pain, and only one of four athletes who did not stretch had back pain.[54] Interestingly, of the study subjects with hyperflexibility of the lumbar spine, the only two who did not have back pain did not stretch. However, it is again unclear whether these athletes became injured because they were stretching, or stretched because they were injured.

In the two other cross-sectional studies that showed that stretching might increase injury rates,[55,56] the authors did not control for any other factor such as training distance, experience, etc. In summary, recommendations based on these studies should be very guarded.

Equivocal studies. There have been seven studies—three randomized controlled trials (RCTs), two prospective studies, and two cross-sectional studies—that found no difference in injury rates between people who stretch before exercise and those who do not.[57–62,66]

In the most recent large RCT, Pope and colleagues randomly assigned 1538 military recruits to either warm-up and then stretch immediately before exercise, or simply warm-up and exercise.[62] The hazard ratio (equivalent to an odds ratio, but taking into account different follow-up times) after adjusting for height, weight, day of enlistment, age, and 20-m shuttle run test score, suggested no benefit. This study was consistent with a previous study by the same authors that used only calf stretching immediately before exercise.[63] With respect to sports injury prevention, the main limitation of this study is that it occurred in military recruits, who may not be doing the same type of activity as recreational or elite athletes, and may experience a sudden increase in activity that is not typical of recreational or elite athletes.

Van Mechelen randomly assigned 421 persons to an intervention group that included 6 min of warm-up and 10 min of stretching.[61] The relative risk for injury for those in the intervention group was 1.12 in comparison with controls. Notably, only 47% of those in the intervention program actually stretched according to the instructions outlined in the study. In addition, many of the runners in the control group also performed some type of pre-exercise stretching. This type of non-compliance (or "misclassification") would be expected to "bias towards the null" and minimize the odds ratio obtained. However, it should not reverse the direction of the odds ratio, which showed more injuries in the group randomized to stretch. Although one could reanalyze the data according to whether the actual intervention was performed, most statistical consultants believe the intention-to-treat analysis (as was done in the paper) is more appropriate.

In a prospective cohort study by Walter *et al.*,[59] the authors found that stretching was unrelated to injury after adjusting for previous injuries and mileage. Macera *et al.*[66] found that stretching before exercise increased the risk of injury, but the differences were not statistically significant. Although not RCTs, these were good studies with few limitations.

Finally, two cross-sectional studies showed no protective effect of pre-exercise stretching.[57,60] In fact, Brunet *et al.* reported that non-stretchers had fewer injuries, even though they had higher mileage per week and fewer previous injuries.[60] The cross-sectional design limits the conclusions that can be drawn from these studies.

Summary of clinical evidence

Even though the studies have very different methodologies, one can perform a meta-analysis for qualitative purposes. In this case, the overall effect is estimated at 0.82 (95% CI, 0.65 to 1.03). However, if one omits the studies that included other interventions besides stretching immediately before exercise,[6,52,64] the overall effect is estimated at 0.97 (95% CI, 0.79 to 1.19). Thus, the clinical evidence available does not support the hypothesis that pre-exercise stretching prevents injury.

Does stretching after or outside periods of exercise prevent injuries?

There have only been two studies that isolated the effect of stretching after or outside periods of exercise on injury risk. Both studies suggested a clinically relevant decrease in injury risk, but the results did not reach statistical significance in one. A third study, previously mentioned, examined stretching before and after exercise and also found a non-statistically significant but clinically relevant decrease in risk.[6] More research is needed in this area before definitive conclusions can be drawn.

Positive studies (Fig. 3.2, Table 3.4). In support of the hypothesis that regular stretching prevents injury, a recent study using basic training for military recruits found that the companies of soldiers who stretched three times per day besides their normal pre-exercise stretching regimen had fewer injuries than a control group who stretched only before exercise.[67] However, there were problems with baseline comparisons and there was no adjustment for previous injuries, fitness levels, etc.

Hilyer *et al.* randomly assigned firefighters from two of four fire districts to perform 12 daily stretches for 6 months, while the firemen from the other two districts were instructed not to stretch (total 469 firemen).[68] Although the change in flexibility was greater in the experimental group, this was due to loss of flexibility in the control group and not a gain in flexibility in the experimental group, even though exercise physiologists visited the various stations during the first month to correct improper technique. Although the number of injuries was not statistically different between groups, there was a clinically relevant decrease in risk for the group that stretched (relative risk 0.82; 95% CI, 0.59 to 1.13). Further, the costs due to lost time from work were also less in the group that stretched ($950/injury vs. $2828/injury).

Finally, Amako *et al.* randomly assigned subjects to stretching before and after exercise or a control group and found an overall relative risk of injury of 0.77 (95% CI, 0.54 to 1.08)

Study or sub-category	log[OR or RR or HR] (SE)	OR or RR or HR (random) 95% CI	Weight %	OR or RR or HR (random) 95% CI	Year
Hilyer (68)	−0.1985 (0.1654)		43.93	0.82 [0.59, 1.13]	1990
Hartig (67)	−0.5551 (0.2180)		25.29	0.57 [0.37, 0.88]	1999
Amako (6)	−0.3011 (0.1976)		30.78	0.74 [0.50, 1.09]	2003
Total (95% CI)			100.00	0.73 [0.59, 0.90]	

Test for heterogeneity: $Chi^2 = 1.71$, df = 2 (P = 0.42), $I^2 = 0\%$
Test for overall effect: Z = 2.92 (P = 0.003)

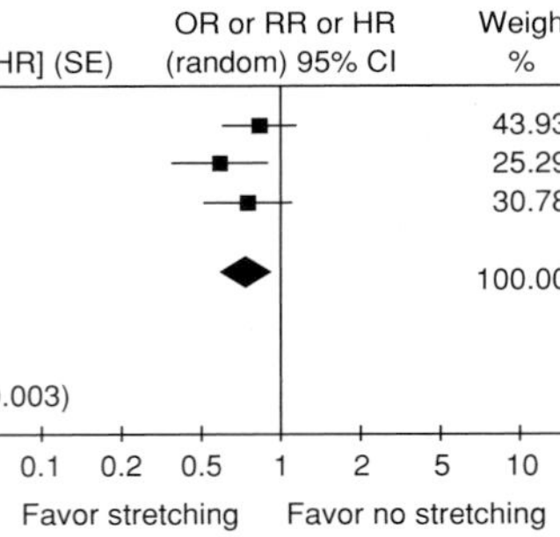

Figure 3.2 A Forrest plot of the relative risks or odds ratios (±95% confidence intervals) from three studies that examined the intervention of stretching regularly not immediately prior to exercise. The test of heterogeneity suggests the studies show similar magnitudes of effect.

for the intervention group.[6] There were some limitations to this study, the most important being that allocation to the stretch or non-stretch group was carried out by the company commander, and different companies may train at different intensities, different levels of fatigue, etc.

Although all three studies have limitations and only one has statistically significant results, they all show clinically relevant decreases in injury risk. In addition, if stretch-induced hypertrophy occurs, as suggested by the basic science evidence,[44–46] one would expect a benefit from regular stretching. These results represent a good beginning, and the area requires further research.

Discussion

A review of the clinical evidence strongly suggests that pre-exercise stretching does not prevent injury, and that the evidence on stretching at other times suggests that it may be beneficial but is too limited to make definitive recommendations at this time. Considering that these results are contrary to many people's beliefs, it seems prudent to review why some people ever believed stretching before exercise was so beneficial. There appear to be six general arguments that have been proposed in the past.

First, paraphrasing an old Chinese saying, "that which does not bend, breaks." However, when a tree bends, the force (i.e., the wind) changes from a perpendicular force to a longitudinal force; it is much easier to break a stick by applying a perpendicular force to the middle in comparison with longitudinal forces at the end. In stretching a muscle prior to activity, we do not alter the direction of force at the time of injury, and the analogy is inappropriate.

Second, compliance refers to the length change that occurs when a force is applied, but is not necessarily related to a tissue's resistance to injury. For example, even though a balloon will stretch before it bursts (high compliance), a sphere made of metal with the same thickness as the balloon might never stretch (low compliance) and still withstand extremely high pressures.

Table 3.4 Brief summary of the clinical studies that suggest stretching not immediately before exercise may prevent injury. For the relative risk (RR) or odds ratios (OR), a value above 1 means a higher rate of injury in people who stretch

Reference	Population	Study Design	Results	Comments
Hilyer *et al.*[68]	469 firefighters	Cluster randomization by fire district. Stretching at work; obviously not possible immediately before fire	48/251 injuries in stretching group and 52/218 injuries in control group (RR 0.82, 95% CI, 0.57 to 1.14). $950 per injury for lost time in stretching group and $2838 in control group ($P = 0.026$)	Reviewed exercises with subjects but not clear how closely. Medical cost difference also greater in control group, but not significantly ($P = 0.19$) Because medical costs more similar than lost time costs, total cost not significantly different (0.56)
Hartig *et al.*[67]	298 basic training recruits	Cluster randomization by company	25/150 injuries in stretching group and 43/148 in control group (RR 0.57, 95% CI, 0.37 to 0.88)	Stretching group more flexible prior to training and not controlled for in analysis. Almost twice the no. lost to follow-up in stretch group, which means less people available to be injured. This would make stretching appear more effective
Amako *et al.*[6] (study also included in Table 3.2)	901 military recruits	Prospective, exposure decided by company commander. Intervention: 4 upper extremity stretches, 7 lower extremity stretches, 7 trunk stretches. Static stretch for 30 s pre- and post-exercise	Risk of injury 11.2% in stretching group and 14.1% in control group ($P = 0.12$)	The company commanders chose whether their group would be exposed to the intervention, and groups may train differently. Further, non-stretch group was not prevented from stretching. Finally, group also stretched before activity, so not purely post-exercise stretch intervention

Third, if muscle compliance is increased with warming from 25 °C to 40 °C, the muscle ruptures at a longer length but absorbs less energy.[69] Which is more important, length or energy absorbed? Although muscles are sometimes injured when stretched beyond their normal length of motion, most authors believe that the majority of injuries occur within the normal ROM during eccentric activity, and that the most important variable with respect to muscle injury is the energy absorbed by the muscle.[65,70,71] For example, the hamstring muscle contracts to slow the forward movement of the lower leg during the swing phase of gait (i.e., as the leg moves forward). If the energy is not absorbed, the leg will continue to move forward in the presence of a compliant tissue until it exceeds the tissue's maximum length, whatever that maximum length happens to be. If the muscle absorbs the energy, the lower leg is stopped from extending and the maximum length is never reached. Finally, the reader must remember that the damage occurs at the level of the sarcomere and not the whole muscle.[72] Therefore, if there is excessive sarcomere lengthening so that the actin and myosin filaments no longer overlap, the force is transmitted to the cytoskeleton of the muscle fiber, and damage occurs. This occurs within the normal ROM, because sarcomere length within the muscle is heterogeneous; some sarcomeres lengthen during a contraction at the same time as others are shortening.[72–76] Therefore, it appears that it is the sarcomere length that is related to most exercise-related muscle strains, rather than the total muscle length. Under this hypothesis, an increase in total muscle compliance is irrelevant.

In support of the above argument, ligaments that have been immobilized are also more compliant but absorb less energy.[77] In addition, resting muscle is more compliant than a contracting muscle,[40,41] but again absorbs less energy.[70,78] Finally, sarcomeres directly attached to the tendon are the least compliant and remain undamaged, but adjacent sarcomeres are stretched beyond actin–myosin overlap and become injured.[75,76,79] These results are consistent with Garrett's whole-muscle studies, in which the sarcomeres attached to the tendon remained intact, but the more compliant adjacent sarcomeres ruptured.[70] Taken together, this evidence suggests that increased compliance is associated with an inability to absorb as much energy, which may increase the risk of injury during an eccentric load.

Fourth, overstretching a muscle can certainly produce damage. However, even strains as little as 20% beyond resting fiber length, as one would expect with "correct" stretching techniques, can produce damage in isolated muscle preparations.[71] Therefore, the basic science evidence suggests that "correct" stretching techniques may be more difficult to define than previously thought.

Fifth, we have seen that the increased ROM with stretching is partly due to an analgesic effect.[28,29,32,35] This may explain some preliminary findings that muscle aches and pains are reduced in pre–post testing,[80–82] but does not mean that the risk of injury is decreased. Nor does it mean that stretching shortens rehabilitation time and prevents re-injury following an injury. In two clinical studies comparing stretching with strengthening after injury,[83,84] both found that a strengthening program was superior to stretching. In one study,[83] 23 of 34 male athletes with more than 2 months of groin pain who participated in a strengthening program returned to pre-activity levels within 4 months, in comparison with only four of 34 of athletes who participated in a stretching program (OR_{adj} 12.7; 95% CI, 3.4 to 47.2). Neither study examined acute injuries, nor the potential benefit/harm of adding stretching to a strengthening program; these remain to be determined.

Sixth, some argue that stretching may prevent tendon or other injuries, even though there is no effect on total injuries. First, in the Australian military, tendon injuries occurred in 20 of 735 subjects (2.7%) who stretched and 16 of 803 (2.0%) who did not stretch.[62] Others have suggested that stretching one area reduces the risk of injury in a different area (e.g., stretch the hamstrings to reduce stress on the back), but have not put forth any data. Finally, even if stretching does prevent one specific type of injury, because overall injury rates among stretchers and non-stretchers are not different, any protection against one type of injury would mean an increased risk of other types of injuries in order to balance the equation. It would therefore only be appropriate to generally advise stretching prior to activity if the severity and long-term consequences were greater for the injury that has a decreased risk with stretching in comparison with the injury that has an increased risk with stretching.

In conclusion, the clinical evidence is consistent with the basic science evidence and theoretical arguments; stretching before exercise does not reduce the risk of injury and stretching at other times may be beneficial. Future research should evaluate high-intensity sports and the effects of stretching on recovery following injury.

Key messages

- Stretching immediately before exercise is different from stretching at other times.
- Stretching immediately before exercise does not appear to prevent injury.
- Regular stretching that is not done immediately before exercise may prevent injury.

Acknowledgments

Some of the material in this chapter has previously been published in the *Clinical Journal of Sport Medicine* 1999; **9**: 221–7, and in *Physician and Sportsmedicine* 2000; **28** (8): 57–63.

Sample examination questions

Multiple-choice questions (answers on page 602)

1 The original study by Ekstrand *et al.*[52] suggested that stretching immediately prior to exercise is associated with a decrease in injuries. Which of the following interventions that are likely to prevent injury were also included in the experimental group as co-interventions?

A Shin guards
B Supervised rehabilitation
C Warm-up
D Education
E All or none of the above

2 With regard to the number of studies examining whether stretching outside periods of exercise prevent injury or minimize the severity of injury:

A 3 found it does and 3 found it does not
B 0 found it does and 3 found it does not
C 3 found it does and 0 found it does not
D All studies used a cohort design
E All or none of the above

3 Theoretical reasons why stretching prior to exercise would not decrease injuries include all of the following *except*:
   A Tissues that are more compliant are associated with a decreased ability to absorb energy
   B The compliance of active muscle is related to the compliance of muscle during normal stretches
   C Most injuries occur during eccentric activity of the muscle, within its normal range of motion
   D Overstretching a muscle is known to be a cause of muscle injury
   E All or none of the above

Essay questions

1 Discuss the evidence for and against the use of stretching immediately prior to exercise as an intervention to prevent injuries.
2 Explain the theoretical reasons why stretching immediately prior to exercise was thought to prevent injuries, and why they do not apply to regular exercise such as jogging.
3 Describe how stretching increases range of motion.

Summarizing the evidence

Comparison	Results	Level of evidence*
Does stretching before exercise prevent injury?	5 RCTs, 4 prospective cohorts, 1 historical cohort, 6 cross-sectional studies. Conflicting results are explained in Tables 3.2 and 3.3. *Overall, stretching before exercise does not prevent injury.* There was an additional prospective cohort study, but it used an intervention of pre- and post-exercise stretching. Note that most studies done on recreational athletes or military personnel. According to the basic science of injury, there is no reason why elite athletes would be expected to have different results. The only study examining high intensity sport was a cohort study on ankle injuries in basketball and suggested a protective effect	A1
Does stretching outside periods of exercise prevent injury?	2 RCTs (n = 300–470) with weaknesses in follow-up and differences in baseline characteristics. *One study suggested a decreased injury rate and the other only decreased severity of injury.* There was an additional prospective cohort study, but it used an intervention of pre- and post-exercise stretching	A1

* A1: evidence from large randomized controlled trials (RCTs) or systematic review (including meta-analysis).†
A2: evidence from at least one high-quality cohort.
A3: evidence from at least one moderate-sized RCT or systematic review.†
A4: evidence from at least one RCT.
B: evidence from at least one high-quality study of nonrandomized cohorts.
C: expert opinions.
† Arbitrarily, the following cut-off points have been used: large study size: ≥ 100 patients per intervention group; moderate study size ≥ 50 patients per intervention group.

References

1 Thacker SB, Gilchrist J, Stroup DF, Kimsey CD. The impact of stretching on sports injury risk: a systematic review of the literature. *Med Sci Sports Exerc* 2004; **36**:371–378.

2 Herbert RD, Gabriel M. Effects of stretching before and after exercising on muscle soreness and risk of injury: systematic review. *Br Med J* 2002; **325**:468.

3 Weldon SM, Hill RH. The efficacy of stretching for prevention of exercise-related injury: a systematic review of the literature. *Man Ther* 2003; **8**:141–150.

4 Ingraham SJ. The role of flexibility in injury prevention and athletic performance: have we stretched the truth? *Minn Med* 2003; **86**:58–61.

5 Johnston CA, Taunton JE, Lloyd-Smith DR, McKenzie DC. Preventing running injuries: practical approach for family doctors. *Can Fam Physician* 2003; **49**:1101–1109.

6 Amako M, Oda T, Masuoka K, Yokoi H, Campisi P. Effect of static stretching on prevention of injuries for military recruits. *Mil Med* 2003; **168**:442–446.

7 McKay GD, Goldie PA, Payne WR, Oakes BW. Ankle injuries in basketball: injury rate and risk factors. *Br J Sports Med* 2001; **35**:103–108.

8 Malliaropoulos N, Papalexandris S, Papalada A, Papacostas E. The role of stretching in rehabilitation of hamstring injuries: 80 athletes follow-up. *Med Sci Sports Exerc* 2004; **36**:756–759.

9 Sherry MA, Best TM. A comparison of 2 rehabilitation programs in the treatment of acute hamstring strains. *J Orthop Sports Phys Ther* 2004; **34**:116–125.

10 Best TM. Muscle–tendon injuries in young athletes. *Clin Sports Med* 1995; **14**:669–686.

11 Garrett WE Jr. Muscle strain injuries: clinical and basic aspects. *Med Sci Sports Exerc* 1990; **22**:436–443.

12 Safran MR, Seaber AV, Garrett WE. Warm-up and muscular injury prevention: an update. *Sports Med* 1989; **8**:239–249.

13 Shellock FG, Prentice WE. Warming-up and stretching for improved physical performance and prevention of sports-related injuries. *Sports Med* 1985; **2**:267–278.

14 Beaulieu JE. Developing a stretching program. *Physician Sportsmed* 1981; **9**:59–65.

15 Stamford B. Flexibility and stretching. *Physician Sportsmed* 1984; **12**:171.

16 Bandy WD, Irion JM, Briggler M. The effect of static stretch and dynamic range of motion training on the flexibility of the hamstring muscles. *J Orthop Sports Phys Ther* 1998; **27**:295–300.

17 Shrier I. Does stretching improve performance? A systematic and critical review of the literature. *Clin J Sport Med* 2004; **14**:267–273.

18 Caro CG, Pedley TJ, Schroter RC, Seed WA. *The Mechanics of the Circulation.* New York: Oxford University Press, 1978.

19 Taylor DC, Dalton JD Jr, Seaber AV, Garrett WE Jr. Viscoelastic properties of muscle–tendon units. *Am J Sports Med* 1990; **18**:300–309.

20 Magnusson SP, Simonsen EB, Aagaard P, Kjaer M. Biomechanical responses to repeated stretches in human hamstring muscle in vivo. *Am J Sports Med* 1996; **24**:622–628.

21 Magnusson SP, Aagaard P, Larsson B, Kjaer M. Passive energy absorption by human muscle–tendon unit is unaffected by increase in intramuscular temperature. *J Appl Physiol* 2000; **88**:1215–1220.

22 Borms J, van Roy P, Santens JP, Haentjens A. Optimal duration of static stretching exercises for improvement of coxo-femoral flexibility. *J Sports Sci* 1987; **5**:39–47.

23 Madding SW, Wong JG, Hallum A, Medeiros JM. Effect of duration of passive stretch on hip abduction range of motion. *J Orthop Sports Phys Ther* 1987; **8**:409–416.

24 Henricson AS, Fredriksson K, Persson I, Pereira R, Rostedt Y, Westlin NE. The effect of heat and stretching on the range of hip motion. *J Orthop Sports Phys Ther* 1984; **6**:110–115.

25 Feland JB, Myrer JW, Schulthies SS, Fellingham GW, Measom GW. The effect of duration of stretching of the hamstring muscle group for increasing range of motion in people aged 65 years or older. *Phys Ther* 2001; **81**:1110–1117.

26 Bandy WD, Irion JM. The effect of time on static stretch on the flexibility of the hamstring muscles. *Phys Ther* 1994; **74**:845–852.

27 Halbertsma JPK, Mulder I, Goeken LNH, Eisma WH. Repeated passive stretching: acute effect on the passive muscle moment and extensibility of short hamstrings. *Arch Phys Med Rehabil* 1999; **80**:407–414.

28 Magnusson SP, Simonsen EB, Aagaard P, Dyhre-Poulsen P, McHugh MP, Kjaer M. Mechanical and physiological responses to stretching with and without preisometric contraction in human skeletal muscle. *Arch Phys Med Rehabil* 1996; **77**:373–378.
29 Halbertsma JPK, van Bolhuis AI, Goeken LNH. Sport stretching: effect on passive muscle stiffness of short hamstrings. *Arch Phys Med Rehabil* 1996; **77**:688–692.
30 Markos PD. Ipsilateral and contralateral effects of proprioceptive neuromuscular facilitation techniques on hip motion and electromyographic activity. *Phys Ther* 1979; **59**:1366–1373.
31 Tanigawa MC. Comparison of the hold–relax procedure and passive mobilization on increasing muscle length. *Phys Ther* 1972; **52**:725–735.
32 Moore MA, Hutton RS. Electromyographic investigation of muscle stretching techniques. *Med Sci Sports Exercise* 1980; **12**:322–329.
33 Osternig LR, Robertson R, Troxel R, Hansen P. Muscle activation during proprioceptive neuromuscular facilitation (PNF) stretching techniques. *Am J Phys Med* 1987; **66**:298–307.
34 Ferber R, Osternig L, Gravelle D. Effect of PNF stretch techniques on knee flexor muscle EMG activity in older adults. *J Electromyogr Kinesiol* 2002; **12**:391–397.
35 Halbertsma JPK, Goeken LNH. Stretching exercises: effect on passive extensibility and stiffness in short hamstrings of healthy subjects. *Arch Phys Med Rehabil* 1994; **75**:976–981.
36 Magid A, Law DJ. Myofibrils bear most of the resting tension in frog skeletal muscle. *Science* 1985; **230**:1280–1282.
37 Horowits R, Kempner ES, Hisher ME, Podolsky RJ. A physiological role for titin and nebulin in skeletal muscle. *Nature* 1986; **323**:160–164.
38 Rack PMH, Westbury DR. The short range stiffness of active mammalian muscle and its effect on mechanical properties. *J Physiol (Lond)* 1974; **240**:331–350.
39 Huxley AF, Simmons RM. Mechanical properties of the cross-bridges of frog striated muscle. *J Physiol (Lond)* 1971; **218**:59P–60P.
40 Wilson GJ, Wood GA, Elliott BC. The relationship between stiffness of the musculature and static flexibility: an alternative explanation for the occurrence of muscular injury. *Int J Sports Med* 1991; **12**:403–407.
41 Sinkjar T, Toft E, Andreassen S, Hornemann BC. Muscle stiffness in human ankle dorsiflexors: intrinsic and reflex components. *J Neurosci* 1988; **60**:1110–1121.
42 Garrett WE, Jr. Muscle strain injuries. *Am J Sports Med* 1996; **24**:S2–S8.
43 Magnusson SP, Simonsen EB, Aagaard P, Soukka A, Kjaer M. A mechanism for altered flexibility in human skeletal muscle. *J Physiol (Lond)* 1996; **497**:291–298.
44 Goldspink DF, Cox VM, Smith SK, Eaves LA, Osbaldeston NJ, Lee DM, *et al.* Muscle growth in response to mechanical stimuli. *Am J Physiol* 1995; **268**:E288–E297.
45 Alway SE. Force and contractile characteristics after stretch overload in quail anterior latissimus dorsi muscle. *J Appl Physiol* 1994; **77**:135–141.
46 Yang S, Alnaqeeb M, Simpson H, Goldspink G. Changes in muscle fibre type, muscle mass and *IGF-I* gene expression in rabbit skeletal muscle subjected to stretch. *J Anat* 1997; **190**:613–622.
47 Black JD, Freeman M, Stevens ED. A 2 week routine stretching programme did not prevent contraction-induced injury in mouse muscle. *J Physiol* 2002; **544**:137–147.
48 Rutherford O, Jones DA, Newham DJ. Clinical and experimental application of the percutaneous twitch superimposition technique for the study of human muscle activation. *J Neurol Neurosurg Psychiatry* 1986; **49**:1288–1291.
49 Cross KM, Worrell TW. Effects of a static stretching program on the incidence of lower extremity musculotendinous strains. *J Athl Train* 1999; **34**:11–14.
50 Wilber CA, Holland GJ, Madison RE, Loy SF. An epidemiological analysis of overuse injuries among recreational cyclists. *Int J Sports Med* 1995; **16**:201–206.
51 Bixler B, Jones RL. High-school football injuries: effects of a post-halftime warm-up and stretching routine. *Fam Pract Res J* 1992; **12**:131–139.
52 Ekstrand J, Gillquist J, Liljedahl SO. Prevention of soccer injuries. *Am J Sports Med* 1983; **11**:116–120.
53 Biros MH, Lewis RJ, Olson CM, Runge JW, Cummins RO, Fost N. Informed consent in emergency research. *JAMA* 1995; **273**:1283–1287.
54 Howell DW. Musculoskeletal profile and incidence of musculoskeletal injuries in lightweight women rowers. *Am J Sports Med* 1984; **12**:278–282.

55 Jacobs SJ, Berson BL. Injuries to runners: a study of entrants to a 10,000 meter race. *Am J Sports Med* 1986; **14**:151–155.

56 Kerner JA, D'Amico JC. A statistical analysis of a group of runners. *J Am Pod Assoc* 1983; **73**:160–164.

57 Blair SN, Kohl HW III, Goodyear NN. Relative risks for running and exercise injuries: studies in three populations. *Res Q* 1987; **58**:221–228.

58 Macera CA, Pate RP, Powell KE, Jackson KL, Kendrick JS, Craven TE. Predicting lower-extremity injuries among habitual runners. *Arch Intern Med* 1989; **149**:2565–2568.

59 Walter SD, Hart LE, McIntosh JM, Sutton JR. The Ontario cohort study of running-related injuries. *Arch Intern Med* 1989; **149**:2561–2564.

60 Brunet ME, Cook SD, Brinker MR, Dickinson JA. A survey of running injuries in 1505 competitive and recreational runners. *J Sports Med Phys Fit* 1990; **30**:307–315.

61 Van Mechelen W, Hlobil H, Kemper HCG, Voorn WJ, de Jongh R. Prevention of running injuries by warm-up, cool-down, and stretching exercises. *Am J Sports Med* 1993; **21**:711–719.

62 Pope RP, Herbert RD, Kirwan JD, Graham BJ. A randomized trial of preexercise stretching for prevention of lower-limb injury. *Med Sci Sports Exerc* 2000; **32**:271–277.

63 Pope RP, Herbert R, Kirwan J. Effects of ankle dorsiflexion range and pre-exercise calf muscle stretching on injury risk in army recruits. *Aust J Physiother* 1998; **44**:165–177.

64 Ekstrand J, Gillquist J, Moller M, Oberg B, Liljedahl SO. Incidence of soccer injuries and their relation to training and team success. *Am J Sports Med* 1983; **11**:636–7.

65 Mair SD, Seaber AV, Glisson RR, Garrett WE. The role of fatigue in susceptibility to acute muscle strain injury. *Am J Sports Med* 1996; **24**:137–143.

66 Macera CA, Croft JB, Brown DR, Ferguson JE, Lane MJ. Predictors of adopting leisure-time physical activity among a biracial community cohort. *Am J Epidemiol* 1995; **142**:629–635.

67 Hartig DE, Henderson JM. Increasing hamstring flexibility decreases lower extremity overuse injuries in military basic trainees. *Am J Sports Med* 1999; **27**:173–176.

68 Hilyer JC, Brown KC, Sirles AT, Peoples L. A flexibility intervention to reduce the incidence and severity of joint injuries among municipal firefighters. *J Occup Med* 1990; **32**:631–637.

69 Noonan TJ, Best TM, Seaber AV, Garrett WE. Thermal effects on skeletal muscle tensile behavior. *Am J Sports Med* 1993; **21**:517–522.

70 Garrett WE, Safran MR, Seaber AV, Glisson RR, Ribbeck BM. Biomechanical comparison of stimulated and nonstimulated skeletal muscle pulled to failure. *Am J Sports Med* 1987; **15**:448–454.

71 Macpherson PCD, Schork MA, Faulkner JA. Contraction-induced injury to single fiber segments from fast and slow muscles of rats by single stretches. *Am J Physiol* 1996; **271**:C1438–C1446.

72 Morgan DL, Proske U. Popping sarcomere hypothesis explains stretch-induced muscle damage. *Clin Exp Pharmacol Physiol* 2004; **31**:541–545.

73 Horowits R, Podolsky RJ. The positional stability of thick filaments in activated skeletal muscle depends on sarcomere length: evidence for the role of titin filaments. *J Cell Biol* 1987; **105**:2217–2223.

74 Edman KAP, Reggiani C. Redistribution of sarcomere length during isometric contraction of frog muscle fibres and its relation to tension creep. *J Physiol (Lond)* 1984; **351**:169–198.

75 Julian FJ, Morgan DL. Intersarcomere dynamics during fixed-end tetanic contractions of frog muscle fibers. *J Physiol (Lond)* 1979; **293**:365–378.

76 Julian FJ, Morgan DL. The effect of tension of non-uniform distribution of length changes applied to frog muscle fibres. *J Physiol (Lond)* 1979; **293**:379–393.

77 Noyes FR. Functional properties of knee ligaments and alterations induced by immobilization. *Clin Orthop* 1977; **123**:210–242.

78 Brooks SV, Zerba E, Faulkner JA. Injury to muscle fibers after single stretches of passive and maximally stimulated muscles in mice. *J Physiol (Lond)* 1995; **488**:459–469.

79 Higuchi H, Yoshioka T, Maruyama K. Positioning of actin filaments and tension generation in skinned muscle fibres released after stretch beyond overlap of the actin and myosin filaments. *J Muscle Res Cell Motil* 1988; **9**:491–498.

80 Valim V, Oliveira L, Suda A, Silva L, de Assis M, Barros NT, *et al.* Aerobic fitness effects in fibromyalgia. *J Rheumatol* 2003; **30**:1060–1069.

81 Peters S, Stanley I, Rose M, Kaney S, Salmon P. A randomized controlled trial of group aerobic exercise in primary care patients with persistent, unexplained physical symptoms. *Fam Pract* 2002; **19**:665–674.

82 Jones KD, Burckhardt CS, Clark SR, Bennett RM, Potempa KM. A randomized controlled trial of muscle strengthening versus flexibility training in fibromyalgia. *J Rheumatol* 2002; **29**:1041–1048.
83 Holmich P, Uhrskou P, Ulnits L, Kanstrup IL, Nielsen MB, Bjerg AM, *et al.* Active physical training for long-standing adductor-related groin pain. *Lancet* 1999; **353**:439–443.
84 Svernlov B, Adolfsson L. Non-operative treatment regime including eccentric training for lateral humeral epicondylalgia. *Scand J Med Sci Sports* 2001; **11**:328–334.

CHAPTER 4

What effect do core strength and stability have on injury prevention and recovery?

Bryan Heiderscheit and Marc Sherry

Introduction

Over the past decade, the focus in sports rehabilitation and performance training has been on core strengthening and stability. Despite the recent gain in popularity, the concept of core strength is not new. As early as the 1920s, Joseph Pilates talked about developing a girdle of strength by recruiting the deep trunk muscles. Additionally, educational programs of various rehabilitation professions have historically taught the concept that stability of proximal segments is required for effective mobility of distal segments (e.g., a stable pelvis and trunk are needed for controlled movement at the knee and ankle).

Hodges and Richardson[1] popularized the term *core stability* in the late 1990s. They described the spine as inherently unstable and requiring active support from intra-abdominal pressure and tensioning of the thoracolumbar fascia and deep lumbar stabilizers. Thus, core strength is considered to be the muscular support about the lumbar spine necessary to achieve and maintain functional stability.[2] More recently, this has been expanded by some to include muscles of the hip[3] and even the scapulothoracic musculature as well.[4] Good core strength contributing to adequate core stability has been suggested to be necessary in maintaining the correct lumbar and pelvic posture and alignment during movement and sport, allowing for powerful extremity movements. Similarly, inadequate core strength leading to poor core stability may decrease biomechanical efficiency and increase the risk for injury.

With the incorporation of core strengthening exercises into injury prevention and rehabilitation programs, scientific investigation of its effects is beginning to grow. In this chapter, we will review the clinical and scientific evidence pertaining to core strengthening as it relates to two specific questions:

- Does core strength prevent injury?
- Does core strengthening enhance recovery from injury?

Methods

A comprehensive search of the peer-reviewed literature was conducted using the following databases: MEDLINE on PubMed (1966–May 2005), Cumulative Index to Nursing and Allied Health (CINAHL) on Ovid (1982–May 2005), SportDiscus on Ovid (1830–May 2005), Science Citation Index (1970–May 2005), HealthSTAR on Ovid (1975–May 2005),

Table 4.1 Search strategy of text words and subject headings for the MEDLINE (1966–2005) and CINAHL (1982–2005) databases. MEDLINE was accessed using the PubMed search engine. All searches (limited to human studies) were conducted in February 2005

Item	Search	Results					
		MEDLINE	CINAHL	SportDiscus	Cochrane reviews	Science Citation Index	HealthSTAR
1	Core OR lumbar OR trunk	156993	8351	3804	461	> 100,000	49645
2	Strength OR stability OR stabilization	243574	12342	24815	802	> 100,000	83318
3	Injury	571250	21321	34163	670	> 100,000	84240
4	1 AND 2 AND 3	722	47	23	52	98	130

and the Cochrane Database of Systematic Reviews on Ovid (volume 2, 2005) (Table 4.1). Due to the variety of terms that are used synonymously with *core strengthening* and *stability*, a comprehensive search strategy was developed (Table 4.1). Identified articles that used strengthening of core muscles as an intervention, involved a comparison group and assessed either risk of injury or recovery from injury were included for this analysis. Finally, reference lists of relevant articles were reviewed to identify any additional citations not found in our search of the databases.

Results

Of the identified references (Table 4.1), the majority investigated the effect of core strengthening and stabilization exercises on specific aspects of muscle physiology and function. As these studies were unrelated to injury prevention or recovery, they were excluded. Only 16 articles were directly related to injury prevention or rehabilitation and were therefore included in this review.

Does core strength prevent injury?

Several correlational studies have been conducted to establish a relationship between core muscle weakness and the likelihood of injury. In their frequently cited paper, Hodges and Richardson[1] observed a significant delay in the activation of the transversus abdominis muscle among individuals with low back pain (LBP) when performing simple reaching tasks while standing. The authors suggested that this delay was a motor control deficit resulting in inefficient muscular stabilization of the lumbar spine, possibly preceding the onset of LBP. A similar delay in activation of the obliquus internus abdominis, multifidus and gluteus maximus was observed on the symptomatic side of individuals with sacroiliac joint pain.[5] Further, Iwai and colleagues[6] demonstrated that trunk extensor isokinetic strength was significantly correlated to the disability level of LBP among collegiate wrestlers without radiological abnormalities in the lumbar region. With regard to lower extremity injury, Ireland *et al.*[7] identified a positive correlation between hip muscle weakness and patellofemoral pain in females. Subjects with patellofemoral pain demonstrated 26% less hip abduction isometric strength and 36% less hip external rotation isometric strength in comparison with age-matched women who were not symptomatic. Unfortunately, the study design utilized by the four investigations cited above does not allow one to determine if the delayed timing or muscle weakness was present prior to symptom onset.

The prospective design employed by two of the identified studies does allow such conclusions to be made. Over a 5-year prospective study, Lee *et al.*[8] identified trunk muscle weakness as a risk factor for LBP. On the basis of isokinetic strength testing (60°/s) performed at the start of the investigation, individuals who developed LBP displayed an imbalance between trunk extensor and flexor strength. Specifically, the trunk extension/flexion strength ratio was approximately 25% less in females who developed LBP in comparison with those who did not. Similar findings were present for males, in whom a 20% deficit was noted.

Using a 1-year prospective design, Nadler *et al.*[9] demonstrated a bilateral imbalance in isometric strength of the hip extensors was related to the development of LBP among females. This relationship did not exist among males, as no significant change in side-to-side strength was evident in males who developed LBP. Further, no significant association was noted between the development of LBP and hip abductor strength for either gender. Although this study involved 163 collegiate athletes (100 males and 63 females), only 13 developed LBP (eight males and five females) over the subsequent year, indicating that caution is necessary in generalizing these findings.

On the contrary, Leetun *et al.*[3] prospectively determined that athletes with greater hip abduction and external rotation strength were less likely to experience LBP or injury to the lower extremities. Core muscle strength and performance (isometric strength of hip abduction and external rotation, endurance of back extension and side-bridging and abdominal performance) was assessed in 139 college basketball and cross-country athletes (79 females and 60 males). After which, they were monitored for injury throughout their respective season. Of the 139 athletes, a total of 41 sustained back or lower extremity injuries. The injured athletes displayed significantly less hip abduction and external rotation strength in comparison with those who did not incur an injury. On the basis of a regression analysis, hip external rotation weakness was the only useful predictor of lower extremity or low back injury over the course of an athletic season.

While the findings from this article are important, it should be noted that the muscle groups traditionally considered as compromising the core (i.e., the abdominals and trunk extensors) were consistent between athletes whether they did or did not sustain an injury. Further, the authors equate core strength to that of core stability. The ability of the lumbopelvic region to resist perturbations (core stability) is not accurately represented through isometric strength testing of associated musculature. Although isometric testing does provide a measure of muscle strength, it does not reflect how or if that strength is used in a stabilizing manner. Thus, conclusions regarding the relationship between core stability and injury may be limited. Testing procedures utilized to measure core strength and stability need continued development in relationship to dynamic movements and sport specific positions. These developments could potentially bolster the early results found in this study.

On the basis of the correlational evidence that activation delay or weakness of the core muscles is related to LBP and lower extremity injury, interventions aimed at restoring core strength should therefore reduce the risk of injury. One study was identified that prospectively determined the effects of core strengthening and injury prevention. Nadler *et al.*[10]

concluded that the incorporation of a core strengthening program among Division I college athletes did not reduce the incidence of LBP. Injury incidence data among these athletes were compared between two academic years, 1998–1999 and 1999–2000. A core strengthening program was instituted at the start of the 1999–2000 academic year, with the injury data from the 1998–1999 academic year used as the control comparison. The incidence of LBP did not differ with the inclusion of the core strengthening program, as 8.5% of the athletes (14 of 164) developed LBP during the 1998–1999 year in comparison with 6% (14 of 236) during the 1999–2000 year. Additionally, the strengthening program had a similar response across genders, as neither the male or female athletes displayed a reduction in LBP incidence.

However, given the study design, caution should be used when considering the results. Of most concern is the lack of reporting of statistical power or sample size estimation. In addition, the inconsistent subject pools between academic years may have confounded the results. Although all athletes participated in core strengthening as it became part of each sport's conditioning program, subject participation in the study remained voluntary, with the number of subjects from the different sports not controlled. Thus, sports having a greater incidence of LBP may have been unequally represented between academic years. Confounding variables such as weather, game and practice schedules, game and practice planning and strategy, or other strength and conditioning programs instituted by the coaching staff may also limit the strength of the findings. Finally, there is some question as to whether the selected exercises constitute a core strengthening program. Only two of the seven exercises focused on strengthening the abdominal and back muscles, with all seven exercises limited to movement in the sagittal plane.

Two additional articles that investigate the effects of core strengthening and stabilization exercises in preventing injury recurrence were identified.[11,12] While likely having implications for injury prevention, these two articles will be discussed in the next section of this chapter.

Summary of key points

- Delay in activation of core muscles, especially the transversus abdominis, has been retrospectively correlated with LBP.
- Imbalance of the trunk flexors/extensors and/or bilateral hip extensors has been prospectively correlated with LBP.
- Weakness of the hip external rotators has been prospectively correlated with lower extremity injury.
- The use of a core strengthening exercise program to prevent LBP in college athletes was not supported.

Does core strengthening enhance recovery from injury?

Most of the evidence available for the use of core strength and stabilization during rehabilitation is related to the treatment of acute and chronic LBP. As the multifidus muscle weakness and inhibition has a known relationship to LBP, Hides *et al.*[13] employed a prospective experimental design to determine if the recovery of the multifidus muscle can be enhanced with core stabilizing exercises. Subjects experiencing acute, first-episode LBP were randomized into either a medical management group or a group receiving medical management and exercise therapy. The medical management included advice on bed rest, absence from work and prescription of medication, while the exercise therapy involved stabilization exercises designed to reeducate the multifidus muscle in combination with the transversus abdominis. While both groups achieved symptom remission in a similar time period, the multifidus muscle recovery was more rapid and complete in the exercise therapy group. Even with a return to full activity, the medical management group continued to show decreased multifidus muscle size at 10 weeks after the onset of symptoms.

The authors[13] suggested that persistent muscle atrophy was related to the high recurrence rate of LBP. Through continued monitoring of subjects over the subsequent 3 years, Hides *et al.*[12] demonstrated that the LBP recurrence rate was 30% in subjects receiving the core stabilization therapy, in comparison with 84% of those who only received the medical management. On the basis of the experimental design, the use of core stabilization exercise is certainly more beneficial in the management of acute LBP than without exercise. However, the relative effectiveness of core stabilization exercise in comparison with other commonly prescribed exercise therapies was not determined.

O'Sullivan *et al.*[14] performed such a comparison in the management of patients with chronic LBP secondary to spondylosis and spondylolisthesis. Subjects were randomized into either a core stabilization exercise group or a group receiving general exercise treatment. The core stabilization exercises involved contraction of the deep abdominal muscles and facilitation of co-activation of the lumbar multifidus muscle above the level of the pars interarticularis defect. Initially, these exercises were performed statically and then progressively incorporated into postures and activities previously known to aggravate the patient's symptoms. The general exercise treatment involved walking, swimming, and care under other medical providers, such as pain-relieving interventions (e.g., heat, massage, ultrasound) and supervised exercise programs.

In comparison with the general exercise treatment group, the core stabilization exercise group had a significant reduction in pain intensity and functional disability immediately after the 10-week intervention. More importantly, this group was able to maintain these levels over a 30-month follow-up period. The general exercise treatment group did not show a significant reduction in these factors at either the 10-week or 30-week follow-ups. The authors concluded that even when the basic morphology of the lumbar spine is compromised, as is the case with spondylosis and spondylolisthesis, the neuromuscular system can be trained to create dynamic stability.[14]

In another investigation comparing exercise programs among individuals with chronic LBP, Danneels *et al.*[15] suggested that a 10-week core stabilization exercise program offered no advantage over a more traditional progressive resistive exercise program of the same duration in increasing the cross-sectional area of the multifidus muscle. However, concern has been raised with both the performance of the core stabilization exercises and the technique employed to characterize the multifidus cross-sectional area.[16] Unfortunately, Danneels and colleagues[15] did not report the recurrence rate of LBP or the changes in either symptoms or functional disability levels, as improvement in all is the ultimate purpose of increasing the size of the multifidus muscle.

On the basis of data from Yilmaz *et al.*,[17] lumbar stabilization exercises were more effective in reducing pain and functional disability levels than traditional flexion–extension exercises among patients following lumbar microdiscectomy. However, it is important to note that the stabilization exercises were supervised by a physiotherapist, while the flexion–extension exercises were performed as an unmonitored home exercise program. Thus, observed differences may not be secondary to the specific exercises, but rather to the level of supervision and compliance.

In comparison to manual therapy alone, a 6-week stabilization exercise program was found to be more effective in reducing low back pain and improving function in patients with either acute or chronic LBP.[18] As others have noted,[12] the recurrence rate of LBP among those receiving core stabilization exercises was also lower.

With regard to the treatment of lower extremity injuries, core strengthening and stabilization was involved in two articles. Holmich *et al.*[19] demonstrated that individuals with long-standing adductor pain had less pain and improved sports performance after undergoing an active rehabilitation program that aimed at improving strength and coordination of the muscles acting on the pelvis, in comparison with individuals who completed a rehabilitation program consisting of modalities and stretching.

Sherry and Best[11] employed a prospective randomized clinical trial to compare two rehabilitation programs in the treatment of acute hamstring strain injuries. The rehabilitation program incorporating core stabilization exercises was found to be protective against the recurrence of hamstring strain injury. In the first 2 weeks after return to sports, none of the 13 athletes (0%) who had received the progressive agility and trunk stabilization exercises during the rehabilitation of their initial injury experienced a hamstring injury recurrence, in comparison with six of the 11 athletes (54.5%) who received isolated hamstring stretching and strengthening exercises. One year after the return to sports, the re-injury rate remained significantly lower.

While this study supports the view that the incorporation of core strengthening and stability can be effective in preventing recurrent hamstring strain, the mechanism for this reduction is not known. As measurements related to the assessment of trunk stabilization and neuromuscular control were not made, it is not possible to conclude that the results were due to changes in trunk stability, coordination, or other aspects of motor control. More research is needed to quantify changes in muscle activation and response times of the trunk and pelvis that may occur from these types of rehabilitation programs.

Summary of key points

- Core stabilization exercises are effective in restoring the size and activation of the multifidus muscles in patients with acute LBP.
- Treatment programs including core stabilization were found to be more effective than manual therapy alone, medical management alone, and other common exercise programs in reducing pain and improving functional disability associated with acute and chronic LBP.
- Core stabilization exercises are more effective in reducing the recurrence of LBP and hamstring strain injuries in comparison with other exercise programs.

Discussion

The objective of this chapter was to review the clinical and scientific evidence pertaining to core strengthening as it relates to injury prevention and recovery. On the basis of our search strategies, 16 articles were identified and discussed, with seven of the 16 comparing core strengthening and stabilization exercises with other common types of exercise. Given our search of multiple databases, we believe it to be unlikely that we missed any prominent articles that would have significantly added to our findings. However, relevant articles not referenced in these databases may have been excluded from our review.

On the basis of the reviewed articles, LBP was the primary injury of concern with respect to core strengthening and stabilization. This is certainly not surprising, given the muscular control deficits observed with LBP and the related focus of these exercises. The clinical trials show strong promise for rehabilitation programs incorporating core strengthening exercise, both from an injury recovery and recurrence perspective. However, the studies investigating the use of these exercises in *preventing* LBP were predominantly observational in design and did not directly involve an intervention. Instead, subjects with known injuries were descriptively compared with control subjects with regard to specific strength and performance measures in the lumbar spine, pelvis and lower extremities. While such designs are useful in directing future studies, they do not allow for conclusions to be made regarding cause and effect.

As stated in the introduction to this chapter, the arguable success these exercises have had in treating LBP has led many to expand their use to treating injuries of the extremities. On the basis of the fact that biomechanically correct and efficient extremity movement cannot exist in the presence of an unstable pelvis and spine, core stabilization has been advocated for the treatment of such injuries as patellofemoral pain, iliotibial band syndrome, hamstring strain and postoperative rehabilitation of ligamentous reconstruction. While this appears to have theoretical merit, evidence addressing this application of core strengthening exercises was limited to two randomized controlled trials, both of which showed favorable results in treating acute hamstring strain[11] and hip adductor muscle pain.[19] Investigations involving the effects of core strengthening exercises on injuries more distal to the lumbopelvic region (e.g., patellofemoral pain) need to be conducted.

Certainly, it stands to reason that specific interventions may be more effective with specific patient types. It has been suggested that the equivocal or conflicting results observed in various investigations of exercise programs for nonspecific LBP may be related to the assumed homogeneity of the subjects. This has led others to investigate exercise treatment efficacy in defined subgroups within a particular diagnosis.[20,21] That is, not all patients with LBP can be grouped and treated uniformly. A patient experiencing LBP secondary to lumbar instability will likely respond favorably to different interventions than one with LBP secondary to hypomobility. It would be somewhat naïve to expect all individuals with LBP and lower extremity injury to require and benefit from a core strengthening and stabilization program. Thus, future studies may wish to identify the characteristics of those most likely to respond to core strengthening exercises.

The overall evidence either for or against the use of core strengthening exercises for injury prevention or rehabilitation is rather limited. While clinical experience appears to be providing motivation for the continued use of such exercises, systematically designed investigations are paramount in order to determine their effectiveness. In the end, this will allow the development of successful and efficient rehabilitation, injury prevention, and sports performance programs.

Sample examination questions

Multiple-choice questions (answers on page 602)

1 The primary injury investigated with respected to core strengthening and stabilization exercises is:
  A Iliotibial band syndrome
  B Patellofemoral pain syndrome
  C Low back pain
  D Hamstring strain injury

Table 4.2 Summary of clinical investigations involving core strength and injury prevention

Study	Design	Sample	Intervention	Results
Hodges and Richardson[1]	Case–control	Case: 15 patients with LBP Control: 15 age- and sex-matched healthy subjects	Not applicable	Transversus abdominis muscle activation was significantly delayed in patients with LBP
Hungerford *et al.*[5]	Case–control	Case: 14 males with sacroiliac joint pain Control: 14 age-matched healthy males	Not applicable	Activation onset of obliquus internus abdominis, multifidus and gluteus maximus was delayed on the symptomatic side of subjects with sacroiliac joint pain
Ireland *et al.*[7]	Case–control	Case: 15 females with patellofemoral pain Control: 15 asymptomatic age-matched females	Not applicable	Subjects with patellofemoral pain demonstrated 26% less hip abduction strength and 36% less hip external rotation strength
Iwai *et al.*[6]	Case–control	53 college wrestlers with LBP Case: 35 with radiologic abnormality Control: 18 without radiologic abnormality	Not applicable	Trunk extensor strength characteristics were correlated ($r = 0.28–0.73$) with the level of disability in the group of wrestlers without radiologic abnormality

Lee *et al.*[8]	5-yr prospective cohort	67 subjects without history of LBP	Not applicable	The 18 subjects that developed LBP had significantly reduced trunk extension/flexion strength ratio at baseline
Leetun *et al.*[3]	Prospective cohort	139 college basketball and cross-country athletes (79 females; 60 males)	Not applicable	Hip external rotation weakness was the only useful predictor for lower extremity or spine injury (OR 0.86)
Nadler *et al.*[9]	1-yr prospective	163 Division I college athletes cohort (63 females; 100 males)	Not applicable	13 athletes developed LBP. Bilateral asymmetry of hip extensor strength was predictive of LBP in females
Nadler *et al.*[10]	2-yr prospective cohort	164 Division I college athletes as a control group and 236 Division I college athletes the following year as an intervention group	Strengthening program performed 4–5 x/week (pre-season) and 2–3 x/ week (season). Exercises included: abdominal crunches, pelvic tilts, squats, lunges, leg press, hang cleans, dead lifts, isolated back extensions	No statistically significant reduction in the incidence of LBP among those participating in the core strengthening program (14/236) in comparison with those that did not (14/164)

LBP, low back pain.

Table 4.3 Summary of clinical investigations using core strengthening and stabilization exercises as part of the recovery from injury

Study	Design	Sample	Intervention	Results
Danneels *et al.*[15]	RCT	59 patients with chronic LBP	Subjects randomly assigned to: 1–10 weeks of stabilization exercises 2–10 weeks of stabilization exercises combined with dynamic resistance training 3–10 weeks of stabilization exercises combined with dynamic–static resistance training	Cross-sectional area of the multifidus muscle at L3 and L4 vertebral levels was significantly increased in group 3 only
Hides *et al.*[13]	RCT	39 patients with acute, first-episode, unilateral LBP and unilateral segmental inhibition of the multifidus	Subjects randomly assigned to: 1 medical management only 2 medical management and exercise therapy group involving stabilization exercises designed to re-educate the multifidus muscle in combination with the transversus abdominis muscle	Symptom remission occurred in a similar time period between groups, but the multifidus muscle recovery was more rapid and complete in the exercise therapy group
Hides *et al.*[12] (follow-up to Hides *et al.*[13])	3-yr prospective cohort	Case: subjects with LBP who received medical management and exercise therapy Control: subjects with LBP who were medically managed only	Same as Hides *et al.*[13]	LBP recurrence rate was 30% in subjects receiving the stabilization exercise therapy in comparison with 84% in the medical management only group

Holmich *et al.*[19]	RCT with blinded investigator	68 male athletes aged 18–50 with long-standing adductor pain	Subjects randomly assigned to: 1, active rehabilitation program aimed at improving strength and coordination of the muscles acting on the pelvis 2, rehabilitation program consisting of modalities and stretching	23/34 patients in the active rehabilitation group returned to sport without groin pain in comparison with 4/34 patients in the group receiving modalities and stretching
O'Sullivan *et al.*[14]	RCT with blinded investigator	44 subjects aged 16–49 with LBP secondary to spondylosis and spondylolisthesis greater than 3 months' duration	Subjects randomly assigned to: 1, core stabilization exercise group (abdominal and multifidus co-contraction) 2, general exercise treatment (swimming, walking, modalities and home exercise program)	Statistically significant reduction in pain intensity and functional disability levels, maintained up to a 30-month follow-up, in the core stabilization group
Sherry and Best[11]	RCT	24 athletes with an acute hamstring strain (6 females; 18 males)	Subjects randomly assigned to: 1, progressive agility and trunk stabilization program (n = 11) 2, isolated hamstring stretching and strengthening program (n = 13)	Significant decrease in hamstring injury recurrence at 2 weeks (0% vs. 54.5%) and 1 y (7.7% vs. 70%) following return to sport for subjects that received the progressive agility and trunk stabilization exercises. Early return to sport in the progressive agility and trunk stabilization group was not statistically significant
Yilmaz *et al.*[17]	RCT	42 patients aged 20–60 who had undergone first-time micro-discectomy for unisegmental lumbar disc herniation	Subjects randomly assigned to: 1, physical therapist–supervised dynamic lumbar stabilization exercises 2, written home exercise program of range-of-motion and trunk/abdominal strengthening exercises 3, no-exercise control group	Both exercise groups demonstrated improvements in pain, functional capacity, body strength, mobility and weight-lifting capacity. However, the gains were greater in those performing the lumbar stabilization exercise program.

LBP, low back pain; RCT, randomized controlled trial.

2 In the treatment of patients with low back pain, which muscle(s) is (are) frequently targeted through core stabilization exercises?
   A Multifidus
   B Erector spinae
   C Transversus abdominis
   D Both A and B
   E Both A and C
3 Which of the following statements is true concerning the evidence for core strength and lower extremity injury?
   A Weakness of the hip external rotators may be a useful predictor of lower extremity injury.
   B Females with patellofemoral pain often demonstrate hip abductor and external rotator weakness.
   C Incorporation of core stabilization exercises into the rehabilitation of acute hamstring strain injuries may significantly reduce the likelihood of re-injury.
   D All of the above.

Essay questions

1 Discuss the limitations associated with case–control design studies in determining the contribution of core strength to low back or lower extremity injury.
2 Create a list of exercises that would be considered core stabilization exercises. Each exercise must involve a stabilization component and not merely strengthening. Place in order of easiest to most difficult.
3 When considering the mechanism by which core stabilization exercises are beneficial, theorize whether it is predominantly due to gains in muscle force output or improved activation and coordination between muscles.

Case study 4.1

Joe Smith is a 16-year-old male diagnosed with plica syndrome of the left knee, who presented to physical therapy for evaluation and treatment. He is 1.93 m tall, weighs 117.5 kg, and has a body mass index of 31.5 kg/m^2. He reports that he gradually developed medial knee pain during the past basketball season. He denies any trauma, instability, swelling or locking episodes in his left knee. Magnetic resonance imaging (MRI) performed by the referring physician was read as normal. He does complain of some clicking/snapping medially, but very intermittent. On physical examination, he had a full knee range of motion, with 12° of hyperextension with tenderness to palpation over the superior medial plica. The ligament examination was negative, with mild patellar hypermobility without apprehension noted. Although he was well-developed for his age, manual muscle testing revealed slight weakness of the medial and lateral hip rotators and hip abductors. A McGill side-bridge position with proper alignment was maintained for 10 s. Mild to moderate medial deviation at the knee was observed in an attempt to stabilize his posture during single leg balance, single leg squat, and single leg landing.

After his initial evaluation, a rehabilitation program was initiated, emphasizing static core strength and stabilization, along with static balance exercises. This program included the McGill side bridge, supine bridging with hip external rotation resistance, four-point multifidus leg lift, prone planks, and single leg balance with the knee and hip slightly flexed.

When Joe was re-evaluated after 2 weeks he had improved his core strength and endurance. He could now hold the side bridge position for 20 s, his hip external and internal rotation strength was normal on single repetition testing but still fatigued quickly. He could control a single leg balance position for 20 s with minimal postural sway. The program was progressed to include single-leg half-squats, single-leg balance on an uneven surface, alternate leg lifting with his prone planks and side bridges, and trunk rotations in standing with band resistance.

After 3½ weeks of therapy, Joe was able to easily maintain the plank and side bridge alignment with alternate leg lifting for greater than 20 s. He had also significantly improved his alignment control with his single-leg squats, and now demonstrated good strength and endurance of the hip rotators. At this time, his program was transitioned to more dynamic sport-specific core strengthening and stabilization exercises, such as medicine-ball rotation throw and catch off the wall, medicine-ball lunge chops with trunk rotation, medicine-ball figure of eight, medicine-ball rotations in a half-squat and multiplanar leap–land balance drills.

After 5 weeks of therapy, Joe was not experiencing pain with his activities of daily living, rehabilitation exercises, or limited basketball shooting drills. He demonstrated excellent postural control with single-leg activities, along with improved timing and speed in the medicine-ball core drills. He was gradually returned to team practices over the next week, with eventual return to competitive basketball without medial knee pain. He continues to incorporate principles of core strengthening and stabilization into his independent strength and conditioning program for basketball.

Summarizing the evidence

Comparison	Results	Level of evidence
Core strength deficits and injury occurrence	6 case–control or cohort studies, 4 of moderate size, 3 prospective, core muscle weakness present in individuals who currently had or developed LBP or lower extremity injury	B
Core deficits and LBP prevention	1 prospective cohort study, moderate size, exercises did not reduce incidence of LBP	B
Core strengthening exercises and LBP rehabilitation	5 RCTs, 1 of moderate size, results in favor of exercises	A3
Core strengthening exercises and lower extremity injury rehabilitation	2 RCTs, 1 of moderate size, results in favor of exercises.	A3

LBP, low back pain; RCT, randomized controlled trial.

* A1: evidence from large randomized controlled trials (RCTs) or systematic review (including meta-analysis).†

A2: evidence from at least one high-quality cohort.

A3: evidence from at least one moderate-sized RCT or systematic review.†

A4: evidence from at least one RCT.

B: evidence from at least one high-quality study of nonrandomized cohorts.

C: expert opinions.

† Arbitrarily, the following cut-off points have been used: large study size: ≥ 100 patients per intervention group; moderate study size ≥ 50 patients per intervention group.

References

1 Hodges PW, Richardson CA. Inefficient muscular stabilization of the lumbar spine associated with low back pain: a motor control evaluation of transversus abdominis. *Spine* 1996; **21**:2640–2650.

2 Akuthota V, Nadler SF. Core strengthening. *Arch Phys Med Rehabil* 2004; **85**:S86–92.

3 Leetun DT, Ireland ML, Willson JD, Ballantyne BT, Davis IM. Core stability measures as risk factors for lower extremity injury in athletes. *Med Sci Sports Exerc* 2004; **36**:926–934.

4 Quinn E. Sports medicine: core stability training. How to build a strong foundation. Available at: http://www.sportsmedicine.about.com/cs/conditioning/a/aa052002a.htm. Accessed September 3, 2006.

5 Hungerford B, Gilleard W, Hodges P. Evidence of altered lumbopelvic muscle recruitment in the presence of sacroiliac joint pain. *Spine* 2003; **28**:1593–1600.

6 Iwai K, Nakazato K, Irie K, Fujimoto H, Nakajima H. Trunk muscle strength and disability level of low back pain in collegiate wrestlers. *Med Sci Sports Exerc* 2004; **36**:1296–1300.

7 Ireland ML, Willson JD, Ballantyne BT, Davis IM. Hip strength in females with and without patellofemoral pain. *J Orthop Sports Phys Ther* 2003; **33**:671–676.

8 Lee JH, Hoshino Y, Nakamura K, Kariya Y, Saita K, Ito K. Trunk muscle weakness as a risk factor for low back pain: a 5-year prospective study. *Spine* 1999; **24**:54–57.

9 Nadler SF, Malanga GA, Feinberg JH, *et al.* Relationship between hip muscle imbalance and occurrence of low back pain in collegiate athletes: a prospective study. *Am J Phys Med Rehabil* 2001; **80**:572–577.

10 Nadler SF, Malanga GA, Bartoli LA, *et al.* Hip muscle imbalance and low back pain in athletes: influence of core strengthening. *Med Sci Sports Exerc* 2002; **34**:9–16.

11 Sherry MA, Best TM. A comparison of 2 rehabilitation programs in the treatment of acute hamstring strains. *J Orthop Sports Phys Ther* 2004; **34**:116–125.

12 Hides JA, Jull GA, Richardson CA. Long-term effects of specific stabilizing exercises for first-episode low back pain. *Spine* 2001; **26**:E243–248.

13 Hides JA, Richardson CA, Jull GA. Multifidus muscle recovery is not automatic after resolution of acute, first-episode low back pain. *Spine* 1996; **21**:2763–2769.

14 O'Sullivan PB, Phyty GD, Twomey LT, Allison GT. Evaluation of specific stabilizing exercise in the treatment of chronic low back pain with radiologic diagnosis of spondylolysis or spondylolisthesis. *Spine* 1997; **22**:2959–2967.

15 Danneels LA, Vanderstraeten GG, Cambier DC, *et al.* Effects of three different training modalities on the cross sectional area of the lumbar multifidus muscle in patients with chronic low back pain. *Br J Sports Med* 2001; **35**:186–191.

16 Jemmett RS. Rehabilitation of lumbar multifidus dysfunction in low back pain: strengthening versus a motor re-education model. *Br J Sports Med* 2003; **37**:91.

17 Yilmaz F, Yilmaz A, Merdol F, *et al.* Efficacy of dynamic lumbar stabilization exercise in lumbar microdiscectomy. *J Rehabil Med* 2003; **35**:163–167.

18 Rasmussen-Barr E, Nilsson-Wikmar L, Arvidsson I. Stabilizing training compared with manual treatment in sub-acute and chronic low-back pain. *Man Ther* 2003; **8**:233–241.

19 Holmich P, Uhrskou P, Ulnits L, *et al.* Effectiveness of active physical training as treatment for long-standing adductor-related groin pain in athletes: randomised trial. *Lancet* 1999; **353**:439–443.

20 Long A, Donelson R, Fung T. Does it matter which exercise? A randomized control trial of exercise for low back pain. *Spine* 2004; **29**:2593–2602.

21 Fritz JM, Delitto A, Erhard RE. Comparison of classification-based physical therapy with therapy based on clinical practice guidelines for patients with acute low back pain: a randomized clinical trial. *Spine* 2003; **28**:1363–1371; discussion 1372.

CHAPTER 5

Do foot orthoses prevent injury?

Karl B. Landorf and Anne-Maree Keenan

Introduction

Foot orthoses (orthotics, orthotic devices, insoles, shoe inserts) are commonly prescribed to prevent and treat injuries associated with sports and exercise. The two primary goals of orthotic therapy are (i) to realign skeletal structures and (ii) to alter movement patterns of the foot and lower extremity. Both of these goals relate to anomalies in foot posture, which have long been suggested to cause a variety of sports injury including plantar fasciitis,[1–3] medial tibial stress syndrome,[4–6] patellofemoral pain,[7,8] iliotibial band friction syndrome,[9] and back pain.[10–13] However, the evidence is contradictory with regard to the relationship between foot posture and injury;[6,12,14–29] several excellent reviews have been written dealing with this issue.[30–36] Moreover, the efficacy of foot orthoses in the management of sporting injuries—particularly the prevention of injuries—is still far from certain. Although there have been rigorous systematic reviews evaluating interventions for preventing lower limb soft tissue injuries in runners,[37,38] shin splints in sports,[35] and for preventing and treating stress fractures and stress reactions of bone in the lower limbs of young adults,[39] none have specifically focused on foot orthoses.

The aim of this chapter is to review the evidence surrounding the use of foot orthoses in the prevention of sporting injuries. The first part of this chapter will explore the terminology and classification of foot orthoses and include an overview on how orthoses are thought to work. The second part is a systematic review of the literature using key databases in order to identify evidence associated with the use of orthoses in sporting injury prevention.

How are foot orthoses classified?

"Foot orthosis" is a term that has been used to describe any type of shoe insert that is designed to alter the function of the foot. However, given the broad definition of orthotic therapy, there are many complexities associated with their prescription and manufacture, such as:

- Variability in the patient profile and the subsequent rationale for orthotic prescription.
- Diversity in the philosophy of orthotic function.
- Discrepancy in the manufacture of the devices, including the type of material used.[40]

Historically, the development of orthotic therapy has often been in response to new theories or assumptions associated with various paradigms of foot function. In addition, the type of device prescribed is often governed by subjective clinician influences including practitioners' previous clinical experience, both positive and negative. Consequently, there is considerable variation in the types of orthoses prescribed by practitioners.[41] This is further compounded by a lack of good-quality research evaluating the effects that different types of foot orthoses have on skeletal pathologies.[40,42] Clearly, it is difficult to develop a consistent terminology for and prescription of foot orthoses when conclusive scientific evidence is not available and practitioners prescribe different devices, often even for the same condition.

A universal terminology for orthotic prescription has been identified as problematic when attempting to discuss almost any aspect of orthotic therapy.[43] Orthoses have previously been categorized in a number of ways, the two most common being: (i) soft/flexible, semirigid and rigid[44,45] and (ii) accommodative and functional.[46] These categories are defined in part by the type of materials used when manufacturing the device. Orthotic materials can be simply categorized as either soft/flexible (generally shock-absorbing) or hard/rigid (generally motion-controlling).[47] However, the characteristics of the materials are generally not as simple as being soft or hard, but relate to more complex variables such as density, compression set, hardness, and the ability to store energy,[48] which further complicates the classification of foot orthoses.

While groups have attempted to address this confusion by producing guidelines and descriptions, it has proved difficult to gain acceptance of these among professional groups with differing philosophies of orthotic fabrication.[43,49] At this stage, there is, unfortunately, no widely adopted international classification of foot orthoses.

How do foot orthoses work?

Evaluating the mechanism of action of foot orthoses is complex and has provided many challenges for researchers. Despite advances in technology, there is still a great deal to learn.[50–52] Most studies investigating the biomechanical effect of foot orthoses have generally utilized one of three investigative techniques: (i) kinematic, (ii) kinetic or plantar pressure, and/or (iii) electromyographic assessment. In addition, neurophysiological effects have been postulated.[53,54] Recently, there has also been a push to include more patient-orientated outcomes in musculoskeletal research.[55–57] Clearly, there is a need to assess patient outcomes in orthotic therapy, not only to determine whether they are effective, but also to ascertain whether surrogate outcome measures, such as kinematic changes, translate into positive outcomes for the patient. This is particularly relevant when the effect of foot posture on injury is still not certain. Nevertheless, surrogate outcome measures appear to be important in understanding how orthoses work, and as such require discussion.

With regard to the *first* investigative technique, kinematics, the majority of research has focused on changes in position/movement of the arch of the foot, the rearfoot and the tibia. Specific variables that have been evaluated that represent changes in foot posture include two-dimensional changes in sagittal plane arch or navicular height, frontal plane calcaneal position, or tibial transverse plane rotation.[58–65] In early studies, much of the research was static in nature; however, dynamic studies are far more common now. More recently still, changes in three-dimensional motion have been assessed, as this better represents the complex movement patterns of the joints of the foot—particularly the amount and rate of pronation and supination of the subtalar joint or rearfoot.[53,66–78] Overwhelmingly, investigators have found that foot orthoses produce only small changes in position or motion. Changes in calcaneal position and tibial rotation are generally in the order of 1–4° (less pronated) and less than 2–4 mm for arch height (increased arch height). These changes tend to be highly variable—that is, not systematic—for each individual,[79] and are greater in magnitude higher up the limb in comparison with the foot with some types of orthoses.[76] Many of these findings are statistically significant, but it is still unknown whether they are clinically worthwhile.

In addition to the motion-based investigations, cadaver-based studies[80,81] have found a decrease in plantar fascial strain with certain types of foot orthoses, which may be of benefit when treating plantar fasciitis. Plantar fascial strain is increased with foot pronation; hence, a decrease in strain is representative of a decrease in pronation (i.e., a more supinated foot posture).[82] Modeling studies have also been performed in an attempt to link the effect of foot orthoses on patellofemoral pain. One study[83] simulated patellofemoral loads, finding that foot orthoses significantly decreased *average* load at this joint. This may be due to changes in skeletal alignment leading to changes in the direction of force created by muscles, or it may be due to altered synergistic muscle activity coordinating the patellar.

Secondly, foot orthoses have also been evaluated using kinetics, predominantly using force and plantar pressure systems. Findings from these studies[84–86] convincingly demonstrate that foot orthoses—particularly ones shaped to the arch and heel—alter both the amount and timing of force and pressure underneath the foot. On average, these changes appear to be significant; however, one center-of-pressure study[79] found that, like the kinematic studies, they were not consistent across individuals. Shock attenuation has also been shown to be significantly reduced by foot orthoses, particularly with certain orthotic materials.[87–89] Attenuation of the shock created when the foot strikes the ground during activity has been hypothesized to decrease low-back pain[87] and stress fractures of the lower limb.[90]

Thirdly, there have been five studies that have evaluated the effects of foot wedging and orthoses on electromyographic activity of muscles.[91–95] Statistically significant changes in electromyographic *activity* of the tibialis anterior, peroneus longus, gastrocnemius, quadriceps, biceps femoris, gluteus medius and erector spinae muscles have been demonstrated. These studies have used different electromyographic variables to assess the effect of wedging and orthoses, including amplitude, timing, and frequency of the electromyographic signal. This area of research is still relatively new. Whether an increase or decrease in these variables is positive in relation to injury has yet to be established, so the meaning of these findings is still unclear.

Finally, Mundermann and colleagues[96] evaluated the effect of foot orthoses on all three of the aforementioned biomechanical variables; kinematics, kinetics and electromyographic activity. However, the authors were specifically concerned with whether changes in these variables influenced orthotic *comfort*. In a highly selected sample, changes in kinematic, kinetic and electromyographic variables did explain comfort of the foot orthoses tested. Therefore, orthotic comfort may be an important variable that helps explain how orthoses work.

In summary, while there is no consensus on how orthoses work, there is evidence to suggest small, yet significant changes to the mechanical function of the lower limb with a variety of orthotic devices. Given that the kinematic changes are relatively small, further research on kinetic, electromyographic and comfort may help explain how orthoses work. The remainder of this chapter will focus on a systematic review, exploring the evidence of orthotic therapy in preventing sporting injuries.

Methodology

Search strategy

Databases searched were MEDLINE (1966-present)/PubMed, CINAHL, EMBASE (1988–present), SportDiscus, and the Cochrane Central Register of Controlled Trials (CENTRAL). The search was initially conducted on 30 November 2005 and updated on 8 February 2006; all databases were searched using OVID. The search strategy included:

1. Search (orthos$s OR orthotic$ OR insole$) AND injury
2. Search (orthos$s OR orthotic$ OR insole$) AND prevention

The search was limited to the English language, as no funds were available for translation services. Only journal articles were accepted. In CINAHL, the search was also limited to systematic reviews and clinical trials. In MEDLINE, the search was limited to randomized and randomized controlled trials, where available. Checking of bibliographies was also carried out for additional references not identified in the initial searches.

Inclusion and exclusion criteria

Trials were included if they evaluated foot orthoses (foot orthotic devices) using a randomized or quasi-randomized trial methodology. Trials were not included if they compared orthoses or orthotic devices that were not foot orthoses (e.g., ankle or knee orthoses).

Quality of trials

Quality ratings are included for readers to gauge the strength of each study's findings. The quality of the trials was assessed by both authors using the PEDro scale[97,98]—a scale for rating the methodological quality of clinical trials. A lower score on the scale is indicative of a poorer quality trial that is more open to bias. Variations within scoring of identified studies were resolved through further exploration of the trials and consensus re-rating of the studies. There were no studies in which consensus was not achieved.

Results

Twelve randomized or quasi-randomized trials met the inclusion and exclusion criteria. The majority (11 of the 12) used military personnel, primarily recruits participating in basic training. One study evaluated soccer referees taking part in a soccer tournament.[99] Although most studies provided little data on baseline characteristics of participants, they were predominantly young, healthy adults, with the vast majority being males. All samples undertook relatively high amounts of physical training and apart from the study on soccer referees,[99] would have had a mix of fitness levels. It is difficult to make any other assessments of activity levels or fitness with the data provided in the published studies.

The definition of injury varied from study to study. Some evaluated injury broadly (i.e., any overuse injury), while some focused on specific injuries such as stress fractures or medial tibial stress syndrome. The impact of the injury was taken into account in a few trials by assessing days off duty due to injury, and one study assessed quality-of-life issues. Because of the multitude of injuries measured and the different types of foot orthoses used in the trials, a meta-analysis was not performed.

The types of foot orthosis used in the trials varied. Orthoses included shock-absorbing insoles,[100–103] heel pads[104] or inserts,[99] or devices that were molded in some way to the shape of the plantar surface of the foot.[105–110] Orthoses shaped to the plantar surface of the foot were either prefabricated or customized. Prefabricated orthoses are made to an "average" foot shape and are available in different sizes. Customized orthoses are generally manufactured from a plaster cast or mold of the individual's foot.

Because different types of foot orthosis were used, the results of this review were grouped into those trials that evaluated shock-absorbing insoles (or inserts) and those that investigated orthoses designed to alter motion of the foot ("biomechanical" orthoses). The findings from both the trials evaluating shock-absorbing insoles and motion-controlling orthoses will now be discussed. Following the discussion on each type of orthosis, a summary of the quality of the trials identified in the systematic search will be presented, with conclusions about the strength of the evidence to date.

Shock-absorbing foot orthoses

Six trials[99–104] identified in the systematic search evaluated shock-absorbing insoles or heel pads for the prevention of injury. Four of the trials demonstrated that shock-absorbing foot orthoses had no significant effect on the prevention of injury (three evaluated insoles[100,102,103] and one heel pads[104]). Two trials found significantly lower injury rates for shock-absorbing foot orthoses (one evaluated a heel insert[99] and one an insole[101]).

The two positive trials used very different samples and suffered from methodological weaknesses. Fauno and colleagues[99] investigated the effectiveness of a shock-absorbing heel insert on injury rate in soccer referees at a soccer tournament (n = 91). They found a significantly lower rate of soreness in the Achilles tendon, calf, and back in the group that used the heel insert. However, this trial was of low quality (see the next section on the quality of trials), scoring very poorly on the PEDro scale.

The other positive trial conducted by Schwellnus and co-workers[101] in the South African military found that a shock-absorbing (neoprene) insole significantly reduced overuse injuries and tibial stress syndrome. This study had a very large sample size (n = 1511) but also had a number of methodological issues that could have introduced bias. Consequently, it too scored poorly from a quality perspective, although it was of slightly better quality than the heel insert trial discussed above.

Importantly, a recent trial by Withnall and colleagues[103] that evaluated two different shock-absorbing insoles (Sorbothane and Poron) against a no-intervention group was of high quality—the highest-quality trial among those identified in the systematic search. This trial found that the insoles did not significantly reduce the incidence of lower limb injury. As this trial is vastly better in quality in comparison with the other trials evaluating shock-absorbing foot orthoses, its results provide the best evidence to date that shock-absorbing insoles do not prevent injury. However, the generalizability of this finding needs to be tempered by the fact that the participants were military recruits undergoing basic training. That is, the recruits were predominantly young and male; would have likely been of mixed fitness levels at the start of training; and would have experienced a period of intense exercise over the 9 weeks they were studied.

When all of the identified randomized or quasi-randomized trials that evaluated shock-absorbing foot orthoses are assessed, the evidence suggests that they do not prevent injury. Table 5.1 summarizes each trial, including information on the participants, interventions, and primary outcomes. Incorporated into this table are specific details regarding injury rates for the primary outcomes of each trial.

Table 5.1 Summary of randomized trials evaluating shock-absorbing foot orthoses for the prevention of injury

First author (ref.)	Participants	Interventions	Intervention period	Primary results
Andrish (1974)[104]	United States naval midshipmen	(i) No intervention (control) (ii) Heel pad (iii) "Heel cord stretches" (iv) Heel pad and heel cord stretches (v) Graduated running program	Not stated ("summer training program")	No significant differences in incidence of shin splints between groups. Incidence of shin splints in each group was (i) 3% for control, (ii) 4% for heel pad, (iii) 4% for heel cord stretches, (iv) 3% for heel pad and heel cord stretches and (v) 6% for graduated running program
Fauno (1993)[99]	Soccer referees	(i) Prefabricated "shock-absorbing heel insert" (Action*) (ii) No intervention	5-day soccer tournament	The insert (orthosis) group experienced a significantly lower rate of soreness in the Achilles tendon, calf and back ($P < 0.05$). No overall incidence rates of injury were provided; however, on days 3 and 4, 63% of the insert group experienced soreness, versus 93% in the group that did not receive the insert
Gardner (1988)[100]	United States marines	(i) Prefabricated "viscoelastic polymer (Sorbothane†)" orthosis (ii) Control group (standard mesh insole)	12 weeks	No significant difference between insoles in preventing stress fractures. In the polymer insole group, 1.4% experienced a stress fracture in comparison with 1.1% in the control group (relative risk 1.2; 95% CI, 0.6 to 2.2)
Schwellnus (1990)[101]	South African military recruits	(i) Neoprene "shock-absorbing flat insole" (ii) No intervention	9 weeks	The insole (orthosis) group experienced a significantly lower rate of overuse injuries and tibial stress syndrome ($P < 0.05$). The incidence of injury in the insole group was 22.8%, compared with 31.9% in the no-intervention (control) group

Sherman (1996)[102]	United States army recruits	(i) Prefabricated "cushioning" (Spenco‡) orthosis (ii) No intervention *A third group developed when a large number of recruits randomly assigned to "no intervention" purchased the orthosis of their own accord*	Basic training (exact no. of weeks not stated)	No significant differences found between groups in the incidence of lower limb pain problems. In the orthosis group, 37.6% experienced lower limb pain problems compared to 29.4% in the no intervention (control group). The incidence of lower limb pain problems in those recruits who were not originally allocated orthoses but purchased their own was 38.4%
Withnall (2006)[103]	Royal Air Force recruits (United Kingdom)	(i) Shock-absorbing (Sorbothane†) insole (ii) Shock-absorbing (Poron§) insole (iii) Non-shock-absorbing (standard issue Saran) insole	9 weeks	There was no significant difference between the shock-absorbing insoles and the non shock-absorbing insole in reducing lower limb injury (odds ratio 1.04, 95% CI 0.75 to 1.44; $P = 0.87$). The incidence of lower limb injury was approximately 18%. There was also no significant difference between the shock-absorbing insoles (17.3% for Sorbothane and 19.8% for Poron) in reducing lower limb injury (odds ratio 0.85; 95% CI, 0.58 to 1.23; $P = 0.37$)

CI, confidence interval.

* Action: manufactured by Action Products Inc., Hagerstown, MD, United States of America.

† Sorbothane: manufactured by Sorbothane Incorporated, Kent, OH, United States of America.

‡ Spenco: the orthosis used was the Spenco Polysorb walker–runner, manufactured by Spenco Inc., Waco, TX, United States of America.

§ Poron: manufactured by Rogers Corporation, Rogers, CT, United States of America.

Quality of randomized trials evaluating shock-absorbing foot orthoses

The median PEDro score for all trials was 3.5 (range 2–7), indicating that the trials included in the systematic review were generally of poor quality. However, one trial[100] scored 6 points and the trial by Withnall and colleagues,[103] the most recent of the trials included, scored 7 points—the highest score of all trials assessed. Given that blinding in trials such as this is difficult (lack of blinding leads to a lower score on the PEDro rating scale), a score as high as 7 indicates a trial of high quality. Table 5.2 presents a methodological comparison between the trials assessed, including the PEDro score. Only one trial[103] reported findings as recommended by the CONSORT guidelines,[111] which have been developed to assist in ensuring transparency of trials. It can be concluded that better-quality trials are needed in order to reduce bias and establish a more precise estimate of the effect of foot orthoses in preventing injury. This will allow the findings by Withnall and colleagues to be confirmed or refuted.

Motion-controlling foot orthoses

Six trials identified in the systematic search evaluated motion-controlling foot orthoses for the prevention of injury. One recent trial performed in the Australian Air Force[110] found that a prefabricated orthosis ("AOL") did not significantly decrease injury. However, this trial was not premised on an a priori sample size calculation, and with the sample size reached (n = 47) was likely to be underpowered—due to this, the authors refer to it as a pilot study. In addition, although an intention-to-treat analysis was performed, difficulties were experienced with compliance (only half the group assigned the orthoses wore them most or all of the time).

In contrast to this negative trial, four trials[105–108] found that motion-controlling orthoses do reduce injury rates. Three of these studies were performed in the Israeli military and one in the Danish military. One further trial[109] investigated the effectiveness of different types of orthosis in reducing injury; that is, the investigators were interested in comparing different orthoses, rather than an orthosis against no intervention.

The Israeli military trials[105–107] that found that foot orthoses did prevent injury all had large sample sizes (between 295 and 874 participants), but were generally of low methodological quality (see the next section on the quality of trials). One trial[107] evaluated semirigid and soft "biomechanical" orthoses against a simple shoe insole. They found that both the "biomechanical" orthoses reduced stress fractures compared to a simple shoe insole. The other two trials evaluated a prefabricated semirigid "military stress" orthosis against a no-intervention group. Milgrom and colleagues[105] found a significant reduction in femoral stress fractures in the orthosis group. Simkin and co-workers[106] evaluated the effect of the orthosis in comparison with no intervention in both high-arched and low-arched feet. They found a significant reduction in femoral stress fractures in recruits with high-arched feet and metatarsal stress fractures in recruits with low-arched feet.

The concerted efforts of the Israeli military to reduce injuries in recruits culminated in a recent study[109] that evaluated different types of foot orthoses (this time with no control group due to the positive findings for foot orthoses in the earlier studies). In this study, the emphasis was on whether one type of foot orthosis performed better than another. Four types of device were investigated including soft and semirigid devices, and prefabricated and customized. All were motion-controlling or "biomechanical" foot orthoses. There were no significant differences in the incidence of stress fractures, ankle sprains or foot problems. The authors concluded, therefore, that there was no justification for prescribing

Table 5.2 A methodological comparison of randomized trials evaluating shock-absorbing foot orthoses for the prevention of injury

First author, ref.	PEDro quality rating* (score out of 10)	Prospective power analysis/sample size calculation	Participants at beginning of trial (n)	Loss to follow-up (%)	Appropriate randomization†	Allocation concealment	Participants blinded to intervention	Assessors blinded to treatment	Intention-to-treat analysis
Andrish (1974)[104]	2	No	2777	0% (not reported)	Yes	No	No	No	No
Fauno (1993)[99]	2	No	91	25%	No (quasi-randomized, by date of birth)	No	No	No	No
Gardner (1988)[100]	6	No	3025	0% (not reported)	Yes	No	Yes	No	Yes (but not stated)
Schwellnus (1990)[101]	4	No	1511	8%	Yes	Not stated	Not stated (probably not)	No	No
Sherman (1996)[102]	3	No	1132	6% (but not clear)	Yes	No	Yes‡	No	No
Withnall (2006)[103]	7	Yes	1205	8%	Yes	Yes	No	No	Yes

* PEDro quality rating—a higher score reflects a better trial that is less prone to bias.

† Although most trials indicated that orthoses (or interventions) were "randomly allocated," it was often difficult to assess how investigators achieved this. Some trials allocated by platoon or unit. We elected to classify these as "randomized" rather than "quasi-randomized," because this would have had little influence on baseline characteristics.

‡ Blinding of the "no-intervention" group was contaminated after approximately one-third of the participants were recruited. Many recruits in this group learnt about the study aims and purchased the orthosis of their own accord.

semirigid biomechanical (customized) orthoses because of their high cost. Although slightly better from a quality point of view in comparison with the other Israeli military trials, this trial still had methodological issues that could have introduced bias.

Finally, the Danish military study[108] had a smaller sample size (n = 146) but was of better quality than the Israeli trials. This study evaluated a prefabricated orthosis ("Formthotic") against a no-intervention group. In an intention-to-treat analysis, it was found that there was a significant decrease in shin splints for the group using the orthosis. This study provides the best evidence to date that motion controlling foot orthoses can reduce injury. Although the intention-to-treat analysis provides superior evidence, the authors also conducted an actual-use analysis, finding that the orthosis, in addition to reducing shin splints, reduced back and lower extremity problems and number of off-duty days. It should be emphasized that an actual-use analysis can introduce bias, as the characteristics of the analyzed groups may be different from those at baseline when initially randomized. This may overestimate the effectiveness of the treatment.

Assessing all identified randomized trials that evaluated motion-controlling foot orthoses, there is evidence from large randomized trials that they reduce the incidence of lower limb stress fractures, particularly femoral stress fractures. The incidence of shin splints also appears to be reduced. Again, similar to the results from the shock-absorbing orthoses trials, the generalizability of these findings needs to be viewed in the light of the fact that the participants were military recruits undergoing basic training.

Table 5.3 summarizes each trial, including information on the participants, interventions, and primary outcomes. Incorporated into this table are specific details regarding injury rates for the primary outcomes of each trial.

Quality of randomized trials evaluating motion-controlling foot orthoses

The median PEDro score for the trials was 3.5 (range 2–6), indicating that the trials included in the systematic review were generally of poor quality. However, two trials[108,110] scored 6 points, although the trial by Esterman and Pilotto, finding no significant reduction in injury rates, was likely to be underpowered. Given that blinding in trials such as this is difficult (lack of blinding leads to a lower score on the PEDro rating scale), a score of 6 indicates a trial of moderately high quality. Table 5.4 presents a methodological comparison between the trials assessed in the review, including the PEDro score. There was little difference in quality between those trials that focused on shock-absorbing foot orthoses (median 3.5, range 2–7) versus those that focused on motion-controlling foot orthoses (median 3.5, range 2–6). No trials reported findings as recommended in the CONSORT guidelines.[111] Although the trials mostly used large sample sizes, better-quality trials are needed in order to reduce bias and establish a more precise estimate of the effect of motion-controlling foot orthoses in preventing injury.

Conclusions

The ability of foot orthoses to prevent injury has received relatively wide attention, particularly in basic training in the military, where high rates of injury have significant cost implications. Although no universally accepted terminology for foot orthoses currently exists, studies evaluating their effectiveness in injury prevention can be divided in two: those that have investigated shock-absorbing insoles or heel pads and those that have evaluated motion controlling "biomechanical" foot orthoses.

Table 5.3 Summary of randomized trials evaluating motion-controlling foot orthoses for the prevention of injury

First author (ref.)	Participants	Interventions	Intervention period	Primary results
Esterman (2005)[110]	Australian Air Force recruits with flat feet	(i) Prefabricated (AOL*) orthosis (ii) No intervention	8 weeks	No significant differences between groups in lower limb pain, incidence of training injury, general foot health, quality of life or physical health. However, the authors reported that those who actually wore orthoses all or most of the time (i.e., non-intention-to-treat) demonstrated a trend toward less injury
Finestone (1999)[107]	Israeli infantry recruits	(i) "Semirigid biomechanical" orthosis (ii) "Soft biomechanical" orthosis (iii) "Simple shoe insole"	14 weeks	The "biomechanical" orthoses groups experienced a significantly lower rate of stress fractures ($P = 0.013$). The incidences of stress fractures in the groups were: 15.7% for semirigid biomechanical orthoses, 10.7% for the soft biomechanical orthoses and 27% for the control group. When the "biomechanical orthoses" were combined, the incidence was 12.7% compared to 27% for the control group (odds ratio 0.421; 95% CI, 0.198 to 0.892)
Finestone (2004)[109]	Israeli infantry recruits	(i) "Customized soft" orthosis (ii) "Prefabricated soft" orthosis (iii) "Semirigid biomechanical" orthosis (iv) "Semirigid prefabricated" orthosis	14 weeks	No significant difference between orthoses in the incidence of stress fractures, ankle sprains or foot problems. Across all four groups the incidence of stress fractures was 9–10%; ankle sprains 8–11%; and foot problems 14–20%. "Soft" orthoses had higher comfort scores compared to the "semirigid" orthoses in those recruits who completed training in their assigned orthoses ($P = 0.001$). However, when those who discontinued use of their assigned orthoses were taken into account (i.e., intention-to-treat), comfort scores were significantly worse in the "prefabricated soft" orthosis ($P = 0.002$). The authors concluded that there was no justification for prescribing semirigid biomechanical orthoses because of their higher cost

Continued

Table 5.3 *(Continued)*

First author (ref.)	Participants	Interventions	Intervention period	Primary results
Larsen (2002)[108]	Danish military conscripts	(i) "Biomechanic shoe" (Formthotic[†]) orthosis (ii) No intervention	3 months	The intention-to-treat analysis found that the orthosis group experienced a significantly lower rate of shin splints ($P = 0.005$). In the orthosis group 6% experienced shin splints in comparison with 24% in the control group (relative risk 0.3; 95% CI, 0.1 to 0.7). Although the intention-to-treat analysis is superior, the authors also reported an "actual use" analysis, in which the orthosis group experienced significantly less back or lower extremity problems, shin splints and number of off-duty days ($P < 0.05$)
Milgrom (1985)[105]	Israeli military recruits	(i) Prefabricated semirigid "military stress" orthosis (ii) No intervention	14 weeks	The orthosis group experienced a significantly lower rate (10% vs. 18%) of femoral stress fractures ($P < 0.05$)
Simkin (1989)[106]	Israeli military recruits	(i) Prefabricated semirigid "military stress" orthosis (ii) No intervention *Combined analysis with high-arched and low-arched foot structure*	14 weeks	The orthosis group experienced a significantly lower rate of femoral stress fractures in recruits with high arches ($P = 0.003$) and metatarsal stress fractures in recruits with low arches ($P = 0.02$). The incidence of femoral stress fracture was 5.1% for the orthosis group compared to 15.5% in the no-intervention group. The incidence of metatarsal stress fractures was 0.0% for the orthosis group compared to 6.0% in the no-intervention group

CI, confidence intervals.

* AOL, Australian Orthotics Laboratory.

† Formthotic: manufactured by Foot Science International Ltd, Christchurch, New Zealand.

Table 5.4 A methodological comparison of randomized trials evaluating motion-controlling foot orthoses for the prevention of injury

First author, ref.	PEDro quality rating* (score out of 10)	Prospective power analysis/sample size calculation	Participants at beginning of trial (n)	Loss to follow-up (%)	Appropriate randomization†	Allocation concealment	Participants blinded to intervention	Assessors blinded to treatment	Intention-to-treat analysis
Esterman (2005)[110]	6	No (likely to be underpowered)	47	0% (but not clear)	Yes	Not stated	No	No	Yes
Finestone (1999)[107]	3	No	404	20%	Yes	Not stated	No	No	No
Finestone (2004)[109]	4	No	874	12%	Yes	Not stated	Yes	No	No
Larsen (2002)[108]	6	No	146	11%	Yes	Yes	No	No	Yes
Milgrom (1985)[105]	3	No	312	10%	Yes	Not stated	No	No	No
Simkin *et al.* (1989)[106]	2	No	295	10% (but not clear)	Yes	Not stated	No	No	No

* PEDro quality rating—a higher score reflects a better trial that is less prone to bias.

† Although most trials indicated that orthoses (or interventions) were "randomly allocated", it was often difficult to assess how investigators achieved this.

Twelve randomized or quasi-randomized trials were identified in this systematic review, of which six related to shock-absorbing orthoses and six to motion-controlling orthoses. The trials mostly used large sample sizes, but their quality ratings were generally low. The evidence suggests (i) that shock-absorbing insoles and heel pads do not prevent injury, and (ii) that motion-controlling foot orthoses decrease the incidence of stress fractures (particularly femoral stress fractures) and shin splints. Better-quality trials are required in order to confirm or refute the evidence to date. Future trials should attempt to evaluate commonly used orthoses; should use consistent outcome measures to assist with pooling results for meta-analysis; and the findings should be reported using the CONSORT guidelines[111] to ensure greater transparency.

Summary

- Foot orthoses are widely used to treat and prevent injury.
- Although a considerable amount is known about the biomechanical/functional effects of foot orthoses, less is known about their effectiveness for preventing injury.
- Most trials that have evaluated whether they prevent injury have used military recruits during basic training.
- Although most of these trials have included large sample sizes, they are generally methodologically poor.
- This limited evidence suggests that shock-absorbing insoles and heel pads do not prevent injury.
- Limited evidence suggests that motion-controlling (biomechanical) foot orthoses decrease the incidence of stress fractures (particularly femoral stress fractures) and shin splints.
- Better-quality randomized trials are required in order to provide more precise estimates of the effect of foot orthoses when used to prevent injury.

Key messages

- The term "foot orthoses" covers a wide range of different devices, and there is no universally accepted terminology to classify them.
- Foot orthoses work by causing changes in kinetics and muscle activity, and small changes in kinematics.
- Most studies evaluating foot orthoses for injury prevention have used military recruits during basic training, so the results may not be generalizable to civilians involved in sport.
- The evidence suggests that shock-absorbing insoles and heel pads do not prevent injury.
- The evidence suggests that motion-controlling (biomechanical) foot orthoses decrease the incidence of stress fractures (particularly femoral stress fractures) and shin splints.
- Further good-quality trials are needed in order to add to the evidence base.

Sample examination questions

Multiple-choice questions (answers on page 602)

1 Which of the following statements are true?

A The majority of randomized trials evaluating the effect of foot orthoses for the prevention of injury have utilized military recruits

B Universal terminology for orthotic therapy has generally been accepted across professional groups

   C Electromyographic studies evaluating the effects of foot orthoses have demonstrated no changes in the activity of any of the foot or leg muscles
   D Semirigid orthoses are indicated only for use with soft tissue injuries
   E Shock-absorbing insoles have never been found in randomized trials to be effective for sports injuries
2 Many of the randomized trials evaluating foot orthoses have methodological problems, including:
   A Lack of allocation concealment
   B Insufficient sample sizes
   C Participants not blinded to treatment
   D Both (a) and (c)
   E Both (b) and (c)
3 In kinematic studies, foot orthoses have consistently been shown to:
   A Increase shock reaching the lower back
   B Increase compression forces at the patellofemoral joint
   C Reduce frontal plane calcaneal movement by a few degrees
   D Reduce tibial rotation by up to 10°
   E Increase strain in the plantar fascia

Essay questions

1 Discuss the evidence for and against using foot orthoses to prevent injury.
2 Discuss how foot orthoses work from a biomechanical perspective.
3 Many of the randomized trials evaluating foot orthoses for the prevention of injury suffer from methodological weakness. With reasoning, outline the most rigorous foot orthosis trial that you can.

Case study 5.1

Adam, a 38-year-old teacher, wants to increase his running distance for fitness reasons. Previously, he has experienced shin splints when he increased his distance to more than 20 km per week. He generally does not have a well-thought-out plan for his running training. He is now seeking advice as to whether he should purchase foot orthoses to use when he runs. What advice would you give Adam?

Case study 5.2

Kathy, a 23-year-old track athlete, has a history of tibial stress fractures. She is now increasing her running training on the track and is again beginning to experience shin soreness. She is concerned about another stress fracture forming, thus interrupting her training. She already wears prefabricated foot orthoses, but now wants customized (biomechanical) foot orthoses that provide more motion control. How would you manage Kathy?

Case study 5.3

Tien, a 15-year-old, has secured a place in a football training camp over the summer. While he has played football with a local team for the past 8 years, he has heard that summer camp is demanding and that a lot of players get injured. He has also had a lot of problems with his feet and legs before, and he is concerned that he will become injured over the summer and not be able to complete the training. He consults you regarding whether foot orthoses would be a good option for him to prevent injury during his training camp. How should Tien be managed?

Summarizing the evidence

Type of orthosis	Results	Level of evidence*
Shock-absorbing	5 RCTs with military recruits and 1 quasi-randomized trial with soccer referees—evidence suggests that shock-absorbing insoles or heel pads do not prevent injury	A1
Motion-controlling	6 RCTs with military recruits—evidence suggests motion-controlling foot orthoses decrease the incidence of stress fractures (particularly femoral stress fractures) and shin splints. Cheaper prefabricated foot orthoses appear to be as effective as customized orthoses, but further good-quality trials are needed to confirm this	A1

* A1: evidence from large randomized controlled trials (RCTs) or systematic review (including meta-analysis).†
A2: evidence from at least one high-quality cohort.
A3: evidence from at least one moderate-sized RCT or systematic review.†
A4: evidence from at least one RCT.
B: evidence from at least one high-quality study of nonrandomized cohorts.
C: expert opinions.
† Arbitrarily, the following cut-off points have been used: large study size: ≥ 100 patients per intervention group; moderate study size ≥ 50 patients per intervention group.

References

1 Taunton JE, McKenzie DC, Clement DB. The role of biomechanics in the epidemiology of injuries. *Sports Med* 1988; **6**:107–120.
2 Kibler WB, Goldberg C, Chandler TJ. Functional biomechanical deficits in running athletes with plantar fasciitis. *Am J Sports Med* 1991; **19**:66–71.
3 Taunton JE, Ryan MB, Clement DB, McKenzie DC, Lloyd-Smith DR. Plantar fasciitis: a retrospective analysis of 267 cases. *Phys Ther Sport* 2001; **2**:1–9.
4 Viitasalo JT, Kvist M. Some biomechanical aspects of the foot and ankle in athletes with and without shin splints. *Am J Sports Med* 1983; **11**:125–130.
5 Sommer HM, Vallentyne SW. Effect of foot posture on the incidence of medial tibial stress syndrome. *Med Sci Sports Exerc* 1995; **27**:800–804.
6 Yates B, White S. The incidence and risk factors in the development of medial tibial stress syndrome among naval recruits. *Am J Sports Med* 2004; **32**:772–780.
7 Clement DB, Taunton JE, Smart GW, McNicol KL. A survey of overuse running injuries. *Phys Sports Med* 1981; **9**:47–58.
8 Tiberio D. The effect of excessive subtalar joint pronation on patellofemoral mechanics: a theoretical model. *J Orthop Sports Phys Ther* 1987; **9**:160–165.
9 Orchard JW, Fricker PA, Abud AT, Mason BR. Biomechanics of iliotibial band friction syndrome in runners. *Am J Sports Med* 1996; **24**:375–379.
10 Voloshin AS, Wosk J. An in vivo study of low back pain and shock absorption in the human locomotor system. *J Biomech* 1982; **15**:21–27.
11 Wosk J, Voloshin AS. Low back pain: conservative treatment with artificial shock absorbers. *Arch Phys Ther Rehabil* 1985; **66**:145–148.
12 Wen DY, Puffer JC, Schmalzried TP. Lower extremity alignment and risk of overuse injuries in runners. *Med Sci Sports Exerc* 1997; **29**:1291–1298.

13 Dananberg HJ, Guiliano M. Chronic low-back pain and its response to custom-made foot orthoses. *J Am Podiatr Med Assoc* 1999; **89**:109–117.

14 Giladi M, Milgrom C, Stein M, *et al.* The low-arch, a protective factor in stress fractures: a prospective study of 295 military recruits. *Orthop Rev* 1985; **14**:709–712.

15 Messier SP, Pittala KA. Etiologic factors associated with selected running injuries. *Med Sci Sports Exerc* 1988; **20**:501–505.

16 Cowan DN, Jones BH, Robinson JR. Foot morphologic characteristics and risk of exercise-related injury. *Arch Fam Med* 1993; **2**:773–777.

17 Nigg BM, Cole GK, Nachbauer W. Effects of arch height of the foot on angular motion of the lower extremities in running. *J Biomech* 1993; **26**:909–916.

18 Cowan DN, Jones BH, Frykman PN, *et al.* Lower limb morphology and risk of overuse injury among male infantry trainees. *Med Sci Sports Exerc* 1996; **28**:945–952.

19 Tomaro J, Burdett RG, Chadran AM. Subtalar joint motion and the relationship to lower extremity overuse injuries. *J Am Podiatr Med Assoc* 1996; **86**:427–432.

20 Kaufman KR, Brodine SK, Shaffer RA, Johnson CW, Cullison TR. The effect of foot structure and range of motion on musculoskeletal overuse injuries. *Am J Sports Med* 1999; **27**:585–593.

21 Hreljac A, Marshall RN, Hume PA. Evaluation of lower extremity overuse injury potential in runners. *Med Sci Sports Exerc* 2000; **32**:1635–1641.

22 Williams DSI, McClay-Davis I, Hamill J. Arch structure and injury patterns in runners. *Clin Biomech* 2001; **16**:341–347.

23 Hogan MT, Staheli LT. Arch height and lower limb pain: an adult civilian study. *Foot Ankle Int* 2002; **23**:43–47.

24 Michelson JD, Durant DM, McFarland E. The injury risk associated with pes planus in athletes. *Foot Ankle Int* 2002; **23**:629–633.

25 Lun V, Meeuwisse WH, Stergiou P, Stefanyshyn D. Relation between running injury and static lower limb alignment in recreational runners. *Br J Sports Med* 2004; **38**:576–580.

26 Wearing SC, Smeathers JE, Yates B, *et al.* Sagittal movement of the medial longitudinal arch is unchanged in plantar fasciitis. *Med Sci Sports Exerc* 2004; **36**:1761–1767.

27 Burns J, Keenan AM, Redmond AC. Foot type and overuse injuries in triathletes. *J Am Podiatr Med Assoc* 2005; **95**:235–241.

28 Esterman A, Pilotto L. Foot shape and its effect on functioning in Royal Australian Air Force recruits. Part 1: prospective cohort study. *Mil Med* 2005; **170**:623–628.

29 Willems TM, De Clercq D, Delbaere K, *et al.* A prospective study of gait related risk factors for exercise-related lower leg pain. *Gait Posture* 2006; **23**:91–98.

30 Brukner P, Bennell K. Stress fractures. *Crit Rev Phys Rehabil Med* 1997; **9**:151–190.

31 Bennell K, Matheson G, Meeuwisse W, Brukner P. Risk factors for stress fractures. *Sports Med* 1998; **28**:91–122.

32 Ilahi O, Kohl HW III. Lower extremity morphology and alignment and risk of overuse injury. *Clin J Sport Med* 1998; **8**:38–42.

33 Jones BH, Knapik JJ. Physical training and exercise-related injuries: surveillance, research and injury prevention in military populations. *Sports Med* 1999; **27**:111–125.

34 Ugalde V, Batt ME. Shin splints: current theories and treatment. *Crit Rev Phys Rehabil Med* 2001; **13**:217–253.

35 Thacker SB, Gilchrist J, Stroup DF, Kimsey CD. The prevention of shin splints in sports: a systematic review of literature. *Med Sci Sports Exerc* 2002; **34**:32–40.

36 Murphy DF, Connolly DAJ, Beynnon BD. Risk factors for lower extremity injury: a review of the literature. *Br J Sports Med* 2003; **37**:13–29.

37 Yeung EW, Yeung SS. A systematic review of interventions to prevent lower limb soft tissue running injuries. *Br J Sports Med* 2001; **35**:383–389.

38 Yeung EW, Yeung SS. Interventions for preventing lower limb soft-tissue injuries in runners. *Cochrane Database Syst Rev* 2001; (3):CD001256.

39 Rome K, Handoll HHG, Ashford R. Interventions for preventing and treating stress fractures and stress reactions of bone of the lower limbs in young adults. *Cochrane Database Syst Rev* 2005; (2):CD000450.

40 Landorf KB, Keenan AM. Efficacy of foot orthoses: what does the literature tell us? *J Am Podiatr Med Assoc* 2000; **90**:149–158.

41 Landorf K, Keenan AM, Rushworth RL. Foot orthosis prescription habits of Australian and New Zealand podiatric physicians. *J Am Podiatr Med Assoc* 2001; **91**:174–183.
42 Landorf KB, Keenan AM, Herbert RD. Effectiveness of different types of foot orthoses for the treatment of plantar fasciitis. *J Am Podiatr Med Assoc* 2004; **94**:542–549.
43 Petchell A, Keenan AM, Landorf K. National clinical guidelines for podiatric foot orthoses. *Australas J Podiatr Med* 1998; **32**:97–103.
44 Jones DC, James SL. Foot orthoses. In: Baxter DE, ed. *The Foot and Ankle in Sport.* St Louis: Mosby, 1995: 369–378.
45 Nawoczenski DA. Orthoses for the foot. In: Nawoczenski DA, Epler ME, eds. *Orthotics in Functional Rehabilitation of the Lower Limb.* Philadelphia: Saunders, 1997: 116–155.
46 Jones L. Prescription writing for functional and accommodative foot orthoses. In: Valmassy RL, ed. *Clinical Biomechanics of the Lower Extremities.* St Louis: Mosby, 1996: 296–306.
47 Philps JW. *The Functional Foot Orthosis.* Edinburgh: Churchill Livingstone, 1995.
48 Rome K. A study of the properties of materials used in podiatry. *J Am Podiatr Med Assoc* 1991; **81**:73–83.
49 Australian Podiatry Council. *Clinical Guidelines for Orthotic Therapy Provided by Podiatrists.* Collingwood, Victoria: Australasian Podiatry Council, 1998 (http://www.apodc.com.au/apodc/orthotic.pdf).
50 Razeghi M, Batt ME. Biomechanical analysis of the effect of orthotic shoe inserts. *Sports Med* 2000; **29**:425–438.
51 Heiderscheit B, Hamill J, Tiberio D. A biomechanical perspective: do foot orthoses work? *Br J Sports Med* 2001; **35**:4–5.
52 Payne C, Chuter V. The clash between theory and science on the kinematic effectiveness of foot orthoses. *Clin Podiatr Med Surg* 2001; **18**:705–713.
53 Nigg BM, Khan A, Fisher V, Stefanyshyn D. Effect of shoe insert construction on foot and leg movement. *Med Sci Sports Exerc* 1998; **30**:550–555.
54 Nigg BM, Nurse MA, Stefanyshyn DJ. Shoe inserts and orthotics for sport and physical activities. *Med Sci Sports Exerc* 1999; **31** (7 Suppl.):S421–428.
55 Altman R, Brandt K, Hochberg M, Moskowitz R. Design and conduct of clinical trials in patients with osteoarthritis. *Osteoarthritis Cartilage* 1996; **4**:217–243.
56 Bellamy N, Kirwan J, Boers M, *et al.* Recommendations for a core set of outcome measures for future phase III clinical trials in knee, hip, and hand osteoarthritis. Consensus development at OMERACT III. *J Rheumatol* 1997; **24**:799–802.
57 Van der Heijde D, Dougados M, Davis J, *et al.* Assessment in Ankylosing Spondylitis International Working Group/Spondylitis Association of American recommendations for conducting clinical trials in ankylosing spondylitis. *Arthritis Rheum* 2005; **52**:386–394.
58 Bates BT, Osternig LR, Mason B, James LS. Foot orthotic devices to modify selected aspects of lower extremity mechanics. *Am J Sports Med* 1979; **7**:338–342.
59 Rodgers MM, Leveau BF. Effectiveness of foot orthotic devices used to modify pronation in runners. *J Orthop Sports Phys Ther* 1982; **4**:86–90.
60 Smith LS, Clarke TE, Hamill CL, Santopietro F. The effects of soft and semi-rigid orthoses upon rearfoot movement in running. *J Am Podiatr Med Assoc* 1986; **76**:227–233.
61 Baitch SP, Blake RL, Fineagan PL, Senatore J. Biomechanical analysis of running with 25 degrees inverted orthotic devices. *J Am Podiatr Med Assoc* 1991; **81**:647–652.
62 Brown GP, Donatelli R, Catlin PA, Wooden MJ. The effect of two types of foot orthoses on rearfoot mechanics. *J Orthop Sports Phys Ther* 1995; **21**:258–267.
63 Cornwall MW, McPoil TG. Footwear and foot orthotic effectiveness research: a new approach. *J Orthop Sports Phys Ther* 1995; **21**:337–344.
64 Stell JF, Buckley JG. Controlling excessive pronation: a comparison of casted and non-casted orthoses. *Foot* 1998; **8**:210–214.
65 Genova JM, Gross MT. Effect of foot orthotics on calcaneal eversion during standing and treadmill walking for subjects with abnormal pronation. *J Orthop Sports Phys Ther* 2000; **30**:664–675.
66 Novick A, Kelley DL. Position and movement changes of the foot with orthotic intervention during the loading response of gait. *J Orthop Sports Phys Ther* 1990; **11**:301–312.
67 McCulloch MU, Brunt D, Vander Linden D. The effect of foot orthotics and gait velocity on lower limb kinematics and temporal events of stance. *J Orthop Sports Phys Ther* 1993; **17**:2–10.

68 Eng JJ, Pierrynowski MR. The effect of soft foot orthotics on three-dimensional lower-limb kinematics during walking and running. *Phys Ther* 1994; **74**:836–844.

69 Nawoczenski DA, Cook TM, Saltzman CL. The effect of foot orthotics on three-dimensional kinematics of the leg and rearfoot during running. *J Orthop Sports Phys Ther* 1995; **21**:317–327.

70 Kitaoka HB, Luo ZP, An KN. Analysis of longitudinal arch supports in stabilizing the arch of the foot. *Clin Orthop Rel Res* 1997; **341**:250–256.

71 Stacoff A, Reinschmidt C, Nigg BM, *et al.* Effects of foot orthoses on skeletal motion during running. *Clin Biomech* 2000; **15**:54–64.

72 Nester CJ, Hutchins S, Bowker P. Effect of foot orthoses on rearfoot complex kinematics during walking gait. *Foot Ankle Int* 2001; **22**:133–139.

73 Kitaoka HB, Luo ZP, Kura H, An KN. Effect of foot orthoses on 3-dimensional kinematics of flatfoot: a cadaveric study. *Arch Phys Med Rehabil* 2002; **83**:876–879.

74 Mundermann A, Nigg BM, Humble RN, Stefanyshyn DJ. Foot orthotics affect lower extremity kinematics and kinetics during running. *Clin Biomech* 2003; **18**:254–262.

75 Nester CJ, van der Linden ML, Bowker P. Effect of foot orthoses on the kinematics and kinetics of normal walking gait. *Gait Posture* 2003; **17**:180–187.

76 Williams DSI, McClay-Davis I, Baitch SP. Effect of inverted orthoses on lower-extremity mechanics in runners. *Med Sci Sports Exerc* 2003; **35**:2060–2068.

77 Branthwaite HR, Payton CJ, Chockalingam N. The effect of simple insoles on three-dimensional foot motion during normal walking. *Clin Biomech* 2004; **19**:972–977.

78 Ferber R, Davis IM, Williams I, Dorsey S. Effect of foot orthotics on rearfoot and tibia joint coupling patterns and variability. *J Biomech* 2005; **38**:477–483.

79 Nigg BM, Stergiou P, Cole G, *et al.* Effect of shoe inserts on kinematics, center of pressure, and leg joint moments during running. *Med Sci Sports Exerc* 2003; **35**:314–319.

80 Kogler GF, Solomonidis SE, Paul JP. Biomechanics of longitudinal arch support mechanisms in foot orthoses and their effect on plantar aponeurosis strain. *Clin Biomech* 1996; **11**:243–252.

81 Kogler GF, Veer FB, Solomonidis SE, Paul JP. The influence of medial and lateral placement of orthotic wedges on loading of the plantar aponeurosis. *J Bone Joint Surg Am* 1999; **81**:1403–1413.

82 Sarrafian SK. Functional characteristics of the foot and plantar aponeurosis under tibiotalar loading. *Foot Ankle* 1987; **8**:4–18.

83 Neptune RR, Wright IC, van den Bogert AJ. The influence of orthotic devices and vastus medialis strength and timing on patellofemoral loads during running. *Clin Biomech* 2000; **15**:611–618.

84 Bennett PJ, Miskewitch V, Duplock LR. Quantitative analysis of the effects of custom-molded orthoses. *J Am Podiatr Med Assoc* 1996; **86**:307–10.

85 Redmond A, Lumb PS, Landorf K. Effect of cast and noncast foot orthoses on plantar pressure and force during normal gait. *J Am Podiatr Med Assoc* 2000; **90**:441–449.

86 Reed L, Bennett PJ. Changes in foot function with the use of Root and Blake orthoses. *J Am Podiatr Med Assoc* 2001; **91**:184–193.

87 Voloshin AS. Shock absorption during running and walking. *J Am Podiatr Med Assoc* 1988; **78**:295–299.

88 Windle CM, Gregory SM, Dixon SJ. The shock attenuation characteristics of four different insoles when worn in a military boot during running and marching. *Gait Posture* 1999; **9**:31–37.

89 Folman Y, Wosk J, Shabat S, Gepstein R. Attenuation of spinal transients at heel strike using viscoelastic heel insoles: an in vivo study. *Prev Med* 2004; **39**:351–354.

90 Ekenman I, Milgrom C, Finestone A, *et al.* The role of biomechanical shoe orthoses in tibial stress fracture prevention. *Am J Sports Med* 2002; **30**:866–870.

91 Tomaro J, Burdett RG. The effects of foot orthotics on the EMG activity of selected leg muscles during gait. *J Orthop Sports Phys Ther* 1993; **18**:532–536.

92 Nawoczenski DA, Ludewig PM. Electromyographic effects of foot orthotics on selected lower extremity muscles during running. *Arch Phys Med Rehabil* 1999; **80**:540–544.

93 Bird AR, Bendrups AP, Payne CB. The effect of foot wedging on electromyographic activity in the erector spinae and gluteus medius muscles during walking. *Gait Posture* 2003; **18**:81–91.

94 Hertel J, Sloss BR, Earl JE. Effect of foot orthotics on quadriceps and gluteus medius electromyographic activity during selected exercises. *Arch Phys Med Rehabil* 2005; **86**:26–30.

95 Mundermann A, Wakeling JM, Nigg BM, Humble RN, Stefanyshyn DJ. Foot orthoses affect frequency components of muscle activity in the lower extremity. *Gait Posture* 2006; **23**:295–302.

96 Mundermann A, Nigg BM, Humble NR, Stefanyshyn DJ. Orthotic comfort is related to kinematics, kinetics, and EMG in recreational runners. *Med Sci Sports Exerc* 2003; **35**:1710–1719.

97 Sherrington C, Herbert RD, Maher CG, Moseley AM. PEDro: a database of randomized trials and systematic reviews in physiotherapy. *Manual Ther* 2000; **5**:223–226.

98 Maher CG, Sherrington C, Herbert RD, Moseley AM, Elkins M. Reliability of the PEDro scale for rating randomized controlled trials. *Phys Ther* 2003; **83**:713–721.

99 Fauno P, Kalund S, Andreasen I, Jorgensen U. Soreness in lower extremities and back is reduced by use of shock absorbing heel inserts. *Int J Sports Med* 1993; **14**:288–290.

100 Gardner LI Jr, Dziados JE, Jones BH, *et al.* Prevention of lower extremity stress fractures: a controlled trial of a shock absorbent insole. *Am J Pub Health* 1988; 78(12):1563–1567.

101 Schwellnus MP, Jordaan G, Noakes TD. Prevention of common overuse injuries by the use of shock absorbing insoles: a prospective study. *Am J Sports Med* 1990; **18**:636–641.

102 Sherman RA, Karstetter KW, May H, Woerman AL. Prevention of lower limb pain in soldiers using shock-absorbing orthotic inserts. *J Am Podiatr Med Assoc* 1996; **86**:117–122.

103 Withnall R, Eastaugh J, Freemantle N. Do shock absorbing insoles in recruits undertaking high levels of physical activity reduce lower limb injury? A randomized controlled trial. *J R Soc Med* 2006; **99**:32–37.

104 Andrish JT, Bergfield JA, Walheim J. A prospective study on the management of shin splints. *J Bone Joint Surg Am* 1974; **56**:1697–1700.

105 Milgrom C, Giladi M, Kashtan H, *et al.* A prospective study of the effect of a shock-absorbing orthotic device on the incidence of stress fractures in military recruits. *Foot Ankle* 1985; **6**:101–104.

106 Simkin A, Leichter I, Giladi M, Stein M, Milgrom C. Combined effect of foot arch structure and an orthotic device on stress fractures. *Foot Ankle* 1989; **10**:25–29.

107 Finestone A, Giladi M, Elad H, *et al.* Prevention of stress fractures using custom biomechanical shoe orthoses. *Clin Orthop Rel Res* 1999; **360**:182–190.

108 Larsen K, Weidich F, Leboeuf-Yde C. Can custom-made biomechanic shoe orthoses prevent problems in the back and lower extremities? A randomized, controlled intervention trial of 146 military conscripts. *J Manipulative Physiol Ther* 2002; **25**:326–331.

109 Finestone A, Novack V, Farfel A, *et al.* A prospective study of the effect of foot orthoses composition and fabrication on comfort and the incidence of overuse injuries. *Foot Ankle Int* 2004; **25**:462–466.

110 Esterman A, Pilotto L. Foot shape and its effect on functioning in Royal Australian Air Force recruits. Part 2: pilot, randomized, controlled trial of orthotics in recruits with flat feet. *Mil Med* 2005; **170**:629–633.

111 Moher D, Schulz KF, Altman DG, CONSORT Group. The CONSORT statement: revised recommendations for improving the quality of reports of parallel-group randomized trials. *JAMA* 2001; **285**:1987–1991 (http://www.consort-statement.org/).

CHAPTER 6
Who should retire after repeated concussions?

Paul McCrory

Introduction

The decision to medically retire an athlete following repeated concussive injuries remains a complex and controversial area. For the most part, there are no evidence-based recommendations to guide the practitioner, and the published "guidelines" have little or no scientific validity.[1] This view has been reinforced by the recent Vienna and Prague Consensus conferences, which emphasized the need to individualize clinical management and avoid reliance on anecdotal recommendations.[2,3]

In situations in which the athlete has suffered a life-threatening severe brain injury, has persistent neurological symptoms, or has a residual neurologic deficit, the decision to retire is straightforward. At the end of the day, good clinical judgment and common sense remain the mainstay of management.

In the broadest sense, an athlete who is closely monitored with stable neuropsychological testing throughout his or her career, and who has no ongoing postconcussive symptoms, has little to be concerned about even after sustaining a number of concussive injuries.

Methodology

The relevant literature was searched by using MEDLINE (1966–2005) and SportDiscus (1975–2005) searches, hand searches of journals and reference lists, and discussions with experts and sporting organizations worldwide. In addition, a keyword search was carried out on the author's EndNote database of over 6000 articles on sport-related concussive injuries. The keywords and Medical Subject Headings (MeSH) terms used in all searches included concussion, brain injury, head injury, head trauma, brain trauma, sports injuries, and brain commotion.

Background

There is no scientific evidence that sustaining several concussions over a sporting career will necessarily result in permanent damage. Part of the neuromythology surrounding concussion is the "three-strike rule"—namely, if an athlete has three concussions, then he or she should be ruled out of competition for an arbitrary period of time. On occasions, the athlete's sports participation is permanently curtailed. This anecdotal approach was originally attributed to Quigley in 1945 and subsequently adopted by Thorndike, who suggested that if any athlete suffered "three concussions, which involved loss of consciousness for any period of time, the athlete should be removed from contact sports for the remainder of the season."[4] This approach has no scientific validity, but it continues to be the anecdotal rationale underpinning most of the current return-to-play guidelines.

The unstated fear behind this approach is that an athlete suffering repeated concussions would suffer a gradual cognitive decline similar to the so-called "punch-drunk" syndrome or chronic traumatic encephalopathy seen in boxers.[5–7] On the basis of published evidence, this fear is largely unfounded, and recent developments suggest that the risk of traumatic encephalopathy in this setting may be largely genetically based, rather than being simply a manifestation of repeated concussive injury.[8]

The issue becomes further confused when well-known athletes suffering from recurrent head trauma appear in the media or lay press. In some cases, the injuries suffered by such athletes are more severe than the typical sports-related concussive injuries, but no distinction is made in the mind of the public. In such injuries, long-term symptoms are not wholly unexpected. In other cases, the so-called "postconcussive" symptoms experienced are mostly headache. This symptom is nonspecific and can be the result of a variety of causes other than concussion.[9]

Adding to the difficulty is the fact that when professional athletes suffer repeated concussions, they are not banned from sport, as may be the advice given to less elite athletes. Whilst it is true that many professional athletes are monitored more closely than other sporting participants, nevertheless the variation in management advice between elite and recreational athletes is often seen as hypocritical, resulting in a situation in which recreational athletes prematurely return to sport after concussion and as a result suffer ongoing problems.

Much of the concern in relation to the management of repeated concussive injury relates to the absence of consensus in the grading of the severity of concussion injury and the lack of scientifically valid return-to-play guidelines. Until these central issues are resolved, it is unlikely that a clear answer to the problem of retirement due to chronic symptoms will emerge.

Definition of concussion

Until recently, there was no universal agreement on the standard definition or nature of sports concussion.[2,3] Historically, the term has been used to refer to a transient disturbance of neurological function caused by the "shaking" of the brain that accompanies low-velocity brain injuries.[10]

The definition published by the Committee on Head Injury Nomenclature of the Congress of Neurological Surgeons was widely used to define concussive injuries until 2001. This definition states that concussion is "a clinical syndrome characterized by the immediate and transient post-traumatic impairment of neural function, such as alteration of consciousness, disturbance of vision or equilibrium, etc., due to brainstem involvement."[11] Over time, however, it had become clear that this definition really did not adequately define the clinical entity, and as a result an expert consensus conference on sports concussion was held in Vienna in 2001, with a second meeting being held in Prague in 2004.[2,3] The Prague meeting redefined sports concussion as follows:

• Sports concussion is defined as a complex pathophysiological process affecting the brain, induced by traumatic biomechanical forces. Several common features that incorporate clinical, pathological, and biomechanical injury constructs that may be used in defining the nature of a concussive head injury include:

— Concussion may be caused either by a direct blow to the head, face, neck, or elsewhere on the body, with an "impulsive" force transmitted to the head.

— Concussion typically results in the rapid onset of short-lived impairment of neurological function, which resolves spontaneously.

— Concussion may result in neuropathological changes, but the acute clinical symptoms largely reflect a functional disturbance rather than structural injury.

— Concussion results in a graded set of clinical syndromes that may or may not involve loss of consciousness. Resolution of the clinical and cognitive symptoms typically follows a sequential course.

— Concussion is typically associated with grossly normal structural neuroimaging studies.

One of the key developments of the Prague Conference was the understanding that concussion may be categorized for management purposes as either *simple* or *complex*.[3] These categories were defined as follows:

• In *simple concussion*, an athlete suffers an injury that progressively resolves without complications over 5–10 days. In such cases, apart from limiting playing or training whilst the patient is symptomatic, no further intervention is required during the period of recovery, and the athlete typically resumes sport without further problem. This form of concussion represents the most common form of this injury, and can be easily managed by primary-care physicians or by certified athletic trainers working under medical supervision.

• *Complex concussion* encompasses cases in which athletes suffer persistent symptoms, specific sequelae, or prolonged cognitive impairment following the injury. This group may also include athletes who suffer multiple concussions over time, or in whom repeated concussions occur with progressively less impact force. In this group, there may be additional management considerations beyond simple return-to-play advice, and it is envisaged that such athletes would be managed in a multidisciplinary manner by physicians with specific expertise in the management of concussive injury, such as a sports neurologist or neurosurgeon.

Whilst this distinction remains a speculative and as yet scientifically unvalidated approach, it reflects the clinical situation, in which the majority of athletes recover quickly after concussion and return to sport without further difficulty; however, there is a small percentage of athletes who suffer persistent symptoms or persistent disability due to the injury. It was therefore recommended that the latter group should be managed more aggressively by concussion experts.

These proposed concussion subtypes may represent differences in individual clinical phenomenology (confusion, memory problems, loss of consciousness), anatomical localization (e.g., cerebral vs. brainstem), biomechanical impact (rotational vs. linear force), genetic phenotype (ApoE4-positive vs. ApoE4-negative), neuropathological change (structural injury vs. no structural injury), or an as yet undefined difference. These factors may operate independently or interact with each other. It is clear that the variations in clinical outcome with the same impact force require a more sophisticated approach to the understanding of this phenomenon than the approaches currently available.

Published guidelines for return to sport after concussion

The published guidelines recommending termination of all contact sport following three concussions during the course of an athletic season need to be considered by clinicians extremely carefully. In the absence of documented objective evidence of brain injury or clinical evidence of persistent postconcussive symptoms, there is no scientific support for this generalization, and the abandonment of such anecdotal approaches has been recommended by two international expert consensus conferences.[2,3]

It is also worth considering that athletes excluded from competition on such a basis may consider a medicolegal appeal that would be impossible to defend in a court of law.

The principal anecdotal guidelines are outlined below for discussion purposes, and—as mentioned above—these are not supported by published scientific evidence and should be considered management "opinions" at best.

The main guidelines on returning to sport after repeated concussive injury are those published by Cantu[12–14] and the Colorado Medical Society.[15] The American Academy of Neurology guidelines[16] are derivative from the latter (Tables 6.1, 6.2).

It can be seen that there are many superficial similarities between the two scale systems. Although the criteria for the severity of injury differ, the mandatory requirement is that two grade 3 injuries or three injuries of any grade should result in termination of the athlete's season. As a Cantu Grade 2 is equivalent to a Colorado Grade 3, it is evident that the scales give differing recommendations for the same injury.

The physiology of concussion

At present, there is no existing animal model or other experimental model that accurately reflects a sporting concussive injury. It has been noted in experimental models of more severe injury that a complex cascade of biochemical, metabolic, and membrane gene-expression changes occur.[17] Whether similar metabolic changes occur in sports concussion, however, is still currently speculative.[18]

Table 6.1 Return-to-sport guidelines: Cantu system (adapted from Cantu 1986[12])

Severity grade	1st concussion	2nd concussion	3rd concussion
Grade 1 No LOC, PTA < 30 min	RTP after 1 week if asymptomatic	RTP in 2 weeks if asymptomatic for at least 1 week	Terminate season. RTP next season if asymptomatic
Grade 2 LOC < 5 min, PTA > 30 min	RTP after 1 week if asymptomatic for at least 1 week	Minimum of 1 month off sport. RTP if asymptomatic for at least 1 week. Consider terminating season	Terminate season. RTP next season if asymptomatic
Grade 3 LOC > 5 min, PTA > 24 h	Minimum of 1 month off sport. RTP if asymptomatic for at least 1 week	Terminate season. RTP next season if asymptomatic	

LOC, loss of consciousness; PTA, post-traumatic amnesia; RTP, return to play.

Table 6.2 Return-to-sport guidelines: the Colorado guidelines (adapted from Kelly *et al.* 1991[15])

Severity grade	1st concussion	2nd concussion	3rd concussion
Grade 1 No LOC, confusion, no amnesia	RTP after 20 min if asymptomatic	RTP if asymptomatic for at least 1 week	Terminate season. RTP next season if asymptomatic
Grade 2 No LOC, confusion, amnesia	RTP after a minimum of 1 week with no symptoms	RTP after a minimum of 1 month with no symptoms for at least 1 week	Terminate season. RTP next season if asymptomatic
Grade 3 LOC	RTP after a minimum of 2 weeks with no symptoms.	Terminate season. RTP next season if asymptomatic	Terminate season. RTP next season if asymptomatic

LOC, loss of consciousness; RTP, return to play.

Although experimental research has enhanced our understanding of the physiological changes to the brain following severe head trauma, there is still uncertainty as to what is happening to the human brain following minor concussive injuries, and in particular in sport-related concussion.

The neuropathology of concussion

The nature of transient loss of cerebral function following a blow to the head has excited much speculation over the centuries regarding whether microscopic neuropathological changes occur, or whether other cerebral pathophysiological processes manifest the clinical symptoms of concussion. At this stage, these important issues remain unresolved. In general terms, although it is well accepted that minor neuropathological changes may occur following concussive brain injury, the clinical symptoms are due to functional disturbance, presumably at the cell membrane level, rather than due to any underlying structural injury. This is supported by experimental evidence demonstrating that mechanical stress can produce a sudden neuronal depolarization followed by a period of nerve-cell transmission failure, in the absence of structural injury.[19]

Human models of concussion are necessarily limited, given that virtually all patients recover without detectable permanent sequelae. In the handful of case reports of individuals dying of other causes after brain injury, scattered neuronal cell death can be demonstrated. However, the findings are generally insufficient to explain the degree of clinical dysfunction, suggesting that the clinical symptoms become manifest through additional functional cell impairment.[20]

The neuropsychology of concussion

The application of neuropsychological testing in concussion has been shown to be of value, and it continues to contribute significant information to the evaluation of concussion.[21–24] It has been demonstrated that cognitive recovery may precede or follow clinical symptom resolution, suggesting that the assessment of cognitive function should be an important component in any return-to-play protocol.

It must be emphasized, however, that neuropsychological assessment should not be the sole basis of a return-to-play decision, but should rather be seen as an aid to clinical decision-making. Although neuropsychological screening may be carried out or interpreted by nonclinicians, the final return-to-play decision should remain a medical one.

It is only in the past few decades that there has been interest in studying the neuropsychological consequences of concussion, and particularly of those injuries seen in sport.[21,25–28] While there is now acceptance that there is an organic basis to the problems associated with concussion, controversy remains regarding the nature of the cognitive deficits, as well as the speed and extent of recovery from them.

A range of neuropsychological deficits has been reported after mild concussive injury. The major areas of deficit include:

- Disturbances of new learning and memory.[29–38]
- Planning and the ability to switch mental "set."[29,35,38,39]
- Reduced attention and reduced speed of information processing.[29,34,35,40–47]

There have also been isolated reports suggesting that impairments may be evident in tasks involving visuospatial constructional ability, language, and sensorimotor function.[29,35]

Recovery of neuropsychological function after concussion in sport

In general terms, there appears to be clear evidence of neuropsychological deficits during the first week after mild concussive injury, but variable findings tend to develop after that period.[1,27,28]

There are a number of methodological issues that may underlie the inconsistencies reported between studies—including test selection, different mechanisms of injury, and varying severities of injury. In the various studies, wide variations in the severity of injury have been included under the rubric of concussion, ranging from no loss of consciousness (LOC) through to LOC for 1 week or more, and mild stunning of the sensorium for a few seconds through to patients with post-traumatic amnesia lasting for 4 months.

In addition, concussive injuries may result from a number of different causes, such as motor-vehicle accidents, sporting injuries, falls, and domestic trauma. This heterogeneity may account for some of the differences between studies, since the magnitude of the head acceleration forces may differ considerably depending on the cause.

With regard to the various neuropsychological test instruments used in the different studies, a number of methodological issues arise, including test selection, lack of sensitivity of various tests, practice effects, inadequate identification of premorbid characteristics influencing test results, inconsistent time points for testing, lack of suitable control groups, small sample sizes, and compensation issues.[48–50]

The postconcussion syndrome

The issue of the constellation of physical and cognitive symptoms that have been labeled as "postconcussive syndrome" (PCS) is as controversial today as when it was first proposed in the 19th century.[51]

PCS may include symptoms such as headache, vertigo, dizziness, nausea, memory complaints, blurred vision, noise and light sensitivity, difficulty in concentrating, fatigue, depression, sleep disturbance, loss of appetite, anxiety, incoordination, and hallucinations.[36,52–55]

Table 6.3 Postconcussion symptoms scale (adapted from Lovell and Collins 1998[26])

	Rating						
	None	Moderate			Severe		
Headache	0	1	2	3	4	5	6
Nausea	0	1	2	3	4	5	6
Vomiting	0	1	2	3	4	5	6
Drowsines	0	1	2	3	4	5	6
Numbness or tingling	0	1	2	3	4	5	6
Dizziness	0	1	2	3	4	5	6
Balance problems	0	1	2	3	4	5	6
Sleeping more than usual	0	1	2	3	4	5	6
Sensitivity to light	0	1	2	3	4	5	6
Sensitivity to noise	0	1	2	3	4	5	6
Feeling slowed down	0	1	2	3	4	5	6
Feeling like "in a fog"	0	1	2	3	4	5	6
Difficulty concentrating	0	1	2	3	4	5	6
Difficulty remembering	0	1	2	3	4	5	6
Trouble falling asleep	0	1	2	3	4	5	6
More emotional than usual	0	1	2	3	4	5	6
Irritability	0	1	2	3	4	5	6
Sadness	0	1	2	3	4	5	6
Nervousness	0	1	2	3	4	5	6
Other	0	1	2	3	4	5	6

Various PCS scales are widely used in sports-concussion assessment (Table 6.3). Although debate continues regarding the relative contribution of organic versus psychological factors in the genesis of PCS, the critical factor that clinicians need to be aware of is that these symptoms are nonspecific in nature and are not confined to concussion. It has been demonstrated that up to 60% of uninjured individuals may report PCS symptoms, and similarly high scores have been demonstrated in various medical and psychological illnesses.[56]

The risk of repeat concussions in sport

It has become a widely held belief that after sustaining a concussive injury, one is then more prone to future concussive injury. The evidence for this is limited at best. In a widely quoted study by Gerberich *et al.*, which involved self-reported questionnaires concerning a history of head injury in high-school gridiron footballers, an increased risk of subsequent concussions was reported in players with a history of concussion.[57] This study is flawed by significant methodological problems. Not least is the fact that the authors included cases of catastrophic brain injury. Furthermore, the reliability of a self-diagnosis of concussion is questionable, given that only 33% of those with loss of consciousness and 12% of those with other symptoms were medically assessed. The majority of the diagnoses of "concussion" were made by the coach, other team-mates, or by the players themselves.

It would seem obvious that in any collision sport, the risk of concussion is directly proportional to the amount of time for which a participant plays the sport. In other words, the more games played, the greater the chance of an injury occurring. The likelihood of a repeat injury may therefore simply reflect the level of exposure to injury risk.

In addition, Gerberich acknowledges that the observed increased likelihood of concussion could also be explained by a player's style of play. The player's risk of injury may be increased by using dangerous game strategies and illegal tackling techniques. Similar criticisms can also be leveled at another retrospective study, in which it was reported that once an initial concussion was sustained, the probability of incurring a second concussion greatly increases.[58]

Does repeat concussion result in cumulative damage?

Apart from boxing-related head injuries, the most widely cited studies on the cumulative effects of concussion have included patients with injuries sustained in motor-vehicle accidents that were severe enough to warrant hospital treatment. Generally, concussive injuries suffered in collision sports such as football involve lesser degrees of acceleration–deceleration forces than those experienced in motor-vehicle accidents.[34,43,59–61]

The limitations of retrospective studies in concussion, such as the widely cited motor-vehicle accident studies by Gronwall and Wrightson, include diagnostic uncertainty, relying on both self-reported injury recall, as well as the lack of medically validated injury diagnosis. For example, some head injuries in the cited studies were retrospectively assessed up to 8 years after their occurrence.[34,43,59–61]

It is widely acknowledged that boxing carries a high risk of neurological injury. However, boxing should not be considered as a model for cumulative head injury seen in other sports, since it presents unique risks to the athlete in terms of the frequency of repetitive head trauma.[7,62] Recently, specific genetic abnormalities have been reported as the major risk factor for the development of traumatic encephalopathy.[63,64]

In another series of retrospective studies involving retired Scandinavian soccer players, cognitive deficits were noted.[65–68] In these studies, significant methodological problems flaw the results. The problems include a lack of pre-injury data, selection bias, lack of observer blinding, and inadequate control subjects. The authors conclude that the deficits noted in the former soccer players were explained by repetitive trauma such as that caused by heading the ball. However, the pattern of deficits is equally consistent with alcohol-related brain impairment, a confounding variable that was not controlled for. To date, there has been no replication of these findings by other independent groups.[69–74]

In other retrospective studies involving a wide range of traumatic brain injury, loss of consciousness was associated with evidence of permanent change in fine motor control.[75] The significance of this symptom in isolation from other cognitive domains is questionable. Other studies have suggested that this may be an effect of environmental factors rather than being due to the effect of injury.[76] More recent prospective studies have failed to find any adverse prognostic features in individuals who suffered a loss of consciousness with concussion in comparison with those who did not.[35,77,78]

In animal studies of experimental concussion, animals have been repeatedly concussed 20–35 times during the same day and within a 2-hour period. Despite these unusually high numbers of injuries, no residual or cumulative effect was demonstrated.[79]

Is there a genetic susceptibility to brain injury in sports?

Recent research in boxers has suggested that chronic traumatic encephalopathy, or the so-called "punch-drunk syndrome," in boxers may be associated with a particular genetic predisposition. The apolipoprotein E epsilon-4 (ApoE) gene, a susceptibility gene for late-onset familial and sporadic Alzheimer's disease, may be associated with an increased risk of chronic traumatic encephalopathy in boxers.[63,80,81] In a nonboxing population, ApoE polymorphism was significantly associated with death and adverse outcomes following acute traumatic brain injury, as seen in a neurosurgical unit.[82] In a recent prospective study, ApoE genotypes were tested for their ability to predict days of unconsciousness and functional outcome after 6 months.[83] A strong association was demonstrated between the ApoE allele and a poor clinical outcome.

Furthermore, ApoE-deficient (knockout) mice have been shown to have memory deficits, neurochemical changes, and diminished recovery from closed head injury in comparison with controls.[84] It is suggested that ApoE plays an important role in both neuronal repair[85] and antioxidant activity,[84] resulting in ApoE knockout mice exhibiting an impaired ability to recover from closed head injury. Although we are only in the early stages of understanding these issues, an interaction between genetic and environmental factors may be critical in the development of postconcussive phenomena or concussive sequelae.

Return to sport after life-threatening head injury

The return to sport following a severe or potentially life-threatening brain injury is controversial, and there are few guidelines for the clinician to follow. There are some situations in which the athlete might place himself or herself at an unacceptably high risk of sustaining further injury and hence should be counseled against participating in collision sports. In such situations, common sense should prevail.

Although sports physicians should keep an open mind when assessing neurological recovery from severe brain injuries, it is nevertheless recommended that at least 12 months should pass before such a decision is contemplated.

Thoughtful deliberation and analysis of all the available medical evidence should occur when such decisions are being taken. It is also recommended that the advice of a neurologist or neurosurgeon experienced in the management of sports head injuries should be sought. This is an important point, because a number of individuals who suffer a moderate to severe traumatic brain injury may be left with a lack of insight and impaired judgment over and above their other neurological injuries. This in turn may make such an individual unreliable in gauging recovery. The use of neuropsychological assessment, as well as information from family and friends, may assist the clinician in his or her deliberation. The assessment of cognitive performance and/or clinical symptoms when the patient is fatigued is often useful.

Returning to collision sport is relatively contraindicated in almost any situation in which a surgical craniotomy is performed. In such situations, the subarachnoid space is traumatized, thus setting up scarring of the pia–arachnoid of the brain to the dura, with both loss of the normal cushioning effect of the cerebrospinal fluid and vascular adhesions that may subsequently bleed if torn during head impact. Even if neurologic recovery is complete, a craniotomy for anything other than an extradural hematoma effectively precludes a return to collision sport (Table 6.4).

When there is an epidural hematoma without brain injury or other condition in which surgery is not required, a return to sport may be contemplated in selected patients, as per the discussion above, after a minimum of 12 months—assuming that neurologic recovery is complete.

Table 6.4 Conditions contraindicating a return to contact sport (adapted from Cantu 1998[13])

- Persistent postconcussional or post-injury symptoms
- Permanent neurological sequelae—hemiplegia, visual deficit, dementia or cognitive impairment
- Hydrocephalus with or without shunting
- Spontaneous subarachnoid hemorrhage from any cause
- Symptomatic neurologic or pain-producing abnormalities around the foramen magnum
- Craniotomy for evacuation of intracerebral or subdural hematoma

Conclusions

Who should retire after recurrent concussive injury? It appears self-evident that athletes with persistent cognitive or neurological symptoms should be withheld from collision sports until such time as their symptoms fully resolve. Following more severe brain injury, persistent neurological deficit, or symptoms, a history of craniotomy or intracranial surgery and spontaneous subarachnoid hemorrhage should preclude further participation.

In a setting of repeated uncomplicated concussive injury with full recovery after each episode, the situation is more difficult. Although published guidelines exist, they do not have any scientific validity and should be seen only as anecdotal suggestions for the clinician. It is the author's practice in professional sport to perform neuropsychological testing routinely on all athletes before the season and serially after concussive injury. More importantly, no athlete returns to sport until he is symptom-free and has returned to his or her neuropsychological baseline performance.

The central issue relates to the nature of the injury. Whilst there is no doubt that severe concussion with persistent symptoms occurs (the "complex concussion" in the Prague guidelines), athletes with typical concussive injuries recover quickly and return to sport without difficulty. In this setting, the scientific evidence that sustaining a number of concussions over the course of a season, or over a career, causes chronic neurological dysfunction is nonexistent. Clinicians should be aware of the neuromythology surrounding this issue and should manage their patients using evidence-based guidelines—or, if guidelines are lacking, then using good common sense.

Key messages

- No evidence-based guidelines exist in relation to the return to sport after repeated concussions.
- Persistent neurological symptoms or cognitive impairment should preclude a return to sport, but once these have resolved, there is no evidence that an athlete is at risk of long-term sequelae from concussive injury.

Sample examination questions

Multiple-choice questions (answers on p. 602)

1 In athletes, the presence of an ApoE4 phenotype (4/4) has been demonstrated to:

A Confer a worse prognosis following traumatic brain injury

B Be associated with chronic traumatic encephalopathy ("punch-drunk syndrome") in boxers

C Be associated with a poorer neuropsychological performance on postinjury assessment
D Be associated with persistent postconcussive symptoms

2 Contraindications to a return to sport after severe traumatic brain injury include:
A Persistent postconcussional or post-injury symptoms
B Permanent neurological sequelae—hemiplegia, visual deficit, dementia, or cognitive impairment
C Craniotomy for evacuation of intracerebral or subdural hematoma
D Spontaneous subarachnoid hemorrhage from any cause
E Symptomatic abnormalities about the foramen magnum

3 The *common* neuropsychological deficits noted following acute concussive injury in sport include:
A Disturbances of new learning and memory
B Reduced ability to switch mental "set"
C Reduced speed of information processing
D Impairment in visuospatial constructional ability
E Language disturbance

4 Are these statements regarding simple concussion from the Prague guidelines true or false?
A In simple concussion, concussion symptoms lasts less than 7–10 days
B Simple concussion can be managed by primary-care physicians
C Simple concussion includes cases in which a concussive convulsion has occurred
D Approximately 95% of concussions fall into this category

Essay questions

1 A 30-year-old professional American football quarterback suffers the 10th concussion of his career during a midseason game. His team is due to make the play-offs, and his presence is crucial for the success of the team. How would you monitor his recovery and determine whether he should return to play?

2 A rugby player suffers a severe head injury in a fight at a club one evening. As a result, he is taken to the regional neurosurgical center, where a craniotomy for intracranial pressure control is required. He recovers, and the skull defect is closed successfully. He comes to see you for advice on return to play. His Glasgow Coma Scale (GCS) score is 15 and he has no focal neurological signs. How do you approach the problem, and what advice would you give?

3 A 24-year-old professional soccer player sees you because of persistent headaches from "heading" the ball. He is worried that repeated heading may cause him to be "punch-drunk" in later life. What advice do you give him? Are there any tests that could assist you in advising him?

Case study 6.1

An Australian-Rules footballer gives a history of sustaining one or two episodes of concussion with loss of consciousness, as well as having four or five minor (no LOC) concussions per season. Despite this, he has no ongoing symptoms or neurological signs. Following each episode, he is withheld from sport until he is symptom-free and his neuropsychological tests have returned to baseline. During his 8-year professional career, no decrement in cognitive performance has been noted. His neuroimaging studies are normal, and his

ApoE4 status is negative (i.e., heterozygous allele). Despite the history of multiple concussions, there is no evidence of ongoing or permanent neurological injury.

Summarizing the evidence

Guidelines	Results	Level of evidence*
Definition	2 published papers	C
Injury severity guidelines	42 published guidelines	C
Return-to-play recommendations	5 published guidelines	C/D
Vienna/Prague guidelines	2 published papers	C
Retirement	3 published guidelines	C
Injury prevention		
Helmets	2 RCTs—helmets not protective	A1
Mouthguards	1 RCT—mouthguards not protective	A3
Rule change	2 published papers	C

* A1: evidence from large randomized controlled trials (RCTs) or systematic review (including meta-analysis).†
A2: evidence from at least one high-quality cohort.
A3: evidence from at least one moderate-sized RCT or systematic review.†
A4: evidence from at least one RCT.
B: evidence from at least one high-quality study of nonrandomized cohorts.
C: expert opinions.
D: case series.
† Arbitrarily, the following cut-off points have been used: large study size: ≥ 100 patients per intervention group; moderate study size ≥ 50 patients per intervention group.

References

1 Johnston K, McCrory P, Mohtadi N, Meeuwisse W. Evidence-based review of sport-related concussion: clinical science. *Clin J Sport Med* 2001; **11**:150–160.
2 Aubry M, Cantu R, Dvorak J, *et al.* Summary and agreement statement of the First International Conference on Concussion in Sport, Vienna 2001. Recommendations for the improvement of safety and health of athletes who may suffer concussive injuries. *Br J Sports Med* 2002; **36**:6–10.
3 McCrory P, Johnston K, Meeuwisse W, *et al.* Summary and agreement statement of the 2nd International Conference on Concussion in Sport, Prague 2004. *Br J Sports Med* 2005; **39**:196–204.
4 Thorndike A. Serious recurrent injuries of athletes. *New Engl J Med* 1952; **246**:554–556.
5 Martland HS. Punch drunk. *JAMA* 1928; **19**:1103–1107.
6 Jordan BD. Boxer's encephalopathy. Neurology 1990; **40**:727.
7 Jordan BD. Chronic traumatic brain injury associated with boxing. *Semin Neurol* 2000; **20**:179–185.
8 Jordan BD, Relkin NR, Ravdin LD, *et al.* Apolipoprotein E epsilon4 associated with chronic traumatic brain injury in boxing. *JAMA* 1997; **278**:136–140.
9 McCrory P. Headaches and exercise. *Sports Med* 2000; **30**:221–229.
10 McCrory P, Berkovic S. Concussion: Historical development of clinical and pathophysiological concepts and misconceptions. *Neurology* 2001; **57**:2283–2289.
11 Congress of Neurological Surgeons Committee on Head Injury Nomenclature. Glossary of head injury. *Clin Neurosurg* 1966; **12**:386–394.
12 Cantu RC. Guidelines for return to contact sports after cerebral concussion. *Phys Sportsmed* 1986; **14**:75–83.
13 Cantu RC. Return to play guidelines after a head injury. *Clin Sports Med* 1998; **17**:45–60.
14 Cantu RC. When to allow athletes to return to play after injury? *J Neurol Orthrop Surg* 1992; **13**:30–34.

15 Kelly JP, Nichols JS, Filley CM, *et al.* Concussion in sports: guidelines for the prevention of catastrophic outcome. *JAMA* 1991; **266**:2867–2869.

16 Kelly J, Rosenberg J. Diagnosis and management of concussion in sports. *Neurology* 1997; **48**:575–580.

17 Hovda D, Lee S, Smith M, *et al.* The neurochemical and metabolic cascade following brain injury: moving from animal models to man. *J Neurotrauma* 1995; **12**:903–906.

18 McIntosh TK, Smith DH, Meaney DF, *et al.* Neuropathological sequelae of traumatic brain injury: relationship to neurochemical and biomechanical mechanisms. *Lab Invest* 1996; **74**:315–342.

19 Shetter A, Demakis J. The pathophysiology of concussion: a review. *Adv Neurol* 1979; **22**:5–14.

20 McCrory P, Johnston K, Meeuwisse W, Mohtadi N. Evidence based review of sport related concussion: basic science. *Clin J Sport Med* 2001; **11**:160–166.

21 Grindel S, Lovell M, Collins M. The assessment of sport-related concussion: the evidence behind neuropsychological testing and management. *Clin J Sport Med* 2001; **11**:134–144.

22 Lovell MR, Collins MW, Iverson GL, *et al.* Recovery from mild concussion in high school athletes. *J Neurosurg* 2003; **98**:296–301.

23 Collie A, Maruff P. Computerised neuropsychological testing. *Br J Sports Med* 2003; **37**:2–3.

24 Collins MW, Grindel SH, Lovell MR, *et al.* Relationship between concussion and neuropsychological performance in college football players. *JAMA* 1999; **282**: 964–970.

25 Grindel SH. Neuropsychological testing: problems with research, validity and clinical use. [Paper presented at American College of Sports Medicine, 30 May 2002.]

26 Lovell MR, Collins MW. Neuropsychological assessment of the college football player. *J Head Trauma Rehabil* 1998; **13**:9–26.

27 Binder L. A review of mild head trauma. Part 2: clinical implications. *J Clin Exp Neuropsychol* 1997; **19**:432–457.

28 Binder LM, Rohling ML, Larrabee J. A review of mild head trauma. Part 1: meta-analytic review of neuropsychological studies. *J Clin Exp Neuropsychol* 1997; **19**:421–431.

29 Barth JT, Macciocchi SN, Giordani B, *et al.* Neuropsychological sequelae of minor head injury. *Neurosurgery* 1983; **13**:529–533.

30 Dikmen S, McLean A, Temkin N. Neuropsychological and psychological consequences of minor head injury. *J Neurol Neurosurg Psychiatry* 1986; **49**:1227–1232.

31 Ewing R, McCarthy D, Gronwall D, Wrightsom P. Persisting effects of minor head injury observable during hypoxic stress. *J Clin Neuropsychol* 1980; **2**:147–155.

32 Gronwall D, Sampson H. *The Psychological Effects of Concussion.* Auckland: Oxford Univeristy Press, 1974.

33 Gronwall D, Wrightson P. Memory and information processing capacity after closed head injury. *J Neurol Neurosurg Psychiatry* 1981; **44**:889–895.

34 Gronwall D, Wrightson P. Delayed recovery of intellectual function following minor head injury. *Lancet* 1974; **ii**:605–609.

35 Leninger B, Gramling S, Farrell A, Kreutzer J, Peck E. Neuropsychological deficits in symptomatic minor head injury patients after concussion and mild concussion. *J Neurol Neurosurg Psychiatry* 1990; **53**:293–296.

36 Levin HS, Grafman J, Eisenberg HM, editors. *Neurobehavioral Recovery from Head Injury.* Oxford: Oxford University Press, 1987.

37 Yarnell P, Lynch S. Retrograde amnesia immediately after concussion. *Lancet* 1970; **i**:863–864.

38 Yarnell P, Rossie G. Minor whiplash head injury with major debilitation. *Brain Inj* 1988; **2**:255–258.

39 Rimel RW, Giordani B, Barth JT. Moderate head injury: completing the clinical spectrum of brain trauma. *Neurosurgery* 1982; **11**:344–351.

40 Barth JT, Alves WM, Ryan TV, *et al.* Mild head injury in sports: neuropsychological sequelae and recovery of function. In: Levin HS, Eisenberg HM, Benton AL, eds. *Mild Head Injury.* New York: Oxford University Press, 1989:257–275.

41 Dencker SJ, Löfving B. A psychometric study of identical twins discordant for closed head injury. *Acta Psychiatr Neurol Scand Suppl* 1958;**122**:1–50.

42 Gentilini M, Nichelli P, Schoenhuber R, *et al.* Neuropsychological evaluation of mild head injury. *J Neurol Neurosurg Psychiatry* 1985; **48**:137–140.

43 Gronwall D, Wrightson P. Cumulative effects of concussion. *Lancet* 1975; **ii**:995–997.

44 Levin H, Eisenberg HM, Benton AL, editors. *Mild Head Injury.* Oxford: Oxford University Press, 1989.

45 Maddocks D, Dicker G. An objective measure of recovery from concussion in Australian rules footballers. *Sport Health* 1989; **7** (Suppl):6–7.

46 Maddocks D, Saling M. Neuropsychological deficits following concussion. *Brain Inj* 1996; **10**:99–103.
47 Ruesch J, Moore B. Measurement of intellectual functions in the acute stages of head injury. *Arch Neurol Psychiatr* 1943; **50**:165–170.
48 Luria AR. *Higher Cortical Functions in Man*, 2nd ed. New York: Basic Books, 1962.
49 Walsh KMA. *Understanding Brain Damage: a Primer of Neuropsychological Evaluation.* 2nd ed. Edinburgh: Churchill Livingstone, 1991.
50 Walsh KW. *Neuropsychology: a Clinical Approach*, 2nd ed. Edinburgh: Churchill Livingstone, 1987.
51 Courville CB. *Commotio Cerebri: Cerebral Concussion and the Postconcussion Syndrome and their Medical and Legal Aspects.* Los Angeles: San Lucas Press, 1953.
52 Binder LM. Persisting symptoms after mild head injury: a review of the postconcussive syndrome. *J Clin Exp Neuropsychol* 1986; **8**:323–346.
53 Rutherford W. Postconcussional symptoms: relationship to acute neurological indices, individual differences and circumstances of injury. In: Levin H, Eisenberg H, Benton A, eds. *Mild Head Injury.* New York: Oxford University Press, 1989:217–228.
54 Rutherford WH, Merret JD, McDonald JR. Sequelae of concussion caused by minor head injuries. *Lancet* 1977; **i**:1–4.
55 Rutherford WH, Merret JD, McDonald JR. Symptoms at one year following concussion from minor head injuries. *Injury* 1979; **10**:225–230.
56 Alexander M. Mild traumatic brain injury. *Neurology* 1995; **45**:1253–1260.
57 Gerberich SG, Priest JD, Boen JR, Straub CP, Maxwell RE. Concussion incidences and severity in secondary school varsity football players. *Am J Public Health* 1983; **73**:1370–1375.
58 Albright J. Head and neck injuries in college football: an eight year analysis. *Am J Sports Med* 1985; **13**:147–152.
59 Gronwall D. Cumulative and persisting effects of concussion on attention and cognition. In: Levin H, Eisenberg H, Benton A, eds. *Mild Head Injury.* New York: Oxford University Press, 1989:153–162.
60 Gronwall D. Minor head injury. *Neuropsychology* 1991; **5**:253–265.
61 Gronwall D, Wrightson P. Duration of post-traumatic amnesia after mild head injury. *J Clin Neurophysiol* 1980; **2**:51–60.
62 Jordan B. Medical and safety reforms in boxing. *J Natl Med Assoc* 1988; **80**:407–412.
63 Jordan BD, Relkin NR, Ravdin LD, *et al.* Apolipoprotein E epsilon4 associated with chronic traumatic brain injury in boxing. *JAMA* 1997; **278**:136–140.
64 Jordan BD, Kanik AB, Horwich MS, *et al.* Apolipoprotein E epsilon 4 and fatal cerebral amyloid angiopathy associated with dementia pugilistica. *Ann Neurol* 1995; **38**:698–699.
65 Tysvaer A, Lochen E. Soccer injuries to the brain: a neuropsychological study of former soccer players. *Am J Sports Med* 1991; **19**:56–60.
66 Tysvaer A, Storli O. Association football injuries to the brain: a preliminary report. *Br J Sports Med* 1981; **15**:163–166.
67 Tysvaer A, Storli O, Bachen N. Soccer injuries to the brain: a neurologic and encephalographic study of former players. *Acta Neurol Scand* 1989; **80**:151–156.
68 Tysvaer AT. Head and neck injuries in soccer the impact of minor head trauma. *Sports Med* 1992; **14**:200–213.
69 Boden B, Kirkendall D, Garrett W. Concussion incidence in elite college soccer players. *Am J Sports Med* 1998; **26**:238–241.
70 Barnes BC, Cooper L, Kirkendall DT, *et al.* Concussion history in elite male and female soccer players. *Am J Sports Med* 1998; **26**:433–438.
71 Green GA, Jordan SE. Are brain injuries a significant problem in soccer? *Clin Sports Med* 1998; **17**:795–809, viii.
72 Kirkendall DT, Garrett WE Jr. Heading in soccer: integral skill or grounds for cognitive dysfunction? *J Athl Train* 2001; **36**:328–333.
73 McCrory PR. Brain injury and heading in soccer. *BMJ* 2003; **327**:351–352.
74 Dvorak J, Junge A, McCrory P. Head injuries in soccer. *Br J Sports Med* 2005; **39** (Suppl 1):1–3.
75 Murelius O, Haglund Y. Does Swedish amateur boxing lead to chronic brain damage? Part 4: a retrospective neuropsychological study. *Acta Neurol Scand* 1991; **83**: 9–13.
76 Bijur P, Haslum M, Golding J. Cognitive outcomes of multiple mild head injuries in children. *J Dev Behav Pediatr* 1996; **17**:143–148.

77 McCrory P, Ariens M, Berkovic S. The nature and duration of acute concussive symptoms in Australian football. *Clin J Sports Med* 2000; **10**:235–239.
78 Lovell M, Iverson G, Collins M, McKeag D, Maroon J. Does loss of consciousness predict neuropsychological decrements after concussion? *Clin J Sports Med* 1999; **9**:193–199.
79 Parkinson D. Concussion is completely reversible: an hypothesis. *Med Hypoth* 1992; **37**:37–39.
80 Saunders A, Strittmatter W, Schmechel D. Association of apolipoprotein E allele epsilon 4 with late onset familial and sporadic Alzheiner's disease. *Neurology* 1993; **43**:1467–1472.
81 Corder E, Saunders A, Strittmatter W. Gene dose of apolipoprotein E type 4 allele and the risk of late onset Alzheimer's disease in families. *Science* 1993; **261**:921–923.
82 Teasdale G, Nicol J, Murray G. Association of apolipoprotein E polymorphism with outcome after head injury. *Lancet* 1997; **350**:1069–1071.
83 Friedman G, Froom P, Sazbon L, *et al.* Apoliporotein E epsilon 4 genotype predicts a poor outcome in survivors of traumatic brain injury. *Neurology* 1999; **52**:244–248.
84 Lomnitski L, Kohen R, Chen Y, *et al.* Reduced levels of antioxidants in brains of apolipoprotein E–deficient mice following closed head injury. *Pharmacol Biochem Behav* 1997; **56**:669–673.
85 Chen Y, Lomnitski L, Michaelson D, Shohami E. Motor and cognitive deficits in apolipoprotein E-deficient mice after closed head injury. *Neuroscience* 1997; **80**:1255–1262.

CHAPTER 7

What recommendations should be made concerning exercising with a fever and/or acute infection?

Christopher A. McGrew

Introduction

Clinicians who care for athletes routinely face difficult decisions concerning what recommendations to make with respect to fever and/or acute infectious diseases. Many of these athletes are reluctant to alter their training schedules, or face external pressures from coaches and team members. For the most part, these common conditions have limited importance with regard to long-term health, but for exercising athletes there are several immediate concerns, ranging from potential impairment of performance to possible catastrophic outcomes, including sudden death.

Upper respiratory infections, infectious mononucleosis, myocarditis, and hepatitis are some of the specific entities that will be addressed in this chapter. Emphasis will be placed on what recommendations to make to athletes concerning exercising while acutely ill and when to return to practice and/or competition.

Methods

A computerized bibliographic database (MEDLINE) was searched from the earliest date until October 2005 using a combination of the following keywords along with Medical Subject Headings (MeSH). Relevant articles were also retrieved from reference lists of pertinent review articles. The keywords used were:

- Exercise
- Physical training
- Fever, infection
- Metabolism
- Acute-phase response
- Viral myocarditis
- Infectious mononucleosis
- Hepatitis
- Gastroenteritis
- Respiratory infections
- Sudden death

Fever and/or acute infectious disease: general considerations

Fever is defined as an oral or rectal temperature of 38 °C or higher. It is associated with acute and chronic infections, muscle trauma, neoplasms, heat-related illness, prolonged exercise, and some medications. It is difficult to differentiate some of the effects of fever from the effects of the condition causing it; however, in general, it is recognized that fever impairs muscle strength,[1] mental cognition, and pulmonary perfusion. Additionally, fever increases insensible fluid loss and increases overall systemic metabolism.[2] These factors, alone or in combination, are potentially detrimental to athletic performance. Additionally, decreased muscle strength could be seen as a potential factor for increased risk of injury, although there are no studies to support this theory.

The aerobic exercise capacity, as determined from submaximal exercise studies, is decreased during fever. On the other hand, the observed maximal oxygen uptake has been shown to be unaffected during short-lasting, experimental pyrogen-induced fever, as well as in conditions of thermal dehydration. There do not appear to be any studies in which maximal oxygen uptake has been measured during ongoing infection and fever (most likely for ethical reasons). Therefore, the rate and magnitude of decrease of the maximal aerobic power during ongoing febrile infections in humans is unknown.[3]

The innate immune system includes anatomic and physiologic barriers (e.g., skin, mucous membranes, temperature, pH), specialized cells (natural killer cells and phagocytes, including neutrophils, monocytes, and macrophages), and inflammatory barriers. When the innate immune system fails to effectively combat an invading pathogen, the body mounts an acquired immune response. The acquired immune system includes special cells called B- and T-lymphocytes, which are capable of secreting specialized chemicals such as antibodies and cytokines to regulate the immune response. T-lymphocytes can also engage in direct cell-on-cell warfare. Acute episodes of vigorous activity have the following effects on the immune system (lasting 3–72 hours): stress hormone-induced neutrophilia and lymphopenia, decreases in natural killer (NK) cell cytotoxic activity, decreases in the delayed-type hypersensitivity response, increases in plasma cytokines, decreases in nasal and salivary IgA concentrations and nasal neutrophil function, and blunted major histocompatibility complex (MHC) II expression and antigen presentation in macrophages. Chronic exercise effects have been more difficult to document. Attempts thus far to compare resting immune function in athletes and nonathletes have failed to provide evidence that athletic endeavor is linked to many specific changes in the immune system, even though epidemiologic studies have shown decreased upper respiratory infections in some groups of regular exercisers in comparison with nonexercisers (the "J-curve" theory). Of all immune measures, only NK cell activity has emerged as a somewhat consistent indicator differentiating the immune systems of athletes and nonathletes. NK cell activity has been reported be higher in athletes in comparison with nonathletes in several studies.[4,5]

Acute infections are associated with a variety of immune-system responses that are triggered by cytokines and are correlated to fever, malaise and anorexia, along with other signs and symptoms. Acute viral illness (most commonly presenting as an upper respiratory infection) can potentially hinder exercise capabilities by affecting multiple body systems, including cardiac, pulmonary, muscular, fluid status, and temperature regulation.[6–9] Heir *et al.* examined the influence of respiratory tract infection and bronchial responsiveness in elite cross-country skiers in comparison with inactive controls. The study found that on a methacholine challenge test, there was a transient increase in bronchial responsiveness in athletes who undertook physical exercise during the symptomatic period of their respiratory tract infections, but not in the inactive controls. The authors concluded that exercise during the symptomatic period of respiratory illness many intensify or generate mechanisms leading to enhanced bronchial responsiveness, or asthma.[10] Conversely, Weidner *et al.* found no significant change in pulmonary function tests, $\dot{V}O_2max$, or duration of cold symptoms during repeated submaximal exercise testing in symptomatic young adults infected with a strain of rhinovirus compared with controls.[11,12] One distinguishing factor may be the presence or absence of a fever. In the study by Weidner *et al.*, the participants did not have a fever.[13]

Muscle protein catabolism, tissue wasting, and negative nitrogen balance may all occur with acute infection. Skeletal muscle is the source of most of the amino acids that are released, but the heart muscle also contributes.[14] A large percentage of these amino acids are taken up by the liver and used for new synthesis of acute-phase proteins, participating in the fight against the infection, along with energy production through gluconeogenesis. After the resolution of fever and other signs of active infection, the muscle protein is gradually replenished. The time required for replacement is related to the amount of the accumulated nitrogen loss. In general, the time for replenishment may be four to five times the length of the acute illness. This is also known as the muscle convalescence period.[15] It should be recalled that exercise during an acute viral illness may also be a risk factor for rhabdomyolysis.[16,17]

Recommendations

Given all of the above potential detrimental effects, it has seemed logical to some authors that exercising/training for sport during an acute infection would impart fewer fitness gains than when working out while healthy;[18] however, there are no studies to confirm this supposition. Although unstudied, an intuitive "neck check" approach is attractive.

- If the athlete has symptoms limited to locations above the neck, such as nasal congestion, runny nose, and sore throat, then he or she can probably continue to exercise at a "reduced" level of intensity. The athlete may try a 10-min test period of exercise. If the athlete feels better or symptoms do not worsen, then he or she may work out at a submaximal intensity with a gradual to full intensity over a few days.
- If the athlete has symptoms below the neck, such as chest congestion, hacking cough, vomiting, diarrhea, or lymphadenopathy, or if the athlete has systemic symptoms such as fever or myalgias, then abstinence from exercise (particularly intense exercise) is recommended.[18]

Additionally, a distinction should be made between the various types of sport, as well as types of training for a sport, and competition. For example, training for American football may involve 2–4-h sessions of continuous activity at a high workload. On the other hand, playing in a football game may only require 10–15 min of actual true playing time for a "first-string" player, given the limited time actually spent playing compared to the amount of time in the huddle or off the field while the offense and defense are switched. Soccer, in contrast to American football, does not have these built-in "down times"—it is a continuous game, and a player may not stop moving for 45 min. Also, the time of day or year may make a difference with regard to heat injury susceptibility when the athlete has a fever. Many sports have specific skills practice that may not be totally incompatible with having a fever—for example, baseball batting practice or putting in golf. Obviously, most athletes with fever and systemic symptoms from acute infections will probably not feel like doing most training activities. However, understanding the specific activity is essential for making recommendations to athletes who are inclined to do some training, regarding what they should and should not do during an acute illness.

Myocarditis

Myocarditis is an inflammatory condition of the myocardial wall. Most acute infectious myocarditis is caused by viruses, with *coxsackievirus B* being the most common agent, although numerous other viruses have been implicated. Myocarditis is a rare cause of reported sudden death in athletes in whom a diagnosis is made.[19] Coxsackie infections usually occur in epidemics, most often in summer and early autumn. Animal data suggest that exercise during experimentally induced septicemic viral infections may increase the risk for the development of acute myocarditis.[20,21] No such studies have been performed in humans. As usual, the degree to which animal data can be transferred to humans is unclear.

Systemic signs and symptoms at the time of a typical viral infection can include fever, headache, myalgia, respiratory/gastrointestinal distress, exanthema and lymphadenopathy. Less frequent, but still possible, are splenomegaly, meningitis, and hepatitis. Typically, symptoms are mild and nonspecific. There are no clinical predictors for which patients with these symptoms are likely to develop myocarditis. Additionally, no clear historical or physical findings can confirm the early diagnosis of myocardial involvement, although retrospectively, myalgia may be a significant clue. A typical clinical picture of myocarditis consists of fatigue, chest pain, dyspnea and palpitations, yet except for palpitations, one might have the same symptoms with the acute phase of a general, systemic viral illness. In myocarditis, however, these manifestations rarely occur at the height of the infectious illness, but instead become evident during the convalescent phase if the acute systemic viral illness subsides. Not all patients who are diagnosed with viral myocarditis recall having a viral illness. Additionally, the majority of myocarditis episodes are subclinical (i.e., the patient is asymptomatic). In the face of all these nonspecific scenarios, one can certainly appreciate the incredible difficulty in management decisions for the clinician, especially one dealing with teams/institutions where numerous athletes present in a short period of time with nonspecific acute infections. There is no research that can offer clear evidence-based guidelines about exercise during viral infections. For the time being, the clinician's advice to athletes with an acute, nonspecific infection will be dependent on common sense and collaboration with the athlete.

Return to activity with myocarditis

At present, there are no clinically accurate predictors of sudden death risk in patients with myocarditis.[22] The 26th Bethesda Conference made the following recommendations for the athlete with regard to return to activity.[23]

- The athlete should be withdrawn from all competitive sports and undergo a prudent convalescent period of about 6 months after the onset of clinical manifestations ("prudent" is not defined). Before the athlete may return to competitive athletic training, an evaluation of cardiac status should be undertaken, including assessment of ventricular function at rest and with exercise.

• An athlete should be allowed to return to competition when ventricular function and also cardiac dimensions have returned to normal, and clinically relevant arrhythmias are absent on ambulatory monitoring.
• Sufficient clinical data are not available to justify a strong recommendation to perform endomyocardial biopsy as a precondition for return to athletic competition after the proposed 6-month period of deconditioning. The role of invasive electrophysiologic testing in assessing the eligibility of athletes with myocarditis remains to be defined.

Viral hepatitis

Acute infections with viral hepatitis are predominantly caused by one of five viruses (hepatitis A, B, C, D, and E viruses). Viral hepatitis can present as a broad spectrum of clinical syndromes, ranging from asymptomatic disease to fulminant and fatal acute infections. (Chronic infections are not discussed in this chapter.) Common presenting symptoms of acute hepatitis include anorexia, nausea, myalgia, and fatigue. These symptoms typically develop 7–14 days before the onset of jaundice. Other common symptoms include headache, arthralgias and, in children, diarrhea. These symptoms are virtually the same in all forms of acute hepatitis, no matter what the cause. Symptoms will persist for a few weeks.

Hepatitis A is usually self-limited and does not result in a chronic carrier state or cirrhosis. Progression to chronic hepatitis is primarily a feature of HBV, HCV and HDV. One of the most feared complications of acute hepatitis is fulminant hepatitis, which has a very high mortality rate. It is primarily seen in adults infected with hepatitis B, D, and E, and only rarely occurs in A and C.

Acute liver insult with viral hepatitis predisposes to hypoglycemia and altered lipid metabolism, compromising energy availability during exercise. Additionally, liver dysfunction results in altered protein synthesis and metabolism, which cause a variety of physiologic disturbances, including coagulopathy and hormonal imbalances.

It has been shown that exercise can significantly alter the hemodynamics of the liver in normal subjects. One study demonstrated decreases in the portal vein cross-sectional area and in portal venous velocity and flow. The decreases were transient and completely reversible. No problems were noted in normal subjects, but theoretically these changes could cause complications in subjects with liver dysfunction associated with acute hepatitis.[24] Given the above parameters—including fatigue symptoms, altered physiology, and the potential for fulminant complications—the traditional recommendation for the athlete with acute hepatitis to comply with a regimen of rest and refraining from exertion seems intuitively reasonable.[25,26] However, experience from several studies challenges this conservative approach.[27–30]

Recommendations

When should the athlete return to training and competition after acute viral hepatitis? Available data suggest that exercise can be safely permitted as tolerated in the previously healthy individual with an episode of acute viral hepatitis. This training should be guided by the clinical condition of the patient. This approach is consistent with position statements/guidelines from the Medical Society for Sports Medicine, the American Orthopedic Society for Sports Medicine, and the American Academy of Pediatrics.[31,32] There are no data on exercise training at an extreme exertion or competitive level. It seems prudent to avoid extreme exercise and competition until liver tests are normal and hepatomegaly (if present) resolves.

Infectious mononucleosis

Infectious mononucleosis (glandular fever) is caused by the Epstein–Barr virus (EBV) and is characterized by a variety of symptoms and signs which occur to varying degrees and are summarized in Table 7.1.[33]

A diagnosis of infectious mononucleosis is made by taking into account the clinical picture, along with a peripheral blood examination and serology for EBV. Once the diagnosis is made, return-to-play considerations are related to the general condition of the athlete and concerns about complications. The spectrum of patient responses to this illness ranges widely; many have significant malaise, weakness, and inability to perform hard physical exertion—obviously their activities will be self-restricted. In contrast, around 50% of EBV infections occur prior to adolescence, and are generally mild and do not prompt a visit to a health-care provider.[34]

Welch and Wheeler examined the aerobic capacity after the subject had contracted infectious mononucleosis.[35] The authors studied 16 cadets at a United States military academy who were recovering from infectious mononucleosis. The aerobic capacity was determined at the point at which the subjects became afebrile ($\dot{V}o_2max$ approximately 60 mL/kg/min for males and 50 mL/kg/min for females). Nine of the cadets were allowed to do a low-intensity exercise programme for 2 weeks, while the other seven remained inactive. After 2 weeks, all were allowed to exercise ad lib. Aerobic capacity was remeasured at this time, and no differences between the groups were found. Additionally, no detrimental effects were found in either group. The authors concluded that athletes recovering from infectious mononucleosis could begin a noncontact exercise program as soon as they become afebrile.[35] Another study suggested that athletes recover faster than other students, although the finding was not considered significant because of the small sample size.[36]

The more difficult questions about the management of athletes with infectious mononucleosis involve issues concerning potential complications, which are relatively infrequent. Although EBV affects most organ systems, complications occur in less than 5% of cases.[37] Since some of these complications have potentially catastrophic outcomes, they should be considered when decisions for each athlete are made. However, it is important to note that, with the possible exception of splenic rupture, there is no evidence that

Table 7.1 Clinical manifestations of infectious mononucleosis

- Moderate to severe sore throat (frequent)
- Tonsillar enlargement (frequent)
- Exudative tonsillopharyngitis (frequent)
- Lymphadenopathy (frequent)
- Moderate fever (frequent)
- Palpable splenomegaly (frequent)
- Headache (frequent)
- Soft-palate petechiae (less frequent)
- Periorbital edema (infrequent)
- Myalgia (infrequent)
- Jaundice (unusual)

significant complications are either triggered by exercise or more common in those who exercise as tolerated during and after the symptomatic phase of the disease.[33]

Splenic involvement with infectious mononucleosis and potential rupture is the primary concern for most clinicians. Splenic rupture occurs in 0.1–0.5% of cases, and almost all cases of splenic rupture occur within the first 3 weeks from the onset of illness (not from when it was diagnosed).[38] Another point to consider is that splenic rupture usually occurs with routine daily activities such as lifting, bending, and straining at defecation, not in association with direct trauma and/or sports activity. A retrospective survey on splenic rupture in college athletes published in 1978 by Frelinger reported that 36% of 22 cases were associated with infectious mononucleosis. This vague preliminary report gave limited details as to the circumstances surrounding the splenic injury, other than that "17 of the 22 cases occurred while a student athlete was participating in football."[39] Since 1978, no specific cases of splenic rupture associated with infectious mononucleosis and sports participation have been reported.

Although for many it seems intuitive that they go hand in hand, it is not clear what the connection between splenomegaly and splenic rupture is. Splenic rupture is most likely to occur during the first few weeks of illness when the organ is undergoing profuse lymphocyte infiltration. This stretches and weakens the capsule and supporting architecture of the spleen (putting it into in a "fragile state"), and this may be more of a causative factor than the enlargement itself.[40]

It is important to note that physical examination techniques for evaluating spleen size have poor sensitivity and specificity.[41] Although sonography and computed tomography (CT) are very accurate in determining spleen size, recent data describing spleen size in a population of 631 collegiate athletes demonstrated considerable variability in the normal spleen size. Because of this wide variability, a single diagnostic imaging measurement is considered unreliable for providing conclusive proof of splenic enlargement.[42] At present, there is no specific evidence to either definitively support or refute the use of ultrasound or CT assessment of spleen size in the routine management of mononucleosis in athletes. Diagnostic imaging such as ultrasound or CT is indicated in cases of suspected splenic injury.

Corticosteroids may be helpful with some complications (for example, airway obstruction, hemolytic anemia, thrombocytopenia, and neurologic disorders), but is not thought to reduce splenic size or prevent splenic rupture.[43]

Recommendations

There does not appear to be any indication that exercise, carried on within self-set limits, adversely affects the outcome of infectious mononucleosis. Restrictions based on systemic symptoms would be similar to those previously mentioned for general viral infections/fever, again with the caveat that there is very little evidence published to support or contradict those recommendations. Fatigue will probably be the most common problem for the athlete, with a wide spectrum of presentations. Some athletes will be completely unable to train, while others may have only a mild drop-off in performance. Obviously, management must be tailored to each case.

Since splenic rupture usually occurs in the first 3 weeks, a prudent course to follow could be to use relative restrictions during that time—these could include avoidance of resistance training or other forms of training that require a strong Valsalva maneuver, as well as contact activities. The athlete can then progress through conditioning over the next week if he or she feels well, with a return to full activity in the following week. The athlete (and guardians if the athlete is under-age) should be informed that splenic rupture has very rarely been reported up to 8 weeks after the onset of illness, and they should take this into account in their return-to-play considerations.

The American Academy of Pediatricians has recommended that "a patient with an acutely enlarged spleen should avoid all sports because of risk of rupture. A patient with a chronically enlarged spleen needs individual assessment before playing collision, contact or limited contact sports."[44] (In the document making this recommendation, no specific references or data are presented that specifically support this recommendation.) If a clinician chooses to use spleen enlargement as a criterion for the return to play, there are no clear-cut guidelines on whether to use palpation or an imaging technique (for example, ultrasound) as the point of reference. Again, given the poor results of studies of physical examinations and the lack of evidence for the use of imaging, neither is recommended by this author at present.

If the patient is well past 3–4 weeks into the illness (past the point of virtually all splenic ruptures) and still has splenic enlargement, it is not known whether extra protection (for example, a "flak jacket") would be useful in such cases. (This possibility is raised because one of the main clinical points about assessing the size of the spleen on physical examination is determining whether or not it is palpable beyond the rib cage. As stated before, the spleen may be enlarged even when it cannot be palpated. Determining the return to play has been based by some authors on a criterion of not being able to palpate the spleen. This would imply that the ribcage can adequately protect an enlarged spleen from trauma if the enlarged spleen is still "under cover." There is no specific evidence for or against this assumption.)[45]

In the case of an athlete with splenic rupture (whether or not it is associated with mononucleosis, and whether or not it is associated with sports-related or other trauma), urgent splenectomy has been suggested as a pragmatic approach.[33] Nonsurgical treatment of splenic rupture[46] would delay a return to athletic activity for up to 6 months, in contrast to the usual return to full activity 4–8 weeks after splenectomy. This is certainly an issue that must be carefully discussed with the athlete, and careful patient selection is essential.

Conclusions

Unfortunately, there is not a large amount of published evidence-based medicine data for making return-to-play decisions for most infections/febrile illnesses. Countless episodes of these illnesses occur on a daily basis in people performing at a high level of physical exertion while at home, at their jobs, or while involved in recreational and competitive sports. Despite this huge population exposure, catastrophic complications are rare and could even be described as random. However, when such catastrophes occur, they cause a great deal of distress for all those involved, along with a ripple effect of medicolegal implications. For now, we depend on limited research and anecdotal data, along with a large dose of what appears to be "cautious common sense" in making recommendations to patients on when to return to play. For the foreseeable future, this is as good as it gets.

Key messages

- Fever and acute infection can have effects on exercise and performance that theoretically could be detrimental, yet conclusive studies are lacking.

• The athlete with myocarditis should be withdrawn from competition for at least 6 months.
• Splenic rupture associated with infectious mononucleosis and sports participation is an extremely rare event.
• Assessment of spleen size in most (if not all) cases of infectious mononucleosis is unwarranted for decisions on returning to play.

Sample examination questions

Multiple-choice questions (answers on p. 602)

1 Acute infection may be associated with
   A Muscle protein catabolism
   B Negative nitrogen balance
   C Tissue wasting
   D Rhabdomyolysis
   E All of the above
2 Athletes with a diagnosis of viral myocarditis should:
   A Be withdrawn from all competitive sports for at least 2 months
   B Always have ventricular function evaluated before return to competitive athletic training
   C Always have an endomyocardial biopsy
   D Always have electrophysiologic testing done prior to return to activity
   E Not have ambulatory monitoring for arrhythmias
3 The most common return-to-play issue for the athlete with infectious mononucleosis concerns:
   A Airway obstruction
   B Epididymitis
   C Sore throat
   D Spleen enlargement
   E Encephalitis

Essay questions

1 How should return to play for an athlete with infectious mononucleosis be managed?
2 What are the primary effects of fever on physiologic function that might affect exercise negatively?
3 What are the key issues concerning measuring spleen size in a patient with infectious mononucleosis?
4 How should return to play for an athlete with myocarditis be managed?

Case study 7.1

Sam is a 15-year-old wrestler who became ill 24 h ago. He has a temperature of 39.5 °C, along with myalgias, chills, sinus congestion, sore throat, nausea, and vomiting. The regional championships are tomorrow. What are the return to play issues for this athlete?

Case study 7.2

Sarah is a 22-year-old college student who within the last 3 months has had two body piercings and three tattoos. Within the last week she has been feeling fatigued, along with experiencing nausea, anorexia, headache, myalgias and right upper abdominal discomfort. She is going out of town tomorrow for a 3-day ultimate Frisbee tournament. What recommendations can you make to this patient concerning participating in this event?

Case study 7.3

John is a 17-year-old football player with a girlfriend with infectious mononucleosis (diagnosed 2 months ago). He presents with moderate fatigue of 2 weeks' duration, sore throat, cervical adenopathy, and a palpable spleen. His monospot test is positive. The last game of the season is 5 days from now. Should this athlete be cleared to play for this final game?

Summarizing the evidence

Recommendations for return to activity	Results	Level of evidence*
Fever/acute infection		
"Neck check" criteria for return to play	–	C
Modification of activity according to sport	–	C
Myocarditis		
Prevention of development of myocarditis by restriction of activities during acute viral infection	–	C
Return to play with myocarditis	–	C
Hepatitis		
Return to play based on patient's symptoms/ clinical condition	–	C
Infectious mononucleosis		
Return to play criteria based on time since onset of illness (3 weeks)	–	C
Use of ultrasound assessment of spleen size for return-to-play decisions	–	C

* A1: evidence from large randomized controlled trials (RCTs) or systematic review (including meta-analysis).†
A2: evidence from at least one high-quality cohort.
A3: evidence from at least one moderate-sized RCT or systematic review.†
A4: evidence from at least one RCT.
B: evidence from at least one high-quality study of nonrandomized cohorts.
C: expert opinions.
† Arbitrarily, the following cut-off points have been used: large study size: ≥ 100 patients per intervention group; moderate study size ≥ 50 patients per intervention group.

References

1 Alluisi EA, Beisel WR, Caldwell LS. Effects of sandfly fever on isometric muscular strength, endurance, and recovery. *J Mot Behav* 1980; 12:1–11.

2 Brenner I, Shek P, Shephard R. Infection in athletes. *Sports Med* 1994; 17:86–107.

3 Friman G, Ilback NG. Acute infection: metabolic responses, effects on performance, interaction with exercise, and myocarditis. *Int J Sports Med* 1998; 19(Suppl. 3): S172–182.

4 Niemen D. *Does Exercise Alter Immune Function and Respiratory Infections?* Washington, DC: President's Council on Physical Fitness and Sports, 2001 (President's Council on Physical Fitness and Sports Research Digest Series 3, No. 13).

5 Shephard R, Shek P. Exercise, immunity and susceptibility to infection. *Physician Sportsmed* 1999; **27**:47–52.

6 Friman G, Wright J, Ilback N. Does fever or myalgia indicate reduced physical performance capacity in viral infections? *Acta Med Scand* 1985; **217**:353–361.

7 Montague TJ, Marrie TJ, Bewick DJ. Cardiac effects of common viral illnesses. *Chest* 1988; **94**:919–925.

8 Cate T, Roberts J, Russ M, *et al.* Effects of common colds on pulmonary function. *Am Rev Respir Dis* 1973; **108**:858–865.

9 Daniels W, Vogel J, Sharp D, *et al.* Effects of virus infection on physical performance in man. *Mil Med* 1985; **150**:8–14.

10 Heir T, Aanestad G, Carlsen K, Larsen S. Respiratory tract infection and bronchial responsiveness in elite athletes and sedentary control subjects. *Scand J Med Sci Sports* 1995; **5**:94–99.

11 Weidner TG, Cranston T, Schurr T, *et al.* The effect of exercise training on the severity and duration of viral upper respiratory illness. *Med Sci Sports Exerc* 1998; **30**:1578–1583.

12 Weidner TG, Anderson BN, Kaminsky LA, *et al.* Effect of a rhinovirus-caused upper respiratory illness on pulmonary function test and exercise responses. *Med Sci Sports Exerc* 1997; **29**:604–609.

13 Hosey RG, Rodenberg RE. Training room management of medical conditions: infectious diseases. *Clin Sports Med* 2005; **24**:477–506.

14 Ilback NG, Friman G, Beisel WR. Biochemical responses of the myocardium and red skeletal muscle to *Salmonella typhimurium* infection in the rat. *Clin Physiol* 1983; **3**:551–563.

15 Beisel WR, Sawyer WK, Ryll ED, Crozier D. Metabolic effects of intracellular infections in man. *Ann Intern Med* 1967; **67**:744–779.

16 Walsworth M, Kessler T. Diagnosing exertional rhabdomyolysis: a brief review and a report of 2 cases. *Mil Med* 2001; **166**:275–277.

17 Line R, Rust, G. Acute exertional rhabdomyolysis. *Am Fam Physician* 1995; **52**: 502–506.

18 Primos WA. Sports and exercise during acute illness: recommending the right course for patients. *Physician Sportsmed* 1996; **24**:44–54.

19 Maron B, Shirani J, Poliac L, *et al.* Sudden death in young competitive athletes. *JAMA* 1996; **276**:199–204.

20 Ilback N, Fohlman J, Friman G. Exercise in coxsackie B3 myocarditis: effects on heart lymphocyte subpopulations and the inflammatory reaction. *Am Heart J* 1989; **117**:1298–1302.

21 Gatmaitan B, Chason J, Lerner A. Augmentation of the virulence of murine coxsackie virus B-3 myocardiopathy by exercise. *J Exp Med* 1970; **131**:1121–1136.

22 Portugal D, Smith J. Myocarditis and the athlete. In: Estes N, Dame D, Wong P, eds. *Sudden Cardiac Death in the Athlete*. Armonk, NY: Futura, 1998: 349–71.

23 Maron B, Isner J, Mckenna W. Hypertrophic cardiomyopathy, myocarditis, and other myopericardial diseases and mitral valve prolapse. *Med Sci Sports Exerc* 1994; **26**(Suppl.):S261–S267.

24 Ohnishi K. Portal venous hemodynamics in chronic liver disease: effects of posture change and exercise. *Radiology* 1985; **155**:757–761.

25 Krikler DM, Zilberg B. Activity and hepatitis. *Lancet* 1996; **ii**:1046–1047.

26 De Celis G, Casal J, Latorre X, Angel J. Hepatitis A and vigorous physical activity. *Lancet* 1998; **352**:325.

27 Chalmers TC, Eschkardt RD, Reynolds WE, *et al.* The treatment of acute infectious hepatitis: controlled studies of the effects of diet, rest and physical reconditioning on the acute course of the disease and on the incidence of relapses and residual abnormalities. *J Clin Invest* 1955; **34**:1163–1194.

28 Chalmers TC. Rest and exercise in hepatitis. *N Engl J Med* 1969; **281**:1421–1422.

29 Edlund A. The effect of defined physical exercise in the early convalescence of viral hepatitis. *Scand J Infect Dis* 1971; **3**:189–196.

30 Repsher LH, Freeborn RK. Effects of early and vigorous exercise on recovery from infectious hepatitis. *N Engl J Med* 1969; **281**:1393–1396.

31 American Medical Society for Sports Medicine and American Orthopedic Society for Sports Medicine. Joint Position Statement: human immunodeficiency virus and other blood-borne pathogens in sports. *Clin J Sport Med* 1995; **5**:199–204.

32 American Academy of Pediatrics, Committee on Sports Medicine and Fitness. Medical conditions affecting sports participation. *Pediatrics* 2001; **107**:1205–1209.

33 Howe W. Infectious mononucleosis in athletes. In: Garrett W, Kirkendall D, Squire D, eds. *Principles and Practice of Primary Care Sports Medicine*. Philadelphia: Lippincott, Williams and Wilkins, 2001; 239–246.

34 Schooley RT. Epstein–Barr virus infections, including infectious mononucleosis. In: Isselbacher K, Wilson J, Braunwald E, *et al.*, eds. *Harrison's Principles of Internal Medicine*, 13th ed. New York: McGraw-Hill, 1994: 790–793.
35 Welch MJ, Wheeler L. Aerobic capacity after contracting infectious mononucleosis. *J Orthop Sports Phys Ther* 1986; **8**:199–202.
36 Dalrymple W. Infectious mononucleosis: relation of bed rest and activity to prognosis. *Postgrad Med* 1964; **35**:435–439.
37 Doolittle R. Pharyngitis and infectious mononucleosis. In: Fields KB, Fricker PA, eds. *Medical Problems in Athletes*. London: Blackwell Science, 1997: 11–20.
38 Haines JD. When to resume sports after infectious mononucleosis. *Postgrad Med* 1987; **81**:331–333.
39 Frelinger DP. The ruptured spleen in college athletes: a preliminary report. *J Am Coll Health Assoc* 1978; **26**:217.
40 Ali J. Spontaneous rupture of the spleen in patients with infectious mononucleosis. *Can J Surg* 1993; **153**:283–290.
41 Tamayo SG, Rickman LS, Mathews WC, *et al.* Examiner dependence on physical diagnostic test for the detection of splenomegaly: a prospective study wit multiple observers. *J Gen Intern Med* 1993; **8**:69–75.
42 Hosey RG, Quarles JD, Kriss VM, Mattacola CG. Spleen size in athletes: a comparison of BMI, gender, race, and past history of mononucleosis. *Med Sci Sports Exerc* 2004; **36**: S312.
43 Cheesman SH. Infectious mononucleosis. *Semin Hematol* 1988; **25**:261–268.
44 American Academy of Pediatrics Committee on Sports Medicine and Fitness. Medical conditions affecting sports participation. *Pediatrics* 2001; **107**:1205–1209.
45 Eichner R. Infectious mononucleosis: recognizing the condition, "reactivating" the patient. *Physician Sportsmed* 1996; **24**:49–54.
46 Guth AA, Pachter HL, Jacobowitz GR. Rupture of the pathologic spleen: is there a role for nonoperative therapy? *J Trauma* 1996; **41**:214–218.

CHAPTER 8

Should you play sport with a congenital or acquired abnormality of a solid abdominal organ?

Abel Wakai and John M. Ryan

Introduction

Ten percent of abdominal injuries are reported to result from sports-related trauma.[1] The spleen and liver are the organs most commonly injured in blunt abdominal trauma, with each accounting for one-third of the injuries.[2] Meanwhile, approximately one in 1500 children or adolescents has either a congenital or acquired solitary kidney.[3] The decision on whether or not an individual should play sport when it is known that he or she has only one kidney, or he has only one testis, is a difficult and controversial one. High-grade kidney injuries (grades IV and V) caused by sports activities have a significant potential to result in partial to complete renal loss. A devastating high-grade renal injury in a child with a solitary kidney could ultimately result in the need for chronic dialysis and transplantation.[4] In a child with a solitary testis, injury to the testis may result in anorchia, which produces sterility and necessitates testosterone supplementation. Ideally, therefore, the decision on restricting children with a solitary kidney or testis from participating in contact sports should be evidence-based.

Such a decision may often need qualifying. For example, "What is sport?" Clearly, the risks for participating in snowboarding far exceed the risks involved in noncontact sports such as bowling, or minimal-contact sports such as fencing. An individual cannot be expected to make a decision without appropriate advice. Physicians involved in a sport need to understand the consequences as well as being able to explain them in a structured manner which the athlete and others understand. This advice must be evidence-based, with any risk being determinable if possible. It is the responsibility of the physician to assist an individual in making an informed, evidence-based decision, but the decision should be a shared one.

Some individuals will have to take the decision on whether or not to continue with a sport following an injury or loss of an organ, or perhaps the discovery of a congenitally absent organ. On these occasions, the physician should not neglect the psychological trauma that may be suffered by athletes discontinuing in sport, particularly those who participate at a high level. Physicians should be prepared to offer counseling or direct an athlete for appropriate support.

For many, participation in sporting activities with peers is one of the formative events in a child's development, and this fact should not be ignored. Ultimately, the individual or his or her parent or guardian will take a risk-versus-benefit decision, which should be based on the current best evidence. In searching for the evidence, one should look for the reported incidence of adverse outcomes for athletes with a congenital or acquired abnormality of a solid abdominal organ who sustain sports-related injuries to these organs. Intuitively, there is an associated risk for people with solitary organs playing sport. The consequences of the worst-case scenario of acute renal failure, infertility, and the ensuing multisystem pathology that can arise following injury are patently obvious. But what is the incidence of such devastating outcomes? Or can we deduce the incidence so that we can inform physicians and patients in assisting them in making their decisions?

This chapter aims to examine the incidence, mechanism, and characteristics of abnormalities of solid abdominal organs in sport. In addition, it aims to produce evidence-based advice on whether or not athletes with a congenital or acquired abnormality of a solid abdominal organ should be allowed to participate in sport.

Methods

MEDLINE (PubMed interface; 1966 to the present) was searched for literature relating to sports-related solid abdominal organ trauma, along with cross-referencing from the reference lists of major articles on the subject. No language restrictions were applied.

Search strategy for liver trauma

#9 Search #3 AND #7 AND #8
#8 Search "Wounds and Injuries" (MeSH)
#7 Search #4 OR #5 OR #6
#6 Search sports medicine
#5 Search sports
#4 Search sport
#3 Search #1 OR #2
#2 Search liver diseases
#1 Search liver

Search strategy for splenic trauma

#9 Search #3 AND #7 AND #8
#8 Search "Wounds and Injuries" (MeSH)
#7 Search #4 OR #5 OR #6
#6 Search sports medicine
#5 Search sports
#4 Search sport
#3 Search #1 OR #2
#2 Search spleen diseases
#1 Search spleen

Search strategy for renal trauma

#9 Search #3 AND #7 AND #8
#8 Search "Wounds and Injuries" (MeSH)
#7 Search #4 OR #5 OR #6
#6 Search sports medicine

#5 Search sports
#4 Search sport
#3 Search #1 OR #2
#2 Search kidney diseases
#1 Search kidney

Search strategy for testicular trauma

#9 Search #3 AND #7 AND #8
#8 Search "Wounds and Injuries" (MeSH)
#7 Search #4 OR #5 OR #6
#6 Search sports medicine
#5 Search sports
#4 Search sport
#3 Search #1 OR #2
#2 Search kidney diseases
#1 Search kidney

Incidence

Liver trauma

The liver is the most frequently injured abdominal organ.[5,6] Liver injury accounts for a third of solid organ injuries in blunt abdominal trauma.[2] While the majority of adult liver injuries are due to motor-vehicle accidents, liver injury in children is predominantly due to bicycle and pedestrian injuries.[7,8] However, there is a lack of information about the incidence of liver injuries in children, because of inadequate pediatric-injury surveillance systems.[7] There are no epidemiological data in the literature on sports-related liver injuries in children, except for the implication of cycling.[7,8]

Regarding participation in sports for a child with hepatomegaly, the current recommendation of the American Academy of Pediatrics (AAP) Committee on Sports Medicine and Fitness is a "qualified yes" if the liver is acutely enlarged, noting that "participation should be avoided because of risk of rupture."[9] The recommendation for a child with a chronically enlarged liver is "an individual assessment is needed before collision, contact, or limited-contact sports are played."[9]

Splenic trauma

Sports injuries account for 10% of abdominal injuries, with the spleen being the most commonly injured organ.[10] Though the liver is the most frequently injured abdominal organ, the spleen is the most frequently injured organ in sport, and the most common cause of death due to abdominal trauma in athletes.[11] Splenic rupture may be spontaneous or traumatic. Traumatic splenic rupture usually occurs as a result of a direct blow to the left lower chest wall or left upper quadrant of the abdomen. Acute enlargement of the spleen, most commonly in infectious mononucleosis, results in an increased incidence of splenic trauma in young males, due to their greater participation in contact sports.[12]

Nonsurgical management and splenic preservation have become standards of care for the management of pediatric blunt splenic trauma.[13] The full risks of allowing early return to vigorous activity following splenic rupture treated with or without splenectomy are not fully known.[14] However, it is possible to return successfully to vigorous sporting activity within 3 weeks of splenic rupture, but the athlete has to be closely monitored during the early phase of return to activity.[14]

Infectious mononucleosis is a common cause of hepatosplenomegaly in physically active young adults.[15] No strong evidence base exists to support the use of a single parameter to predict the safe return to sports participation for athletes recovering from infectious mononucleosis.[12] Current consensus supports that athletes be afebrile, well hydrated, and asymptomatic with no palpable liver or spleen. Clinical judgment incorporating these criteria 1 month after diagnosis has been suggested as a safe predictor for gradual return to competition.[12]

The current recommendation of the American Academy of Pediatrics (AAP) Committee on Sports Medicine and Fitness is a "qualified yes" if the spleen is acutely enlarged, noting that "a patient with an acutely enlarged spleen should avoid all sports because of risk of rupture."[9] The recommendation for a child with a chronically enlarged spleen is a "qualified yes," noting "needs individual assessment before playing collision, contact, or limited-contact sports."[9]

Renal trauma

The kidney is one of the most commonly injured visceral organs following blunt abdominal trauma. Children are more susceptible to major renal injury from blunt trauma than adults.[16] In the pediatric population, recreational sports activity is the mechanism of renal injury in 2–28% of cases.[4] These findings have resulted in the controversial restriction of many children with a solitary kidney from participating in contact sports, although there are no reports in the published literature of a child injuring a solitary kidney, with resultant renal loss, while participating in a contact sport.[4,17]

The majority of renal injuries in children associated with kidney loss (21 of 28) have occurred as a result of motor-vehicle accidents, pedestrians being struck by a vehicle or other objects, and falls.[17] Johnson *et al.* reported no kidneys lost in any contact sports in a retrospective data base analysis of 49,651 pediatric trauma cases.[17] From a survey sent to pediatric urologists, Sharp *et al.* reported that American football, hockey and martial arts are the sports associated with the greatest risk for renal injury.[3] In contrast, from a retrospective chart review, Gerstenbluth *et al.* reported bicycling, rather than contact sports, as the most common recreational activity to cause renal injury, and more than half of these injuries were high-grade.[4] Another retrospective chart review reported 113 cases of blunt renal trauma and found that bicycling accounted for 24% of renal injuries, while team sports were responsible for only 5%.[18] In another retrospective chart review of 15 grade IV renal injuries, two resulted from bicycling and none from team sports.[19]

Compensatory hypertrophy of the solitary kidney, with resultant increased surface area, may increase the risk of major injury during sports activity.[4] Of 37 children with kidney injuries due to various causes, two had injury to a solitary kidney, including a low-grade renal contusion from playing American football.[20] A retrospective study of 240 cases of blunt renal trauma included four with a solitary kidney.[21]

The current recommendation of the American Academy of Pediatrics (AAP) Committee on Sports Medicine and Fitness for a child with a solitary kidney is for an "individual assessment for contact, collision, and limited-contact sports."[9] Some institutions caution patients with a solitary kidney regarding the risk of major kidney trauma from bicycling and recommend they avoid racing or stunt riding, but place no restriction on participation in team sports, except for ice hockey with body checking.[4]

Testicular trauma

Testicular trauma is rare. No testicular injuries were reported in a retrospective review of 81,923 cases, of which 5439 were sports-related, in the National Pediatric Trauma Registry from 50 United States pediatric trauma centers.[22] No testicular injuries were reported by Wan *et al.* in a retrospective review of 4921 children in a pediatric trauma registry.[23] McAleer *et al.* reported 16 patients (7.7%) with a testicular injury in a retrospective review of 14,763 patients.[18]

Although the incidence of solitary testis (undescended and absent) is unknown, maldescent of the testis occurs in 0.8% of boys.[24] In a retrospective review of 14,763 pediatric trauma patients, no patient injured in team sports had a solitary testis.[18] Regarding participation in sports for a child with one testicle (undescended or absent), the current recommendation of the American Academy of Pediatrics (AAP) Committee on Sports Medicine and Fitness is an unqualified "yes," noting that a protective cup may be required in some cases.[9]

Implications

Clearly, patients who knowingly have one kidney or one testis need to present early for consultation if they suffer an injury to the flank or scrotum. This is all the more important nowadays, given the ready availability of advanced diagnostic procedures such as computed tomography, magnetic resonance imaging, and ultrasound. There is also some evidence that early repair can help preserve hormonal function as well as fertility.

The physiological consequences of testicular trauma are difficult to quantify and are largely unknown.[25] Nolten *et al.*, in one paper, reported an unexpectedly high incidence of remote blunt testicular trauma among a cohort of infertile men.[26]

On rare occasions, sports participants need to consider the medical implications of participating in sport, given the coexisting problems that one can find with solitary kidneys. Rugiu *et al.* reported a higher incidence of proteinuria and diastolic hypertension in patients with a solitary kidney.[27] All athletes with solitary organ disorder should have a thorough preparticipation physical examination to look for evidence of other congenital anomalies or for the presence of comorbidity.

Assessing risk

So who gets injured? It is worth bearing in mind that the risk of injuring a kidney is paradoxically reduced by 50% in an individual with a solitary kidney in comparison with someone with both kidneys, as injury is almost always unilateral and the chances of injury occurring to the side with or without the kidney are equal. A review of the literature reveals that blunt renal trauma remains an uncommon problem[17] and that renal trauma with significant consequences is even less common. As for testicular injuries, the majority are sustained in motor-vehicle collisions or assaults and not sport.[22]

There are few reports of sports-related trauma to the kidney or testis. Considering the numbers of people who participate in sporting activities, this is perhaps surprising. Thus, one could suggest that the incidence of renal or testicular damage in sport is very rare.

One needs to perform an extensive review of the literature to find evidence of significant renal trauma sustained in sport, and a review of English-language journals alone is not sufficient. For instance, one Czechoslovakian paper reported on 102 cases of renal trauma over a 22-year period, of which 19.5% were sustained in sport. In 5% of cases, a nephrectomy had been performed.[28]

Unofficial participation, training, and "back yard" leisure sport have the same likelihood of injury as participation in organized competitive contact sports. Athletes need to be informed of the risks of taking part in unscheduled sporting activity where the risks of injury may be just as high as in competitive sporting activity. The same precautions may need to be taken in many aspects of daily life. Indeed, it may be that leisure activities are more likely to produce major blunt renal trauma than supervised controlled sporting activity, as has been reported in one paper from Japan. Sekiguchi *et al.* reported two cases of major blunt renal trauma, one sustained by a 13-year-old-girl in a fall from a bicycle and the other by a 12-year-old boy in a fall from a tree.[29]

It may also be that the incidence and potential for significant renal trauma increases with age. The force that may cause injury is proportionate to the speed and the mass involved in an injury, which are clearly small in children. This hypothesis is supported by the findings described in a review of genitourinary trauma in a pediatric population, which found that surgery was rarely indicated.[30]

The literature on blunt abdominal trauma sustained during the more common sporting activities such as football, skiing, cycling and cricket yields specific findings. A New Zealand paper reporting cricket injuries in children described 66 cases of injury treated at a children's emergency department over 5 years. However, only two of these cases were severe.[31] In reporting a series of renal trauma sustained from skiing injuries over a 19-year period, Skowvron *et al.* reported that 91% of the patients were male, with a mean age of 27.5 years.[32] Thus, within some sports there appears to be an age-related and sex-related predilection to injury. This may of course be proportionate to the age and sex of participants in that sport, but this biased incidence of renal trauma among males should be pointed out to athletes and their families.

It should be remembered that significant injuries may be sustained by the renal vasculature, which in turn may have significant implications for the viability of a kidney, as shown by Borrero, who described a left renal artery dissection caused by a football injury.[33]

There are few reviews of testicular injury in sport. One study by Lawson reported the occurrence of testicular injuries among rugby league and rugby union football players in Australia. Eleven players sustained loss of a testis and three sustained partial loss of one or both testes over a 16-year period, in a state where an average of 100,000 players per year are registered. The causes of the testicular injuries were kicking and kneeing, usually during tackles. At least three injuries appeared to have been intentional. However, the incidence of significant testicular injury is clearly very small in rugby union and rugby league football, given the number of participants involved in these games. Furthermore, given that the incidence of people with single testicles is also small, it would appear that the chances of someone sustaining a serious testicular injury playing rugby football are very small indeed.

The low incidence of sports-related testicular injuries may be due to the position of the testicles, being free and mobile, making them less vulnerable to crush injury and disruption.[22] Furthermore, the use of specific cups design to protect the testis may contribute to the low incidence of sports-related testicular injuries.[22]

A review of blunt testicular injury was carried out by Cass and Luxenberg, who reported a low incidence of orchiectomy and anorchidism during the follow-up.[34] In another study in 1991, Cass *et al.* reported a loss of the testis in 21% of cases treated conservatively, versus 6% of those explored promptly—reinforcing the importance of presenting early for evaluation.[35]

Sparnon *et al.* reported two cases of severe scrotal injury in BMX bicycle riding and suggested that scrotal protection should be worn when participating in jumping sports.[36] Indeed, all athletes need to be vigilant if they decide to participate in contact sports and should wear appropriate protective shields during training and not just during competitive fixtures, as the risk of injury may be at least as great.

Calculating risk

While reviewing the incidence of sports-related solid abdominal organ injuries is relevant, it is also important to attempt to quantify the risk associated with individual sporting activities, particularly as all sports do not present the same risk of injury. For example, the risk of sustaining an injury of the spleen resulting from blunt abdominal trauma while snowboarding is significantly greater than the risk while downhill skiing.[37] Wan *et al.* calculated the mean number of kidney injuries per annum as two (16 injuries per 8 years) and the kidney injury incidence per year per million children as 6.9 (two injuries per 290,264.25 × 1 million children).[23] However, the retrospective nature of the published studies does not permit easy calculation of the degree of sports-related risk.[22] The number of injuries for each sport alone is insufficient. The total number of participants and factors such as the number of games played and number of hours spent playing and practicing are relevant variables in the true calculation of risk.[22] Ideally, one would need to follow a large number of players prospectively and compute the injuries after several sessions to derive a "player-game" or "player-hour-played/practiced" risk ratio.[22] The nature of this type of study and the low number of reported injuries in retrospective surveys suggest that this would be a costly and lengthy project that might not necessarily yield any more insightful data.[22]

Specific risks

In some sports, consideration needs to be given to the overuse consequences of athletes with a single participation sport. One paper reported ultrasound findings of a 94% incidence of scrotal abnormalities in extreme mountain bikers.[38]

Athletes who have undergone renal transplantation may require advice. Because the transplanted organ is in a vulnerable position, usually located in the right or left iliac fossa, it is reasonable to advise against participation in contact sport. If an athlete chooses to continue to participate, then he or she should be supported in achieving the goal and advised to use appropriately protective garments, as some standard equipment may be dangerous. Welch has described the dangers of climbing harnesses that come into contact with the superficially placed transplanted kidney.[39] Interestingly, some nephrologists encourage participation in the majority of sports following renal transplantation, although they counsel against sports such as rugby football, boxing, and Asian martial arts.[40]

In a paper on the emergency management of blunt testicular trauma, Mulhall *et al.* showed that many patients present late.[41] "At-risk" patients must be strongly encouraged to attend early following injury.

In attempting to define risk, there has been some attempt to differentiate contact sports. One paper has classified sporting activities into the following categories:

- High to moderate dynamic and static demands
- High to moderate dynamic and low static demands
- High to moderate static and low dynamic demands

It is possible for physicians to discuss with athletes and their relatives the dangers associated with particular sports. There is also some evidence that within a sport, playing in a particular position may expose one to less injury.[42] In providing athletes with solutions, the physician must incorporate a risk analysis. Solutions should also be suggested as to which sporting activities may be more suitable. The benefits of sport and exercise are well described, so participation in low-risk sports may be advisable. Thus, while it may not be considered appropriate to participate in contact or collision sports, a physician should be able to advise an athlete on a sport which is suitable. The concept of nonparticipation in all sporting activities is rarely indicated for any illness, injury, or deprivation. The tradition of excluding the disabled athlete has now been replaced by the concept of facilitation and support for the athlete who may be challenged or "disabled."

Consideration should be given to advising young athletes with one testis to store semen before taking up or continuing in contact or collision sport.

The viewpoint of the advising physician must be respected. While there is no documented case of a successful lawsuit against a physician for advice to compete in sport with one kidney or one testis, there remains a theoretical risk that a physician could be sued. In particular, the sometimes suggested "apparent waiver of entitlement to sue" by an athlete may not stand up to scrutiny in a court of law.

Making the decision

Decisions should be participatory and informed, not unilateral or uninformed as has so often been the case in the past. Strategies in coping with this problem include matching the missing organ with a sport which might be safest. Furthermore, it could be suggested that we should now be looking for inclusion in sport for athletes, providing information about risk and utilizing protective equipment to facilitate the process, rather than the historical blanket exclusion which was previously so prevalent.

When making a decision, there are a number of groups who must be advised, including the athlete, his or her coach, families, and sometimes schools. On occasions, one needs to consider the rights of the handicapped as well as those of children. There is the child for whom the solitary organ diagnosis is already known, and there is the individual who has already succeeded in a sport by the time the diagnosis is made. With regard to protection of a solitary organ in a child, it has been questioned whether or not it is appropriate to spare an organ but spoil a child with overprotection. The implications and stigmatization of nonparticipation or wearing of a shield are not insignificant for a child, particularly in children's sports, where the forces involved are not very great. Finally, there is the individual who has lost an organ through injury or illness and who has to reevaluate a decision about continuing in sport.

For some, the advice is clear. For example, patients with a single polycystic, pelvic, iliac, or horseshoe kidney have too great a risk to participate in contact or collision sports, where the organ is dangerously vulnerable to blunt trauma.

It may be helpful in making the decision to use a classification as described by The Committee on Sports Medicine and Fitness in the United States and classify sports into contact/collision, limited-contact, and noncontact sports.[9] Contact or collision sports include those in which athletes purposely hit or collide with each other or inanimate objects, including the ground, with great force. Limited-contact sports include those in which athletes routinely make contact with each other or inanimate objects, but usually with less force than in collision sports. In noncontact sports, contact with other athletes or inanimate objects is either occasional or inadvertent, such as in softball or squash.

Ethics

It is not surprising that the question about participation will not be answered by randomized controlled trials. Who would willingly volunteer to compete in a trial in which the outcome is end organ injury or failure as a consequence of participating in sport?

What evidence do we need to enable us to answer the question of who should play sport? A randomized controlled trial involving two groups of patients who play sport would be ideal, but is impracticable. Furthermore, on an intention-to-treat basis alone, the power required for such a study would be too great, given the infrequency with which renal or testicular trauma is sustained in sport.

One possible study would be to design a trial of patients with a single kidney or testis and compare the injury rate with another cohort with normal anatomy. However, because of the large number of variables involved in sustaining an injury, such a study would be largely impractical. The variables are likely to be too great, as the study would need to encompass a wide variety of sports and so, to reach statistical significance, it is unlikely that one would be able to recruit enough people for the study, even before the issue of ethics is considered.

Benefits of sport

In making a decision about participation, it is important not to deemphasize the value of sport and assign the same risk to all sports. It is evident that the risks of renal injury will be greater with sports such as skiing, horse-riding and some sports with missiles such as hockey and cricket, but many sports do not have the same risk and could probably be encouraged.

There is a body of opinion which suggests that the greatest cause of significant renal trauma is sustained in motor-vehicle collisions. But as individuals with a solitary kidney or testicle are not advised against automobile travel, similarly perhaps individuals should not be advised against sport.

One should weigh up the value of participation in sport, including the physical and psychological well-being that accompanies it versus the risk of organ damage. Clearly, the balance will be tilted against participation in sports such as horse-riding, skiing, and other collision sports. More appropriate sports may include those in which value is attributed to an individual from the benefits of exercise and other aspects such as team building for youngsters involved in team sports.

One must also consider the forces involved. Simple formulae have major significance: force $\times$ mass $\times$ velocity. The risk of damage to single organs in sport is associated with the force of the injury. In cases of blunt trauma, it is clear that the relative risk to a kidney and testis will increase with age as the components of force increase, for example: size (mass) and the speed at which participants move, or indeed the speed at which individuals can project a missile such as a cricket ball or hockey ball.

Discussion

Given the rarity of solitary kidneys or testes in participating athletes, it is not surprising that the evidence on which to base advice about participation is thin. The available evidence is low in terms of the hierarchy of clinical evidence, consisting of retrospective surveys and chart reviews. The easy advice for the physician to offer is not to play sport. Such advice implies that an athlete will not suffer any injury and that the physician will not incur any medicolegal consequences in the future. However, the physician has a duty of care to advise the athlete in consultation and to offer advice based on evidence. The focus in encouraging sport should be to look at the opportunities that certain "low-risk" sports provide, rather than defending the at-risk organ.

Physicians are much more likely to be required to provide advice about return to sports in patients with an enlarged liver or spleen, because infectious mononucleosis is a relatively common cause of hepatosplenomegaly in physically active young adults. Again, the evidence base to support this advice is limited. The current recommendation of the American Academy of Pediatrics (AAP) Committee on Sports Medicine and Fitness for children with an enlarged liver or enlarged spleen is limited by the frequency with which it recommends individual assessment when a "qualified yes" appears. The physician's clinical judgment is, therefore, essential for applying these recommendations to a specific patient.[9] This judgment involves the available published information on the risks of participation, the advice of knowledgeable experts, the current health status of the athlete, level of competition, the position played, the sport in which the athlete participates, the maturity of the competitor, the availability of effective protective equipment that is acceptable to the athlete, the availability and efficacy of treatment, whether treatment (for example, rehabilitation of an injury) has been completed, whether the sport can be modified to allow safe participation, and the ability of the athlete and parents to understand and accept risks involved in participation. [9]

It is clear that physicians do not always follow the evidence when advising athletes. Indeed, there is some evidence that the advice currently offered by physicians remains dichotomous and indeed may be biased. For instance, Anderson, in a questionnaire sent to the 1994 membership of the American Medical Society for Sports Medicine, found that 54.1% of respondents indicated they would allow participation in collision and contact sports for an athlete with a single kidney after discussion of the possible risks. However, the percentage allowing participation decreased to 41.6% if the athlete was the respondent's own son or daughter.[43]

The evidence for participation or nonparticipation in sport in the presence of a solitary kidney is largely related to anecdotal reports. There are few papers in which we are able to judge the incidence. Three points are clear from the literature in favor of participation:

- Blunt renal trauma in sport is rare.[17–19]
- When it occurs, it can usually be managed conservatively and the outcome is usually satisfactory, with no long-term complications.[2]
- Trauma to a side without a kidney will clearly cause no renal damage, though there is some evidence to suggest that single kidneys may hypertrophy and therefore be at greater chance of injury.[4]

Consideration should be given to the aim of participation in sport. For instance, if the intention for a child to participate in a sport is purely for recreational reasons, the decision about participation will not be as difficult to make as with an adult for whom the sport is a central part of his or her life or livelihood.

Liability and medicolegal aspects of health care are becoming pervasive in today's society. Physicians asked for their opinion, particularly where they agree to a patient with an abnormality of a solid abdominal organ participating in sport, should ensure they have kept a proper record of advice given.

In advising children on participation in sport when the absence of a testis or kidney is known, it may be that at an early age children can be directed to sports with a low incidence of potential renal or testicular trauma. Goldberg has suggested that medical, orthopedic and fitness factors should be carefully evaluated so that interventions can be developed which will reduce the possible adverse effects of participation.[45] He argues that children should not be excluded from sports unless specific risk-to-benefit ratios are firmly established.

It could be hoped that in the future, protection will have a greater role for athletes with a congenital or acquired abnormality of a solid abdominal organ. Improving compounds and designs may provide easier-to-produce shields that will be more effective and more user-friendly.

Conclusions

The evidence base to support the decision on whether or not to participate in sport with a congenital or acquired abnormality of a solid abdominal organ remains limited. In making the decision, one must have an understanding of the forces involved in any sporting activity, the mechanisms by which an injury can occur, and the anatomy of a vulnerable area. One must understand the reliability and practicality of protective shields and finally balance the desire to participate in a chosen sport with the associated risk.

Summary

- The spleen is the most frequently injured solid abdominal organ in sports.
- Renal and testicular injury is uncommon in sport.
- A decision on participation in sport should be based on evidence from the literature.
- Protective equipment for solitary organs will have an increasingly important role.

Key messages

- It is possible to return to sport within 3 weeks of splenic rupture, under close monitoring.
- Gradual return to sports is possible 1 month after diagnosis of acute liver or spleen enlargement.
- Renal and testicular trauma in sport is uncommon.
- Blunt renal trauma sustained in sport is rarely serious.
- Blunt renal trauma can usually be managed conservatively.
- Patients with a transplanted kidney need specific advice about participating in sport.

Sample examination questions

Multiple-choice questions (answers on p. 602)

1 A 15-year-old youth with one kidney wishes to play rugby at school.

A He should not be allowed to participate
B There is no need for a preparticipation medical examination
C The kidney will usually be smaller than a normal kidney
D The wishes of his coach should take precedence in making a decision
E Should not be allowed to play any contact sports

2 Athletes with a solitary testicle:
   A Should wear a scrotal guard when participating in contact sport
   B Have normal endocrine function
   C Require advice about sperm banks
   D Are particularly vulnerable to penetrating trauma
   E Should have a thorough preparticipatory medical examination
3 Athletes with a solitary kidney:
   A Are more likely to suffer blunt trauma to a kidney than someone who has both kidneys
   B Usually have a larger than normal kidney
   C May be more likely to suffer from hypertension than someone with both kidneys
   D Should not participate in contact sport if the kidney is a transplanted one
   E Always require surgery when gross hematuria is present following trauma

Essay questions

1 Describe the consequences of loss of function of a solitary kidney or testicle injured in sport.
2 Classify contact sports according to risk of injury to a solitary kidney or testicle.
3 What strategies are available to athletes with a single kidney or testicle who are determined to participate in sport?

Case study 8.1

Robert, an ambitious 24-year-old semiprofessional rugby player, was recently involved in a motorcycle accident when he sustained a significant scrotal injury. His scrotum had been damaged by a front tank carrier. A clinical diagnosis of a ruptured right testicle was made and confirmed at surgery. Attempted repair was unsuccessful, and an orchiectomy was performed. He made an excellent recovery from the soft-tissue injuries. At the start of a new football season, he is now seeking advice about continuing in sport, as someone suggested to him that this was not advisable given the risks associated with injury to his remaining testicle.

Case study 8.2

Michelle, a 20-year-old student, was injured while skiing off-piste. She struck a tree at high speed and hurt her back. She was airlifted to the nearest hospital for emergency medical treatment. In the hospital, she was noted to have microscopic hematuria in association with right flank tenderness. An ultrasound examination was performed, which showed a normal right kidney but an absent left kidney. She was advised not to ski again because of the risk to her single kidney, but is seeking confirmation of the appropriateness of this advice.

Case study 8.3

Mr. and Mrs. Smith have brought James, their 6-year-old son, along for advice about participating in sport. At a 6-month check, he was noted to have an undescended testicle on the right side. This was investigated further, and he was found to have testicular agenesis on that side. They were advised that he should not play sport in the future. His father was an international athlete, and his parents were keen for James to attend a sporting school. They are now reconsidering this if he would not be able to participate in sport. They are looking for guidance on how to proceed.

Summarizing the evidence[44]

Recommendation	Grade of recommendation	Level of evidence
For a child with an acutely enlarged liver or spleen, participation in sports should be avoided because of the risk of rupture	D	5
For a child with a chronically enlarged liver or spleen, individual assessment is needed before collision, contact, or limited-contact sports are played	D	5
1 month after diagnosis of infectious mononucleosis, athletes can gradually return to competitive sports on the basis of clinical judgment incorporating the following criteria: afebrile, well-hydrated, and asymptomatic with no palpable liver or spleen	D	5
For a child with a solitary kidney, individual assessment is needed before collision, contact, or limited-contact sports are played	D	5
For a child with one testicle (undescended or absent), individual assessment is needed before collision, contact, or limited-contact sports are played	C	4

Grade of recommendation	Level of evidence	
A	1a	SR (with homogeneity*) of inception cohort studies; CDR validated in different populations
A	1b	Individual inception cohort study with > 80% follow-up; CDR validated in a single population
A	1c	All or none case series
B	2a	SR (with homogeneity*) of either retrospective cohort studies or untreated control groups in RCTs
B	2b	Retrospective cohort study or follow-up of untreated control patients in an RCT; derivation of CDR or validated on split-sample only
B	2c	"Outcomes" research
B	3a	
B	3b	
C	4	Case series (and poor-quality prognostic cohort studies)
D	5	Expert opinion without explicit critical appraisal, or based on physiology, bench research, or "first principles"

CDR, clinical decision rule; RCT, randomized controlled trial.

References

1 Bergqvist D, Hedelin H, Karlson G, *et al.* Abdominal trauma during thirty years: analysis of a large case series. *Injury* 1981; **13**:93–99.

2 Stylianos S. Outcomes from pediatric solid organ injury: role of standardized care guidelines. *Curr Opin Pediatr* 2005; **17**:402–406.

3 Sharp DS, Ross J, Kay R. Attitudes of pediatric urologists regarding sports participation by children with a solitary kidney. *J Urol* 2002; **168**:1811–1815

4 Gerstenbluth RE, Spirnak JP, Elder JS. Sports participation in high grade renal injuries in children. *J Urol* 2002; **186**:2575–2578.

5 Parks RW, Chrysos E, Diamond T. Management of liver trauma. *Br J Surg* 1999; **86**:1121–1135.

6 Wemyss-Holden SA, Bruening M, Launois B, *et al.* Management of liver trauma with implications for the rural surgeon. *ANZ J Surg* 2002; **72**:400–404.

7 Wakeman C, Beasley S, Pearson S, *et al.* Liver injury in children: causes, patterns and outcomes. *N Z Med J* 2003; **116**: U515.

8 Halman SI, Chipman M, Parkin PC, *et al.* Are seat belt restraints as effective in school children as in adults? A prospective crash study. *BMJ* 2002; **324**:1123.

9 American Academy of Pediatrics, Committee on Sports Medicine and Fitness. Medical conditions affecting sports participation. *Pediatrics* 2001; **107**:1205–1209.

10 Flik K, Callahan LR. Delayed splenic rupture in amateur hockey player. *Clin J Sport Med* 1998; **8**:309–310.

11 Rifat SF, Gilvydis RP. Blunt abdominal trauma in sports. *Curr Sports Med Rep* 2003; **2**:93–97.

12 Waninger KN, Harcke HT. Determination of safe return to play for athletes recovering from infectious mononucleosis: a review of the literature. *Clin J Sport Med* 2005; **15**:410–416.

13 Potoka DA, Schall LC, Ford HR. Risk factors for splenectomy in children with blunt splenic trauma. *J Pediatr Surg* 2002; **37**:294–299.

14 Terrell TR, Lundquist B. Management of splenic rupture and return-to-play decisions in a college football player. *Clin J Sport Med* 2002; **12**:400–402.

15 Auwaerter PG. Infectious mononucleosis: return to play. *Clin Sports Med* 2004; **23**:485–497.

16 Brown SL, Elder JS, Spirnak JP. Are pediatric patients more susceptible to major renal injury from blunt trauma? A comparative study. *J Urol* 1998; **160**:138–140.

17 Johnson B, Christensen C, DiRusso S, *et al.* A need for reevaluation of sports participation recommendations for children with a solitary kidney. *J Urol* 2005; **174**:686–689.

18 McAleer IM, Kaplan GW, LoSasso BE. *J Urol* 2002; **168**:1805–1807.

19 Russell RS, Gomelsky A, McMahon DR, *et al.* Management of grade IV renal injury in children. *J Urol* 2001; **166**:1049–1050.

20 Linke CA, Frank IN, Young LW, *et al.* Renal trauma in children: diagnostic work-up and management. *N Y State J Med* 1972; **72**:2414–2420.

21 Kuzmarov IW, Morehouse DD, Gibson S. Blunt renal trauma in the pediatric population: a retrospective study. *J Urol* 1981; **126**:648–649.

22 Wan J, Corvino TF, Greenfield SP, DiScala C. Kidney and testicle injuries in team and individual sports: data from the National Pediatric Trauma Registry. *J Urol* 2003; **170**:1528–1533.

23 Wan J, Corvino TF, Greenfield SP, DiScala C. The incidence of recreational genitourinary and abdominal injuries in the Western New York pediatric population. *J Urol* 2003; **170**:1525–1527.

24 MacKinnon AE. The undescended testis. *Indian J Pediatr* 2005; **72**:429–432.

25 Kukadia AN, Ercole CJ, Gleich P, *et al.* Testicular trauma: potential impact on reproductive function. *J Urol* 1996; **156**:1643–1646.

26 Nolten WE, Voisca SP, Korenman SG, *et al.* Association of elevated estradiol with remote testicular trauma in young infertile men. *Fertil Steril* 1994; **62**:143–149.

27 Rugiu C, Oldrizzi L, Lup A, *et al.* Clinical features of patients with solitary kidneys. *Nephron* 1986; **43**:10–15.

28 Base J, Navratilova J, Zborilova I, Urbanova E. Blunt injury of the kidney: personal experience and present views on its therapy [in Czech]. *Sb Ved Pr Lek Fak Karlovy Univerzity Hradci Kralove Suppl* 1995; **38**:81–86.

29 Sekiguchi Y, Miyai K, Noguchi K, *et al.* Non-operative management of major blunt renal lacerations with urinary extravasation; report of 2 cases. *Acta Urologica Japonica* 1998; **44**:875–878.

30 McAleer IM, Kaplan GW, Scherz HC, *et al.* Genitourinary trauma in the pediatric patient. *Urology* 1993; **42**:563–567.
31 Upadhyay V, Tan A. Cricketing injuries in children: from the trivial to the severe. *N Z Med J* 2000; **113**:81–83.
32 Skowvron O, Descotes JL, Frassinetti E, *et al.* Kidney injuries due to skiing. *Prog Urol* 1995; **5**:361–369.
33 Borrero E. Left renal artery dissection caused by a football injury. *N Y State J Med* 1991; **91**:550–552.
34 Cass AS, Luxenberg M. Testicular injuries. *Urology* 1991; **37**:528–530.
35 Cass AS, Ferrara L, Wolpert J, *et al.* Bilateral testicular injury from external trauma. *J Urol* 1988; **140**:1435–1436.
36 Sparnon T, Moretti K, Sach RP. BMX handlebar: a threat to manhood? *Med J Aust* 1982; **29**:587–588.
37 Geddes R, Irish K. Boarder belly: splenic injuries resulting from ski and snowboarding accidents. *Emerg Med Australas* 2005; **17**:157–162.
38 Frauscher F, Klauser A, Stenzl A, *et al.* US findings in the scrotum of extreme mountain bikers. *Radiology* 2001; **219**:427–431.
39 Welch TR. Climbing harness fit in kidney transplant recipients. *Wilderness Environ Med* 1999; **10**(1):3–5.
40 Heffernan A, Gill D. Sporting activity following kidney transplantation. *Pediatr Nephrol* 1998; **12**:447–448.
41 Mulhall JP, Gabram SG, Jacobs LM. Emergency management of blunt testicular trauma. *Acad Emerg Med* 1995; **2**:639–643.
42 Ryan J, McQuillan RF. A survey of rugby injuries presenting to an accident & emergency department. *Ir Med J* 1992; **85**:72–73.
43 Anderson CR. Solitary kidney and sports participation. *Arch Fam Med* 1995; **49**:885–888.
44 Centre for Evidence-based Medicine (Oxford, UK). Levels of Evidence (May 2001). http://www.cebm.net/levels_of_evidence.asp#levels (accessed 22 August 2006).
45 Goldberg B, Boiardo R. Profiling children for sports participation. *Clin Sports Med* 1984; **3**(1): 153–69.

CHAPTER 9

What type of exercise reduces falls in older people?

M. Clare Robertson and A. John Campbell

Introduction

A third of people aged 65 years and older fall each year, and half of those in their eighties fall at least once a year.[1] Falls are the most common cause of injury in people aged 65 years and older and may result in institutionalization and death.[2,3] Falls are the costliest category of injury among older people, and the health-care costs increase with fall frequency and injury severity.[4] Although guidelines for the prevention of falls in older people are available,[5,6] the importance of these common events is often overlooked.

Muscle weakness and poor balance have been well established as risk factors for falls in prospective cohort studies.[7–10]

Appropriately targeted exercise programs of sufficient intensity will increase and improve muscle strength, balance, and endurance in older people.[11,12] Exercises to improve strength and balance have therefore been central to most falls prevention programs.

The purpose of this systematic review of randomized controlled trials is to examine the evidence for the value of exercise in preventing falls and injuries resulting from falls in older people. Grade A evidence relates to all the studies reviewed in this chapter. This review updates an earlier publication by the authors[13] and the one in the previous edition of this book, both of which included falls prevention trials with exercise as an intervention, either used alone or as one component of a multifactorial intervention.

Methods

Search methods

The search included:

- The Cochrane Musculoskeletal Group specialized register (January 2005)
- Cochrane Controlled Trials Register (The Cochrane Library, Issue 4, 2004)
- MEDLINE (1966 to January 2005)
- EMBASE (1988 to 2005 Week 8)
- CINAHL (1982 to January 2005)
- The National Research Register, Issue 4, 2004
- Current Controlled Trials (http://www.controlled-trials.com, accessed January 2005)
- Reference lists of articles

No language restrictions were applied for the trials identified until 2001, but resources since then have allowed only articles published in English. This search strategy was developed and used during a systematic review of interventions to prevent falls in elderly people for the Cochrane Library.[14]

Data extraction

Studies were reviewed if they met the following criteria:

- Participants were randomly allocated to intervention and control groups.
- Participants were aged 60 years or older.
- An exercise program was tested as a separate intervention.
- Details were provided on exercise type, frequency, and duration.
- Prevention of falls and/or fall-related injuries was an aim.
- Falls or falling were reported as an outcome of the study.

The following factors were considered in each study: study design; eligible population; population agreeing to be randomized; age distribution; setting; inclusion and exclusion criteria; type, frequency, and duration of the exercise program; co-intervention or contamination; adherence to the exercise program; adverse effects; qualifications of instructors; measurement of fall events; use of blinding; numbers lost to follow-up; effects of the intervention and the strength of this evidence; generalizability; costs and cost-effectiveness of the intervention, and effect on health-care resources.

Quality assessment

The quality of the methodology used in each trial was assessed by two reviewers independently, using a predetermined scoring system.[14] Reviewers were not blinded to author and source institutions, and authors did not review their own studies. Disagreement was resolved by consensus or third-party adjudication. In addition, we considered the power of the study and statistical methods used for analysis of fall events.

Results

Thirty articles reporting results from 27 randomized controlled trials meeting the inclusion criteria were identified and reviewed.[15–44] The results of one trial were reported both at 1 year and after 2 years of follow-up,[17,18] and a separate article reported an economic evaluation of the intervention.[19] We excluded MacRae *et al.*,[29] as the results reported in this article are for a subset of the sample in the trial reported by Reinsch *et al.*[34] We did not include trials reported in abstract form only. One study was excluded because all the participants took part in the same exercise program.[45] We also excluded a controlled, but not randomized, New Zealand trial[46] of the Otago Exercise Programme, the same home exercise program used in three of the included trials.[17,18,20,36] These four trials were further investigated in a meta-analysis of individual-level data.[47] Three of the trials[16,31,43] contributed to data reported in a preplanned meta-analysis of the Frailty and Injuries: Cooperative Studies of Intervention Techniques (FICSIT) trials.[48]

Table 9.1 summarizes the study aims, sample, exercise programs used, adherence to the exercise program, and intervention effects, and gives relevant comments based on the review of each of the 27 included studies. Four of the trials included costs of the intervention, cost-effectiveness, or costs of health-care resource use as outcome measures (see Table 9.2).

Table 9.1 Summary of randomized controlled trials on exercise interventions for falls prevention

Article, study aims, sample, number in study, duration	Interventions	Adherence to exercise programs	Intermediate and other effects	Effect on falls and fall injuries	Comments
• Barnett *et al.* 2003[15]: • To determine whether a weekly group exercise program plus home exercises improves physical functioning or health status and prevents falls in at risk community living older people • ≥ 65 years, ≥ 1 risk factor on standardized assessment by general practitioner or hospital based physiotherapist • n = 163, 150 (92%) completing the trial included in falls analysis • 1 year	• Intervention group: supervised group exercise program (mean 9 per group) for 1-hour weekly for 1 year (warm up then functional, balance, co-ordination, and strengthening exercises, fast walking, cool down, all to music) with ancillary home exercises (based on class content) plus information on strategies for avoiding falls • Control group: provided with written falls prevention material only	• Intervention participants attended a median of 23 exercise classes (range 0 to 36, 37 offered) • 91% of those still attending classes at 1 year (total not provided) were performing home exercise sessions at least weekly, 13% were performing the exercises daily	At 6 months: • Exercise group performed better in tests of postural sway and coordinated stability • No difference in measures of strength, reaction time, walking speed, and fear of falling or on short-form 36 and physical activity scale for the elderly scores	• Number of falls reduced by 40% (incidence rate ratio 0.60; 95% CI, 0.36 to 0.99) • Trend for lower rate of falls injuries (incidence rate ratio 0.66; 95% CI, 0.38 to 1.15)	• Although relatively low-intensity, program targeted group with reduced physical functioning • "Considerable emphasis" on balance exercises
• Buchner *et al.* 1997[16]: • To determine the effect of strength and endurance training on gait, balance, physical health status, falls risk, and use of health services • 68–85 years, with at least mild deficits in strength and balance • n = 105, 100 (95%) included in falls analysis • Up to 25 months (median 18 months)	Interventions were center-based, supervised 1-hour sessions 3 × week for 24–26 weeks, then unsupervised: • Intervention group 1: strength training using weights machines • Intervention group 2: endurance training using stationary bicycles • Intervention group 3: combination of strength + endurance training • Control group: instructed to maintain usual activity levels	• Exercise participants remaining at 6 months (71%) attended 95% of scheduled sessions • At 9 months, 58% of participants reported carrying out the exercises 3 × week, 24% 2 ≥ week, and 5% not at all	At 6 months: • Improvement in hip and knee strength in strength-training group (knee strength only in combination training group) • No effect of exercise on measures of gait, balance or physical health status	• Exercise (3 groups combined) increased time to first fall compared with control group (relative hazard 0.53; 95% CI, 0.30 to 0.91) • Exercise groups had a lower fall rate (relative risk 0.61; 95% CI, 0.39 to 0.93)	• Evidence for exercise other than balance to lower falls risk in older people • Evidence for lack of improvement in gait and balance with short-term strength and endurance training in people with minor deficits in gait and balance

Continued

Table 9.1 *(Continued)*

Article, study aims, sample, number in study, duration	Interventions	Adherence to exercise programs	Intermediate and other effects	Effect on falls and fall injuries	Comments
• Campbell *et al.* 1997[17] (see also Campbell *et al.* 1999[18]): • To determine the effectiveness of an individually tailored home exercise program in preventing falls and injuries in elderly women • Women ≥ 80 years, enrolled through general practices • n = 233, all included in falls analysis, 213 (91%) completed trial • 1 year	• Intervention group: muscle strengthening and balance retraining exercises (≥ 3 × week, 30 minutes), plus walking plan (≥ 2 × week, 30 minutes), individually prescribed and progressed over 4 home visits by a physiotherapist then monthly telephone contact for 1 year (Otago Exercise Programme[56]) • Control group: equivalent number of social visits by nurse, and usual care	At 2 months: • (4 home visits): • 77% exercised ≥ 3 × week At 1 year (4 home visits, 10 phone calls): • 63% had exercised ≥ 2 × week and 42% had exercised ≥ 3 × week	At 6 months: • Balance score and chair stand test improved in exercise group At 1 year: • Exercise group maintained physical activity level and falls self-efficacy score (self-confidence for daily activities without falling)	• Relative hazard for first 4 falls for exercise group 0.68; 95% CI, 0.52 to 0.90 • Relative hazard for a fall resulting in moderate or severe injury 0.61; 95% CI, 0.39 to 0.97	• Targeted high-risk group for falling • Program was most effective in the prevention of recurrent falls • Designed for wider implementation
• Campbell *et al.* 1999[18] (see also Campbell *et al.* 1997[17]): • To assess the effectiveness of an individually tailored home exercise program in preventing falls and injuries over two years • Women ≥ 80 years, enrolled through general practices • n = 233 year 1, n = 152 year 2, all 233 (100%) included in falls analysis, 103 of 152 (68%) completed 2 years • 2 years	• Intervention group: home-based exercise program (Otago Exercise Programme,[56] see above) established in year 1*; in year 2 participants were phoned every 2 months by the physiotherapist and encouraged to maintain/increase exercise sessions • Control group: no active intervention in year 2	At 2 years: • 31 of 71 (44%) of the exercise participants had carried out the exercises ≥ 3 × week	• No intermediate variables assessed in year 2	• Adjusted relative hazard for all falls for exercise group 0.69; 95% CI, 0.49 to 0.97 • Relative hazard for a fall resulting in moderate or severe injury 0.63; 95% CI, 0.42 to 0.95	• Evidence that fall rate reduction was sustained over 2 years

• Campbell *et al.* 1999[20]: • To determine the effectiveness of gradual withdrawal of psychotropic medication and a home-based exercise program in reducing falls • ≥ 65 years and currently taking psychotropic medication • n = 93, all included in falls analysis, 72 (77%) completed trial • 44 weeks	2 × 2 factorial design: • Intervention 1: psychotropic medication withdrawal, active ingredient gradually withdrawn over 14-week period • Control group for medication withdrawal intervention: continue with original medication • Intervention 2: exercise program (Otago Exercise Programme[56])* for 44 weeks • Control group for exercise program: no active intervention	• 20 of 32 (63%) exercise participants completing the trial were carrying out the exercises ≥ 3 times a week at 44 weeks[73] • 23 of 32 (72%) exercise participants were walking twice a week at 44 weeks[73]	At 6 months[73]: • Exercise group improved in tests of balance and strength: functional reach ($P <$ 0.015), knee extensor strength ($P < 0.004$), chair stand test ($P < 0.010$) • Exercise group improved in SF-36 mental component summary score	• No evidence that exercise program reduced the risk of falling • Relative hazard for falling in medication withdrawal group compared with original medication group 0.34; 95% CI, 0.16 to 0.74)	• Very large reduction in falls by psychotropic medication withdrawal • Small sample size and high dropout rate
• Day *et al.* 2002[21]: • To test effectiveness of, and explore interactions between, 3 interventions to prevent falls in older people • ≥ 70 years, living at home • n = 1090, all included in falls analysis, 971 (89%) completed trial • 18 months	Full factorial design (8 groups defined by presence or absence of each intervention): • Intervention 1: group exercise (flexibility, leg strengthening, and balance exercises) 1-hour weekly class for 15 weeks supplemented with home exercise for up to 12 months • Intervention 2: home hazard checklist then management by participant or local authority home maintenance program • Intervention 3: vision improvement (referral to eye care provider or general practitioner), control group for this intervention received a brochure on eye care	• 401 of 541 (74%) started an exercise class • Mean number of sessions attended 10.0 (SD 3.8) • 328 attended > 50% of their sessions • Mean number of home exercise sessions 9 a month	At final exercise class (first 177 participants): • Improvements in strength and balance (mean number of errors made during coordinated stability testing, maximal balance range, quadriceps strength in both weaker and stronger legs) After 18 months (442 randomly selected participants): • Maintenance of maximal balance range • No difference in other strength and balance measures	• Exercise reduced risk of first fall by 18% (relative hazard 0.82; 95% CI, 0.70 to 0.97) • Home hazard management alone and vision improvement alone did not show a significant effect, but both were effective in combination with exercise • Strongest effect on first fall was with all 3 interventions (relative hazard 0.67; 95% CI, 0.51 to 0.88)	• Low acceptance rate for study (1090 of 11 120 invited to participate, 9.8%) • Analysis included first fall only, therefore reduction in the number of falls not known • No interaction shown between interventions (effects were additive) • Transport to classes provided when necessary

Continued

Table 9.1 *(Continued)*

Article, study aims, sample, number in study, duration	Interventions	Adherence to exercise programs	Intermediate and other effects	Effect on falls and fall injuries	Comments
• Donald *et al.* 2000[22]: • To compare 2 types of flooring in the bed areas and 2 modes of physiotherapy in avoiding falls in an elderly care rehabilitation ward of a community hospital • Consecutive patients, mean age 83 years • n = 54, all included in falls analysis, 32 (59%) completed study • 9 months (falls monitored for duration of hospital stay, mean 29 days)	2 × 2 factorial design: • Intervention 1: carpet vs. vinyl flooring in bed area • Intervention 2: conventional functional based physical therapy (once or × 2 daily, tailored to patient, e.g., transfers, walking exercises, dynamic balance) vs. conventional therapy plus additional leg strengthening exercises (3 sets of 10 lifts using hip flexors, the same using ankle dorsiflexors, with ankle cuff weights, performed while seated, × 2 daily)	• Additional exercises "tolerated" by 73% of allocated patients	13 (54%) of conventional therapy group and 20 (66%) of conventional plus additional exercises group at discharge: • Hand grip strength improved in conventional plus additional exercises group • No significant differences between groups for ankle flexor, hip flexor strength, or timed up and go test	• No difference in number of patients receiving conventional vs. conventional plus additional exercises who fell • Trend for more people to fall on carpet (RR 8.3; 95% CI, 0.95 to 73)	• Low number of events (8 patients fell a total of 11 times recorded on incident report forms) • 8 of the 54 (15%) patients were not given physiotherapy (refused, too frail)
• Hauer *et al.* 2001[23]: • To determine safety and efficacy of exercises to improve strength, mobility, and balance and to reduce subsequent falls in geriatric patients with a history of injurious falls • Women, history of recurrent or injurious falls, recruited after acute	• Intervention group: group exercise (4–6 participants) warm up on stationary cycles 10 minutes, progressive resistance training 1.5 hours (with breaks) using exercise machines, progressive static and dynamic balance training plus group games, basic forms of	• Adherence to intervention was 85% (intervention 85% (SD 28%) vs. control 84% (SD 29%)) • All participants could follow the intensive, individually adjusted regimen	At 3 months: • Exercise improved performance and strength scores for all muscles trained in trial • Intervention group more than doubled total physical activity and sports activity At 6 months:	• Nonsignificant 25% reduction in number of fallers in intervention group (relative risk 0.75; 95% CI, 0.46 to 1.25)	• Study underpowered for fall outcome • Syncopal falls were excluded • Training started immediately after discharge • Minor problems of cramping, tenderness,

care or inpatient rehabilitation, mean age 82.0 (SD 4.8) years • n = 57, 56 (98%) included in falls analysis • 6 months	dance and tai chi (when performance allowed) 45 minutes, 3 × weekly for 12 weeks • Control group: placebo group met for 1 hour 3 × weekly for 3 months (flexibility exercises, callisthenics, ball games, and memory tasks while seated)		• Differences between groups for muscle strength still significant • Functional performance still significantly higher than baseline levels • Physical activity level returned to baseline levels		and knee pain at first, all improved during training • Transport was provided
• Helbostad *et al.* 2004[24]: • To determine the effectiveness of home training and whether group training in addition to home training enhances the effect • ≥ 75 years living at home, fall(s) in previous year, uses walking aid • n = 77, 68 (88%) included in falls analysis • 1 year	• Intervention: combined training (as below but with 1 hour group sessions 2 × week for 12 weeks, 5–8 per group, consisting of warm up, progressive strength training using ankle weights, functional balance training, relaxation), • Control: home training (functional aspects of balance and strength, delivered by local physiotherapist) twice a day for 12 weeks plus 3 group meetings to learn the exercises, motivate and gain knowledge on importance of preventing functional decline and falls	• Combined training: 21 of the 24 training sessions (14–24); home training: average 2.5 of the 3 group meetings attended (range 0–3) • At 3 months combined training group 1.35 (SD 0.51) sessions a day; home training group reported completing on average 1.29 (SD 0.54) per day	At 3 months: • Improvements but no group differences for walking speed, figure of eight, timed up and go, maximum step length, timed pick up, and sit to stand tests • No improvement in posturography and quadriceps strength At 9 months: • Function was equivalent to baseline level	• No group differences in number of falls, rate of falls, number of fallers, or time to first fall • No difference between number of fallers in the previous year and number of fallers during the trial	• Individualized group exercises did not have an additional effect on daily home exercises • Study underpowered to compare falls between the 2 groups • Transport provided to group sessions

Continued

Table 9.1 *(Continued)*

Article, study aims, sample, number in study, duration	Interventions	Adherence to exercise programs	Intermediate and other effects	Effect on falls and fall injuries	Comments
Latham *et al.* 2003[25]: • To determine effectiveness of vitamin D and home-based quadriceps resistance exercise on reduction of falls and improving physical health of frail older people after hospital discharge • ≥65 years, considered frail according to simple clinical measures of frailty, admitted to 5 geriatric rehabilitation units (inpatient or day ward) • n = 243, 222 (91%) completed trial and included in falls analysis • 6 months	2 × 2 factorial design: • Intervention 1: single oral dose of vitamin D (1.25 mg calciferol, 300 000 IU) • Control group for intervention 1: matching placebo tablets • Intervention 2: instructed individually to perform high-intensity quadriceps resistance exercise (knee extensions aimed at 60% to 80% of the person's 1 repetition maximum using ankle cuff weights) 3 sets of 8, 3 × week for 10 weeks, first 2 sessions in hospital, remainder at home • Control group for intervention 2: frequency matched telephone calls and home visits	• Participants adhered to 82% of prescribed exercise sessions (mean 24.6 of 30 sessions) • Protocol modified to 30% to 40% of 1 repetition maximum for first 2 weeks due to complaints of muscle soreness, back pain and difficulty applying heavy ankle weights • Only 25% were able to reach > 60% of their 1 repetition maximum • Average training weight increased from 5.8 (SD 2.9) lb to 11.2 (SD 5.5) lb	At 3 months: • More improvement in timed up and go test for nonexercisers At 6 months: • No effect of exercise on quadriceps strength, timed walking test, timed up and go, or Berg balance test • Exercise control group scored better in vitality domain of short form 36 • No differences in activities of daily living scores	• No effect on fall rate, number of fallers or time to first fall with resistance exercise • Fall-related injuries did not differ between the 2 groups • No effect of exercise in participants with high adherence to resistance program	• Exercises increased musculoskeletal injury that required medical attention and self reported fatigue • Good evidence for caution when prescribing high-intensity quadriceps exercises to frail older people • Clear definition and good monitoring of adverse events • Efficacy of outcome assessor blinding confirmed

• Li *et al.* 2004[26]: • To determine whether improved physical functional balance through tai chi is related to subsequent reductions in falls among elderly persons • > 70 years inactive (not involved in regular moderate or strenuous physical activity program in previous 3 months) • n = 256, all included in comparison of faller status from month 6 through month 12, falls data in same 6 months available for 188 (73%) • 1 year	• Intervention group: tai chi (24 form, classical Yang style), experienced tai chi instructors, 1 hour classes 3 × week for 6 months • Control group: stretching (trunk and upper body) 1 hour classes 3 × week for 6 months	• 34 did not start the exercise classes • A further 47 (24 in tai chi and 23 in control group) withdrew during the trial • Median compliance 61 sessions for both groups, range 30–77 for tai chi and 35–78 for control group • 92 of 115 (80%) tai chi group and 87 of 107 (81%) attended ≥ 50 sessions	Comparison of baseline, 3 and 6 month values: • Tai chi group performed better in Berg balance scale, dynamic gait index, and functional reach tests; no changes observed for control group Comparison of 6 and 12 month values: • Functional balance showed overall decline in both groups, but slower deterioration in tai chi group	During post intervention phase (month 6 through month 12): • Fewer fallers in tai chi group (27 of 125 vs. 68 of 131; $P < 0.001$)	• Comparison of falls during 6 months of intervention reported elsewhere: fewer falls, fallers, and injurious falls in tai chi compared with control group 74 • High withdrawal rate (81 of 256, 32% did not start exercise classes or withdrew during the intervention period) • Tai chi participants with improved functional balance scores at 1 year were less likely to fall in post intervention phase than control group participants
• Lord *et al.* 1995[27]: • To determine whether a 12-month program of regular exercise would improve physical function and reduce the rate of falling in older women • Women ≥ 60 years • n = 197, falls monitored for 1 year in 169 (86%) and included in falls analysis • 1 year	• Intervention group: exercise classes (warm up; aerobic and strengthening exercises; activities for balance, flexibility, endurance, and hand eye and foot eye coordination; stretching; relaxation), 1 hour 2 days a week for 4 10–12 week terms for 1 year • Control group: no active intervention	• Participants attended 26–82 (32%–100%) classes • On average, 60 (73%) classes were attended by the 75 participants who completed the year	At 1 year: • Exercise group improved in reaction time, lower limb muscle strength, neuromuscular control and body sway measures	• No difference in the proportion of people falling at least once or recurrently at 1 year	• Good objective evidence of improvements in physical function risk factors for falls • Authors considered exercise program may be more effective in higher risk group

Continued

Table 9.1 *(Continued)*

Article, study aims, sample, number in study, duration	Interventions	Adherence to exercise programs	Intermediate and other effects	Effect on falls and fall injuries	Comments
• Lord *et al.* 2003[28]: • To determine whether a 12-month program of group exercise could improve physical functioning and reduce falls in frail older people • 62 to 95 years, resident in self and intermediate care retirement villages • n = 551, 508 (92%) completed study and included in falls analysis • 1 year	• Intervention group: exercise classes (warm up, aerobic, strengthening, balance, hand eye and foot eye coordination, cool down) 1 hour 2 days a week for 12 months • Control group: n = 90 flexibility and relaxation program 1 hour 2 days a week for 12 months; n = 181 no active intervention	• Mean number exercise classes attended 39.4 (SD 28.7), 42% of available classes	After 6 months: • Choice stepping reaction time ($P < 0.01$), 6-minute walking distance tests ($P < 0.05$) performed better by intervention group	• Number of falls 22% lower in intervention group (adjusted incidence rate ratio 0.78, 95% CI, 0.62 to 0.99)	• Exercise classes individualized to functional capabilities of participant • Exercises designed to address known major risk factors for falls and to improve ability to perform activities of daily living
• Morgan *et al.* 2004[30]: • To evaluate the effect of an easily implemented, low-intensity exercise program on time to first fall in a clinically defined population of elderly people • ≥ 60 years, with either a hospital admission or bed rest for ≥ 2 days within previous month • n = 294, 49 (17%) lost between randomization and baseline assessment, 229 (78%) with complete data and included in falls analysis • 1 year	• Intervention group: exercise sessions (SAFE-GRIP program: strengthening, flexibility, postural, balance, and gait training exercises), up to 5 in group, 45 minutes 3 days a week for 8 weeks (24 sessions), instructed to exercise at home until 1 year • Control group: no active intervention	• Average of 70%[75] exercise group sessions completed, mean 18.8 (SD 8.4) • Those who did not drop out of study (n = 229, 78% of randomized sample) completed 83%, mean 19.9 (SD 6.2) group sessions	At 6 month[75]: • Exercise program improved strength, gait, balance, and mobility measures	• No difference in risk of a first fall using time to first fall • Risk of a fall decreased for those with low self rated physical function (SF-36 physical function component score < 55) at baseline (hazard ratio 0.51; $P \leq 0.03$), but increased for those with high physical function (score ≥ 55) at baseline (hazard ratio 3.51; $P \leq 0.02$)	• This low-intensity exercise program may reduce risk of a fall for people with low levels of physical functioning • No cardiovascular distress during sessions, all participants tolerated the activity levels and workload

• Mulrow *et al.* 1994[31]: • To investigate the effectiveness of physical therapy on physical function (including falls) and self perceived health in frail long-stay nursing home residents • $\geq$60 years, dependent in $\geq$2 activities of daily living • n = 194, 180 (93%) completed trial • 4 months	• Intervention group: one on one 30–45-min sessions with physical therapist (addressing 3 to 5 of highest ranked of 17 assessed deficits) 3 times a week for 4 months • Control group: one on one friendly visits 3 times a week for 4 months	• 89% of scheduled physical therapy sessions were attended	• No improvement in physical disability index, sickness impact profile or activities of daily living scores • Improvement in mobility subscale of the physical disability index (15.5%; 95% CI, 6.4% to 24.7%) • Physical therapy group less likely to use assistive devices and wheelchairs for locomotion ($P < 0.005$)	• No difference in proportion of falls compared with hypothesized value (50% of total number of falls experienced by both groups)	• No evidence to support implementation of one on one physical therapy in this group of frail long-stay nursing home residents to prevent falls • Short follow-up time • Falls not reduced, but modest improvements in function
• Nitz *et al.* 2004[32]: • To determine whether a specific balance strategy training program delivered in a work station format was superior to a community based exercise class program for reducing falls • > 60 years living independently, fall(s) in previous year • n = 73, 45 (62%) included in analysis • 6 months	1-hour session a week for 10 weeks in groups of up to 6 (ratio 2 or 3 participants to 1 trainer): • Intervention: progressive exercise program with workstation focus (sit to stand to sit; stepping forwards, side and back; reaching to limits of stability; step up and down; balance strategies; ball games; card treasure hunt) • Control exercise intervention: community class, progressive exercises (warm up; marching; arm flexing, hip extension, abduction, flexion; warm down)	• Not reported	At 3 months: • Specific balance strategy group showed more improvement in functional ability (clinical outcomes variable scale score) • No differences between the 2 groups for both clinical and laboratory balance measures (both groups improved on some clinical balance measures)	• Reduction in falls in both groups ($P = 0.001$), no difference between the 2 groups	• Pretest/post-test study design (comparing number of falls in previous one year with number of falls during the trial) • High dropout rate and low event rate for falls (12 and 13 falls in 6 months in the exercise and control groups respectively) • No adverse events, even though participants were very frail

Continued

Table 9.1 *(Continued)*

Article, study aims, sample, number in study, duration	Interventions	Adherence to exercise programs	Intermediate and other effects	Effect on falls and fall injuries	Comments
• Nowalk *et al.* 2001[33]: • To use 2 different exercise programs over a 2 year period to reduce falls in residents of 2 long term care facilities • Residents capable of ambulating and following simple instructions, mean age 85 years • n = 110, 74 (67%) included in falls analysis, 69 (63%) completed 2 years • 2 years	• Intervention 1: individualized, progressive strength training and conditioning exercises (Fit NB Free), 3 × week for 2 years plus basic enhanced programming (team management, 3 educational quality of life programs) • Intervention 2: tai chi 3 × week, "Living and learning" program (goal setting, role playing, to modulate fear of falling) once per month plus basic enhanced training • Intervention 3: basic enhanced training only	• Overall adherence declined from 50.0% (SD 37.5) during the first 6 months to 31.2% (SD 37.7) during the last 6 months • Intervention 1 had higher overall adherence than Intervention 2 (55.8% (SD 29.4) vs. 24.2% (SD 30.8), $P < 0.001$)	• "Small changes" in some of the measures of functional capacity (chair stand, 20 feet walk, grip, quadriceps, and hip flexor strength) but no differences between groups, data not provided	• No difference for time to first fall or number of fallers between the 3 groups • No difference between adherers and nonadherers in number of fallers in the 2 years	• Authors acknowledge sample size too small for adequate power to detect differences in rate of falls between exercise and control groups • Falls determined from incident reports • First fall only used in analyses • Adherence clearly defined (as attending > 67% of all possible exercise sessions)
• Reinsch *et al.* 1992[34]: • To investigate the effectiveness of exercise and cognitive behavioral programs compared with a discussion control group in reducing falls and injuries • > 60 years • n = 230, 184 (80%) completed trial • 1 year	2 × 2 factorial design: • Intervention 1: exercise classes (stand up/step down procedure) 1 hour 3 days a week for 1 year • Intervention 2: cognitive behavioral group sessions 1 hour once a week for 1 year (health and safety curriculum to prevent falls, relaxation and video game playing) • Control group: discussion sessions 1 hour once a week for 1 year covering health topics of interest to seniors (and not specifically related to falls)	• Not reported	• No difference in balance, strength, fear of falling inside the home, self rated present health between the 4 groups In a subset of 80 women (MacRae *et al.* 1994[29]): • Control group declined in knee and ankle strength ($P < 0.002$), both groups declined in hip strength ($P < 0.002$) • No difference in balance and gait	• No difference between the 4 groups in the number of fallers, time to first fall, fall rate or level of severity of fall-related injury	• No evidence that the exercise program or cognitive behavioral approach should be implemented to prevent falls in older people • Analysis compared the 4 groups (rather than each intervention with its control group) and for first fall only • Authors suggest exercise intervention of insufficient intensity and focus to lower falls risk

• Resnick *et al.* 2002[35]: • To test the feasibility of the WALC intervention and test its effects on self efficacy and outcome expectations, exercise and free living activity, physical and mental health status, and falls and fall-related injuries • Women resident in continuing care community, sedentary lifestyle, mean age 88 (SD 4) • n = 20, data for 17 available for analysis • 6 months	• Intervention group: walking on own or in walking group, address pain, fear and fatigue on exercise, education on exercise and verbal encouragement, visual aids (WALC), 20 minutes 3 × week for 6 months • Control group: routine care	• 7 of 10 adhered to walking program • 1 of 10 did no regular exercise	At 2 and 6 months: • Exercise group scored higher on score for self efficacy expectations related to exercise	• No difference between the 2 groups in the number of falls ($P > 0.05$) • No falls during the study resulted in injuries	• Pretest/post-test design (number of falls in 2 months prior to study compared with number of falls in trial period, self report) • Authors acknowledge power was low for all analyses • Main focus was for nurses to initiate and help adherence to a walking program (to increase physical activity) • Both physical and psychological adverse events noted
• Robertson *et al.* 2001[36]: • To assess the effectiveness of a trained district nurse individually prescribing a home exercise program to reduce falls and injuries • ≥ 75 years, recruited through general practices • n = 240, all included in falls analysis, 211 (88%) completed trial • 1 year	• Intervention group: muscle strengthening and balance retraining exercises, walking plan (Otago Exercise Program[56])* individually prescribed and progressed over 5 home visits and monthly telephone contact for 1 year by trained district nurse supervised by a physiotherapist • Control group: no active intervention	• 49 of 113 (43%) participants completing trial exercised ≥ 3 × week for 1 year • 72% exercised ≥ 2 × week for 1 year • 71% walked ≥ 2 × week for 1 year	• Exercise group had improved in 4-test balance scale score (difference 0.3, 95% CI, 0.0 to 0.5)[73] • Higher proportion in exercise group had improved in chair stand and one foot stand tests[73]	• Number of falls reduced in exercise group by 46% (incidence rate ratio 0.54; 95% CI, 0.32 to 0.90) • Fewer in exercise group had serious injury from a fall ($P < 0.033$)	• This home exercise program is effective in reducing falls and injuries when delivered by trained nurse in usual health-care service setting • Now tested in four controlled trials, total 1016 participants[17–20,36,46,47,57] • Program manual available for health professionals[56]

Continued

Table 9.1 *(Continued)*

Article, study aims, sample, number in study, duration	Interventions	Adherence to exercise programs	Intermediate and other effects	Effect on falls and fall injuries	Comments
• Rubenstein *et al.* 2000[37]: • To study the effects of a low to moderate intensity group exercise program on strength, endurance, mobility, and fall rates in fall prone elderly men with chronic impairments • Men ≥ 70 years with leg weakness, impaired gait or balance or previous falls • n = 59, 52 (88%) completed study and included in falls analysis • 3 months	• Intervention group: 90-minute strength, endurance, and balance training sessions 3 × week for 12 weeks led by exercise physiology graduate students • Control group: asked to continue usual activities	• Exercise group participants attended 84% of sessions • Exercise group participants who completed the trial attended 91% of exercise sessions	• Improvements in endurance, strength, gait, and function measures	• No difference in proportion of fallers in the 2 groups • Fall rate (adjusted for activity level) lower in exercise group (6 falls/1000 hours of activity vs. 16.2 falls/1000 hours, $P < 0.05$)	• Generalizable only to similar fall-prone men because of small sample size and short follow-up period
• Schoenfelder 2000[38]: • To assess the effectiveness of an ankle strengthening and walking program to improve balance, ankle strength, and walking speed and reduce number of falls and fear of falling • ≥ 65 years, resident in 2 nursing homes • n = 16, 14 completed study • 6 months	• Intervention group: supervised exercise (progressive ankle strengthening, accompanied walking for 10 minutes progressing distance and gait speed) total 20 minutes 3 × week for 3 months • Control group: not reported	• Exercise program was "well received and tolerated" by participants who "did not voice physical complaints" or "express reluctance to do the exercises"	At 3 months: • Balance stand scores did not change, number of heel raises increased, 6 metre walk time improved, falls efficacy score improved in exercise group (results not significant)	• 12 falls in previous year, 42 in 6 months in exercise group; 7 falls in previous year, 12 in 6 months for the control group	• Pretest/post-test design, analysis compared falls in previous 1 year and number of falls recorded during the trial from incident reports

• Shimada *et al.* 2004[39]: • To determine the effectiveness of a perturbed walking exercise in physically disabled elderly people • 66 to 98 years, resident of long term care facility or outpatient of geriatric health service • n = 32, 26 (81%) included in analysis) • 6 months	• Intervention group: individually tailored treadmill gait exercise, (continuously and randomly generates unexpected perturbations) from 1 to 3 × week, up to 600 minutes over 6 months, in addition to usual exercise program (see control group) • Control group: usual exercise program (individually tailored stretching exercises, resistance training, gait training over level surfaces, outdoor walking, balance training, stair climbing, and group exercise designed to improve lower limb function) details of frequency and duration of sessions not reported	• 15 of 18 (83%) completed the treadmill exercise program	• Functional reach test and reaction time during perturbed treadmill walking improved in treadmill exercise group compared with usual exercise program group	• No difference between groups in number of falls (8 vs. 11, $P = 0.384$), number of fallers (5 vs. 6, $P = 0.425$), or time to first fall (mean 147 vs. 120 days, $P = 0.275$)	• Inadequate sample size for falls
• Steadman *et al.* 2003[40]: • To evaluate an enhanced balance training program to improve mobility and reduce falls in elderly patients • > 60 years, attendees at a falls clinic, Berg balance scale score < 45 • n = 198, 133 (67%) completed study • 6 months	• Intervention group: individual enhanced balance training sessions (conventional therapy plus additional progressive balance activities) up to 45 minutes by physiotherapists, 2 × week for 6 weeks • Control group: conventional physiotherapy sessions (no defined repetition of tasks or progressive grading in complexity) 2 × week for 4 weeks then 2 weeks of telephone follow-up	• Structured observation schedules (random selection of participants) showed that the protocol was being adhered to in all 48 receiving enhanced balance training and 55 receiving conventional therapy	• Both groups showed improvement in 10 metre timed walk test, Berg balance scale, Frenchay activities index, falls handicap inventory, and EuroQol scores • More people reported increased confidence in walking indoors and outdoors in the enhanced balance training group	• No difference between the 2 groups in number of falls in the previous month at baseline compared with 6 weeks, or baseline compared with 6 months • Significant reduction in number of falls per month for both groups	• Pretest/post-test analysis of falls

Continued

Table 9.1 *(Continued)*

Article, study aims, sample, number in study, duration	Interventions	Adherence to exercise programs	Intermediate and other effects	Effect on falls and fall injuries	Comments
• Suzuki *et al.* 2004[41]: • To examine the effectiveness of an intervention designed to improve overall function as a means of preventing falls • Women aged 73 to 90 years, living at home, attended a geriatric health check • n = 52, 44 (85%) included in analysis • 20 months	• Intervention group: exercise class (warm up and stretching; muscle strengthening of legs, waist and abdomen; balance and gait training; resistance; 24-form Yang tai chi) 10 1-hour sessions every 2 weeks for 6 months plus individualized home program (2 or 3 sets of the 15 exercises learned in the last session mailed monthly for 8 months) 3 × week, 30 minutes per day • Control group: pamphlet and advice on falls prevention	• Average rate of attendance at exercise classes was 64% (range 64% to 86%) • 15 (54%) attended all group sessions, 21 of 22 attended more than 7 sessions • Home exercise session monitoring not mentioned	At 8 months: • Improvements in tandem walk, functional reach, and knee extension power, and enhanced self confidence (before and after comparison for intervention group only)	• Fewer fallers in exercise group (3 of 22 vs. 12 of 22, $P = 0.0097$)	• Low sample size and event rate
• Toulotte *et al.* 2003[42]: • To examine the effects of a general physical training program on the physical capacity of frail elderly people who were demented and had a history of falls, with the aim of preventing falls • Mean age 81.4 (SD 4.7) years, Residents of institution, fall(s) during previous 3 months, Mini-Mental state score < 21 • n = 20, no analysis of falls • 16 weeks	• Intervention group: 2 supervised 1-hour sessions a week for 16 weeks (5 per group, exercises for muscle strengthening, proprioception, static and dynamic balance, and flexibility) • Control group: no active intervention	• A participant occasionally refused to take part in an exercise during a session, although agreeing to do the same exercise in a previous session	• Significant improvements in tests for walking, mobility, flexibility, and static balance in the exercise group but not in control group	• Numbers of falls in the 2 groups provided (no falls in intervention group, 6 falls in control group) but too few for statistical comparison	• Promising improvement of static balance in elderly patients with dementia with a program of physical training

• Wolf *et al.* 1996[43]: • To evaluate the effects of tai chi and computerized balance training on specified indicators of frailty and the occurrence of falls • ≥ 70 years, living independently in the community • n = 200, all included in falls analysis • From 7 to 20 months	• Intervention group 1: group tai chi 45-minute classes 2 × week for 15 weeks; also instructed to practise tai chi 2 × day for 15 minutes • Intervention group 2: one on one computerized balance training one day a week for 15 weeks • Control group: 1-hour discussion of topics of interest to older people once a week for 15 weeks	• Participants who missed class were rescheduled for next session or to make them up individually • Tai chi home practice sessions not monitored	At 4 months: • Grip strength declined in all groups ($P = 0.025$) • People in tai chi group were less afraid of falling than control group ($P = 0.046$)	• Tai chi (n = 72) reduced risk of all falls by 47.5% compared with remainder (n = 64 balance training, n = 64 control group) (adjusted relative hazard ratio 0.525; 95% CI, 0.321 to 0.860)	• Authors considered tai chi warranted further investigation as an exercise treatment to improve the health of older people
• Wolf *et al.* 2003[44]: • To determine whether an intense tai chi program could reduce the risk of falls more than a wellness education program in older adults transitioning to frailty • ≥ 70 years from congregate living facilities, use of 10 attributes to define not "vigorous" and not "frail" • n = 311, 286 (92%) included in analysis • 48 weeks	• Intervention group: "intense" tai chi (6 of the 24 forms) 60-minute progressing to 90-minute sessions ("work" time increased from 10 to 50 minutes) 2 × week for 48 weeks • Control group: wellness education (general advice about falls prevention, exercise and balance, diet and nutrition, pharmacological management, legal issues relevant to health, changes in body function, and mental health issues) 1 hour per week for 48 weeks (comparable contact time to intervention group)	• 69 of 286 (24%) did not complete the intervention (37 from tai chi and 32 from control group) • Average attendance in tai chi group was 76% (SD 19%), range 6–100% of sessions; control group 81% (SD 17%), range 10–100% of sessions	• Not reported	• No difference in risk of falling (all falls, relative hazard adjusted for center 0.75; 95% CI, 0.52 to 1.08) • Tai chi group had a lower risk of falls from month 5 through month 12 (relative hazard adjusted for center 0.61; 95% CI, 0.40 to 0.94)	• Effectiveness of "intense" tai chi in frail people may not reach the level seen in robust older adults taking part in less intense tai chi (Wolf *et al.* 1996[43]) • No adverse events occurred during either intervention • Wellness education program may have motivated participants to become more physically active and make other lifestyle changes affecting falls risk

* Same home exercise program (Otago Exercise Programme[56]) as in Campbell *et al.* 1997.[17]

Table 9.2 Results from studies reporting costs of intervention and health-care resource use

Article, study sample, length of time falls monitored	Interventions and number being compared, length of intervention phase	Type of currency, year of costs, time period costs measured	Cost items measured	Intervention costs	Health-care service costs	Measures of cost-effectiveness
• Buchner *et al.* 1997[16]: • Patients from a HMO, mild deficits in strength and balance, mean age 75 years • Up to 25 months	• Center-based endurance training and/or strength training (n = 75) vs. no active intervention (n = 30) • Supervised for 24–26 weeks then self supervised	• US dollars • Randomization 1992–1993 • Period 7–18 months after randomization	• Hospital costs, ancillary outpatient costs (from HMO computerized records)		• Hospitalized control participants more likely to have hospital costs > $5000 ($P < 0.05$)	
• Mulrow *et al.* 1994[31]: • Residents (≥ 3 months) from 9 nursing homes; dependent in ≥ 2 activities of daily living; mean age intervention group 79.7 (SD 8.5) years, control group 81.4 (SD 7.9) years • 4 months	• One on one sessions with physical therapist (n = 97) vs. friendly visits (n = 97) • 4 months	• US dollars • Participants recruited 1992 • 4 months from study entry	• Intervention charges (wages and fringe benefits for personnel time, travel expenses, equipment based on annual depreciation, overhead costs) • Nursing home, hospitalization, physician, and other health professional visits, emergency department visits, procedures, and medication charges (estimated from reimbursement fees, reference prices, and prevailing allowable charges)	• Mean charge per intervention participant $1220 (95% CI, $412 to $1832) • Mean charge per control participant $189 (95% CI, $80 to $298)	• Mean per participant (excluding intervention costs) $11,398; 95% CI, $10,929 to $11,849, no difference between groups	

• Robertson *et al.* 2001[19] (effectiveness of the intervention is reported in Campbell *et al.*[17] and Campbell *et al.*[18]): • Women from 17 general practices, mean age 84.1 (SD 3.3) years • Up to 2 years	• Specific set of muscle strengthening and balance retraining exercises individually prescribed at home* by physiotherapist during 4 visits plus monthly phone calls (n = 116) vs. social visits and usual care (n = 117) • Up to 2 years	• New Zealand dollars • 1995 prices • During participation in trial	• Intervention costs (recruitment, program delivery, overheads) • Health-care costs resulting from falls during trial (actual costs of hospital admissions and outpatient services, estimates of general practice and other costs) • Total health-care resource use during trial (actual costs of hospital admissions and outpatient services)	In research setting: • $173 per person in year 1 • $22 per person in year 2	• No difference between the 2 groups for health-care costs resulting from falls or for total health-care costs • 27% of hospital admission costs resulted from falls during trial	For 1 year: • $314 per fall prevented (program implementation costs only) For 2 years: • $265 per fall prevented (program implementation costs only)
• Robertson *et al.* 2001[36]: • From 17 general practices, community living, mean (SD) age 80.9 (4.2) years • 1 year	• Specific set of muscle strengthening and balance retraining exercises individually prescribed at home* by trained district nurse during 5 visits plus monthly phone calls, supervised by physiotherapist (n = 121) vs. usual care (n = 119) • 1 year	• New Zealand dollars • 1998 prices • During participation in trial	• Intervention costs (training course, recruitment, program delivery, supervision of exercise instructor, overheads) • Hospital admission costs resulting from fall injuries during trial (actual costs of hospital admissions)	In community health service setting: • $432 per person for 1 year	• 5 hospital admissions due to fall injuries in control group, none in exercise group (cost savings of $47,818)	• $1803 per fall prevented (program implementation costs only) • $155 per fall prevented for 2 years (program implementation costs and hospital admission cost savings)

HMO, health maintenance organization.
*Same home exercise program (Otago Exercise Programme[56]) as in Campbell *et al.* 1997.[17]

Study designs

All 27 trials stated that either individuals, local districts, hospital wards, senior centers, retirement villages, or long-term care facilities were randomly allocated to intervention or control groups, but in only seven trials were details provided to describe random number sequence generation and to indicate that the sequence was concealed until after group assignment. In 12 trials, there was no mention of the randomization process. Most (23 of the 27) trials had a parallel-group prospective design, with falls recorded at least monthly by self-reporting or incident forms. The four trials with a pretest/post-test analysis compared the number of falls either in the month, 2 months, or 12 months before baseline with those during the trial.[32,35,38,40] Since recall of falls is known to be inaccurate,[49,50] diaries or postcard calendars filled in daily are recommended.

There were a variety of definitions of a fall used in the trials, while nine of the trials did not provide a definition. One trial used two different definitions[43] and one trial cited references for two conflicting definitions.[23] Length of monitoring of falls varied from three of 25 months. In 10 studies, the period of falls monitoring extended past the end of the intervention phase of the study; the length of the postintervention phase ranged from 3 of 16 months.[23–26,30,32,38,40,41,43] One study reported falls for the second 6 months (postintervention phase) of the study only.[26] The incidence rate of falls can be seasonal, so that at least 1 year is regarded as the optimum time for monitoring falls in intervention studies.

In 22 studies, the control group was involved in an activity not likely to reduce falls, or received routine care. Two trials compared conventional physiotherapy with a physical therapy program designed to enhance strength[22] or balance,[40] one compared participants receiving a home program with those who attended additional group sessions,[24] and two tested exercises in a workstation format[32] or the addition of treadmill gait exercises[39] compared with traditional community based exercise classes.

Study samples and settings

The total number of participants in the 27 trials was 5169 with sample sizes ranging from 16 to 1090 participants. Four studies investigated the effect of exercise in women only[17,18,23,27,35] and one included men only.[37] Eleven studies reported including people aged 60–70 years,[15,16,20,25,27,28,30,31,34,38,40] and in one study participants were aged 80 years and older.[17,18]

The majority of studies (16 of the 27) involved independent, community-dwelling older people, three were in those living in retirement or congregate living facilities,[28,35,44] and three in long-term care residents.[31,33,38] Other trials recruited participants from hospital wards,[22] a falls clinic,[40] a geriatric rehabilitation outpatient unit,[23] or participants were a combination of long-term care residents or outpatients and those living independently in their own homes.[39,42] In 17 studies, one or more risk factors for falls, such as reporting a fall in the previous year or assessment scores indicating impaired physical function, were used as entry criteria, whereas the remaining 10 studies recruited a more general sample. One study each recruited consecutive hospital patients,[22] participants who had previously been selected randomly for an ongoing epidemiological study,[27] or a random selection from a health-maintenance organization.[12]

Analysis and reporting of results

The formal quality assessment summary scores for the 27 trials ranged from 0.55 to 0.88 of the possible total score. In addition, we noted that a prestudy sample size calculation was reported for only 12 of the trials, so that it was sometimes unclear whether the trial was considered powered for falls or an intermediate outcome. It was common for all falls to be recorded during the trial, but only the first fall for each participant to be used in analyzing for efficacy of the exercise program, thus wasting useful information. The aim of a falls prevention program is to reduce the number of falls, so that the use of time to first fall, or the proportion of fallers versus nonfallers as outcomes, limits the value of the study.

Statistical approaches used for testing the efficacy of the exercise program and the manner in which the results were reported differed. Although use of an intention-to-treat analysis was often stated, data from all the study participants were not always included in the analysis. It is important to take into account variable individual follow-up times since bias will result if the total time falls are monitored in the exercise and control groups differs. Statistical techniques are available for including all falls in the analysis right up until the time the person withdraws from the study, dies, or completes the study.[51] These techniques take into account individual follow-up times, the nonnormal (Poisson type) distribution of falls, and can adjust for clustering in the study design.

A checklist for reporting randomized controlled trials is available from CONSORT,[52] and recommendations for reporting and analyzing factorial[53] and cluster-randomized[54] trials are available. The international collaborative group Prevention of Falls Network Europe (ProFaNE) has published recommendations for measuring outcomes and reporting results in falls prevention trials.[55] It is important to consider these recommendations and appropriate analytical techniques at the trial design stage.

In the following sections, we have concentrated our comments particularly on the efficacy of the exercise program in reducing falls, on the 19 studies reporting an analysis of fall events during the complete trial period for more than 50 participants, in order to avoid undue emphasis on studies perhaps more correctly described as pilot trials.

Effects of exercise programs on falls and injuries

A significant reduction in the number of all falls during the study was demonstrated in six of the nine studies with analysis of multiple falls and adjustment for variable monitoring time of individuals in the trial.[15–18,28,36,43] The relative reduction in the number of falls achieved for those receiving the exercise program compared with the control group ranged from 22% to 47.5%. The remaining 10 trials with an analysis of fall data for more than 50 participants, presented results based on the first fall per person during the trial. One of these 10 studies showed a significant, 18% reduction in the risk of having at least one fall during the trial as a result of the exercise program.[21] All seven successful trials involved independent, community living people, with selection criteria based on falls risk used in three of the trials.[15–18] In two successful trials, the exercise program (the Otago Exercise Programme[56]) was delivered individually at home by a physiotherapist or a community nurse trained and closely supervised by a physiotherapist,[17,18,36] and the remaining five successful exercise programs were center based.[15,16,21,28,43] Improvements in scores for physical function assessments, when reported, did not guarantee a reduction in falls.

Owing to the low number of serious fall injury events such as fractures, the studies, even in meta-analyses, lacked sufficient power to determine whether exercise had a beneficial effect on serious fall injury risk.[47,48] One study reported a significant reduction in moderate injuries in the exercise group compared with the control group at 1 year[17] and 2 years,[18] and one reported a reduction in serious injuries.[36]

Exercise program components

The interventions included muscle strengthening or resistance, balance and gait training, aerobic, endurance, coordination, functional task training, flexibility, stretching, and relaxation exercises; computerized balance platform or treadmill training; tai chi; the "stand up/step down" procedure; and walking, as well as combinations of these activities. Most were a specific set of exercises beginning with a warm up, with a set number of repetitions or time allocated for each exercise. Two programs were described as "high-intensity,"[23,25] one as "intense,"[44] and one as "low-intensity."[34] In the group exercise programs, class sizes were generally small (five to nine participants). The qualifications or training of the instructors were not always reported, but included physiotherapists, "trained" exercise physiologists, postgraduate exercise physiology students, "experienced" tai chi instructors, physicians, and nurses, with specific training programs of up to a week.

The exercise programs in the seven successful studies can all be described as "moderate" intensity.[15–18,21,36,43] Successful programs included at least four of the following seven features:

1 Strengthening exercises carried out against resistance (ankle cuff weights, Thera-Bands, weights machines).
2 Dynamic balance exercises and/or tai chi.
3 Endurance or aerobic exercises or walking outside.
4 At least some exercises based on activities of daily living (chair stands, stair climbing, reaching, weight transference).
5 Coordination activities (dance steps, ball games).
6 Individual tailoring of exercises to the person's functional ability.
7 Progression in the difficulty and complexity of the set of exercises.

The frequency of the successful group exercise sessions ranged from 1 hour per week with participants also encouraged to exercise at home,[21] to 1 hour, three times a week.[16] In the three randomized controlled trials of the Otago Exercise Programme, participants were expected to exercise at least three times a week (about 30 min per session) and to walk, if walking outside could be done safely, at least twice a week for 30 minutes.[17,18,20,36]

Adherence to exercise programs

An exercise program may be designed to address the common risk factors for falls, but adherence to the program is critical for its success. Most studies reported adherence although some did not give specific details; there was no standard definition of adherence or standard method of measurement. Adherence was measured using exercise calendars filled in daily by the participant, or by recording the number of group sessions attended. One study reported the average increase of weight training loads at 6 months as an indication of adherence[16] and another assessed a random selection of participants using a structured observation schedule.[40] Adherence after exercising for 1 and 2 years will provide a better indication of program acceptability than measures after shorter time periods. One trial reported 27% (31 of 116) of participants from the original sample of 233 still carrying out exercise sessions at least three times a week at 2 years.[18]

Programs should be acceptable to older people to ensure adherence, and this needs to be considered at the exercise program design stage.[57] One program included both exercise calendars and monthly telephone contact from the instructor as part of the program protocol with the aim of maintaining motivation.[56] It is not known whether a home-based or group approach is more acceptable to older people and it may differ from individual to individual. Offering a choice of both approaches may enhance adherence.

Adverse effects of exercise

Several studies briefly addressed adverse events.[16,23,27,31,32,36–38,44] Examples included statements that "exercise-related injuries were infrequent and not an important cause of dropouts"[16] and that "The exercise program was found to be safe, with no medical incidents occurring [during group exercise]."[27]

Only two studies included an in-depth investigation of potential adverse events in the study design. Adverse effects of exercise in long-term care residents were monitored by research assistants, blinded to group assignment.[31] There were no significant differences in severe soreness, bruising, and fatigue between participants receiving physical therapy and those in the control group. Intervention participants reported moderate muscle soreness at 7% of the physical therapy sessions, but physical therapists reported no injuries during the exercises. In the home-based study of high-intensity strength training by Latham *et al.*, coding of adverse events was by blinded assessors.[25] All participants were also asked to rate their degree of pain every week using a four-point Likert scale. After the 10-week intervention of quadriceps exercise against resistance, participants in the exercise group had more episodes of back or knee pain which was directly attributable to the exercises, a significant increase in self reported fatigue, and lower scores in the vitality component of the SF-36, compared with controls. Exercise programs of *moderate* intensity can be carried out safely in older people with moderate disability and intact cognitive functioning, and also in frail institutionalized older people with intact cognitive functioning, under careful supervision from a physiotherapist.

Economic evaluation within the studies

Three of the studies reviewed reported the cost of the intervention in the article[31,36] or in a subsequent publication.[19] One study reported hospital admission costs as a result of fall injuries during the trial,[19] and three studies included total health-care service costs as outcome measures in the trial.[16,19,31] For two of the trials, a comprehensive economic evaluation was carried out and the cost-effectiveness of the intervention established.[19,36] The authors limited the time horizon to the duration of the trials and did not attempt to forecast costs or consequences of the intervention into the future. Table 9.2 provides a summary of the results.

One study reported the charge for the physical therapy intervention delivered to nursing home residents and estimated health-care costs for all participants during the four month trial.[31] Buchner *et al.*[16] estimated health-care use and costs after the first 6 months of the trial because exercise participants (but not controls) were asked to delay elective procedures until the end of the supervised exercise period. Hospital use was similar in both exercise and control groups, but control participants were more likely to spend more than three days in hospital. One study showed that fall-related injuries accounted for a substantial proportion (27%) of all hospital admission costs for study participants during the two year trial.[19]

The cost-effectiveness of the Otago Exercise Programme has been established in the research setting,[19] and in two routine health-care settings—a community health service[36] and general practices.[46] In the trial of this intervention in those aged 75 years and older in a community health-service setting, this program was shown to be more cost-effective in a higher risk group.[36] There were fewer serious injuries in the exercise group resulting from a fall during the trial ($P = 0.033$), and this resulted in health-care cost savings for those 80 years and over receiving the program.

Discussion

We reviewed published results of randomized controlled trials of exercise programs used alone as an intervention aimed at reducing falls, or reducing the risk of falls and falls-related injuries. We found 27 trials meeting our criteria, 19 of which reported analysis of fall data from more than 50 participants. Seven of these 19 trials reported a statistically significant reduction in the number of falls (rate or risk of falls reduced by 22% to 47.5%) or fallers (18%) in the exercise compared with the control group during the trial. Our findings update those of previous systematic reviews of falls prevention interventions by other authors, but the overall findings concerning exercise programs are similar.[5,14,58,59]

Implications of the evidence

We found good evidence that appropriate exercise programs can decrease the number of falls both in carefully selected and general groups of older people. The study by Latham *et al.* provides a cautionary message here.[25] More harm than benefit resulted from prescribing a high-intensity quadriceps strengthening exercise to patients leaving hospital. In all other studies, the exercise program appeared safe and acceptable to participants. In one study, effectiveness continued for a second year in those who continued to exercise.[18]

There is a need to identify which components of an exercise program are most effective in lowering falls risk. A wide variety of types of exercise interventions have been tested using different combinations of frequency and duration of sessions. Studies successfully lowering falls have used a home-based strength and balance retraining program, a center based endurance and strengthening program with individual supervision, and small groups or community exercise classes carrying out combinations of strength, balance, and functional activities, or tai chi. A meta-analysis of the seven FICSIT exercise trials suggests balance may be more effective in lowering falls risk than the other exercise components.[48]

The Otago Exercise Programme[56] has now been tested in four controlled trials, and a total of 608 men and women from 64 general practices in nine centers in New Zealand have received the program.[17,18,20,36,46] A meta-analysis showed that overall in the four trials, both the number of falls and the number of injuries (serious and moderate combined) were reduced by 35%.[47] This moderate intensity program resulted in the greatest absolute reduction in falls and injuries in those aged 80 or over with a previous fall.

The authors consider that the following factors contribute to the success of the program:

- The program is individually tailored and prescribed by a trained health professional.
- The specific set of exercises stress both strength and balance (ankle cuff weights from 1 to 8 kg are used for resistance; dynamic balance exercises are used).
- The exercises progress in difficulty and complexity.
- The exercises include functional activities and a walking plan is included if appropriate.
- Supervision of instructors by an experienced physiotherapist maintains the quality of program delivery.
- Participants were invited to take part by their general practitioner.
- Exercise calendars, and monthly phone calls throughout the year from the instructor, help to maintain motivation.
- Clients can include home-bound frail people, who have more to gain from the program than fitter people in terms of improving strength and balance above critical thresholds required for stability in carrying out daily activities.

We suggest that researchers make their successful exercise program details available for those running falls prevention programs in both community and institutional settings. The Otago Exercise Programme, our home program of muscle strengthening and balance retraining exercises, has now been published in manual form and can be ordered by health professionals from the ACC New Zealand web site (www.acc.co.nz).[56] Publication of successful programs in a practical, low-cost format may go some way to discourage the current widespread use of programs with no evidence for effectiveness.

Study factors diminishing benefit

Twelve of 19 studies reported no statistically significant reduction in falls compared with the control activity, although reductions in falls from 1% to 79% were reported in nine of these 12 trials. We consider that the following factors contributed to effectiveness not reaching statistical significance. Most negative studies lacked sufficient power to detect a reduction in falls, even in some that stated falls were a primary outcome measure. In several trials, the study numbers were low, particularly in those in which the control group activity was also likely to reduce falls, or where follow-up time was short and therefore the number of falls was low. Some studies extended the time for monitoring falls long after any beneficial effects of the intervention would be expected. The exercise programs used may have been of inadéquate intensity to modify falls risk factors, as demonstrated by the lack of a significant change in intermediate variables. Exercise may be less effective in fall prevention when there are other significant risk factors for falls present that are not influenced by exercise. For example, in a younger sample of men and women on psychotropic drugs, exercise was less effective in reducing falls than in older, frailer populations.[20,36] One study reported modest improvements in physical function following one on one physical therapy targeted at frail nursing home residents, but with no effect on falls.[31] While intermediate outcomes improve in frail institutionalized elderly people following high-intensity strength training,[60] falls may not decrease because other risk factors may not improve. Lastly, study compliance or exercise adherence may have been too low across the sample as a whole when analyzed on an intention-to-treat basis. Using the first fall only for each participant in the analysis did not optimize power in these studies.

Exercise as a component of multifactorial interventions

There is good evidence that exercises are of value in falls prevention when part of a comprehensive package, in the community, long-term care settings, and hospital wards.[61–63] The components of these exercise programs are the same as in successful exercise programs used as the only intervention. However if a multifactorial intervention is successful in reducing falls, it is not possible to determine which of the components contributed to the success. Tinetti *et al.* investigated the effectiveness of a multifactorial intervention program on the number of falls risk factors and concluded that a change in balance score of 1 (possible scores ranged from 0 to 12) was associated with an 11% reduction in the fall rate.[64] It is probable that in this particular trial, the exercise program would have had the greatest effect on balance.

One particular group of elderly people, those with cognitive impairment or dementia, remain a challenge. One multifactorial study aimed the intervention specifically at this group and recorded improved gait speed, reduced environmental hazards and carotid cardioinhibitory sinus hypersensitivity, but there was no reduction in the number of falls.[65]

Health-care resource use

We would encourage researchers to report the cost-effectiveness of their falls prevention interventions. It is important that decision-makers and health-care providers take into account both costs of delivery and the benefits of the program when considering various possible fall prevention initiatives. If exercise programs are effective in reducing falls and injuries resulting from falls, it follows that a reduction in health-care service use could result, but studies reporting health-care costs lacked adequate power to demonstrate cost savings. However, two studies did report a reduction in health-care use as a result of the intervention.[16,36] Reductions in falls should reduce the number of fall-related injuries but there may be a difference in the degree of reduction. An exercise program may improve protective responses at the time of the fall. A long-term exercise program may improve bone mineral density. On the one hand, a fitter, quicker group of elderly people may fall at greater speed while about their daily activities.[66] On the other hand, active older people may spend less time in hospital.[16]

Conclusions

The wide variety of exercise interventions tried does enable us to draw some conclusions. Appropriate exercise programs can decrease the number of falls and fall risk in randomized controlled trials of community dwelling people but certain conditions need to be met. For maximum effect the population needs to be right—not too fit and not too frail. With increasing age, there is a progressive loss of muscle strength and stability, but the weakness needs to reach a certain point or threshold before daily functions are affected. It is possible that around this threshold small increases in strength have a disproportionate effect on function, and exercise programs are most effective. There is trial evidence that the same exercises used in younger populations have not been as effective as in older groups.[47]

Exercise interventions used on their own have not yet been shown to lower the risk of falling in people in institutions, but have been a component of successful multifactorial interventions in long-term care and in a hospital setting.[62,63,67]

Although the most common components of successful exercise programs to reduce falls were moderate-intensity strength training against resistance and dynamic balance retraining, a similar proportion of unsuccessful programs also included these exercises. The unsuccessful studies were more likely to have a smaller sample size, shorter intervention phase, shorter follow-up time, a higher dropout rate, or recruited younger participants at a lower risk of falling.

The exercises need to be of sufficient intensity to improve muscle strength. We suggest that most investigators, including ourselves, initially underestimated the capacity of older people to manage weights. Balance retraining should be an important component of any exercise program designed to decrease falls. This may consist of specific dynamic balance retraining exercises or be a component of a movement form such as tai chi. Exercising needs to be regular and sustainable. There is no good evidence of benefit beyond the period of the exercises, but continued participation can lead to sustained lower fall risk at least up to 2 years.[18]

Summary

- Seven of the studies reviewed provided good evidence that exercise programs delivered at home or in a group setting can reduce falls in community dwelling older people.

• Successful programs were of moderate intensity and used various combinations of strength and balance retraining exercises, endurance training, tai chi, and activities to improve coordination and reaction time.
• There were no successful exercise programs used alone for falls prevention in long-term care facilities or hospital wards.

The exercises may be performed at a center or at home. Home exercises are suitable for a frail, less mobile population without easy access to transport. They are safe if properly established by a trained instructor, but the supervision is less than with a center-based program. A center-based program does have the additional value of social interaction, which has important beneficial effects in its own right.[68]

If the exercises are part of a public health program to be introduced widely in the community, they should be simple, easily instituted, and low cost. Elderly people involved in falls prevention exercise programs are prone to intercurrent illness, accident, and social change. Programs need to have the resources to reassess and restart. They should also be planned for long term use. If the exercises are part of a program of falls prevention in a person presenting with falls, then the exercises must be part of a full assessment of the person's risk factors and treatment. Exercises are of value in falls prevention when part of a comprehensive package.[61]

Summary

• Negative studies were more likely to be as a result of inadequate power than differences in the exercise program components.
• This makes it difficult to contrast positive and negative studies in order to determine the types of exercises contributing to effectiveness.
• No falls prevention study with an exercise intervention used alone has had sufficient power to demonstrate conclusively a reduction in serious fall injuries such as fractures.
• Two exercise interventions have been associated with reduced health-care resource use.

More trials are required to determine the combination of exercise type, frequency, duration, and intensity most effective in lowering falls risk in different groups of older people. However, the effectiveness of new exercise programs in reducing falls would need to be tested against existing programs and large study numbers would be needed to show any increased benefit from the new program. Alternatively, studies could use intermediate outcomes such as compliance or strength and balance measures, but these were not always predictive of success in reducing falls in the studies included in this review. It is important to establish the cost-effectiveness of new programs and ensure ease of replication beyond the research setting.

Exercise programs designed to prevent falls in older people have two important advantages. Falls are very common, so programs are likely to be cost-effective when compared with other public health measures in this population. Exercise is also beneficial to the participants in additional ways such as decreasing fear of falling, improving functional reserve by increasing strength and in improving other important health areas as varied as cardiovascular health,[69] sleep,[70] depression,[71] mortality,[69] and quality of life.[72]

Summary

• Exercise programs of moderate intensity can be carried out safely by older people living independently in the community and by long term care residents.

• Exercise sessions must be regular and sustained to be effective.
• More quality trials are required to determine the combination of exercise type, frequency, duration, and intensity most effective in reducing falls in different subgroups of older people.

Key messages

• Many different risk factors contribute to falls, but muscle weakness and poor balance underlie most falls.
• The most common components of successful exercise programs to reduce falls are moderate-intensity strength training against resistance and dynamic balance retraining, but there are insufficient good-quality negative studies to determine whether some types of exercises are ineffective.
• Exercise programs that are individually tailored, progress in difficulty, and target carefully selected groups at high risk have so far resulted in the greatest absolute reduction in falls and injuries.
• Those running falls prevention programs in particular settings or subgroups of older people should use evidence-based interventions.
• To facilitate this, researchers should make the necessary program details available.

Acknowledgments

The authors are grateful to Lesley Gillespie for the literature searches and to the Cochrane Collaboration Musculoskeletal Injuries Group for quality assessment of the included trials. We thank the authors who contributed additional information for the review. Melinda Gardner was an author in two previous versions of this review.

The authors were investigators for three of the trials included in the review.

Sample examination questions

Multiple-choice questions (answers on p. 602)

1 Falls prevention exercise programs work on which of the following premises?
  A Muscle strength and balance are common risk factors for falls
  B Exercise must be continued to be effective
  C Only fit elderly people should take part
  D Strength training should be a gentle, optional extra exercise
2 Proven benefits of exercise programs in older people to date include:
  A Decreased fear of falling
  B Reduced admissions to rest home
  C Improved functional independence
  D Reduced hip fractures
3 In a systematic review on falls prevention, which electronic databases would be searched?
  A Web of Science
  B Ovid
  C Generator
  D Cochrane Database of Systematic Reviews

Essay questions

1 Are falls prevention interventions that target multiple risk factors in older people more effective than those that target single risk factors?

2 Discuss the advantages and disadvantages of high-intensity, high-frequency exercise interventions compared with low-intensity to moderate-intensity and frequency programs designed to prevent falls and injuries in older people.
3 Design a program you consider would be successful in reducing falls, and a protocol to assess the effectiveness of the program, for frail institutionalized elderly people. Would this program be suitable for residents with cognitive impairment?

Case study 9.1

P.S., a 65-year-old woman, presents to her general practitioner with a painful wrist. She is normally fit and well and on no medications except for the occasional sleeping tablet. She was on her way to visit the optometrist when she tripped on the kerb and put her hand out to break the fall.

Case study 9.2

A.M., an 83-year-old woman, is admitted from a nursing home following a fall with a resulting fractured neck of the femur. Her history is obtained from the nursing staff, as A.M. suffers from mild dementia. She is normally fit and active and independent with activities of daily living (ADLs). Usual medications include: gliclazide, calcitriol, digoxin, metoprolol, doxepin, and furosemide. According to the staff, A.M. never lost consciousness, but collapsed when trying to rise from a chair using one crutch. She landed on her left hip, immediately complaining of pain, and was unable to walk. She said she was not dizzy or nauseated at the time of the fall.

Case study 9.3

J.K., a 78-year-old man, was found by his wife unconscious on the floor of the bathroom. He had a wound to his forehead. He has a history of angina, heart disease, heart failure, chronic obstructive respiratory disease (CORD), non-insulin-dependent diabetes mellitus (NIDDM), all poorly controlled on maximal therapy. He recently gave up smoking, but still drinks one or two pints of beer a day. His wife has observed that he has been less active of late, with weight loss and reduced appetite for 6 months. Medications include digoxin, furosemide, captopril, temazepam, glyceryl trinitrate (GTN) spray, prednisone, salbutamol (Ventolin) and beclomethasone (Becotide) inhalers, and insulin.

References

1 Campbell AJ, Reinken J, Allan BC, Martinez GS. Falls in old age: a study of frequency and related clinical factors. *Age Ageing* 1981; **10**:264–270.
2 Tinetti ME, Williams CS. Falls, injuries due to falls, and the risk of admission to a nursing home. *N Engl J Med* 1997; **337**:1279–1284.
3 Donald IP, Bulpitt CJ. The prognosis of falls in elderly people living at home. *Age Ageing* 1999; **28**:121–125.
4 Rizzo JA, Friedkin R, Williams CS, *et al.* Health care utilization and costs in a medicare population by fall status. *Med Care* 1998; **36**:1174–1188.
5 American Geriatrics Society, British Geriatrics Society, American Academy of Orthopaedic Surgeons Panel on Falls Prevention. Guideline for the prevention of falls in older persons. *J Am Geriatr Soc* 2001; **49**:664–672.
6 NHS National Institute for Clinical Excellence. Falls: the assessment and prevention of falls in older people. Clinical Guideline 21, November 2004. Available at: http://www.nice.org.uk/CG021NICEguideline (accessed May 2005).

7 Tinetti ME, Speechley M, Ginter SF. Risk factors for falls among elderly persons living in the community. *N Engl J Med* 1988; **319**:1701–1707.
8 Campbell AJ, Borrie MJ, Spears GF. Risk factors for falls in a community based prospective study of people 70 years and older. *J Gerontol Med Sci* 1989; **44**:M112–117.
9 Nevitt MC, Cummings SR, Hudes ES. Risk factors for injurious falls: a prospective study. *J Gerontol Med Sci* 1991; **46**:M164–170.
10 O'Loughlin JL, Robitaille Y, Boivin JF, Suissa S. Incidence of and risk factors for falls and injurious falls among the community-dwelling elderly. *Am J Epidemiol* 1993; **137**:342–534.
11 Fiatarone MA, Marks EC, Ryan ND, *et al.* High-intensity strength training in nonagenarians: effects on skeletal muscle. *JAMA* 1990; **263**:3029–3034.
12 Buchner DM, Beresford SA, Larson EB, LaCroix AZ, Wagner EH. Effects of physical activity on health status in older adults. II: intervention studies. *Annu Rev Public Health* 1992; **13**:469–488.
13 Gardner MM, Robertson MC, Campbell AJ. Exercise in preventing fall and fall related injuries in older people: a review of randomised controlled trials. *Br J Sports Med* 2000; **34**:7–17.
14 Gillespie LD, Gillespie WJ, Robertson MC, *et al.* Interventions for preventing falls in elderly people. *Cochrane Database Syst Rev* 2003; (**4**):CD000340.
15 Barnett A, Smith B, Lord SR, Williams M, Baumand A. Community-based group exercise improves balance and reduces falls in at-risk older people: a randomised controlled trial. *Age Ageing* 2003; **32**:407–414.
16 Buchner DM, Cress ME, de Lateur BJ, *et al.* The effect of strength and endurance training on gait, balance, fall risk, and health services use in community-living older adults. *J Gerontol Med Sci* 1997; **52A**:M218–224.
17 Campbell AJ, Robertson MC, Gardner MM, *et al.* Randomised controlled trial of a general practice programme of home based exercise to prevent falls in elderly women. *BMJ* 1997; **315**:1065–1069.
18 Campbell AJ, Robertson MC, Gardner MM, Norton RN, Buchner DM. Falls prevention over 2 years: a randomized controlled trial in women 80 years and older. *Age Ageing* 1999; **28**:513–518.
19 Robertson MC, Devlin N, Scuffham P, *et al.* Economic evaluation of a community based exercise programme to prevent falls. *J Epidemiol Community Health* 2001; **55**:600–606.
20 Campbell AJ, Robertson MC, Gardner MM, Norton RN, Buchner DM. Psychotropic medication withdrawal and a home-based exercise program to prevent falls: a randomized, controlled trial. *J Am Geriatr Soc* 1999; **47**:850–853.
21 Day L, Fildes B, Gordon I, *et al.* Randomised factorial trial of falls prevention among older poeple living in their own homes. *BMJ* 2002; **325**:128.
22 Donald IP, Pitt K, Armstrong E, Shuttleworth H. Preventing falls on an elderly care rehabilitation ward. *Clin Rehabil* 2000; **14**:178–185.
23 Hauer K, Rost B, Rütschle K, *et al.* Exercise training for rehabilitation and secondary prevention of falls in geriatric patients with a history of injurious falls. *J Am Geriatr Soc* 2001; **49**:10–20.
24 Helbostad JL, Sletvold O, Moe-Nilssen R. Effects of home exercises and group training on functional abilities in home-dwelling older persons with mobility and balance problems: a randomized study. *Aging Clin Exp Res* 2004; **16**:113–121.
25 Latham NK, Anderson CS, Lee A, *et al.* A randomized, controlled trial of quadriceps resistance exercise and vitamin D in frail older people: the Frailty Interventions Trial in Elderly Subjects (FITNESS). *J Am Geriatr Soc* 2003; **51**:291–299.
26 Li F, Harmer P, Fisher KJ, McAuley E. Tai Chi: improving functional balance and predicting subsequent falls in older persons. *Med Sci Sports Exerc* 2004; **36**:2046–2052.
27 Lord SR, Ward JA, Williams P, Strudwick M. The effect of a 12-month exercise trial on balance, strength, and falls in older women: a randomized controlled trial. *J Am Geriatr Soc* 1995; **43**:1198–1206.
28 Lord SR, Castell S, Corcoran J, *et al.* The effect of group exercise on physical functioning and falls in frail older people living in retirement villages: a Randomized, controlled trial. *J Am Geriatr Soc* 2003; **51**:1685–1692.
29 MacRae PG, Feltner ME, Reinsch S. A 1-year exercise program for older women: effects on falls, injuries, and physical performance. *J Aging Phys Activity* 1994; **2**:127–142.
30 Morgan RO, Virnig BA, Duque M, Abdel-Moty E, Devito CA. Low-intensity exercise and reduction of the risk for falls among at-risk elders. *J Gerontol Med Sci* 2004; **59**:1062–1067.
31 Mulrow CD, Gerety MB, Kanten D, *et al.* A randomized trial of physical rehabilitation for very frail nursing home residents. *JAMA* 1994; **271**:519–524.

32 Nitz JC, Choy NL. The efficacy of a specific balance-strategy training programme for preventing falls among older people: a pilot randomised controlled trial. *Age Ageing* 2004; **33**:52–58.
33 Nowalk MP, Prendergast JM, Bayles CM, D'Amico FJ, Colvin GC. A randomized trial of exercise programs among older individuals living in two long-term care facilities: the FallsFREE program. *J Am Geriatr Soc* 2001; **49**:859–865.
34 Reinsch S, MacRae P, Lachenbruch PA, Tobis JS. Attempts to prevent falls and injury: a prospective community study. *Gerontologist* 1992; **32**:450–456.
35 Resnick B. Testing the effect of the WALC intervention on exercise adherence in older adults. *J Gerontol Nurs* 2002; **28**:40–49.
36 Robertson MC, Devlin N, Gardner MM, Campbell AJ. Effectiveness and economic evaluation of a nurse delivered home exercise programme to prevent falls. 1: randomised controlled trial. *BMJ* 2001; **322**:697–701.
37 Rubenstein LZ, Josephson KR, Trueblood PR, *et al.* Effects of a group exercise program on strength, mobility, and falls among fall-prone elderly men. *J Gerontol Med Sci* 2000; **55A**:M317–321.
38 Schoenfelder DP. A fall prevention program for elderly individuals: exercise in long-term care settings. *J Gerontol Nurs* 2000; **26**:43–51.
39 Shimada H, Obuchi S, Furuna T, Suzuki T. New intervention program for preventing falls among frail elderly people: the effects of perturbed walking exercise using a bilateral separated treadmill. *Am J Phys Med Rehabil* 2004; **83**:493–499.
40 Steadman J, Donaldson N, Kalra L. A randomized controlled trial of an enhanced balance training program to improve mobility and reduce falls in elderly patients. *J Am Geriatr Soc* 2003; **51**:847–852.
41 Suzuki T, Kim H, Yoshida H, Ishizaki T. Randomized controlled trial of exercise intervention for the prevention of falls in community-dwelling elderly Japanese women. *J Bone Miner Metab* 2004; **22**:602–611.
42 Toulotte C, Fabre C, Dangremont B, Lensel G, Thevenon A. Effects of physical training on the physical capacity of frail, demented patients with a history of falling: a randomised controlled trial. *Age Ageing* 2003; **32**:67–73.
43 Wolf SL, Barnhart HX, Kutner NG, *et al.* Reducing frailty and falls in older persons: an investigation of Tai Chi and computerized balance training. *J Am Geriatr Soc* 1996; **44**:489–497.
44 Wolf SL, Sattin RW, Kutner M, *et al.* Intense tai chi exercise training and fall occurrences in older, transitionally frail adults: a randomized, controlled trial. *J Am Geriatr Soc* 2003; **51**:1693–1701.
45 Means KM, Rodell DE, O'Sullivan PS, Cranford LA. Rehabilitation of elderly fallers: pilot study of a low to moderate intensity exercise program. *Arch Phys Med Rehabil* 1996; **77**:1030–1036.
46 Robertson MC, Gardner MM, Devlin N, McGee R, Campbell AJ. Effectiveness and economic evaluation of a nurse delivered home exercise programme to prevent falls. 2: Controlled trial in multiple centres. *BMJ* 2001; **322**:701–704.
47 Robertson MC, Campbell AJ, Gardner MM, Devlin N. Preventing injuries in older people by preventing falls: a meta-analysis of individual-level data. *J Am Geriatr Soc* 2002; **50**:905–911.
48 Province MA, Hadley EC, Hornbrook MC, *et al.* The effects of exercise on falls in elderly patients: a preplanned meta-analysis of the FICSIT trials. *JAMA* 1995; **273**:1341–1347.
49 Cummings SR, Nevitt MC, Kidd S. Forgetting falls: the limited accuracy of recall of falls in the elderly. *J Am Geriatr Soc* 1988; **36**:613–616.
50 Hale WA, Delaney MJ, Cable T. Accuracy of patient recall and chart documentation of falls. *J Am Board Fam Pract* 1993; **6**:239–242.
51 Robertson MC, Campbell AJ, Herbison P. Statistical analysis of efficacy in falls prevention trials. *J Gerontol Med Sci* 2005; **60A**:530–534.
52 Moher D, Schulz KF, Altman DG, Group C. The CONSORT statement: revised recommendations for improving the quality of reports of parallel-group randomised trials. *Lancet* 2001; **357**:1191–1194.
53 McAlister FA, Straus SE, Sackett DL, Altman DG. Analysis and reporting of factorial trials: a systematic review. *JAMA* 2003; **289**:2545–2553.
54 Campbell MK, Elbourne DR, Altman DG, CONSORT group. CONSORT statement: extension to cluster randomised trials. *BMJ* 2004; **328**:702–708.
55 Lamb SE, Jorstad-Stein EC, Hauer K, *et al.* Development of a common outcome data set for fall injury prevention trials: the Prevention of Falls Network Europe consensus. *J Am Geriatr Soc* 2005;**53**:1618–1622.

56 Accident Compensation Corporation. Otago Exercise Programme to prevent falls in older adults. August 2003. Available at: http://www.acc.co.nz/otagoexerciseprogramme (accessed November 2006).
57 Gardner MM, Robertson MC, McGee R, Campbell AJ. Application of a falls prevention program for older people to primary health care practice. *Prev Med* 2002; **34**:546–553.
58 Chang JT, Morton SC, Rubenstein LZ, *et al.* Interventions for the prevention of falls in older adults: systematic review and meta-analysis of randomised clinical trials. *BMJ* 2004; **328**:680.
59 Sherrington C, Lord SR, Finch CF. Physical activity interventions to prevent falls among older people: update of the evidence. *J Sci Med Sport* 2004; **7**(1 Suppl):43–51.
60 Fiatarone MA, O'Neill EF, Ryan ND, *et al.* Exercise training and nutritional supplementation for physical frailty in very elderly people. *N Engl J Med* 1994; **330**:1769–1775.
61 Tinetti ME, Baker DI, McAvay G, *et al.* A multifactorial intervention to reduce the risk of falling among elderly people living in the community. *N Engl J Med* 1994; **331**:821–827.
62 Becker C, Kron M, Lindemann U, *et al.* Effectiveness of a multifaceted intervention on falls in nursing home residents. *J Am Geriatr Soc* 2003; **51**:306–313.
63 Haines TP, Bennell KL, Osborne RH, Hill KD. Effectiveness of targeted falls prevention programme in subacute hospital setting: randomised controlled trial. *BMJ* 2004; **328**:676.
64 Tinetti ME, McAvay G, Claus E. Does multiple risk factor reduction explain the reduction in fall rate in the Yale FICSIT trial? *Am J Epidemiol* 1996; **144**:389–399.
65 Shaw FE, Bond J, Richardson DA, *et al.* Multifactorial intervention after a fall in older people with cognitive impairment and dementia presenting to the accident and emergency department: randomised controlled trial. *BMJ* 2003; **326**:73.
66 Speechley M, Tinetti M. Falls and injuries in frail and vigorous community elderly persons. *J Am Geriatr Soc* 1991; **39**:46–52.
67 Jensen J, Lundin-Olsson L, Nyberg L, Gustafson Y. Fall and injury prevention in older people living in residential care facilities: a cluster randomized trial. *Ann Intern Med* 2002; **136**:733–741.
68 Glass TA, de Leon CM, Marottoli RA, Berkman LF. Population based study of social and productive activities as predictors of survival among elderly Americans. *BMJ* 1999; **319**:478–483.
69 U.S. Department of Health and Human Services. *Physical Activity and Health: a Report of the Surgeon General.* Atlanta, GA: U.S. Department of Health and Human Services, Centers for Disease Control and Prevention, National Center for Chronic Disease Prevention and Health Promotion, 1996.
70 Singh NA, Clements KM, Fiatarone MA. A randomized controlled trial of the effect of exercise on sleep. *Sleep* 1997; **20**:95–101.
71 Singh NA, Clements KM, Fiatarone MA. A randomized controlled trial of progressive resistance training in depressed elders. *J Gerontol Med Sci* 1997; **52A**:M27–35.
72 Munro JF, Nicholl JP, Brazier JE, Davey R, Cochrane T. Cost effectiveness of a community based exercise programme in over 65 year olds: cluster randomised trial. *J Epidemiol Community Health* 2004; **58**:1004–1010.
73 Robertson MC. Development of a falls prevention programme for elderly people: evaluation of efficacy, effectiveness, and efficiency [Ph.D. thesis]. University of Otago, 2001.
74 Li F, Harmer P, Fisher KJ, *et al.* Tai Chi and fall reductions in older adults: a randomized controlled trial. *J Gerontol Med Sci* 2005; **60**:187–194.
75 DeVito CA, Morgan RO, Duque M, Abdel-Moty E, Virnig BA. Physical performance effects of low-intensity exercise among clinically defined high-risk elders. *Gerontology* 2003; **49**:146–154.

CHAPTER 10

Is there a role for exercise in the prevention of osteoporotic fractures?

Gladys Onambele-Pearson

Introduction

Loss of balance has previously been associated with increased postural sway[1] and incidence of falls,[2] and subsequently, to fractures.[3] It is in fact estimated that generally speaking, every 3 minutes someone has a fracture due to osteoporosis. Given the apparent interaction between osteoporosis and falls,[4] identifying risk groups for falls is an important factor in relevant public health policies, and determining the main contributors to fractures should be a crucial part of targeted rehabilitation strategies.

What is osteoporosis?

The bones in our skeleton are made of a thick outer shell and a strong inner mesh filled with collagen (protein), calcium salts, and other minerals. The inside looks like honeycomb (holes in effect), with blood vessels and bone marrow in the spaces between bones. Bone is alive and throughout life, it is continually renewing itself through a process known as remodeling or bone turnover. Remodeling is when old, worn out bone is broken down through the activity of cells called osteoclasts and replaced through the activity of cells called osteoblasts. In healthy bone, there is a balance between the rates of bone resorption (i.e., bone breakdown) and osteogenesis (i.e., bone formation) so that bone mass is maintained. Even in the adult skeleton, 10% of the structure is remodeled each year.

Peak bone mass is achieved by the age of 30 years. After skeletal maturity, the rate at which bone is broken down increases and exceeds the rate at which bone is formed, resulting in a rate of bone lost of about 1% per year and often leading to osteoporosis and the associated increased risk of fracture. It should be noted here however that the concept of measuring bone quality relative to a peak bone mass, itself linked to chronological age, is slowly being superseded by a new concept where bone mass should be assessed in relation to bone size or muscle function.[5]

Osteoporosis literally means "porous bones." A systemic skeletal disease characterized by a bone mass lower than the average (i.e., < 2.5 standard deviations below the mean[6]) and microarchitectural deterioration. Osteoporosis is therefore associated with increased bone fragility and liability for bone to break easily. As this condition is symptomless until a bone is broken, it has traditionally been difficult to pinpoint which individuals have fragile bones prior to fracture occurring.

Research has associated certain factors with increased bone loss, including:

- Acute and long-term physical inactivity, as seen during limb immobilization, paralyzed limbs in poliomyelitis and after stroke, and spinal cord injury.

• Space flight (i.e., microgravity) and/or prolonged bed rest.
• Cigarette smoking.
• Poor diet (particularly one low in calcium and vitamin D, and high in alcohol), anorexia nervosa.
• Family history.
• Use of oral contraceptives
• The menopause.
• Hysterectomy, with ovaries removed, before 45 years of age.
• Low testosterone levels in men.
• Endocrine disease—Cushing's syndrome, diabetes, hyperthyroidism.
• Long-term use of drugs—steroids, thyroxine, diuretics.

It should be noted, nevertheless, that low bone density, although it is regularly associated with increased fractures risk,[7] should be considered as a risk factor for fracture and not a foregone conclusion. In other words, there will be people who have low bone density but never experience a fracture,[8] and conversely there are cases where fractures occur despite the patient not having particularly low antecedent BMD measures.[9]

General preventative and treatment guidelines for osteoporosis

The general guidelines to try and prevent the condition include either:
• Optimization of peak bone mass through dietary calcium and bone formation agents (e.g., fluoride, parathyroid hormone), or:
• Reduction of the rate of bone loss through hormonal replacement therapy (HRT, estrogen receptor modulators), bisphosphonates, lifestyle, adoption of moderate alcohol intake, and no smoking (Fig. 10.1).

The value of exercise as an intervention for the prevention of excessive bone loss is a somewhat controversial subject. It is therefore the purpose of this chapter to review the role of exercise in maintaining bone density. The potentially adverse effects to the skeleton of excessive exercise are also considered.

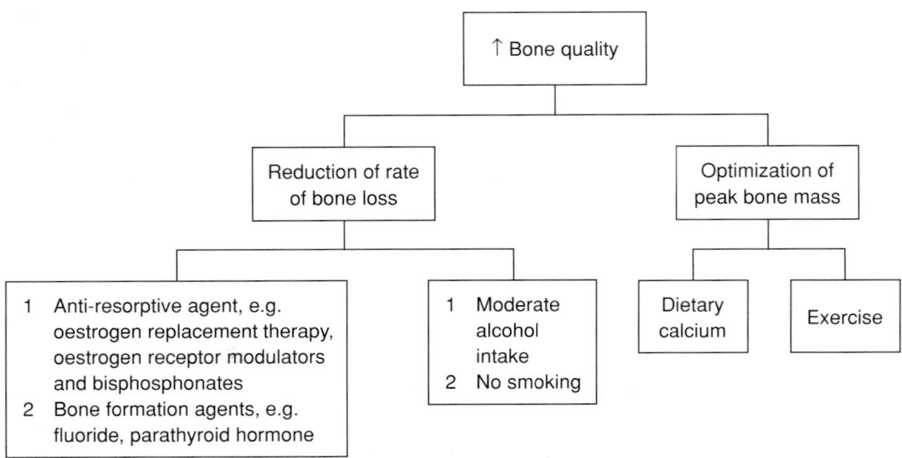

Figure 10.1 General guidelines for preventing/reversing osteoporosis.

Methodology

The studies were selected from MEDLINE and ISI Web of Knowledge (V1.2) searches. The first two searches using the Medical Subject Headings (MeSH) terms "osteoporosis AND exercise AND fractures," and "BMD AND physical activity" returned a great number of hits (601 and 585, respectively). It was beyond the scope of this review to cover all this research. Thus, a more detailed search of "osteoporosis AND exercise AND fractures" with an inclusion limit of "randomized controlled trial" (n = 18) was used. To this we added the results of "osteoporosis AND HRT AND exercise" (inclusion limit of "clinical trial", n = 11, and reviews, n = 20). Intervention studies had to meet the criteria that there was a suitably matched control group and that detail of the exercises were given. In all cases, in addition to the MeSH limits, particular emphasis was given to a) the most recent review papers, b) representative samples of key intervention studies—i.e., the earliest study in a particular subject area. Material already known to the author was also added to the discussions.

Muscle properties in older age

There are many factors other than bone strength that can predispose a person to falls and fractures. These include inadequate strength of the muscle–tendon complex, lower limb asymmetry in strength and power, decreased joint flexibility, slow reaction time, and decreased functional ability owing to lack of practice and/or pain.[10–12]

Age-related muscle atrophy is a primary factor in impaired muscle performance in the elderly.[13] The extent to which deteriorations in muscle performance can be reversed through increments in physical activity levels, has been shown to help in partly reversing the frailty of elderly subjects through neuromuscular adaptations to the training stimulus.[14,15] It was recently shown, in a group of elite weight-lifters as old as 89 years, that even though lifelong muscle-strengthening work does not stop muscle-strength losses—nor indeed does it slow down the normal rate of loss in muscle strength—it still provides a 20-year strength advantage for the trained individuals in comparison with age-matched sedentary peers.[16] These findings thus suggest that, with the appropriate safety precautions (i.e., exercises to be introduced gradually into classes after an initial, progressive, skill-specific training period to allow soft-tissue adaptation and the requisite safe technique to be learnt), older populations are as trainable as their younger counterparts and should therefore not be discounted where training intervention strategies are considered as a possible therapeutic route. Aside from the potential importance of muscle strength in fall risk, a good muscle mass may also be protective against fracture after a fall, as the tissue can act as a cushion absorbing some of the impact forces. Strategies aimed at preventing bone loss should therefore also aim to strengthen muscle.

Exercise and fractures

In response to the question of what kind of exercise is best for keeping bones healthy, the National Osteoporosis Foundation suggests that 20–30 minutes three times a week of weight-bearing exercises (e.g., weight training, stair climbing, walking, running, jogging, dancing, aerobics, racquet sports, court sports and field sports) are the best for keeping bones healthy. What is the evidence behind this recommendation?

Evidently, the recent consensus for the effects of exercise on bone strength appear to be that the type of loading is a major factor in determining whether exercise will have a positive, or a negative impact on bone quality, where this refers interchangeably to bone mineral density (BMD) or bone mineral content (BMC). It would appear, for instance, that whilst endurance cycle training has been associated with up to 10–17% decrement in bone quality, weightlifters and sports boxers on the other hand are reported as exhibiting a higher bone quality in comparison with aged-matched sedentary controls.[17] Similarly, it is not clear whether the "transference" of the benefits of muscle loading (for example, loading the lower limbs) onto the rest of the skeletal mass (example of BMD of the radius) occurs,[18,19] thereby putting into question the systemic value of exercise loading unless all skeletal sites are loaded separately.

The rationale for muscle strength to be involved in bone quality often comes from the observation that the same conditions that are associated with bone loss are also associated with concomitant decrements in muscle strength[20] and size (see factors associated with increased bone risk in the "What is osteoporosis?" section above), thereby increasing the likelihood of a causal relationship between decreased muscle strength and size, and decreased bone quality. Both animal and computer models indicate that when muscle force decreases, significant degradations in bone density occur.[21] In addition, a study of 185 women with an average age of 81 showed that increments in trunk weakness (which is related to vertebral fractures) can be successfully reversed in a structured physical activity regime.[22] The current paradigm is therefore that the most important mechanical feature of load-bearing bones is that they are modeled relative to the amount of customary voluntary loading. In other words, bone quality is intrinsically linked to the level of mechanical stimuli applied by the skeletal muscle.[23] It should be noted here that body weight by itself is not sufficient to create the loading levels necessary for an osteogenic response. Rather, muscle contractions are needed for bone to respond by increasing either their volume or their density. This therefore reinforces the idea that physical exercise might be an option in bone loss prevention measures.[24,25]

A wide range of studies, both longitudinal and cross-sectional in design, have investigated whether exercise does indeed play a role in decreasing the likelihood of a fracture ensuing after a fall.[26,27] It is, however, beyond the scope of this chapter to cover them all. Rather, representative examples of the type of exercise which might be most effective for different types of fractures are summarized. In general terms, exercise types may be grouped into endurance, strength/resistance, high impact, walking, and aerobics training. Whereas in the early days it was believed that endurance exercises were all-round magic wands, not only good for cardiovascular fitness but also for bone strength, it is more apparent from the current literature that this is not necessarily true.

Cross-sectional studies

The best model of exercise effects on BMD are highly trained individuals. In 1971, Nilsson and Westlin[28] measured the femoral bone density of athletes, including weightlifters, throwers, runners, soccer players, swimmers, active nonathletes, and sedentary men. Bone density varied with the amount and extent of loading placed on the femur, with the greatest density occurring in the weightlifters and lowest in the sedentary group. Similar findings have since been shown in more recent studies.[29,30]

The criticism about such comparative studies is that the high bone density may simply reflect a genetically determined strong musculoskeletal system that favors the participation of these individuals in high-level sports, rather than the training itself leading to an increase in BMD. An argument against this comes from studies of asymmetric activities, such as tennis, where the playing arm has a larger bone mass than the nonplaying arm.[31] Other criticisms about cross-sectional studies come from the observations that a) the differences observed in bone density between athletes and nonathletes are often much greater than the changes measured as a result of prospective exercise intervention studies; and b) studies sometimes show spurious differences in BMD in populations, with no real explanation as the cause for the difference. One such study is that in which muscle strength was seen to correlate with BMD in women, but not in men.[32] There are several possible explanations for these observations.

- *Peak bone mass effect.* The bone mass at 30 years of age determines the behavior of the skeleton for the remainder of a lifetime, owing to a decrement in the potential for bone formation.
- *Training duration effect.* The athlete's training history tends to be longer than the duration of intervention studies.
- *Genetic predisposition effect.* The athletes may have a genetic advantage in that their response to training is greater than that of sedentary people.
- *Gender effect.* The axes of sex hormones in both females and males may significantly impact on the structural and mechanical properties of bone

Not all athletic groups, however, show beneficial effects on bone, and this is discussed below.

Exercise intervention

Longitudinal randomized intervention studies are the only true ways in which exercise can conclusively be shown to either decrease bone loss or increase bone formation. Problems arise when trying to compare such studies, as there are large variations in the type (a representative sample of exercises in an older population is shown in Fig. 10.2), intensity, and duration of the training. Additional confounding factors include wide differences in the age range of subjects, concurrent treatments, calcium supplementation, and skeletal sites investigated. Despite these problems, it is becoming evident that specific types of activities can provide benefits for different skeletal sites.

Strengthening the wrist

The Colles fracture of the wrist is debilitating not only because of restricted function immediately after the facture, but also because it will often be followed by carpal tunnel

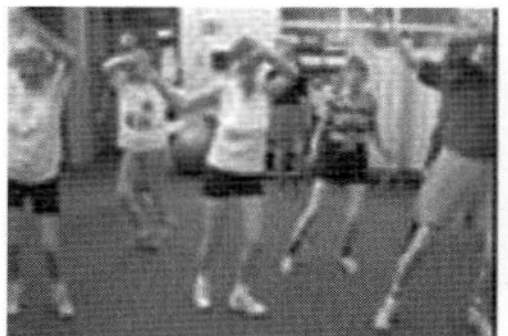
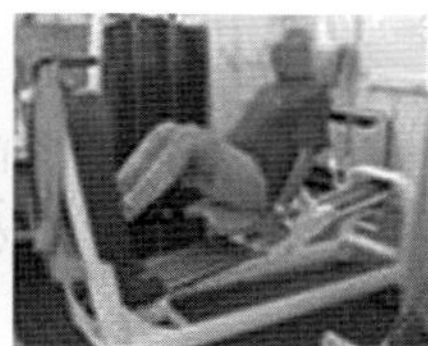
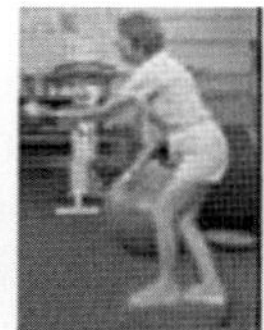
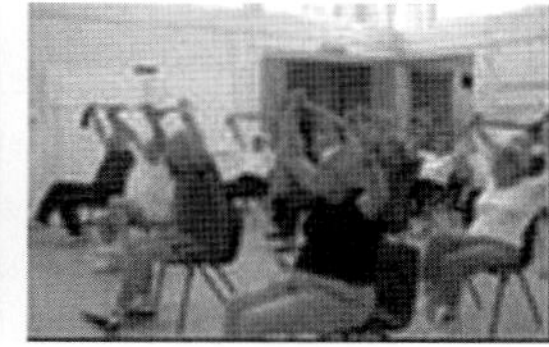

Figure 10.2 Exercise intervention types. Illustrations of high-impact aerobic, muscle-strengthening, balance, and low-impact exercises.

syndrome owing to acute median nerve compression mediated progressive edema and hematoma formation within the carpal tunnel. Whilst 6 weeks of squeezing a tennis ball for 30 seconds a day has significant benefits in the noninjured forearm of women who have already sustained a Colles fracture,[33] a lack of vigorous exercise in the preceding 2 weeks has been associated with an increased risk of wrist fracture.[34]

Increasing the bone density at the spine and hip

More challenging to researchers has been defining the optimal form of exercise that can have significant effects on bone density at the spine and hip. It has been difficult to isolate the type of exercise that places sufficient strain magnitude and of novel distribution to significantly alter bone remodeling.

Walking

Despite significant improvements in aerobic capacity, a yearlong investigation of treadmill walking at 70–85% of maximum heart rate together with calcium supplementation found no effect at the spine or forearm in postmenopausal women.[35] In recently menopausal women, walking appeared to attenuate the loss of bone at the spine when compared with controls. Nelson *et al.*[36] compared supervised walking and either moderate or high calcium diet on BMD of the spine and hip. The spine, but not the hip, showed a moderate improvement independent of calcium intake. A similar exercise regimen, but with no dietary supplementation, showed no effect on trabecular bone density in the spine.[37] In a 7-month trial, Hatori *et al.*[38] compared walking above (high intensity) or below (low intensity) the anaerobic threshold on the BMD of the spine. The moderate intensity group showed a similar loss of bone to the controls, whereas the high intensity group showed a small improvement. The available evidence is therefore inconclusive about whether walking is sufficient to improve BMD at the spine or hip.

Low-intensity repetitive exercise

Chow *et al.*[39] showed that, when compared with that of controls, total body calcium (no site-specific effect detected) is improved in subjects who train at a repetitive low force, as well as in subjects who train at a similar level with the addition of light weights attached to their wrists and ankles during the exercise classes, however, without the group performing with the weights showing any additional benefit compared with the group trained at repetitive low intensity only.

In a randomized study, Dalsky *et al.*[40] used a training protocol which included walking, running, and stair climbing in women aged 55–70. Calcium supplements were given at a dose of 1500 mg/day regardless of dietary intake and subjects were randomly divided into exercise and nonexercise groups. In the first stage of the study, exercise was carried out for 9 months. Some subjects in the exercise group then stopped training and the others continued to train for a further 13 months, after which the exercise was stopped and subjects were followed up after a further 12-month detraining period. The results showed that the first 12 months of exercise resulted in a significant increase of 6% in spine BMC, and this was maintained without further improvements in those who carried on training. Those who had stopped training after the initial 12 months of exercise returned to their baseline BMC. This study highlights many aspects outlined in the general principles for training as summarized by the American College of Sports Medicine. Firstly, within the exercise group some did not benefit from exercise and carried on losing bone, while others had very large increases of up to 15%. This could be due to different intensities of training, differences in initial BMC, or differences in genetic potential to respond to training. As with any intervention treatments, it highlights the need to monitor response and not assume that every person will respond positively. Secondly, it demonstrates the plateau effect in that the response was maintained but not increased in the second training phase. Thirdly, the results show that once exercise is stopped, the normal bone loss continues and the benefits are not maintained, this is in agreement with another recent study.[41]

Strength training

The rationale for strength training as a means to maximize the osteogenic response was based on findings from animal studies which showed that the greatest effects were seen when the magnitude and rate of strain was high, but required few repetitions, and when the strain was novel in magnitude or direction.[42,43] Strength training provides an equivalent loading characteristic. Kerr *et al.*[44] found an effect of high-intensity strength training on BMD of several regions on the hip: trochanter, intratrochanteric area, and Ward's triangle. They found no effect at the neck of femur and no effect of low intensity (endurance) strength training. Both types of exercise improved muscle strength to a similar extent, and these improvements correlated with the bone changes at several sites in the high intensity group. Mitchell *et al.*[45] studied 16 transplant patients with signs of osteoporosis performing 6 months of exercise on a lumbar extensor machine. Bone mineral density (BMD) of the lumbar vertebra (L2–3), was found to have improved by 9.2% after the training period, thereby further supporting the notion that progressive mechanical loading is effective at reducing osteoporotic symptoms. This does indeed make sense if we consider a hypothesis recently put forward[46] that since a) bones adapt to mechanical stimuli and b) the largest forces in the musculoskeletal system arise from muscle pull with the tendon acting as the transmission unit between the muscle and the joint, any intervention that positively affects the material properties of muscle and/or tendon would therefore positively affect BMD. The take-home message here is that the added benefit of increased muscle strength may in the longer term result in a significant effect on fracture risk.

High-impact exercise

Many of the studies so far discussed have been ineffective at increasing BMD at the hip. As this is the most serious fracture site, it is essential that safe, affordable, and accessible exercise is defined. A 1-year study incorporating jumping, stepping, marching, and side stepping into an exercise class[47] showed that there were significant increases in hip, but not in spine, BMD. The increases were in the range 1.6–2.2%, depending on the site on the hip. Some of the subjects continued for a second year, in which the spine BMD increased significantly and the changes in hip BMD were maintained. This type of exercise also completely reversed the age-related loss of muscle strength, with an approximately 20% net benefit in quadriceps strength in the training group. Urinary excretion of pyridinoline and deoxypyridinoline were measured to assess the impact of the exercise on bone resorption. Both markers significantly decreased during the first 6 months of exercise and then returned to baseline values. This suggests that the exercise was suppressing osteoclastic bone resorption. It remains to be determined whether exercise may promote osteogenic responses. Similar findings on the response to high-impact work have been obtained in younger subjects.[29,48] As mentioned earlier, the necessary safety precautions need to be observed, in this group as in any other. In addition, it would be advisable to simultaneously incorporate most exercise types (aerobics or different weight-bearing exercises, weight-lifting and flexibility or coordination exercises) during a training session since the knock-on effect on health, functional capacities, and fall risk may also be positively impacted.[49]

Exercise and the menopause

The time course of the decrease of muscle force in men and women is very different. In general terms, in men the decrease begins at about 60 years of age and is steady. Women reach peak muscle strength in their early twenties and plateau till their mid-forties, then steadily decline with increasing age.[50] A loss of 15–25% of total muscle strength (on top of the decline associated with aging) has been found to coincide with the menopause.[51]

Similarly, at the menopause bone density declines relatively rapidly.[52] It is well established that bone density is substantially improved after hormone replacement therapy (HRT).[53] HRT is also associated with a restoration of muscle strength.[54–56] In osteoporosis, the process of bone remodeling is usually defective.[57,58] Little is known about the pathophysiology of this process at the cellular level, although it is thought to be osteoclast-mediated and that acute estrogen deficiency may make osteoclasts hyperactive. Cytokines that promote bone resorption such as interleukin-1 (IL-1), IL-6, and IL-11 have been implicated in osteoclast activation due to estrogen deficiency,[59,60] and a recent study[61] has recently shown an association between IL-6 gene polymorphism and the magnitude of bone response to HRT.

The high prevalence of osteoporosis in postmenopausal women, and the prevalence of bone fractures among women with osteoporosis, makes prevention of the disease important. The relations and similarities between responses to HRT and to physical activity, sarcopenia, and osteoporosis[62] suggests three possible approaches for the prevention of fractures:

- Through structured supervised physical exercise (since the evidence is that home-based programs are not effective at increasing BMD[63]). Indeed, active women over the age of 50 have a comparatively higher bone mineral content[13,47] and calcaneal stiffness[64] than age-matched sedentary controls.
- Through HRT alone, which has been proved to have beneficial effects on bone (preferentially affecting trabecular bone).[53,61,65]
- Through using a combination of exercise and HRT. This is the most promising therapeutic intervention, since current indications are that weight-bearing exercises and estrogen (in the form of HRT) have additive effects, at least in terms of increasing the bone mineral density[66] of older women, though preliminary results would suggest that the same is not necessarily true for muscle strength.[67]

Studies on the bone effects of exercise with calcium supplementation of 1500 mg/day[66] or 600 mg/day[68] show that in the estrogen-replete state, older women have a greater bone response. There is in fact additional evidence that the effects are truly linked to estrogen, since it was shown that exercise plus estrogen has greater benefits on bone than calcium supplementation plus exercise.[69,70] Again in postmenopausal populations, tai chi chuan exercise has been linked with a significant 2.6-fold to 3.6-fold retardation of bone loss in both trabecular and cortical compartments of the distal tibia compared with a sedentary lifestyle,[71] as well as reducing fall risk (both home-based exercises[72] and tai chi[73] have been recognized as an integral part of multifactorial intervention programs for the reduction of falls and therefore fractures, particularly in older female populations). In addition, a population-based study of 1363 older women showed a high degree of positive correlation between physical activity and hip BMD, further supporting the concept that lifestyle factors play an important role in the maintenance of lower extremity bone mass in older women.[74] The data show that body fat mass is lower in women with trochanteric fracture compared to those with cervical fracture, whereas lean body mass appears to have an effect on the type of hip fracture, contributing to the necessity to consider the target for exercise: increase muscle mass and/or decrease fat mass.[75] Another example of the positive effects of exercise on bone strength after the menopause comes from a study of 320 healthy post-menopausal women, in which it was found that aerobic, weight-bearing activity combined with weightlifting improved femoral neck, trochanteric, and lumbar spine BMD.[76] However, it has to be acknowledged that not all studies are in agreement with the suggestion that physical exercise has a necessarily positive impact on the bone strength of post-menopausal subjects. In fact, a recent study of 1004 women aged 75 years suggested that physical activity only accounted for 1–6% of the variability in bone mass. Instead, they found body weight to be the best predictor of bone mass, accounting as it did for 15–32% (depending on skeletal site) for the variability in this parameter.[77] This observation, however, should be viewed with caution, since gaining excessive weight will have negative knock-on effects on other health-related variables. A long-term high-intensity weight-bearing exercise program has been associated with a slowing down in the mean rate of decrease in hip BMD, but not in lumbar spine BMD, which is another argument both for the effectiveness of exercise but also for the limitation of the extent of the benefits.[78]

A novel type of skeletal loading: whole-body microvibration

Animal studies have given evidence that vibration loading may be an efficient and safe way to improve indices of bone strength, thus providing another potential for either preventing or treating osteoporosis. The effects of vibration on the human body have been documented for many years.

Recently, the use of vibration for improving the training regimes of athletes has been investigated. Vibration has been used during strength-training movements such as elbow flexion, and vibration has also been applied to the entire body by having subjects stand on vibration platforms. Exposure to whole-body vibration has resulted in 10–50% increases in maximal strength (and flexibility).[79] In a group of young people aged 19–38 years, it was found that vibrations at 25–45 Hz, 4 min/day, three to five times per week for a total of 8 months had no effect on mass, structure, or estimated strength of bone at either the lumbar spine, femoral neck, trochanter, calcaneus, or distal radius.[80] In the older subject, it would appear that the type of periodization as well as load intensity might also be a factor in the observed effects. Indeed, it would appear that whole-body vibration, at 30 Hz for < 20 min for 12 months is linked with increased bone strength in 70-year-old women.[81] At 35–40 Hz three times weekly for 24 weeks, vibration has also been associated with significant BMD increments in women aged 58–74.[82] However, at 20 Hz for 4 min once a week for 12 months, microvibrations appeared to have no additional positive bone strength effect (compared with a course of 5 mg daily of alendronate) in women aged 55–88.[83]

Despite the potential benefits of vibration training, there is substantial evidence regarding the negative effects of vibration, not only in laboratory animals but also on the human body. Worryingly, issues include headaches, internal bleeding, and even death. Generally speaking, particular care must be taken to reduce resonance or the transmissibility of vibrations to the head, which is a factor of frequency. Frequency depends on body weight, muscle stiffness, and body position with respect with the vibration platform. Also, there are still uncertainties about the load, training duration, intensity of each training session, frequency, and amplitude of vibration training needed for there to be positive and minimal/no negative effects. It is therefore essential that a thorough understanding of the implications of this type of treatment be acquired through responsible research prior to its use. In other words, future research should be done with the aim of understanding the biological effects of vibration prior to its generalized use in a therapeutic context.

The downside of exercise

A commonly accepted paradigm is that an important determinant of future fracture risk is the bone mass accrued prior to the third decade (note caveat near the beginning of the introductory notes on page 167). This peak bone mass is thought to be influenced by levels of physical activity. An active lifestyle should therefore be encouraged throughout the life span. Studies show that regular physical activity is most efficient at maximizing peak bone mass early in life,[84–86] and this is believed to help in minimizing the age-related bone loss in older adults.[87,88] Yung *et al.*[88] investigated bone properties using heel quantitative ultrasound (QUS) in 55 young males aged 18–22 participating in various sports including football (a high-impact weight-bearing activity), dancing (a low-impact, weight-bearing activity), and swimming (non-weight-bearing), plus a sedentary control group. No significant differences in broadband ultrasound attenuation (BUA) and velocity of sound (VOS) were found between the dominant and nondominant heel. The two weight-bearing groups had significantly higher BUA and VOS values than both swimmers and controls, thus indicating that regular participation in weight-bearing exercise in young people might be beneficial for accruing peak bone mass and optimizing bone structure. Moreover a study of young children showed that jumping at ground reaction forces of eight times body weight is an effective intervention for improving hip and lumbar spine bone mass.[89] However, not all skeletal sites of interest appear to benefit from exercise, at least not in young adults. A case in point is the study of young army trainees in which it was shown that an exercise regime that involved endurance and cardiovascular and strength elements had positive effects on lumbar spine BMD, distal tibia BMD, and total body bone mineral content, but no effect on hip BMD.[90]

Another limitation of exercise is that there are younger people who may compromise the development of bone density by the adoption of extreme levels of exercise. Increased incidences of menstrual disorders have been observed in athletic women and infertility has been reported in amenorrheic athletes. This is a condition known as the athlete triad (or simply the "triad"). It describes the simultaneous presence of three distinct medical conditions in athletic females. It includes eating disorders/disordered eating behavior, amenorrhea/oligomenorrhea (i.e., 0–9 menses per year), and decreased bone mineral density (osteoporosis and osteopenia). Many of the women who develop such disorders have a later than average puberty, which may be associated with the adoption of intense exercise early in life.[91,92] Not only a) are eating disorders strongly related to menstrual irregularity or oligo/amenorrhea for instance in young competitive female distance runners, but also b) menstrual irregularity is linked with low BMD,[93–95] and c) eating disorders have been associated with low BMD even in the absence of menstrual irregularity.[96,97]

In addition, injuries to the musculoskeletal system are much more common in amenorrheic athletes, in particular the development of stress fractures.[98] There has even been a report of an osteoporotic fracture occurring in a young female athlete.[99] At the cellular level, it would appear that the normal osteogenic response to bone loading (e.g., the formation as monitored through osteocalcin and bone-specific alkaline phosphatase, or the resorption as monitored through deoxypyridinoline) is compromised in the estrogen deplete state, be it the amenorrhoeic[95] or the postmenopausal states.[57,58] It is important that athletes are aware of the potential risks to the skeleton of extended periods of menstrual irregularities, as it remains to be shown whether these skeletal deficits can be reversed by the resumption of menses or estrogen replacement.[100]

What are the possible physiological factors involved in the triad? In normally menstruating females, gonadotropin-releasing hormone (GnRH) stimulates the secretion of luteinizing hormone (LH) and follicle-stimulating hormone (FSH), thereby leading to increased estrogen production. The lack of phasic elevations in gonadotropin and steroid hormone patterns in athletic women[101] and the abrupt suppression of LH surge in eumenorrheic women on whom either strenuous athletic exercise and/or dietary restrictions[102] are imposed, results in a reduction in oestradiol and/or a shortening of the luteal phase of the cycle, all of which are evidences of extreme ovarian suppression.

The hormone leptin, a regulator of metabolic rate, is known to have receptors on hypothalamic neurons involved in GnRH secretion. It is in fact suggested that an energy drain incurred by women whose energy expenditure exceeds dietary energy intake may be a factor in the GnRH suppression, which results in compromised fertility and decreased BMD in female athletes.[103] It is thought that this is because not only are leptin levels chronically low in underweight women,[104] but also amenorrhea has been linked to changes in metabolism since cortisol and endorphins levels are raised in this condition.[105] However, the "leanness" theory is inadequate to explain compromised reproductive function in all cases, because it is found that sports that emphasize strength over leanness (e.g., swimming) cause increased androgen rather than decreased estrogen in female athletes.[106] We would therefore suggest that treatment with exogenous estrogen may not always be as effective at curbing these exercise effects as treatment aimed at correcting metabolic abnormalities would be.

The many benefits gained from exercise training should not, however, be sacrificed in the face of the above evidence. It is possible that only certain aspects of exercise are responsible for these side effects. If certain sports adversely affect the female reproductive system more than others (it would appear that weight-bearing athletes exhibit more menstrual irregularities[107,108] compared to their nonweight counterparts such as swimmers),[106] it is important that causes should be explored so that approaches to prevention and therapy can be developed.

Sparse scientific and/or clinical attention has been paid to elite male athletes, even though effects similar to those seen in women could be occurring and leading, in this case, to a reduced production of testosterone. If this were the case, it would indeed be worthy of serious investigation since at least in animal models testosterone levels are linked to bone length and density.[109] A study has found that testosterone levels are significantly lower in male triathletes.[110] In addition, athletic males have been found to not have increased bone density at the spine or total body compared with sedentary controls despite their high levels of activity. The above would therefore suggest that, as in their female counterparts, disturbances in the male hypothalamic–pituitary–gonadal axis also occur in highly active males.

Conclusions

Epidemiological data indicate that a history of physical activity can reduce the incidence of fractures. Weight-bearing activity, including walking, jumping, and stair-climbing, appears to be particularly effective. This effect is probably multifactorial in nature, through improved BMD, muscle strength, and balance. Similarly, studies show that the cessation of activity results in partial loss of BMD benefits, thereby supporting the suggestion that exercise has to be maintained for benefits to be upheld. It is not clear what should be the optimal exercise protocol to maximize benefits whilst at the same time minimizing negative side effects. Particularly in frail populations with a high risk of fracture, safety as well as exercise compliance considerations are highly relevant. Nevertheless, the general recommendation for decreasing the fracture risk would be to practice lifelong weight-bearing physical activities, so as to avoid the development of disproportionately large holes in the trabecular plates, or in the worst case, a total loss of bone, as this is an irreversible stage of skeletal ill-health.

Summary

• Research data indicate that current (rather than simply a history of) weight-bearing activity is particularly effective at reducing fracture incidence and that the cessation of activity results in partial (or complete) loss of BMD benefits previously accrued, thereby supporting the suggestion that exercise has to be maintained for benefits to be upheld.

• Evidently, the consensus on the effects of exercise on bone strength appears to be that the type of loading is a major factor in determining whether exercise will have a positive or a negative impact on bone quality. It would appear, for instance, that whilst endurance cycle training is associated with up to a 17% decrement in bone quality, weight-lifters and sports boxers on the other hand are reported as exhibiting higher bone quality in comparison with aged-matched sedentary controls.

• Strategies aimed at preventing bone loss should also aim to strengthen muscle, since aside from the potential importance of skeletal muscle performance in fall and/or fracture risk, adequate muscle mass may also be protective against fracture after a fall as the tissue can act as a cushion, damping some of the impact forces.

• All things considered, it is advisable to simultaneously incorporate most exercise types (aerobics, weight-bearing exercises, weightlifting, flexibility, and coordination exercises) during a training session, since the knock-on effect on health, functional capacities, and fall risk would also be positively impacted.

Key messages

• A history of physical activity in adolescence/early adulthood is a significant determining factor of bone strength and likelihood of fracture incidences in later life.

• In order to achieve maximal benefit, regular physical activity must a) be specific to a skeletal site, b) sufficiently overload the skeleton through increased intensity and duration.

• Exercise effects on the BMD are reversible, in that values will return to baseline when exercise is discontinued.

• The presence of osteoporotic tendencies, excessive exercise training, low levels of circulating estrogen (in females) and testosterone (in males) are examples in which intensive skeletal loading may be contraindicated.

Sample examination questions

Multiple-choice questions (answers on p. 602)

There may be more than one correct answer.

1 Bone density of 2.5 SD below the mean young reference range means a patient is:
  A Unlikely to have a fracture
  B Certain to have fracture
  C Likely to fracture a bone following a fall or high-impact collision with a solid object
  D Has a greater chance than normal to have spontaneous bone fractures

2 Bone mineral density can by improved:
  A In the spine by swimming and in the total body by moderate-intensity walking
  B By high-impact exercise
  C Only when exercise is combined with HRT
  D More by strength training than endurance training

3 Peak bone mass is a primarily a factor of:
  A Age and activity levels
  B A combination of activity levels and other non-exercise-related life style matters
  C Hormonal status
  D Previous injuries

4 Aside from exercise, the other major determining factors for BMD in later life include:
  A Lifestyle factors (i.e., diet deficient in calcium and/or vitamin D, excessive alcohol and/or caffeine)
  B Being on any medication and smoking
  C Inheritance rather than current health status
  D Gender, ethnicity and peak bone mass

Essay questions

Critically discuss the statements below:

1 Physical activity should be promoted as much as possible in the early years.

2 To be overtrained is as much a handicap for athletes as being completely sedentary for nonathletes.

Case study 10.1

Claire, a middle-aged semiprofessional long-distance female cyclist, has recently had a routine DEXA scan and been told that the BMD of the spine and hip are both 2.5 SD below the young reference normal. She has been borderline underweight since the beginning of her second decade. She has never had a fall, but has a history of fall-related fractures in her family. She does not smoke, nor is she currently receiving any medication/vitamin supplements, as she is against taking pharmacological agents in general.

1 What other information about this woman would you like to know?

2 In the description above, what factors may be important for the BMD result?

3 Considering that the patient is already very active but has an aversion to medication in general, what would you recommend to the patient?

Case study 10.2

Mr. and Mrs. Kaur have brought Kirti, their 9-year-old daughter, along for advice about participating in sport. During a gymnastics class at her school, Kirti fell and broke her arm in several places. Their first reaction was to advise Kirti that she should not participate in high-impact physical activity in the future. Kirti, however, is part of her county's gymnastics team and is keen to carry on with her sport. What advice would you give her?

Case study 10.3

Stephen, is a fit older man who used to believe in working hard and playing even harder. At 76, he is still a strong swimmer, but nevertheless owing to a lifetime of cigarette and alcohol abuse, he has a history of cardiovascular disease, precluding him from participating in heavy resistance training exercises. Stephen slipped and fell on the pavement on a frosty morning, and it was discovered that he had broken his fourth metatarsal on impact with a lamp-post (Stephen is also long-sighted). What are your recommendations for Stephen, either in terms of lifestyle or physical exercise regime?

Summarizing the evidence

Type of activity	Skeletal site	Effect	Level of evidence*
Endurance cycling	Femur	Negative	A2
Exercise + calcium	Spine	Positive	A1
Exercise + hormone replacement therapy	Spine	Positive	A1
	Total body	Positive	A1
	Ward's triangle	Positive	A1
	Distal tibia	Positive	A2
High-impact	Spine	Absent	A2
	Hip	Positive	A2
	Forearm§	Absent	A1
Low-impact	Total body	Positive	A1
Mixed aerobic§	Spine	Positive	A1
	Hip	Positive	A1
	Wrist	Inconclusive	A3
	Whole body	Positive	A2
Resistance/strength	Spine	Positive	A1
	Hip	Positive	A2
	Tibia§	Absent	A3
	Wrist	Positive	A3
	Spine	Absent unless at anaerobic levels	A2
Walking	Hip	Absent	A2
Whole body vibration	Hip	Inconclusive	A4
	Forearm	Inconclusive	A4

* A1: evidence from at least one high quality cohort or systematic review (including meta-analysis)†
A2: evidence from at least one randomized study of moderate size cohort or systematic review (including meta-analysis)†
A3: evidence from small to moderate size studies†
A4: evidence from at least one small randomized study
† Arbitrarily, the following cut-off points have been used; large study size: ≥ 100 patients per intervention group; moderate study size 26–99 patients per intervention group; small study size ≤ 25 patients per intervention group.
§ Transference studied—i.e., whether there is a systemic effect. In other words, whether loading one bone site shows generalized increments in another unrelated skeletal site.

References

1 Liu-Ambrose T, Eng JJ, Khan KM, *et al.* Older women with osteoporosis have increased postural sway and weaker quadriceps strength than counterparts with normal bone mass: overlooked determinants of fracture risk? *J Gerontol Ser A Biol Sci Med Sci* 2003; **58**:862–866.

2 Fernie GR, Gryfe CI, Holliday PJ, *et al.* The relationship of postural sway in standing to the incidence of falls in geriatric subjects. *Age Ageing* 1982; **11**:11–16.

3 Campbell AJ, Borrie MJ, Spears GF, *et al.* Circumstances and consequences of falls experienced by a community population 70 years and over during a prospective study. *Age Ageing* 1990; **19**:136–141.

4 Pfeifer M, Sinaki M, Geusens P, *et al.* Musculoskeletal rehabilitation in osteoporosis: a review. *J Bone Miner Res* 2004; **19**:1208–1214.

5 Schonau E. The peak bone mass concept: is it still relevant? *Pediatr Nephrol* 2004; **19**:825–831.

6 Group TWs. *Assessment of Fracture Risk and its Application to Screening for Postmenopausal Osteoporosis.* Geneva: World Health Organization, 1994: 5–6.

7 Nguyen TV, Center JR, Eisman JA. Femoral neck bone loss predicts fracture risk independent of baseline BMD. *J Bone Miner Res* 2005; **20**:1195–1201.

8 McClung MR. The relationship between bone mineral density and fracture risk. *Curr Osteoporos Rep* 2005; **3**:57–63.

9 Wainwright SA, Marshall LM, Ensrud KE, *et al.* Hip fracture in women without osteoporosis. *J Clin Endocrinol Metab* 2005; **90**:2787–2793.

10 Lord SR, McLean D, Stathers G. Physiological factors associated with injurious falls in older people living in the community. *Gerontology* 1992; **38**:338–346.

11 Lord SR, Sambrook PN, Gilbert C, *et al.* Postural stability, falls and fractures in the elderly: results from the Dubbo Osteoporosis Epidemiology Study. *Med J Aust* 1994; **160**:684–685, 8–91.

12 Skelton DA, Kennedy J, Rutherford OM. Explosive power and asymmetry in leg muscle function in frequent fallers and non-fallers aged over 65. *Age Ageing* 2002; **31**:119–125.

13 Rutherford OM, Jones DA. The relationship of muscle and bone loss and activity levels with age in women. *Age Ageing* 1992; **21**:286–293.

14 Pearson G, Narici M, Maganaris C, *et al.* Isoinertial versus isotonic training for the prevention of sarcopenia. In: International Congress on Sports Rehabilitation & Traumatology, ed. *The Rehabilitation of Sports Muscle & Tendon Injuries.* Milan, Italy: International Congress on Sports Rehabilitation & Traumatology, 2004:**8**.

15 Reeves ND, Narici MV, Maganaris CN. Effect of resistance training on skeletal muscle-specific force in elderly humans. *J Appl Physiol* 2004; **96**:885–892.

16 Pearson SJ, Young A, Macaluso A, *et al.* Muscle function in elite master weightlifters. *Med Sci Sports Exerc* 2002; **34**:1199–1206.

17 Sabo D, Reiter A, Pfeil J, Gussbacher A, Niethard FU. [Modification of bone quality by extreme physical stress. Bone density measurements in high-performance athletes using dual-energy x-ray absorptiometry; in German.] *Z Orthop Ihre Grenzgeb* 1996; **134**:1–6.

18 Kronhed ACG, Knutsson I, Lofman O, *et al.* Is calcaneal stiffness more sensitive to physical activity than forearm bone mineral density? A population-based study of persons aged 20–79 years. *Scand J Public Health* 2004; **32**:333–339.

19 Rittweger J, Frost HM, Schiessl H, *et al.* Muscle atrophy and bone loss after 90 days' bed rest and the effects of flywheel resistive exercise and pamidronate: results from the LTBR study. *Bone* 2005; **36**:1019–1029.

20 Pang MYC, Eng JJ. Muscle strength is a determinant of bone mineral content in the hemiparetic upper extremity: Implications for stroke rehabilitation. *Bone* 2005; **37**:103–111.

21 Be'ery-Lipperman M, Gefen A. Contribution of muscular weakness to osteoporosis: computational and animal models. *Clin Biomech (Bristol, Avon)* 2005; **20**:984–997.

22 Gold DT, Shipp KM, Pieper CF, *et al.* Group treatment improves trunk strength and psychological status in older women with vertebral fractures: results of a randomized, clinical trial. *J Am Geriatr Soc* 2004; **52**:1471–1478.

23 Rubin CT, Lanyon LE. Kappa Delta Award paper. Osteoregulatory nature of mechanical stimuli: function as a determinant for adaptive remodeling in bone. *J Orthop Res* 1987; **5**:300–310.

24 Law MR, Wald NJ, Meade TW. Strategies for prevention of osteoporosis and hip fracture. *BMJ* 1991; **303**:453–459.

25 Joakimsen RM, Magnus JH, Fonnebo V. Physical activity and predisposition for hip fractures: a review. *Osteoporos Int* 1997; **7**:503–513.

26 Ernst E. Exercise for female osteoporosis: a systematic review of randomised clinical trials. *Sports Med* 1998; **25**:359–368.

27 Gutin B, Kasper MJ. Can vigorous exercise play a role in osteoporosis prevention? A review. *Osteoporos Int* 1992; **2**:55–69.

28 Nilsson BE, Westlin NE. Bone density in athletes. *Clin Orthop Relat Res* 1971; **77**:179–182.

29 Heinonen A, Kannus P, Sievanen H, *et al.* Randomised controlled trial of effect of high-impact exercise on selected risk factors for osteoporotic fractures. *Lancet* 1996; **348**:1343–1347.

30 Meyer NL, Shaw JM, Manore MM, *et al.* Bone mineral density of Olympic-level female winter sport athletes. *Med Sci Sports Exerc* 2004; **36**:1594–1601.

31 Jones HH, Priest JD, Hayes WC, *et al.* Humeral hypertrophy in response to exercise. *J Bone Joint Surg Am* 1977; **59**:204–208.

32 Ribom E, Ljunggren O, Piehl-Aulin K, *et al.* Muscle strength correlates with total body bone mineral density in young women but not in men. Scand. *J Med Sci Sports* 2004; **14**:24–29.

33 Beverly MC, Rider TA, Evans MJ, *et al.* Local bone mineral response to brief exercise that stresses the skeleton. *BMJ* 1989; **299**:233–235.

34 Ivers RQ, Cumming RG, Mitchell P, *et al.* Risk factors for fractures of the wrist, shoulder and ankle: the Blue Mountains Eye Study. *Osteoporos Int* 2002; **13**:513–518.

35 Martin D, Notelovitz M. Effects of aerobic training on bone mineral density of postmenopausal women. *J Bone Miner Res* 1993; **8**:931–936.

36 Nelson ME, Fisher EC, Dilmanian FA, *et al.* A 1-y walking program and increased dietary calcium in postmenopausal women: effects on bone. *Am J Clin Nutr* 1991; **53**:1304–1311.

37 Cavanaugh DJ, Cann CE. Brisk walking does not stop bone loss in postmenopausal women. *Bone* 1988; **9**:201–204.

38 Hatori M, Hasegawa A, Adachi H, *et al.* The effects of walking at the anaerobic threshold level on vertebral bone loss in postmenopausal women. *Calcif Tissue Int* 1993; **52**:411–414.

39 Chow R, Harrison JE, Notarius C. Effect of two randomised exercise programmes on bone mass of healthy postmenopausal women. *Br Med J (Clin Res Ed)* 1987; **295**:1441–1444.

40 Dalsky GP, Stocke KS, Ehsani AA, *et al.* Weight-bearing exercise training and lumbar bone mineral content in postmenopausal women. *Ann Intern Med* 1988; **108**:824–828.

41 Nordstrom A, Karlsson C, Nyquist F, *et al.* Bone loss and fracture risk after reduced physical activity. *J Bone Miner Res* 2005; **20**:202–207.

42 Rubin CT, Lanyon LE. Regulation of bone mass by mechanical strain magnitude. *Calcif Tissue Int* 1985; **37**:411–417.

43 Rubin CT, Lanyon LE. Regulation of bone formation by applied dynamic loads. *J Bone Joint Surg Am* 1984; **66**:397–402.

44 Kerr D, Morton A, Dick I, *et al.* Exercise effects on bone mass in postmenopausal women are site-specific and load-dependent. *J Bone Miner Res* 1996; **11**:218–225.

45 Mitchell MJ, Baz MA, Fulton MN, *et al.* Resistance training prevents vertebral osteoporosis in lung transplant recipients. *Transplantation* 2003; **76**:557–562.

46 Rittweger J, Maffulli N, Maganaris CN, *et al.* Reconstruction of the anterior cruciate ligament with a patella–tendon–bone graft may lead to a permanent loss of bone mineral content due to decreased patellar tendon stiffness. *Med Hypotheses* 2005; **64**:1166–1169.

47 Welsh L, Rutherford OM. Hip bone mineral density is improved by high–impact aerobic exercise in postmenopausal women and men over 50 years. *Eur J Appl Physiol Occup Physiol* 1996; **74**:511–517.

48 Vainionpaa A, Korpelainen R, Leppaluoto J, *et al.* Effects of high-impact exercise on bone mineral density: a randomized controlled trial in premenopausal women. *Osteoporosis Int* 2005; **16**:191–197.

49 Scheel AK, Backhaus M, Koziolek M, *et al.* Osteoporosis and exercise. *Aktuelle Rheumatol* 2003; **28**:203–209.

50 Phillips SK, Rook KM, Siddle NC, *et al.* Muscle weakness in women occurs at an earlier age than in men, but strength is preserved by hormone replacement therapy. *Clin Sci (Lond)* 1993; **84**:95–98.

51 Meeuwsen IB, Samson MM, Verhaar HJ. Evaluation of the applicability of HRT as a preservative of muscle strength in women. *Maturitas* 2000; **36**:49–61.

52 Pouilles JM Tremiollieres F, Ribot C. Effect of menopause on femoral and vertebral bone loss. *J Bone Miner Res* 1995; **10**:1531–1536.

53 Shintani M. Which is the better choice, estrogen or SERMs in postmenopausal women? *Clin Calcium* 2004; **14**:105–110.

54 Skelton DA, Phillips SK, Bruce SA, *et al.* Hormone replacement therapy increases isometric muscle strength of adductor pollicis in post-menopausal women. *Clin Sci (Lond)* 1999; **96**:357–364.

55 Onambele NG, Skelton DA, Bruce SA, *et al.* Follow-up study of the benefits of hormone replacement therapy on isometric muscle strength of adductor pollicis in postmenopausal women. *Clin Sci (Lond)* 2001; **100**:421–422.

56 Woods D, Onambele G, Woledge R, *et al.* Angiotensin-I converting enzyme genotype-dependent benefit from hormone replacement therapy in isometric muscle strength and bone mineral density. *J Clin Endocrinol Metab* 2001; **86**:2200–2204.

57 Cicinelli E, Ignarro LJ, Lograno M, *et al.* Acute effects of transdermal estradiol administration on plasma levels of nitric oxide in postmenopausal women. *Fertil Steril* 1997; **67**:63–66.

58 Rosselli M, Imthurn B, Keller PJ, *et al.* Circulating nitric oxide (nitrite/nitrate) levels in postmenopausal women substituted with 17 beta-estradiol and norethisterone acetate. A two-year follow-up study. *Hypertension* 1995; **25**:848–853.

59 Jay PR, Centrella M, Lorenzo J, *et al.* Oncostatin-M: a new bone active cytokine that activates osteoblasts and inhibits bone resorption. *Endocrinology* 1996; **137**:1151–1158.

60 Pfeilschifter J. Role of cytokines in postmenopausal bone loss. *Curr Osteoporos Rep* 2003; **1**:53–58.

61 James L, Onambele G, Woledge R, *et al.* IL-6-174G/C genotype is associated with the bone mineral density response to oestrogen replacement therapy in post-menopausal women. *Eur J Appl Physiol* 2004; **92**:227–230.

62 Walsh MC, Hunter GR, Livingstone MB. Sarcopenia in premenopausal and postmenopausal women with osteopenia, osteoporosis and normal bone mineral density. *Osteoporos Int* 2006; **17**:61–67.

63 Papaioannou A, Adachi JD, Winegard K, *et al.* Efficacy of home-based exercise for improving quality of life among elderly women with symptomatic osteoporosis-related vertebral fractures. *Osteoporosis Int* 2003; **14**:677–682.

64 Welch JM, Rosen CJ. Older women track and field athletes have enhanced calcaneal stiffness. *Osteoporosis Int* 2005; **16**:871–878.

65 Uusi-Rasi K, Sievanen H, Heinonen A, *et al.* Determinants of changes in bone mass and femoral neck structure, and physical performance after menopause: a 9-year follow-up of initially peri-menopausal women. *Osteoporosis Int* 2005; **16**:616–622.

66 Kohrt WM, Snead DB, Slatopolsky E, *et al.* Additive effects of weight-bearing exercise and estrogen on bone mineral density in older women. *J Bone Miner Res* 1995; **10**:1303–1311.

67 Onambélé NGL, Bruce SA, Woledge RC. Oestrogen status in relation to the early training responses in human thumb adductor muscles. *Acta Physiologica* 2006; **188**(1):41–52.

68 Kerr D, Ackland T, Maslen B, *et al.* Resistance training over 2 years increases bone mass in calcium-replete postmenopausal women. *J Bone Miner Res* 2001; **16**:175–181.

69 Kaplan RJ, Vo AN, Stitik TP, *et al.* Rehabilitation of orthopedic and rheumatologic disorders. 1. Osteoporosis assessment, treatment, and rehabilitation. *Arch Phys Med Rehabil* 2005; **86**:S40–S7.

70 Prince RL, Smith M, Dick IM, *et al.* Prevention of postmenopausal osteoporosis: a comparative study of exercise, calcium supplementation, and hormone-replacement therapy. *N Engl J Med* 1991; **325**:1189–1195.

71 Chan KM, Qin L, Lau MC, *et al.* A randomized, prospective study of the effects of Tai Chi Chuan exercise on bone mineral density in postmenopausal women. *Arch Phys Med Rehabil* 2004; **85**:717–722.

72 Campbell AJ, Robertson MC, Gardner MM, *et al.* Randomised controlled trial of a general practice programme of home based exercise to prevent falls in elderly women. *BMJ* 1997; **315**:1065–1069.

73 Wolf SL, Barnhart HX, Kutner NG, *et al.* Reducing frailty and falls in older persons: an investigation of tai chi and computerized balance training. *J Am Geriatr Soc* 2003; **51**:1794–1803.

74 Devine A, Dhaliwal SS, Dick IM, *et al.* Physical activity and calcium consumption are important determinants of lower limb bone mass in older women. *J Bone Miner Res* 2004; **19**:1634–1639.

75 Di Monaco M, Vallero F, Di Monaco R, *et al.* Body composition and hip fracture type in elderly women. *Clin Rheumatol* 2004; **23**:6–10.

76 Going S, Lohman T, Houtkooper L, *et al.* Effects of exercise on bone mineral density in calcium-replete postmenopausal women with and without hormone replacement therapy. *Osteoporosis Int* 2003; **14**:637–643.

77 Gerdhem P, Ringsberg KAM, Akesson K, *et al.* Influence of muscle strength, physical activity and weight on bone mass in a population-based sample of 1004 elderly women. *Osteoporosis Int* 2003; **14**:768–772.

78 De Jong Z, Munneke M, Lems WF, *et al.* Slowing of bone loss in patients with rheumatoid arthritis by long-term high-intensity exercise: results of a randomized, controlled trial. *Arthritis Rheum* 2004; **50**:1066–1076.

79 Mester J, Kleinoder H, Yue Z. Vibration training: benefits and risks. *J Biomech* 2006; **39**: 1056–1065.

80 Torvinen S, Kannus P, Sievanen H, *et al.* Effect of 8-month vertical whole body vibration on bone, muscle performance, and body balance: a randomized controlled study. *J Bone Miner Res* 2003; **18**:876–884.

81 Rubin C, Recker R, Cullen D, *et al.* Prevention of postmenopausal bone loss by a low-magnitude, high-frequency mechanical stimuli: a clinical trial assessing compliance, efficacy, and safety. *J Bone Miner Res* 2004; **19**:343–351.

82 Verschueren SMP, Roelants M, Delecluse C, *et al.* Effect of 6-month whole body vibration training on hip density, muscle strength, and postural control in postmenopausal women: a randomized controlled pilot study. *J Bone Miner Res* 2004; **19**:352–359.

83 Iwamoto J, Takeda T, Sato Y, *et al.* Effect of whole-body vibration exercise on lumbar bone mineral density, bone turnover, and chronic back pain in post-menopausal osteoporotic women treated with alendronate. *Aging Clin Exp Res* 2005; **17**:157–163.

84 Kannus P, Haapasalo H, Sankelo M, *et al.* Effect of starting age of physical activity on bone mass in the dominant arm of tennis and squash players. *Ann Intern Med* 1995; **123**:27–31.

85 Bloomfield SA. Contributions of physical activity to bone health over the lifespan. *Top Geriatr Rehabil* 2005; **21**:68–76.

86 Chan KM, Anderson M, Lau EMC. Exercise interventions: defusing the world's osteoporosis time bomb. *Bull World Health Organ* 2003; **81**:827–830.

87 Ford MA, Bass MA, Turner LW, *et al.* Past and recent physical activity and bone mineral density in college-aged women. *J Strength Cond Res* 2004; **18**:405–409.

88 Yung PS, Lai YM, Tung PY, *et al.* Effects of weight bearing and non-weight bearing exercises on bone properties using calcaneal quantitative ultrasound. *Br J Sports Med* 2005; **39**:547–551.

89 Fuchs RK, Bauer JJ, Snow CM. Jumping improves hip and lumbar spine bone mass in prepubescent children: a randomized controlled trial. *J Bone Miner Res* 2001; **16**:148–156.

90 Armstrong DW, Shakir KMM, Drake AJ. Dual X-ray absorptiometry total body bone mineral content and bone mineral density in 18- to 22-year-old Caucasian men. *Bone* 2000; **27**:835–839.

91 Malina RM. Menarche in athletes: a synthesis and hypothesis. *Ann Hum Biol* 1983; **10**:1–24.

92 Stager JM, Hatler LK. Menarche in athletes: the influence of genetics and prepubertal training. *Med Sci Sports Exerc* 1988; **20**:369–373.

93 Wolman RL, Clark P, McNally E, *et al.* Menstrual state and exercise as determinants of spinal trabecular bone density in female athletes. *BMJ* 1990; **301**:516–518.

94 Rutherford OM. Spine and total body bone mineral density in amenorrheic endurance athletes. *J Appl Physiol* 1993; **74**:2904–2908.

95 Stacey E, Korkia P, Hukkanen MV, *et al.* Decreased nitric oxide levels and bone turnover in amenorrheic athletes with spinal osteopenia. *J Clin Endocrinol Metab* 1998; **83**:3056–3061.

96 Papanek PE. The female athlete triad: an emerging role for physical therapy. *J Orthop Sports Phys Ther* 2003; **33**:594–614.

97 Cobb KL, Bachrach LK, Greendale G, *et al.* Disordered eating, menstrual irregularity, and bone mineral density in female runners. *Med Sci Sports Exerc* 2003; **35**:711–719.

98 Bennell KL, Malcolm SA, Wark JD, *et al.* Skeletal effects of menstrual disturbances in athletes. *Scand J Med Sci Sports* 1997; **7**:261–273.

99 Wilson JH, Wolman RL. Osteoporosis and fracture complications in an amenorrhoeic athlete. *Br J Rheumatol* 1994; **33**:480–481.

100 Keen AD, Drinkwater BL. Irreversible bone loss in former amenorrheic athletes. *Osteoporos Int* 1997; **7**:311–315.

101 Warren MP, Shantha S. The female athlete. *Baillière's Best Pract Res Clin Endocrinol Metab* 2000; **14**:37–53.

102 Loucks AB, Thuma JR. Luteinizing hormone pulsatility is disrupted at a threshold of energy availability in regularly menstruating women. *J Clin Endocrinol Metab* 2003; **88**:297–311.

103 Loucks AB. Physical health of the female athlete: observations, effects, and causes of reproductive disorders. *Can J Appl Physiol* 2001; **26**:S176–185.

104 Kopp W, Blum WF, von Prittwitz S, *et al.* Low leptin levels predict amenorrhea in underweight and eating disordered females. *Mol Psychiatry* 1997; **2**:335–340.

105 Jurkowski JE, Jones NL, Toews CJ, *et al.* Effects of menstrual cycle on blood lactate, O_2 delivery, and performance during exercise. *J Appl Physiol* 1981; **51**:1493–1499.

106 Constantini NW, Warren MP. Menstrual dysfunction in swimmers: a distinct entity. *J Clin Endocrinol Metab* 1995; **80**:2740–2744.

107 Torstveit MK, Sundgot-Borgen J. The female athlete triad: are elite athletes at increased risk? *Med Sci Sports Exerc* 2005; **37**:184–193.

108 Carbon RJ. Exercise, amenorrhoea and the skeleton. *Br Med Bull* 1992; **48**:546–560.

109 Sims NA, Brennan K, Spaliviero J, Handelsman DJ, Seibel MJ. Perinatal testosterone surge is required for normal adult bone size, but not for normal bone remodeling. *Am J Physiol Endocrinol Metab* 2006; **290**:E456–62.

110 Smith R, Rutherford OM. Spine and total body bone mineral density and serum testosterone levels in male athletes. *Eur J Appl Physiol Occup Physiol* 1993; **67**:330–334.

SECTION 2
Acute injury

CHAPTER 11

What is the role of ice in soft-tissue injury management?

Chris Bleakley and Domhnall MacAuley

Introduction

Soft-tissue injuries occur frequently during athletic activity.[1,2] Cryotherapy (the application of ice for therapeutic purposes) is largely accepted as the initial treatment of choice, and is also recommended as an adjunct to functional rehabilitation. Newer techniques have broadened its use for postsurgical patients, and ice is also a common postoperative intervention.[3]

Previous reviews[4–6] have documented a number of shortcomings in the evidence base. It seems that recommendations for the use of ice in sports-medicine textbooks show a lack of consensus, and little is known on the specific physiological effect of ice on injured soft tissue. Few randomized controlled clinical trials could be highlighted, and it is not yet possible to establish an optimal mode, duration or frequency of ice application, although the consensus from the basic sciences seems to support the use of an intermittent protocol. Finally, there are no clear evidence-based guidelines on how best to use compression, elevation, and exercise as an adjunct to ice application.

The main aim of this study was to build on preliminary work undertaken to date[4–6] and further develop the clinical evidence base for cryotherapy. Some of the findings are based on secondary research previously published.[7] The objectives were:

- To undertake a more comprehensive and systematic literature search to identify randomized and controlled studies assessing the effect of cryotherapy on acutely injured human subjects.
- To assess for the presence of confounding concomitant therapies.
- To study the modes, duration, and frequency of cryotherapy treatments employed, and assess for evidence of an optimal treatment protocol.
- To identify when cryotherapy was initiated in relation to the injury, and study the goals of treatment in each study—i.e., for immediate care or rehabilitation.

Methods

Search strategy and selection of studies

A computer-based literature search was undertaken on a total of 11 databases: MEDLINE on Ovid (1966–April 2005), PubMed (1966–April 2005), Proquest (1986–April 2005), ISI Web of Science (1981–April 2005), Cumulative Index to Nursing and Allied Health (CINAHL) on Ovid (1982–April 2005), SportDiscus (1830–April 2005), the Allied and Complementary Medicine Database (AMED) on Ovid (1985–April 2005), Physiotherapy

Evidence Database (PEDro), the Cochrane Database of Systematic Reviews (CDSR), the Cochrane Database of Abstracts of Reviews of Effectiveness (DARE) and the Cochrane Controlled Trials Register (Central/CCTR), last search April 2005—by combining the following MEDLINE subject headings and free-text topic words; "surgery," "orthopedics," "sports injury," "soft-tissue injury," "sprains and strains," "contusion," "athletic injury" "acute" "compression," "cryotherapy," "ice," "RICE" and "cold." The search also included citation tracking of relevant primary and review articles (n = 71), incoming full-text papers (n = 84), and hand searching of a convenience sample of 10 key journals. There was no blinding to study author, place of publication, or results. The primary researcher assessed the content of all full-text articles, making the final inclusion/exclusion decisions.

To be included in the review, studies had to fulfill the following conditions: the study should be a randomized and controlled trial including human subjects; published in English as a full paper; subjects should be recovering from acute soft-tissue injuries or orthopedic surgical interventions; therapy should be in-patient, outpatient, or home-based cryotherapy treatment, used either in isolation or in combination with placebo or other therapies; comparisons should have been made with no treatment, placebo, a different mode or protocol of cryotherapy, or other physiotherapeutic interventions; and outcome measures must have included at least one of the following: function (subjective or objective), pain, swelling, and range of movement (ROM).

Assessment of methodological quality and data extraction

All eligible articles were rated for methodological quality, using the PEDro scale.[8] Disagreement or ambiguous issues arising between the first two raters were resolved by either consensus discussion, or consultation with a PEDro project officer.

Results

Study selection

Figure 11.1 shows the Quality of Reporting of Meta-Analysis (QUORUM) statement flow diagram.[9] This summarizes the process of study selection and the number of studies excluded at each stage, with reasons.

Study characteristics

Patients had a wide variety of acute injuries. Only one study included subjects with muscle contusions or general soft-tissue injuries,[10] and five used subjects with acute ligament sprains.[11–15] The remaining 18 studies used patients recovering from a range of operative procedures.

Table 11.1 summarizes the mode, duration, and frequency of cryotherapy, the total cryotherapy treatment time (overall dosage), the time cryotherapy was initiated in relation to the injury, and the number of days of treatment, for each included study.

In total, seven different modes of cooling were used; cold gel, cold saline, crushed or chipped ice, Cryocuff or cold compressive devices, commercial ice machines, commercial/gel ice packs, and ice submersion. Five studies[12,15–18] simply stated that an ice bag or pack was applied, and eight studies[15–21] used more than one mode of cooling during the trial. Thirteen studies applied cryotherapy continuously after injury, eight studies employed an intermittent protocol, and the remaining six failed to specify the protocol. With such an array of icing protocols, the total treatment time (dosage) subjects received was extremely

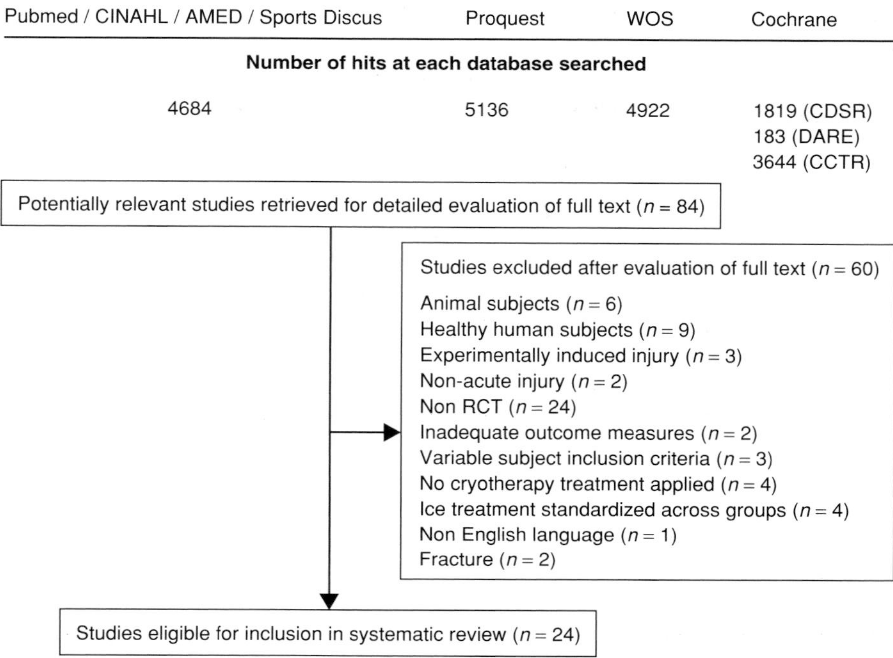

Figure 11.1 Quorum statement flow diagram summarizing the literature search.

diverse. For one group of subjects, the entire course of cryotherapy treatment consisted of just 20 minutes' cooling,[13] in comparison with others whose treatment time ranged from 216[22] to 336 hours.[17]

The time of cryotherapy initiation may be a key factor in dictating its effectiveness, but again this was poorly reported. Three studies[19,23,24] stated that cryotherapy was employed immediately after surgery, but they failed to provide a quantifiable time period. Likewise, others simply stated that cooling began during the operative procedure,[25] prior to tourniquet release,[17] in the recovery room,[26] in the operating room,[16,22,27] or after wound closure and dressing application.[28–31] Most studies including patients with soft-tissue injury or ankle sprain initiated cryotherapy between days 1 and 3 post-injury.[10–14] One study[15] initiated cryotherapy in the acute phases of injury, but again failed to state a definite time period.

Few studies reported the specific goals of cryotherapy, and it is not clear whether cooling was employed for immediate care or for rehabilitative purposes. Only two studies[11,32] stated that cryotherapy was applied in conjunction with exercise, for rehabilitative purposes. It seems that the majority of studies,[16,17,21–24,26,28,30] despite continuing cryotherapy for days and even weeks after the immediate stages of trauma, failed to incorporate functional movements or therapeutic exercises.

Effectiveness of treatment

A total of 10 treatment comparisons were made. Table 11.2 subgroups the studies according to treatment comparison and provides the sample size, overall PEDro score, and effect

Table 11.1 The cryotherapy protocols used in the included studies

First author, ref.	Mode	Treatment duration (h)	Treatments/day (n)	Days treated (n)	Total cryotherapy time (overall damage) (h)	Time/place of cryotherapy initiation
Cote[11]	Water bath + ex's	0.3	1	3	1	Third day post injury
Michlovitz[12]	Ice pack	0.5	1	3	1.5	1–28 h post injury
Lessard[32]	Gel pack + ex's	0.3	4	7	9.3	At home after discharge
Hochberg[24] (a)	Commercial m.	12	1	3	36	Immediately after surgery
Hochberg[24] (b)	Crushed ice Commercial p.	0.3	18	3	18	Immediately after surgery
Healy[20] (a)	Cryocuff	–	–	–	–	Unclear
Healy[20] (b)	Crushed ice	–	–	–	–	Unclear
Schroder[17] (a)	Cryocuff	Continuous	Continuous	14	336	Prior to tourniquet release
Schroder[17] (b)	Ice bags	–	3	–	–	Unclear
Konrath[21](a)	Commercial m.	–	–	3–5 days post discharge	–	Unclear
Konrath[21] (b)	Crushed ice	–	–	–	–	Unclear
Whitelaw[18] (a)	Cryocuff	–	–	–	–	Unclear
Whitelaw[18](b)	–	–	–	–	–	Unclear
Laba[13]	Crushed ice	0.3	1	1	0.3	Day 0–2 since injury
Sloan[14]	Commercial p.	0.5	1	1	0.5	Within 24 h of injury
Edwards[27]	Cryocuff	Continuous	Continuous	1.5	36	In operating room
Cohn[16] (a)	Commercial m.	Continuous	Continuous	4	96	In operating room

Cohn[16] (b)	Ice bag	–	1	1	–	In recovery room
Wilkerson[15] (a)	Ice pack	0.5	1	Acute phase*	1.5	Acute stages*
Wilkerson[15] (b)	Commercial p.	Continuous	Continuous	Acute phase*	64	Acute stages*
Ivey[26]	Commercial m.	Continuous	Continuous	3	64	In recovery room
Scarcella[22] (a)	Commercial m.	Continuous	Continuous	9	216	In operating room
Scarcella[22] (b)	Commercial m.	Continuous	Continuous	9	216	In operating room
Dervin[33]	Cryocuff	Continuous	Continuous	2.5	55–60	Unclear
Barber[30]	Commercial m.	Continuous	Continuous	3 (POD 1–3) 3 (POD 4–6)	64 48 av.	After application of postoperative dressing
Ohkoshi	Commercial m.	Continuous	Continuous	2	48	After surgical wound was covered
Bert[19]	Commercial m/p.	Continuous	Continuous	1–2	27	Immediately post surgery in recovery room
Levy[28]	Cryocuff	Continuous	Continuous	3	64	After skin closure and dressing were applied
Gibbons[23]	Cryocuff	6 (at least)	1	13 (at least)	78	Immediately after the surgical procedure
Brandsson[29]	Cryocuff	Continuous	Continuous	1	24	After surgical wounds were closed
Airaksinen[10]	Cold gel	–	4	14	–	Within 48 h of injury
Fincher[25]	Saline (4 deg C)	–	1	1	–	Continuously during surgery

* "Acute" stage of injury not specified; –, information not reported; Commercial m., commercial icing machine; Commercial p., commercially produced ice pack; + ex's, exercises incorporated with cooling; (specifically stated by the author); POD, postoperative day.

N.b.: (a) and (b) after the study reference indicate that a single study applied more than one cryotherapy protocol.

Table 11.2 Effect size estimates and final PEDro scores for individual studies

Intervention	Injury	n	Effect size (95% CI)				PEDro (10)
			Function	Pain	Swelling	ROM	
Ice vs. heat	Ankle	30	–	–	1.38 (0.35; 2.29)	–	5
Ice vs. contrast	Ankle	30	–	–	2.35 (1.13; 3.37)	–	5
Ice vs. ice + e-stim. (freq. 28 pps)	Ankle	30	–	−0.64 (−1.51; 0.28)	$-0.47(-1.34; 0.44)_{Day\ 1}$ $-0.14\ (-1.01; 0.75)_{Day\ 3}$	$-0.69\ (-1.56, 0.24)_{Day\ 1}$ $-0.58\ (-1.45, 0.24)_{Day\ 3}$	4
Ice vs. ice + e-stim. (freq. 80 pps)	Ankle	30	–	−0.62 (−1.5; 0.3)	$-1.39\ (-2.3; 0.36)_{Day\ 1}$ $-0.09\ (-0.96; 0.8)_{Day\ 3}$	$-1.36(-2.3; -0.3)_{Day\ 1}$ $-0.39\ (-1.3, 0.5)_{Day\ 3}$	4
Ice ex vs. ex	Arthros	45	–	$0.24\ (-0.35; 0.82)_T$ $0.59\ (-0.02; 1.17)_A$	0.35 (−0.24; 0.93)	0.38 (−0.21, 0.97)	5
Ice (continuous) vs. Ice (intermittent)	CTR	48	–	1.09 (0.4; 1.7)	2.2 (1.43; 2.9)	–	4
I/C vs. I/C	TKA	76	–	n/a	n/a	n/a	2
	ACL	44	–	n/a	n/a	n/a	3
	ACL	100	–	n/a	–	n/a	4
	Arthros	102	–	n/a	n/a	n/a	1
I/C vs. no treatment	Ankle	30	n/a *0.88 (0.62; 1.14)*	*1.5 (1.24; 1.76)*	*0.76 (0.5; 1.02)*	–	3
	Ankle	143	–	n/a	n/a	n/a	3
	ACL	63	–	n/a	–	n/a	4
I/C vs. ice	ACL	54	n/a 4.49 (3.41; 5.4)	4.43 (3.3; 5.24)	–	–	4
I/C vs. C (same mode)							
	Ankle	34	−0.14 (−0.97, 0.7)	–	–	–	3
	TKA	90	–	−0.43 (−0.95; 0.1)	–	–	4

	TKA	24	−0.75 (−1.55, 0.1)	–	–	0.39 (−0.44, 1.18)	5
	ACL	100	n/a	n/a	–	n/a	4
	ACL	63	–	n/a	–	n/a	4
	ACL	78	n/a	−0.33 (−0.7; 0.12)$_{VAS}$	–	–	3
				−0.17 (−0.6; 0.3)$_{A/gesic}$	–		
				−0.09 (−0.5; 0.4)$_{IV}$	–		
	ACL	99	–	n/a	–	*1.14 (1.0; 1.28)*	1
	ACL	21	–	−0.6 (−1.64; 0.5)$_{VAS}$	–	1.02 (−0.16; 2.05)	4
				0.3 (−0.75; 1.36)$_{A/gesic}$	–		
	ACL	21	–	1.21 (0; 2.2)$_{VAS}$	0.89 (−0.26; 1.92)	0.8 (−0.27; 1.9)$_{A/gesic}$	4
	THA	50	–	n/a	–	–	5
I/C vs. C (different mode)	LRR	110		Overall score: *0.35 (0.27; 0.42)*			2
	Ankle	34	0.55 (−0.32, 1.38)	–	–	–	3
	TKA	80	–	0.75 (0.3–1.2)$_{VAS(D2)}$	–	0.64 (0.19, 1.08)$_{Day\ 7}$	5
			–	0.41 (−0.04; 0.85)$_{A/gesic}$	–	0.89 (0.42, 1.34)$_{Day\ 14}$	
	TKA	60	–	n/a	–	n/a	3
I/C + P. vs. P. vs I/C and I/A inj.	ACL	50	–	n/a	–	–	4
I vs. no I	Arthros	93	–	n/a	n/a	–	5
	STI	74	n/a	1.03 (0.3–1.83)$_{Day\ 7}$	–	–	8
				0.64 (0.01–1.21)$_{Day\ 14}$			
				0.61 (0.2–1.19)$_{Day\ 28}$			

–, outcome not measured; A/gesic, oral analgesic consumption; A, affective component of McGill questionnaire score; ACL, anterior cruciate ligament reconstruction; Ankle, ankle sprain; Arthros, arthroscopy; C, compression; CI, confidence intervals; CTR, carpal tunnel release; different mode, mode of compression differed across groups; Effect size, relative risk ratio; e-stim, electrical stimulation; Ex, exercise; freq., frequency; I, ice treatment; I/A inj., intra-articular analgesic injection; I/C, simultaneous ice and compression; I/V, intravenous analgesic consumption; LRR, lateral retinacular release; n/a, data not available; P, placebo; Same mode, mode of compression constant across groups; pps, pulse per second; ROM, range of movement; STI, general soft-tissue injury; T, total McGill questionnaire score; THA, total hip arthroplasty; TKA, total knee arthroplasty; VAS, visual analogue scale.

Note: Studies are grouped according to the treatment comparisons employed. A positive standardized mean difference (SMD) or relative risk represents an effect in favor of the treatment group (e.g., group A if the groups are compared as A vs. B).

size estimates for individual studies (standardized mean difference, SMD; relative risk, RR). Effect sizes could not be pooled for statistical analysis due to heterogeneity of the study population, intervention mode and dosage, timing and type of outcome measures, or insufficient reporting of data.

Ice (exercise) versus heat (exercise)/ contrast bath (exercise)

There was some evidence that cryotherapy was more effective than thermotherapy after ankle injury. A single study[11] found that ice submersion with simultaneous exercises was significantly more effective than heat (SMD 1.38; 95% CI, 0.35 to 2.29) and contrast therapy (SMD 2.35; 95% CI, 1.13 to 3.37) plus simultaneous exercises, at reducing swelling between 3 and 5 days after ankle sprain.

Ice versus ice and electrical stimulation

A single study[12] compared the effect of ice alone with that of ice and simultaneous high-voltage electrical stimulation after acute ankle sprains. There was no significant difference when comparing ice alone and ice combined with low-frequency electrical stimulation (28 pulses per second) in terms of swelling (SMD −0.47; 95% CI, −1.34 to 0.44), pain (SMD −0.64; 95% CI, −1.51 to 0.28) and ROM (SMD −0.69; 95% CI, −1.56 to 0.24). Similarly, there was no significant difference comparing ice alone and ice combined with higher-frequency electrical stimulation (80 pulses per second), in terms of swelling (SMD −1.39; 95% CI, −2.3 to 0.36), pain (SMD −0.62; 95% CI, −1.5 to 0.31) and ROM (SMD −1.36; 95% CI, −2.3 to −0.3).

Ice and exercise versus exercise alone

A single study[32] compared the effect of an intermittent icing protocol combined with knee exercises, to exercises alone, after minor arthroscopic knee surgery. The application of ice immediately before a rehabilitation program significantly decreased pain, as measured by the affective component of the McGill pain questionnaire (SMD 0.59; 95 CI, −0.02 to 1.17). The study also reported that subjects applying cryotherapy used significantly less prescription and nonprescription analgesia, and had a significantly better weight-bearing status, but insufficient data are provided for the calculation of an effect size.

Ice versus no ice

Using a group of subjects undergoing arthroscopic knee surgery, Fincher *et al.* opted to use cold in the form of intra-articular saline, applied continuously throughout surgery[25] No significant differences were reported between groups treated with saline at 4 °C and saline at room temperature (18 °C), in terms of pain and knee swelling. In contrast, Airaksinen *et al.* compared the effectiveness of a cold gel to a placebo gel when treating subjects with a range of soft-tissue contusions.[10] Subjects using cold gel over a period of 28 days post-injury experienced significantly less pain both at rest and on movement and significantly less functional disability.

Ice (continuous) versus ice (intermittent)

Using subjects who had undergone carpal tunnel release (CTR), Hochberg compared the effect of continuous cryotherapy to intermittent 20-minute ice applications over the first three postoperative days.[24] Subjects applying continuous cryotherapy had a significantly greater decrease in pain (SMD 1.09; 95% CI, 0.4 to 1.7), and wrist circumference

(SMD 2.2; 95% CI, 1.43 to 2.9), in comparison to those using cryotherapy intermittently. This was the only study to compare the effectiveness of two different cryotherapy protocols, and although it appears that continuous cryotherapy should be the treatment of choice after surgery, the modes of cryotherapy application were not consistent across the two groups.

Ice and compression versus ice and compression

Four studies[17,18,20,21] compared two different methods of applying simultaneous compression and cryotherapy, but few conclusions could be reached. Poor reporting of data meant that individual effect size could not be calculated for any of these studies. Furthermore, two studies[17,18] did not provide adequate information on the mode of cryotherapy, and all failed to specify the duration and frequency of the ice application.

Ice and compression versus no ice

There is marginal evidence that a single simultaneous treatment with ice and compression is no more effective than no cryotherapy, after an ankle sprain. Laba[13] found that a single application of ice and compression, in addition to standard rehabilitation treatment (ultrasound, mobility, and proprioceptive exercises), caused similar levels of swelling (RR 0.76; 95% CI, 0.5 to 1.02) and pain immediately post treatment (RR 1.5; 95% CI, 1.24 to 1.76) and at discharge (RR 0.88; 95% CI, 0.62 to 1.14), in comparison with those receiving standard treatment only. Sloan *et al.*[14] also found that a single application of simultaneous ice and compression was as effective as no treatment in terms of reducing pain, swelling and ROM after ankle sprain. Similarly, Edwards *et al.*[27] found that the continuous use of ice and compression had similar benefits to no treatment, in terms of improving pain and ROM, when applied postsurgically; however, insufficient data were provided in the latter two studies.[14,27]

Ice and compression versus ice

Only one clinical study has compared ice and compression to ice alone.[16] The combination of treatments appeared to be significantly more effective than ice, in terms of reducing the amount of intramuscular (SMD 4.43; 95% CI, 3.3 to 5.24), and oral analgesia (SMD 4.49; 95% CI, 3.4 to 5.4) administered post anterior cruciate ligament (ACL) reconstruction. These results must be interpreted with caution, however, as the mode and duration of ice treatment was not controlled for across groups.

Ice and compression versus compression

The majority of included studies tried to disentangle the effects of ice from those of compression by comparing a variety of treatment combinations. Eight studies strictly controlled for the type of compressive bandages used across comparison groups;[15,21,22,26,27,30,31,33] however, there seemed to be little difference in the effectiveness of ice and compression and compression alone.

In four studies, it was difficult to compare the efficacy of each modality,[15,19,23,28] as the mode of compression differed between the intervention and control groups.

Wilkerson and Horn-Kingery[15] found no significant difference in the time of restricted activity after ankle sprain, in subjects treated with compression alone, and simultaneous ice and compression, (SMD −0.14; 95% CI, −0.97 to 0.7). Using subjects who had undergone ACL reconstruction, others reported no significant differences between groups in terms of function,[21] pain,[21,27] and swelling;[21,27,30] however, insufficient data were reported and effect size could not be calculated for these outcomes. Similarly, Dervin *et al.*[33] found no significant differences in subjective pain scores (SMD −0.33; 95% CI, −0.77 to 0.12), and the amounts of intravenous (SMD −0.09; 95% CI, −0.53 to 0.35) and oral analgesics (SMD, −0.17; 95% CI, −0.62 to 0.27). In a group of subjects who had undergone total knee arthroplasty (TKA), Ivey *et al.*[26] found no significant difference between groups with regard to the amount of injected morphine (SMD −0.43; 95% CI, −0.95 to 0.1) after surgery. Scarcella and Cohn[22] found no significant difference in subjects after TKA in terms of ROM (SMD 0.39; 95% CI, −0.44 to 1.18) and the time to independent ambulation (SMD −0.75; 95% CI, −1.55 to 0.1). The study[22] also reported that the analgesic consumption in each group was almost identical. Correspondingly, in a subgroup of patients recovering from total hip arthroplasty (THA), Scarcella and Cohn[22] reported no significant differences in analgesic consumption after surgery; however, insufficient data were provided and the effect size could not be calculated.

Only two studies reported significant differences between subjects treated with ice and compression and compression alone. Although Barber *et al.*[30] found no differences between groups in knee ROM after ACL reconstruction (RR 1.14; 95% CI, 1.0 to 1.28), a significantly decreased analgesic consumption was reported in favor of the ice and compression group; however, inadequate data were provided. Again using subjects post ACL reconstruction, Ohkoshi *et al.*[31] treated two groups with simultaneous ice and compression and a third with compression only. The ice and compression groups were cooled to slightly different temperatures using a commercial ice machine (5 °C and 10 °C). Subjects using less extreme cooling (10 °C group) with concomitant compression, had significantly lower subjective pain scores (SMD 1.21; 95% CI, 0.00 to 2.2) and analgesic consumption (SMD 0.88; 95% CI, −0.27 to 1.91) in comparison with those using compression alone. In contrast, there were no significant differences in subjects treated with simultaneous cooling (5 °C group) and compression, and those treated with compression only, in terms of subjective pain scores (SMD −0.6; 95% CI, −1.64 to 0.5), and analgesic consumption (SMD 0.3; 95% CI, −0.75 to 1.36). A better improvement in range of movement was observed in the 5 °C (SMD 1.02; 95% CI, −0.16 to 2.05) and 10 °C groups (SMD 0.89; 95% CI, −0.26 to 1.92) in comparison with the compression group, but these differences were not significant.

Therefore, despite eight trials comparing the effectiveness of ice and compression with compression alone, only two[30,31] reported significant differences in favor of ice and compression. The studies by Barber *et al.*[30] and Ohkoshi *et al.*[31] were both of low quality, scoring just 1/10 and 4/10 on the PEDro scoring scale, respectively, and therefore the strength of their conclusions is limited. Generally, there was very little evidence to suggest that the addition of ice to compression has any significant effect. It must be noted, however, that all but one of the studies[15] were undertaken after surgery, and any conclusions are restricted to hospital in-patients with postsurgical wound dressings.

Ice and compression plus placebo injection versus ice and compression plus injection versus placebo injection

Brandsson *et al.* found that ice and compression plus a placebo injection were significantly more effective than a placebo injection alone at reducing postoperative pain.[29] The addition of a pain-killing injection to ice and compression therapy significantly improved the analgesic effect further; again, however, no data were provided and the effect size could not be calculated.

Discussion

Study limitations

This is the first study to systematically review the literature, assessing the clinical evidence base supporting the use of cryotherapy on the basis of the highest-quality research evidence. The review is restricted to English-language publications, however, and as the inclusion criteria for the study population were broad, some of the information contained was difficult to compare and synthesize. The randomized and controlled trials included scored an average PEDro score of 4.9, and the contrast in treatment protocols means that comparison within and across studies is often impossible. Moreover, persistent methodological problems and the failure of the majority of studies to carry out a power analysis may prevent wider extrapolation of evidence.

To date, only one randomized study has assessed the efficacy of ice in the treatment of muscle contusions or strains, and only five studies have assessed the effect of ice on acute ankle sprains. Single applications of combined ice and compression appear to be as effective as "no treatment" after an acute sprain; however, these conclusions must be taken with caution. Aside from the paucity of high-quality studies undertaken, this particular research question may also be subject to a unique set of problems inherent to cryotherapy research. Given the strong empirical evidence base and the popularity of cryotherapy treatment with the layman, it may be difficult to randomize a subject to a "no ice" group. This is particularly evident in Laba's study,[13] in which 60% of subjects randomized to the "no ice" group had already applied ice as a self-treatment prior to recruitment.

Cryotherapy dosage

The basic premise of cryotherapy is to cool injured tissue. It is clearly documented, however, that excessive temperature reduction is harmful, whereas mild cooling may not be of any physiological benefit to the patient. The key aim of a treatment protocol is therefore to strike a balance between safety and efficacy. It has been suggested that intermittent 10-minute ice treatments are most effective at safely cooling injured animal tissue and healthy human tissue.[5] Although the effectiveness of this particular protocol has not yet been tested on injured human subjects, Hochberg[24] found that intermittent 20-minute applications are less effective than continuous ice treatment, after CTR surgery. The strength of the study's conclusions is greatly limited, however, as crucially Hochberg failed to control for the mode of cryotherapy across the continuous and intermittent groups.[24]

Using a novel treatment method, Airaksinen *et al.* found that application of an ethanol/methanol-based gel was superior to placebo gel for up to 2 weeks after mild soft-tissue injury.[10] Although the degree of cooling associated with the topical gel was not reported, it has been postulated that its mechanism of action may be due to more systemic effects, rather than those attributed to traditional cryotherapy. Future study is essential to determine if this mode of cooling is as effective in treating moderate to severe soft-tissue injuries.

In general, no individual study has rigorously compared the efficacy of different modes, durations or frequencies of ice treatment, and preliminary recommendations for an optimal cryotherapy protocol cannot be made.

Barrier effect

The interaction between the cooling surface and the subjects' tissue is vital in determining the effectiveness of treatment. Within this review, the initial consensus from eight

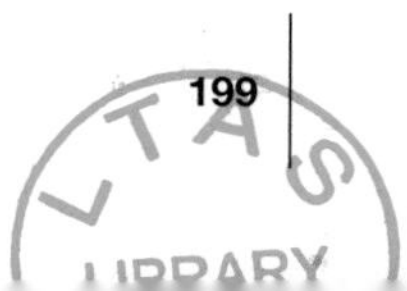

well-controlled studies[15,21,22,26,27,30,31,33] seemed to be that the addition of ice to compression is no more effective than compression alone. However, such a conclusion may be limited, as in all eight of these studies, postsurgical dressings or socks were used to separate the injured area of the body and the cooling device. Although the thicknesses of dressings varied, from gauze[22] to cast padding and an elastic bandage,[26] all such barriers have the potential to mitigate the cooling effect of cold compress.

To maximize the therapeutic effects of cryotherapy, an optimal tissue temperature reduction of 10–15 °C may be necessary.[5] Skin temperature reductions to below 13.6 °C may be needed to achieve local analgesia[34] and perhaps lower tissue temperatures of between 10 °C and 15 °C may be required to maximally lower metabolism.[35,36] Such temperature reductions simply may not be possible due to the barrier effect. Indeed, the only study[21] that monitored skin tissue temperatures during treatment reported a maximum reduction to just 28 °C. Correspondingly, there is evidence from observational studies[37–42] that it is difficult to achieve optimal tissue temperature reductions when cooling is applied over postoperative dressings or towels. Furthermore, the insulating effect of subcutaneous fat has also been well documented,[43,44] and it seems there is a direct relationship between adipose thicknesses and cooling time[45] This could suggest that a universal icing protocol may not be possible and that treatment guidance may be patient-dependent.

Side effects

A number of case studies have reported the occurrence of skin burns[46] and nerve damage[47–50] after as little as 20–30 minutes of cooling. Within this review, there was just one reported case of cold-induced nerve palsy, possibly caused by a continuous 40-minute ice application in the recovery room after surgery.[16] Surprisingly, none of the other studies reported any incidences of skin burns or nerve palsies, despite applying continuous ice treatments for between 6 and 226 hours. This may be due to concomitant compression or wound bandaging mitigating the cooling effect.

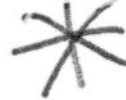

Icing for acute or rehabilitative treatment

Cryotherapy is a versatile modality and has been advocated in the immediate[51–53] and rehabilitative[54,55] phases of injury management. However, a common source of confusion is the basis for its application at each phase. Immediately after injury, ice reduces tissue metabolism, thereby minimizing secondary hypoxic injury, cell debris, and edema. The sooner after injury cryotherapy is initiated, the more beneficial this reduction in metabolism might be.[55] A number of studies[12–14] began cryotherapy between 24 and 48 hours after injury, and therefore may not have optimized this positive physiological effect.

It may be easier to initiate early cryotherapy in studies using surgical patients. Fincher *et al.*[25] initiated cooling during the surgical procedure using intra-articular cold saline irrigation; however, this approach proved to be ineffective. For most subjects, however, cooling was stopped less than 10 minutes after the conclusion of the surgical insult, and the author postulates that an extended protocol, potentially coinciding with the onset of inflammation, might have been more beneficial.

Most other surgical studies stated that cryotherapy was initiated either immediately after surgery, in the operating room, or after dressing and wound closure; however, few significant differences were reported. Again, this may be due to concomitant compression or wound bandaging mitigating the cooling effect and preventing adequate metabolic reduction.

Outside the immediate stages of injury management, cryotherapy may be most effective when combined with exercise.[52,55] Adequate cooling can reduce pain, spasm, and neural inhibition, thereby allowing for earlier and more aggressive exercises. In the current review, many studies[16,17,21–24,26,28,30] continued cryotherapy treatment for days and even weeks after injury, but chose not to integrate therapeutic exercise. In the past, clinical evidence supporting the use of cryotherapy for such rehabilitative purposes was restricted to observational studies.[56,57] There is now more recent evidence from two randomized and controlled studies[11,32] that cooling may be significantly more effective when used in combination with exercises in the subacute phases of injury.

Potentially, cryotherapy enables injured athletes to perform exercises earlier and more aggressively than normal. This had been solely attributed to the analgesic qualities of cryotherapy;[58] however, more recent evidence has inferred that cryotherapy may also have a disinhibiting effect on the musculature surrounding an injured joint, thereby allowing greater activation of the motor neuron pools.[59–61] There is also an increasing body of evidence to refute the common supposition that applying cryotherapy prior to therapeutic exercise should be contraindicated, as it increases the risk of injury.[62,63] Icing does not appear to alter joint positional sense or sensory perception,[64–66] agility,[67] balance,[68] muscle strength endurance,[69–71] ground reaction force,[72] side-stepping performance,[73] or motor control.[71] This new wave of evidence certainly suggests that combining cryotherapy and exercise is a safe and effective approach to managing soft-tissue injury. Future study will be required to suggest an optimal cryotherapy and exercise protocol, and indeed how best to combine them during injury rehabilitation.

Concomitant therapies

The mnemonic RICE—representing rest, ice, compression and elevation—remains the mantra of physiotherapists, clinicians, and athletes in treating any soft-tissue injury.[74] An ongoing problem within research and clinical practice is that all three modalities are applied simultaneously, and the relative efficacy of each is unknown.[51,54,75,76] A number of studies in the current review have compared a wide range of combinations of ice and compression in a bid to try and disentangle their relative efficacy. Most have done little to separate and quantify their individual effects, as the modes and durations of cold and compressive treatments applied across groups were starkly contrasting.

Few studies have been undertaken on elevation, and the research published surrounding the individual use of compression after injury remains poor.[77] Potentially, the development of an optimal mode, duration, and frequency of compressive treatment will be a priority for future study in this area. Clarifying the respective value of each individual modality could provide the basis for an optimal method of combining ice and compression and could further develop the research base for acute soft-tissue injury management.

Summary

- The basic premise of applying ice is to cool skin and deep tissue temperature to a therapeutic level.
- The degree of skin and deep tissue temperature reduction is dependent on the mode, duration, and frequency of ice application.
- Compression bandages and dressing may mitigate the cooling effect, compromising the effectiveness of ice treatments.

• Few studies to date have considered the pathophysiological rationale behind ice application.
• Ice can safely be applied in the acute or rehabilitative phases of treatment.
• There is preliminary evidence that ice is superior to no treatment, heat, and contrast therapy in minimizing pain and swelling after injury.
• There is preliminary evidence that ice can be safely and effectively combined with therapeutic exercise during rehabilitation.

Key messages

• A large number of randomized and controlled trials have been added to our information base regarding the use of ice in the treatment of acute soft-tissue injuries.
• The methodological quality of these studies is generally poor.
• The majority have not fully considered the pathophysiological basis of cryotherapy, and may not have used it to its full potential.
• There is little evidence to suggest that the addition of ice to compression has any significant effect, but this is restricted to treatment of hospital inpatients.
• Few studies assessed the effectiveness of ice on closed soft-tissue injury, and there was no evidence of an optimal mode or duration of treatment.
• There is some preliminary evidence that ice can safely and effectively be combined with therapeutic exercise.

Sample examination questions

Multiple-choice questions (answers on page 602)

1 Following current best evidence, an athlete with a 7-day-old knee medial ligament strain should:
  A Not apply ice
  B Apply ice, but for longer durations
  C Apply ice, but only with compression
  D Apply ice, but only with intermittent exercise
  E Apply with simultaneous elevation
2 Which of the following statements are *true*?
  A Icing before exercise can increase the risk of injury
  B Ice and compression should never be applied simultaneously
  C Ice should always be applied over a compressive bandaging to minimise the risk of skin burns
  D Intermittent ice treatments may minimise the incidence of skin burns
  E Contrast therapy is more effective than ice alone in decreasing swelling
3 Which of the following statements are *false*?
  A Deep tissue temperatures can be reduced to therapeutic levels faster in athletes with a lower percentage of body fat
  B Decreasing secondary hypoxic injury is the most important physiological effect in acute injury management
  C Icing may facilitate therapeutic exercise
  D Icing is only effective when applied immediately after an injury
  E The magnitude of skin temperature reduction is dependent on the mode of icing

Essay questions

1 Describe the potential advantages of applying an intermittent icing protocol after an acute soft-tissue injury.
2 Compare and contrast the physiological aims when applying ice in the immediate and rehabilitative phases of injury management.

Case study 1

Robin, a 28-year-old soccer player, has suffered grade-2 ligament damage to his ankle 2 days ago. His ankle is swollen and he can partially weight-bear. He is aware of the potential benefits of the protection, relative rest, ice, compression, and elevation (PRICE) regime. His friend has advised him that he will no longer benefit from applying ice at this stage, but should continue to wear a compressive bandage. He is seeking guidance on the best way to proceed.

Case study 2

Deborah, a 24-year-old netball player, has just been discharged from hospital after arthroscopic knee surgery. She was advised to apply ice intermittently over the next week to minimize the swelling around her knee. She has also been provided with a series of stretching and strengthening exercises. After 2 days, she is thinking about stopping icing, as there seems to be no difference in the degree of swelling around her knee. She is looking for confirmation on the appropriateness of this.

Summarizing the evidence

Comparison/treatment strategy	Conclusions	Level of evidence
Ice vs. thermotherapy/ contrast therapy	Ice alone is significantly better at minimizing swelling	A6
Ice vs. ice and electrical stimulation	The addition of electrical stimulation to ice has no significant effect	A6
Ice and exercise vs. exercise alone	Therapeutic exercise is most effective when combined with ice	A6
Ice vs. no ice	Cold gel appears to be more effective than placebo Intra-articular cold saline is an ineffective method of cooling tissue during minor knee surgery	A2 A2
Continuous ice vs. intermittent ice	Continuous icing is more effective than intermittent ice applications N.b., mode of icing was not consistent across comparison groups	A6
Ice and compression vs. no treatment	Single applications of ice and compression are ineffective	A3

Continued

Summarizing the evidence *(Continued)*

Comparison/treatment strategy	Conclusions	Level of evidence
Ice and compression vs. ice	Ice and compression is more effective than ice alone N.b., mode and duration of ice treatment was not controlled for across groups	A6
Ice and compression vs. ice and compression	Limited conclusions 2 studies did not provide adequate information on the mode of cryotherapy All 4 studies failed to specify the duration and frequency of the ice application	
Ice and compression vs. compression	6 studies concluded that the addition of ice to compression has no significant effect 2 studies reported that ice and compression was significantly more effective than compression alone The remaining 4 studies failed to control for the type of compressive bandages used across comparison groups NB. Potential mitigation of cooling effect of cold compress, since in all studies (n = 14) postsurgical dressings or socks were used to separate the injured area of the body and the cooling device	A3

A1, evidence from two or more large randomized controlled trials (RCTs; n ≥ 60 per study group); A2, evidence from at least one large RCT (n ≥ 60 per study group); A3, evidence from two or more moderate-sized RCTs (n ≥ 30 per study group); A4, evidence from at least one moderate-sized RCT (n ≥ 30 per study group); A5, evidence from two or more small RCTs (n ≥ 15 per study group); A6, evidence from at least one small RCT (n ≥ 15 per study group).

References

1 Adirim TA, Cheng TL. Overview of injuries in the young athlete. *Sports Medicine* 2003; **33**:75–81.
2 Best TM. Soft tissue injuries and muscle tears. *Clin Sports Med* 1997; **16**:419–434.
3 McDowell JH, McFarland EG, Nalli BJ. Use of cryotherapy for orthopaedic patients. *Orthopaedic Nursing* 1994; **13**:21–30.
4 MacAuley D. Do textbooks agree on their advice on ice? *Clin J Sports Med* 2001; **11**:67–64.
5 MacAuley D. Ice therapy: how good is the evidence? *Int J Sports Med* 2001; **22**:379–384.
6 MacAuley D. What is the role of ice in soft tissue injury management? In: MacAuley D, Best TM, eds. *Evidence-Based Sports Medicine.* London: BMJ/Blackwell Publishing, 2002:45–65.
7 Bleakley CM, McDonough SM, MacAuley DC. The use of ice in the treatment of acute soft tissue injuries: a systematic review of randomized controlled trials. *Am J Sports Med* 2004; **32**:251–262.
8 Moseley A. Evidence for physiotherapy practice: a survey of the Physiotherapy Evidence Database (PEDro). *Aust J Physiother* 2002; **48**:43–49.
9 Moher D, Cook DJ, Eastwood S, *et al.* Improving the quality of reports of meta-analyses of randomized controlled trials: the QUORUM statement. *Lancet* 1999; **354**:1896–1900.
10 Airaksinen O, Kyrklund N, Latvala N, *et al.* Efficacy of cold gel for soft tissue injuries: a prospective randomized controlled trial. *Am J Sports Med* 2003; **31**:680–684.
11 Cote DJ, Prentice WE, Hooker DN, Shields EW. Comparison of three treatment procedures for minimizing ankle sprain swelling. *Phys Ther* 1988; **68**:1064–1076.

12 Michlovitz S, Smith W, Watkins M. Ice and high voltage pulsed stimulation in treatment of acute lateral ankle sprains. *J Orthop Sports Phys Ther* 1988; **9**:301–304.
13 Laba E. Clinical evaluation of ice therapy for acute ankle sprain injuries. *N Z J Physiother* 1989; **17**:7–9.
14 Sloan JP, Hain R, Pownall R. Clinical benefits of early cold therapy in accident and emergency following ankle sprain. *Arch Emerg Med* 1989; **6**:1–6.
15 Wilkerson GB, Horn-Kingery HM. Treatment of the inversion ankle sprain: comparison of different modes of compression and cryotherapy. *J Orthop Sports Phys Ther* 1993; **17**:240–246.
16 Cohn BT, Draeger RI, Jackson DW. The effects of cold therapy in the postoperative management of pain in patients undergoing anterior cruciate ligament reconstruction. *Am J Sports Med* 1989; **17**:344–349.
17 Schroder D, Passler HH. Combination of cold and compression after knee surgery: a prospective randomized study. *Knee Surg Sports Traumatol Arthrosc* 1994; **2**:158–165.
18 Whitelaw GP, DeMuth KA, Demos HA, Schepsis A, Jacques E. The use of cryocuff versus ice and elastic wrap in postoperative care of knee arthroscopy patients. *Am J Knee Surg* 1995; **8**:28–31.
19 Bert JM, Stark JG, Maschka K, Chock C. The effect of cold therapy on morbidity subsequent to arthroscopic lateral retinacular release. *Orthop Rev* 1991; **20**:755–758.
20 Healy WL, Seidman J, Pfeiffer BA, Brown BA. Cold compressive dressing after total knee arthroplasty. *Clin Orthop Rel Res* 1994; **299**:143–146.
21 Konrath GA, Lock T, Goitz HT, Scheidler J. The use of cold therapy after anterior cruciate ligament reconstruction: a prospective randomized study and literature review. *Am J Sports Med* 1996; **24**:629–633.
22 Scarcella JB, Cohn BT. The effect of cold therapy on the postoperative course of total hip and knee arthroplasty patients. *Am J Orthop* 1995; **24**:847–852.
23 Gibbons CER, Solan MC, Ricketts DM, Patterson M. Cryotherapy compared with Robert Jones bandage after total knee replacement: a prospective randomized trial. *Int Orthop* 2001; **25**:250–252.
24 Hochberg J. A randomized prospective study to assess the efficacy of two cold therapy treatments following carpal tunnel release. *J Hand Ther* 2001; **14**:208–215.
25 Fincher L, Woods G, O'Connor D. Intraoperative arthroscopic cold irrigation solution does not affect postoperative pain and swelling. *J Athl Train* 2004; **39**:12–17.
26 Ivey M, Johnston RV, Uchida T. Cryotherapy for postoperative pain relief following knee arthroplasty. *J Arthroplast* 1994; **9**:285–290.
27 Edwards DJ, Rimmer M, Kenne GC. The use of cold therapy in the post operative management of patients undergoing arthroscopic anterior cruciate ligament reconstruction. *Am J Sports Med* 1996; **24**:193–195.
28 Levy AS, Marmar E. The role of cold compression dressings in the postoperative treatment of total knee arthroplasty. *Clin Orthop Rel Res* 1993; **297**:174–178.
29 Brandsson S, Rydgren B, Hedner T, *et al.* Postoperative analgesic effects of an external cooling system and intra-articular bupivacaine/morphine after arthroscopic cruciate ligament surgery. *Knee Surg Sports Traumatol Arthrosc* 1996; **4**:200–205.
30 Barber AF, McGuire DA, Click S. Continuous-flow cold therapy for outpatient anterior cruciate ligament reconstruction. *Arthroscopy* 1998; **14**:130–135.
31 Ohkoshi Y, Ohkoshi M, Nagasaki S, Ono A, Hashimoto T, Yamane S. The effect of cryotherapy on intraarticular temperature and postoperative care after anterior cruciate ligament reconstruction. *Am J Sports Med* 1999; **27**:357–362.
32 Lessard LA, Scudds RA, Amendola A, Vas MD. The efficacy of cryotherapy following arthroscopic knee surgery. *J Orthop Sports Phys Ther* 1997; **26**:14–22.
33 Dervin GF, Taylor DE, Keene GC. Effects of cold and compression dressings on early postoperative outcomes for the arthroscopic anterior cruciate ligament reconstruction patient. *J Orthop Sports Phys Ther* 1998; **27**:403–406.
34 Bugai R. The cooling, analgesic, and rewarming effects of ice massage on localized skin. *Phys Ther* 1976; **55**:11–19.
35 Knight KL. Effects of hypothermia on inflammation and swelling. *J Athl Train* 1976; **11**:7–10.
36 Sapega AA, Heppenstall RB, Sokolow DP, *et al.* The bioenergetics of preservation of limbs before replantation. The rationale for intermediate hypothermia. *J Bone Joint Surg Am* 1988; **70**:1500–1513.
37 La Velle BE, Snyder M. Differential conduction of cold through barriers. *J Adv Nurs* 1985; **10**:55–61.
38 Daniel DM, Stone ML, Arendt DL. The effect of cold therapy on pain, swelling, and range of motion after anterior cruciate ligament reconstructive surgery. *Arthroscopy* 1994; **10**:530–533.

39 Culp RW, Taras JS. The effect of ice application versus controlled cold therapy on skin temperature when used with postoperative bulky hand and wrist dressings: a preliminary study. *J Hand Ther* 1995; **8**:249–251.
40 Levy AS, Kelly B, Lintner S, Speer K. Penetration of cryotherapy in treatment after shoulder arthroscopy. *Arthroscopy* 1997; **13**:461–464.
41 Osbahr DC, Cawley PW, Speer KP. The effect of continuous cryotherapy on glenohumeral joint and subacromial space temperatures in the postoperative shoulder. *Arthroscopy* 2002; **18**:748–754.
42 Janwantanakul P. Different rate of cooling time and magnitude of cooling temperature during ice bag treatment with and without damp towel wrap. *Phys Ther Sport* 2004; **5**:156–161.
43 McMaster WC. A literary review on ice therapy in injuries. *Am J Sports Med* 1977; **5**:124–126.
44 Hocutt, J. Cryotherapy in ankle sprains. *Am J Sports Med* 1982; **10**:316–319.
45 Otte JW, Merrick MA, Ingersoll CD, Cordova ML. Subcutaneous adipose tissue thickness alters cooling time during cryotherapy. *Arch Phys Med Rehabil* 2002; **83**:1501–1505.
46 O'Toole G, Rayatt S. Frostbite at the gym: a case report of an ice pack burn. *Br J Sports Med* 1999; **33**:278–279.
47 Drez D, Faust DC, Evans JP. Cryotherapy and nerve palsy. *Am J Sports Med* 1981; **9**:256–257.
48 Bassett FH, Kirkpatrick JS, Engelhardt DL, Malone TR. Cryotherapy-induced nerve injury. *Am J Sports Med* 1992; **20**:516–518.
49 Malone TR, Engelhardt DL, Kirkpatrick JS. Nerve injury in athletes caused by cryotherapy. *J Athl Train (Dallas)* 1992; **27**:235–237.
50 Moeller JL, Monroe J, McKeag DB. Cryotherapy-induced common peroneal nerve palsy. *Clin J Sports Med* 1997; **7**:212–216.
51 Meeusen R, Lievens P. The use of cryotherapy in sports injuries. *Sports Med* 1986; **3**:398–414.
52 Knight KL. Cryotherapy in sports injury management. *Int Perspect Physiother* 1989; **4**:163–185.
53 Swenson C, Sward L, Karlsson J. Cryotherapy in sports medicine. *Scand J Med Sci Sports* 1996; **6**:193–200.
54 Rivenberg DW. Physical modalities in the treatment of tendon injuries. *Clin Sports Med* 1992; **11**:645–659.
55 Knight KL, Brucker JB, Stoneman PD, Rubley MD. Muscle injury management with cryotherapy. *Athl Ther Today* 2000; **5**:26–30.
56 Grant A. Massage with ice (cryogenics) in the treatment of painful conditions of the musculoskeletal system. *Arch Phys Med* 1964; **45**:233–238.
57 Hayden C. Cryokinetics in an early treatment programme. *Am J Phys Ther* 1964; **44**:990–993.
58 Knight KL. *Cryotherapy in Sport Injury Management.* Champaign, IL: Human Kinetics, 1995.
59 Hopkins JT, Ingersoll CD, Edwards JE, Cordova ML. Changes in motoneurone pool excitability after artificial knee joint effusion. *Arch Phys Med Rehabil* 2000; **81**:1199–1203.
60 Hopkins JT, Ingersoll CD, Edwards JE, Klootwyk TE. Cryotherapy and transcutaneous electric neuromuscular stimulation decrease arthrogenic muscle inhibition of the vastus medialis after knee joint effusion. *J Athl Train* 2001; **37**:25–31.
61 Hopkins JT, Stencil R. Ankle cryotherapy facilitates soleus function. *J Orthop Sports Phys Ther* 2002; **32**:622–627.
62 Oliver RA, Johnson DJ, Wheelhouse WW, Griffen PP. Isometric muscle contraction response during recovery from reduced intramuscular temperature. *Arch Phys Med Rehabil* 1979; **60**:126–129.
63 Cross KM, Wilson RW, Perrin DH. Functional performance following an ice immersion to the lower extremity. *J Athl Train* 1996; **31**:113–116.
64 Ingersoll CD, Knight KL, Merrick MA. Sensory perception of the foot and ankle following therapeutic application of heat and cold. *J Athl Train* 1992; **27**:231–234.
65 LaRiviere JA. The effects of ice immersion on joint positional sense. *J Sports Rehabil* 1994; **3**:58–67.
66 Hopper D, Whittington D, Davies J, Chartier JD. Does ice immersion influence ankle joint positional sense? *Physiother Res Int* 1997; **2**:223–236.
67 Evans TA, Ingersoll C, Knight KL, Worrell T. Agility following the application of cold therapy. *J Athl Train* 1995; **30**:231–234.
68 Elley R. The effect of ice pack application at the ankle joint one-legged balance ability. *N Z J Physiother* 1994; **22**:17–22.
69 Kimura IF, Gulick DT, Thompson GT. The effect of cryotherapy on eccentric plantar flexion peak torque and endurance. *J Athl Train* 1997; **32**:124–126.

70 Shimor T, Akayama S. Effects of short term cold application on moderate muscle force with electromyographic study. In: *Proceedings of the 14th International WCPT Congress, Barcelona, Spain, 7–12 June 2003.* Abstract number: RR PL 0843.

71 Rubley MD, Denegar CR, Buckley WE, Newell KM. Cryotherapy, sensation, and isometric force variability. *J Athl Train* 2003; **38**:113–119.

72 Jameson AG. Lower extremity joint cryotherapy does not effect vertical ground reaction forces during landing. *J Sports Rehabil* 2001; **10**:132–142.

73 Atnip BL, McCrory JL. The effect of cryotherapy on three dimensional ankle kinematics during a sidestep cutting manoeuvre. *J Sports Sci Med* 2004; **3**:82–90.

74 MacAuley D, Best T. Reducing the risk of injury due to exercise. *BMJ* 2002; **325**:451–452.

75 Kerr KM, Daily L, Booth L. *Guidelines for the Management of Soft Tissue (Musculoskeletal) Injury with Protection, Rest, Ice, Compression and Elevation (PRICE) during the First 64 Hours.* London: Chartered Society of Physiotherapy 1999.

76 Thorsson O. Cold therapy of athletic injuries: a literature review. *Lakartidningen* 2001; **98**:1512–1513.

77 Wilson S, Cooke M. Double bandaging of sprained ankles. *BMJ* 1998; **317**:1722–1723.

CHAPTER 12
Compression

Andrew Currie and Matthew Cooke

Ankle sprains are a common injury encountered by medical practitioners, and represent much of the workload in sports medicine, accounting for 19–23% of all sports injuries.[1–3] Ankle sprains commonly damage the lateral ligament complex,[4] which comprises three ligaments—the anterior talofibular, the posterior talofibular, and the calcaneofibular. The anterior talofibular (ATFL) is the most commonly (and sometimes only) affected ligament in an ankle sprain, being damaged in 97% of cases.[5] The ATFL is most commonly injured as it is the weakest component of the lateral ligament complex.[5] Anatomically positioned, the ATFL is horizontal, but when the foot is plantarflexed (as it is when ankle sprains occur), the ligament is in line with the long axis of the leg. The latter position is when the ATFL is damaged, particularly when the foot is inverted.[6,7]

Since the times of Hippocrates, ice has been used to treat injuries. In treating "aches and sprains," health professionals have used a form of the time-honored mantra of the rest, ice, compression, and elevation (RICE) paradigm. Despite being a very extensively used treatment, there is a substantial lack of evidence to back up the use of this intervention.

Rest

In order to reduce the metabolic demands of the injured area and to avoid further increase in blood flow, rest for the injured area is essential at the early stage after injury.[8] Rest can range from minimization of movements of the affected limb to strict immobilization with splintage or plaster slab, depending on the degree of the soft-tissue injury. The duration of rest also depends on the severity of initial injury. Immobilization may lead to disuse atrophy,[9] adhesion formation,[10] and joint stiffness.[11] However, too early mobilization of the injured tissue can exacerbate the inflammatory response.[12] Animal studies showed that controlled mobilization would affect the viscous property of connective tissue and promote healing of dense fibrous tissue.[13] The optimal time of rest should be guided by the degree of initial injury and the inflammatory response of the patient.

Ice

Ice is commonly used to reduce inflammation, hemorrhage, swelling and pain in soft-tissue injuries.[14] The principal effects of ice are to reduce the blood circulation to the injured area by vasoconstriction[15] and to reduce tissue temperature to diminish the metabolic demand and production of metabolites.[16] The effect of cooling on metabolism is vital in limiting the degree of injury. Cell necrosis takes place within a few hours after injury, releasing lysins and inducing local edema, which lead to secondary cell damage.[17]

Cooling, in the initial 2 hours post-injury, will minimize secondary cell necrosis by reducing the metabolic demand.[18] Analgesia attributed to ice treatment can be achieved by several mechanisms:[17]

- Reduction of edema and reduced release of pain-inducing metabolites
- Impaired pain impulse transmission, possibly via Aδ fibers
- Sensory stimuli of cold acting on a pain gate mechanism

It is generally recommended that ice should be given for 20–30 minutes in order to achieve the results of decreased pain, blood flow, and metabolism,[14,19] although it is commented by others that the recommendations are only based on empirical experience rather than on evidence.[20] Flaked or crushed ice is the most common mode of ice application. Chipped ice in a wet towel or plastic bag molded to the surface of the injured area can achieve good contact.[21] The recommendations for the frequency of ice application after a soft-tissue injury vary from every 1–2 hours to several times a day.[20] Again, the scientific evidence for the recommendations is sparse. In the presence of some pathological conditions (such as Raynaud's disease and cryoglobulinemia), ice application would be contraindicated.[17]

Compression

Compression is applied to limit the edema formation caused by the exudation of fluid from the damaged capillaries into the tissue.[22] This will control the amount of inflammatory exudates and reduces fibrin deposition and the subsequent formation of scar tissues. In addition, the osmotic pressure of the tissue fluid over the injured area can also be reduced.[23] It is recognized that compression strapping can reduce inversion of the ankle by 35%, but that tape stability decreases by 14% after 30 minutes.[24]

Elevation

Elevation of the injured limb lowers the pressure in local blood vessels and helps to limit bleeding.[25] It also improves the drainage of inflammatory exudate through the lymph vessels, thus reducing edema.[25] Studies have shown that elevation above the subject's heart level can help to reduce swelling and to increase drainage of the extravascular fluid away from the injured area.[25,26] It is a common practice to combine elevation with compression but care has to be taken to avoid compromising arterial supply in case of arterial insufficiency.[25]

While the whole of the RICE regime merits an in-depth analysis of the evidence base, the purpose of this chapter is to investigate the quality of the evidence for compression. However, the three issues of temperature, rest, and elevation cannot be isolated from compression. Any compressive device may also limit movement, but is often given to enable earlier activity and may therefore reduce rest and elevation. Taping has been confirmed to restrict movements associated with inversion sprains of the ankle.[27] Ice is more difficult to apply with compression in place, and tape may increase the temperature of tissues underlying it, particularly during exercise. Compression implies the primary action to be reduction of swelling, but it is always also associated with support to the joint. Support, in turn, implies restriction of movement. A number of methods exist for exerting a compressive effect around the ankle including taping, elastic bandage, and numerous external ankle supports (such as the Aircast stirrup). Capasso and colleagues[28] evaluated the compressive effect of taping on swelling around the ankles. The investigators found that the nonadhesive taping they tested could only exert a compressive effect sufficient to reduce swelling for 3 days before requiring replacement. The adhesive tape, conversely, could last 5 days before requiring renewal. Viljakka[29] compared taping with elastic bandages and found that both padded adhesive and elastic bandages had a significant compressive effect. Stover[30] investigated the impact on acute ankle edema of an external ankle support with the Aircast stirrup. The support was able to produce a compressive effect of 25 mmHg, which increased to 50 mmHg when the individual was weight-bearing.

Methods

This review was conducted using computerized searches of MEDLINE, EMBASE, and CINAHL for studies published between 1966 and 2005. We only considered studies published in English. The key words used singly or in combination for the literature search were:

- Ankle sprain
- Inversion injury
- Lateral ligament
- Compression
- Immobilization
- Brace
- Elastic bandage
- Ankle support
- Orthosis
- Rehabilitation

Reference lists from the identified articles were also searched for possible relevant studies. The study focused only on the compressive treatments and prophylaxis of ankle sprains.

Compression as treatment (Table 12.1)

It is important to remember that any ankle that is held within a compressive implement like a bandage will be subject to a certain degree of immobilization. Most evidence points to a poorer outcome following a lateral ankle ligament injury with immobilization. A Cochrane review by Kerkhoffs and colleagues[31] evaluated any intervention consisting of immobilization with or without a plaster cast. It reported outcomes from 21 trials on injuries to the lateral ankle ligament complex at short-term, medium-term, and long-term follow-up. The trial found that functional treatments (including strapping, bracing, Tubigrips, and elastic bandages) significantly improved outcome in:

- Increased return to sport
- Quicker return to sport
- Increased return to work at short-term follow-up
- Shorter time taken to return to work
- Reduced objective instability
- Less persistent swelling in the short term
- Increased patient satisfaction

However, when only the "high-quality" trails (> 50% of an accepted rating score) were analyzed, the earlier return to work was a significant difference. The authors concluded that functional treatment was superior to immobilization, but that in general the standard of trial reporting was poor.

Table 12.1 Randomized trials of compression as treatment

First author, ref.	n	Treatments tested	Conclusions
Brooks[32]	102	No treatment/early physiotherapy/ double Tubigrip/cast	No treatment led to better return to work and better early clinical symptom score
Linde[33]	102	4 days compression bandage/ non–weight-bearing splint	No difference
Hedges[36]	93	Elastic bandage and weight-bearing/non–weight-bearing splint	No difference
Dettori[37]	64	Elastic wrap/cast/air stirrup	No difference
Eiff[38]	82	Elastic wrap then air stirrup/ non–weight-bearing splint	Wrap gave better early results, but no difference in late outcomes
Watts[39]	400	Double Tubigrip/no compression	No difference in recovery
Boyce[41]	50	Air stirrup/elastic bandage	Aircast better at 10 days and 1 month
Leanderson[42]	73	Air stirrup/compression	Air stirrup better for early mobilization

Most studies have weaknesses, which are described in the text.

A large randomized controlled trial of severe ankle sprain treatment comparing tubular bandage, Aircast splint, plaster cast and Bledsoe boot is due to report in 2006 (www.warwick.ac.uk/go/ankle).

Brooks *et al.*[32] randomly assigned 102 patients with acute ankle sprain to treatment with either cast immobilization, early physiotherapy, double Tubigrip, or no treatment. Patients placed on the no-treatment arm returned to work earlier and had a lower clinical score. The small numbers of patients studied and the absence of stringent statistical analysis limit the application of this study. There is also a suggestion in the paper that the individuals receiving no treatment had less severe injuries, which significantly reduces the quality of the evidence.

Linde *et al.*[33] included 100 patients in a comparative study of elastic compression bandage, for 4 days, against no treatment for an ankle sprain. They found no significant difference between the two groups for pain, function, swelling, or range of movement. This study was limited by the absence of randomization in the allocation of treatment. Tufft and Leaman recognized that wool and crepe exerts more pressure than an elasticated bandage, but that neither exerted significant pressure on the ankle after a brief period.[34]

It is important to remember that immobilization is not a homogeneous group of interventions. Korkala *et al.*[35] conducted a randomized control trial comparing a semirigid cast with a rigid cast. The return-to-work period was significantly shorter for the semirigid cast (95% CI, 1.66 to 6.44 days). There was no significant difference in pain, swelling, or objective stability at the short-term follow-up point. This study was limited by the fact that the semirigid cast wearers were fully weight-bearing immediately, whereas the rigid cast wearers were not allowed to weight-bear for one week. Such a difference in treatment between the groups reduced the scientific rigor of the report.

Hedges and Anwar[36] conducted a randomized controlled trial (RCT) including 93 patients aged between 15 and 65 years with ankle sprains. These individuals were randomly assigned to either elastic bandage and early weight-bearing vs. a non–weight-bearing splint. No significant differences were found for functional disability, pain, swelling, or recurrent injury. This study had a number of weaknesses, including combining compression and weight-bearing advice—making any differences between the groups difficult to attribute. In addition, the study included many patients who had previous ankle injuries, and the 8-month follow up group had only a 33% attendance.

Dettori *et al.*[37] investigated 64 military personnel with ankle sprains who were randomized to plaster cast, air stirrup, or elastic wrap. Early mobilization was shown to be beneficial in reducing return-to-work and running time, increasing range of motion, and reducing swelling and pain. No significant difference was found between the groups for difficulty in running 1 year post-injury. This study had some flaws, in that it contained only those with moderate and severe sprains, making its application to the numerous grade 1 injuries difficult. Also, the long-term follow-up was conducted using a postal questionnaire, leaving some room for misinterpretation and loss of scientific rigor.

Eiff *et al.*[38] randomized 82 military recruits to elastic wrap for 2 days followed by 8 days with air stirrup or a non–weight-bearing splint for 10 days. Return to work was significantly more likely in the elastic wrap group, as was reduced pain at 3 weeks post-injury. Residual symptoms between the two groups at later follow-up examinations (6 and 12 months) showed no significant difference. The weakness of this study was a combination of two modes of compressive therapy (elastic wrap and air stirrup), which prevents delineation of the proportionately effective intervention.

Watts and Armstrong[39] conducted an RCT of 400 emergency-department attenders to determine the effectiveness of double-layered Tubigrip in grade 1 and 2 ankle sprains. Having been allocated to either double-layer Tubigrip or no compression treatment, the patients completed a standardized telephone questionnaire 1 week later. Of the 197 who completed follow-up, there was no significant difference in time to walking unaided, number of days off work, or whether the patient's sleep was disturbed by the ankle injury. Comparison of the use of analgesia found that those with a double-layered Tubigrip appeared significantly more likely to use analgesia. The authors concluded that the double-layered Tubigrip did not improve functional outcome of grade 1 and 2 ankle sprains and may increase the need for analgesia. The limitations of this study include the 59% drop-out rate (from 400 to 197), which reduces the validity of a controlled trial. The use of a standardized questionnaire, while being easier to administer, can fail to tease out the exact information needed (for instance, the analgesia information was given in response to the question "Did you need analgesia?" rather than "How much analgesia and which forms?"). The use of only a 10-day follow-up period is also insufficient in determining the efficacy of a treatment for ankle sprain.

Kerkhoffs *et al.*[40] conducted another Cochrane review of nine studies (including 892 patients) comparing different functional treatments of acute lateral ankle ligament injuries. They concluded that lace-up ankle supports were better than semirigid ankle supports, elastic bandage, and tape in reducing persistent swelling at the short-term follow-up. Semirigid ankle supports were concluded to be associated with a quicker return to work and sport and less reported instability than an elastic bandage. Comparison of elastic bandages and lace-up ankle supports for return to work, pain, subjective instability, and range of motion found no significant differences. When semirigid and lace-up ankle supports were compared for return to work, pain, subjective instability, objective instability, and range of motion, no significant differences were found. The authors felt that elastic bandages were less preferable to semirigid ankle supports, but overall thought that insufficient data existed for making a determination of the optimal functional intervention.

Boyce *et al.*[41] undertook an RCT comparing elastic support bandages against the Aircast ankle support brace for treatment of inversion ankle injuries in 50 patients at two district general hospitals emergency departments in Scotland. Loss to follow-up was similar in the two groups (eight of 17 with the elastic support bandage and seven of 18 with the Aircast). Using the Karlsson score to evaluate ankle joint function, the investigators found the Aircast brace produced significantly better ankle function at 10 days and 1 month of follow-up. Swelling, as measured by ankle girth, was not significantly different between the two groups. Unfortunately, the authors do not detail their rest, ice, compression, and elevation advice, or determine its use by the individuals in the study, which may have complicated the results. In addition, the exact components of the Karlsson score that were different between the two groups were not specified, which makes drawing specific conclusions difficult. A further limitation exists, in that swelling at the ankle is more accurately and reproducibly measured using water volume displacement, rather than ankle girth. Importantly, the investigators do not detail the use of analgesia, crutches, or other treatment between the two groups. Differences in treatment may have altered the interpretation of the results gained.

Leanderson *et al.* studied 73 patients with grade II and III ankle sprains randomized to an air stirrup splint or compression bandage.[42] Both groups had similar instructions on early motion and weight bearing. Recovery was assessed at 3/5 days, 2, 4, and 10 weeks by clinical examination, Sickness Impact Profile, Karlsson score, and sick-leave records. The group treated with the air stirrup had better early mobilization and shorter sick-leave times.

Most studies involving taping did not describe the application of the tape in detail. The method of applying the taping has important implications, with only full taping and figure of eight taping able to withstand significant angular displacement before failure (on an anatomical model).[43] The Chartered Society of Physiotherapists has suggested guidance on the application of compression strapping.[44]

Other forms of compression?

A review of the literature reveals a paucity of information on any type of compressive therapy for acute sprains other than continuous support devices. Intermittent compression is one possible addition. Airaksinen *et al.*[45] compared the effectiveness of elastic bandages and intermittent compression for the treatment of acute ankle sprains. Subjects who had sustained an inversion injury to the ankle were randomized into two groups; the control group wore elastic bandages, and the experimental group had intermittent compression therapy once per day for 5 days in addition to wearing elastic bandages. At the 1-week and 4-week follow-up measurements, both groups demonstrated improvements in all measures, but the compression group had significantly less edema, less pain, a greater range of movement, and improved function in comparison with the control group. This suggests that a combination of elastic bandage and intermittent compression is better than an elastic bandage alone. Although the study was in the form of a randomized controlled trial, no information was given about advice on elevation, weight-bearing, or the position in which the compression treatment was given (recumbent or elevated), which reduced the quality of evidence in the study.

A study by Rucinski *et al.*[22] compared three treatment protocols in the management of post-traumatic edema in 30 subjects following lateral ligament ankle sprains. Subjects were divided into three groups. One group had the limb elevated at 45° for 30 minutes, the second had the limb elevated at 45° and an elastic wrap applied for 30 minutes, and the third group had the limb elevated to 45° and an intermittent pressure device applied at 40–50 mmHg for 30 minutes. Both of the compression protocols resulted in slightly increased limb volume when measured by water displacement, and the elevation alone resulted in a significantly decreased limb volume, suggesting that elevation alone is the treatment of choice. However, although elevation alone produced the most favorable results, in reality this is difficult to maintain over prolonged periods of time and it may be that compression has its most beneficial effect when the limb is not elevated. Furthermore, the degree of compression (40–50 mmHg in the intermittent compression device) may have caused arteriolar dilation under the area of compression, which on removal of the compressive device caused increased blood flow and an increase in limb volume. This study was limited by the small numbers examined and by the absence of investigation for more than 30 minutes post-injury.

Compression as prophylaxis (Table 12.2)

Ankle injuries, as we have described, are very common, arising with high frequency in a number of sports.[1–3] The majority of lateral ankle ligament injuries are mild and resolve quite easily, but others can be severe and may cause prolonged disability because of the pain they cause or due to some consequential instability.[46] This can significantly affect an individual's quality of life, preventing him or her from competing in sp ort or just carrying

Table 12.2 Randomized trials of compression as prophylaxis in ligament injuries

First author, ref.	n	Treatments tested	Conclusions
Simon[49]	148	Cloth wrap/taping	No difference detected
Ekstrand[50]	180	Training program with strapping/normal care	Program reduced injuries
Surve[51]	504	Aircast/control	Less sprains in Aircast group in those with previous injuries
Sitler[52]	1601	Aircast/control	Aircast reduced injuries
Sharpe[53]	38	No support/lace-up brace/ tape/combination	All groups better than no-support group
Amoroso[54]	777	Aircast/no support	Aircast better than no support
Stasinopoulos[56]	52	Teaching program/proprioceptive program/external support	Support only effective in those with less than four previous injuries; training was more effective

out their day-to-day routine. In this section, we investigate only those studies looking at the impact of compression as a preventative treatment of ankle sprain. A recent Cochrane review has evaluated all available evidence on prophylaxis[47] and should be a stopping-point for those wanting to know more. Handoll and colleagues[47] describe 14 studies (including 8279 participants) investigating the impact of an external ankle support in the form of a semirigid orthosis, Aircast brace or high top shoes with other functional treatments such as physiotherapy on acute lateral ankle ligament injuries. The methodology rating of the trials involved was given as "poor to moderate," having scores between 3/22 and 13/22. The authors concluded there was a significant reduction in the number of ankle sprains in people allocated external ankle support (relative risk 0.53; 95% CI, 0.40 to 0.69). This reduction was greater for those with a prior history of ankle sprain, but still possible for those without previous sprain. Handoll *et al.* concluded that the application of an external ankle support was effective in preventing ankle sprains in those with previous injury, but that there was insufficient evidence to determine the relative effectiveness of the various types of support. In another systematic review, Thacker *et al.* studied cloth and tape wrapping, orthosis, and high top shoes for preventing further ankle sprains.[48] They concluded that athletes suffering a moderate or severe ankle injury should have supervised rehabilitation and use of an orthosis for 6 months after injury.

Simon[49] randomized 148 American college football players to either cloth wrapping or taping over two spring seasons. Each group was to wear the wrapping one season and the taping the other. Each treatment group had four ankle sprains. This study has limited application because of the small numbers treated and the absence of a control group, which prevents knowledge of the injury rate without treatment.

Ekstrand *et al.*[50] randomized 180 football players to either a preventative program (involving training correction, optimum equipment, ankle strapping, controlled rehabilitation, information, and correction and supervision by doctors and physiotherapists) or a control group. The two groups had the same incidence of 2.6 injuries per month before the introduction of the preventative program. Following the introduction of the prophylactic program, the number of injuries in that group fell to an incidence of 0.6 injuries per month, which was a significant reduction ($P < 0.05$). The main limitation of this study is that the prophylactic program contained multiple interventions concurrently, and thus it is difficult to elucidate which intervention was responsible for the difference.

Surve *et al.*[51] conducted a randomized control trial to investigate the effect of a semirigid ankle support of the incidence of ankle sprains in one football season. A total of 504 players from all four divisions were randomly assigned to either an Aircast sport stirrup support or control. The groups were stratified according to their prior injury status, and all groups were of similar number. The incidence of ankle sprains was significantly reduced in those with the semirigid support ($P < 0.001$) in the stratified group who had previous injuries. In the group who did not have prior injuries, there was no significant difference in ankle sprain incidence between the intervention and control group. The authors concluded that a semirigid ankle support was an effective prophylaxis for ankle sprains in players with previous ankle sprains.

Sitler and colleagues[52] randomized 1601 U.S. military cadets with no evidence of ankle instability (from self-report, clinical examination or radiograph analysis) to semirigid Aircast stirrup support (789 subjects, of whom 87 had a prior injury) or a control group (812 subjects, 90 of whom had a prior ankle injury). The recruits were followed over two basketball seasons, on both practice and games. The injury rate was 5.2 per 1000 athlete exposures in the control group, and 1.6 per 1000 in the group wearing the Aircast support, giving a relative risk for the control group approaching three times greater ($P < 0.01$). This reduction was only shown for contact injuries, and not for noncontact ones. In the group with no prior injuries, the effect of wearing the Aircast lowered the injury rate from 4.8 (control) to 1.7 per 1000. In the group with a history of ankle sprain, the impact of the Aircast support was reduced from 8.0 (control) to 1.7 per 1000 athlete exposures. The authors conclude that the Aircast support significantly reduces the rate of ankle injury. This study was successful in attempting to control for variables including shoe type, method of diagnosis, and compliance. However, the study was limited by being too small to statistically analyze the Aircast's effect in subsections of the groups with or without prior injuries.

In a retrospective study, Sharpe *et al.*[53] evaluated medical records of 38 female American college football players (with 56 ankle injuries) to examine the impact of taping and bracing. Looking over five seasons, the players had worn either no external support (n = 17), tape (n = 12), lace-up brace (n = 19), or a combination of taping and bracing (n = 8). The frequency of recurrent ankle sprain was 35% with no external support, 25% with taping, and 25% for the taped and braced group. The authors conclude that support is effective in reducing ankle sprain incidence. This study is limited by the small study numbers, the retrospective nature of the study, and the fact that the interventions were self-selected.

An RCT conducted by Amoroso and colleagues[54] investigated 777 army parachutists during the last week of their training course. The 745 subjects completing the analysis were randomized to wearing an Aircast outside the boot brace (n = 369) or no external support (n = 376). A total of 3674 jumps were made. The incidence of ankle sprains was 1.9% in those with no external support and 0.3% in the intervention group (risk ratio 6.9, $P = 0.04$). The authors concluded that outside-the-boot ankle braces were effective in significantly reducing the incidence of inversion ankle injuries during parachute training. A limitation of this study is that despite asking the subjects about prior ankle injuries (about half of them had such injuries), no results were given on the relative impacts on previously healthy or injured ankles.

Schumacher *et al.*[55] conducted a retrospective cohort study using medical records examining the incidence of ankle sprains, before (7857 jumps) and after (5928 jumps) the mandatory use of an outside the boot brace. Before the brace was introduced, the rate of injury was 4.45 per 1000 jumps, and after the rate was reduced significantly to1.52 per 1000 jumps ($P = 0.002$). This study is limited by its design as a retrospective cohort study, which is very susceptible to surveillance and confounding bias.

Stasinopoulos[56] compared three preventative methods in 52 female volleyball players who had ankle sprains in the preceding season. The subjects were allotted randomly to either a technical training program (n = 18), a proprioceptive program (n = 17), or an external ankle support (n = 17). The players filled out a questionnaire at the end of the season reporting incidence of ankle injuries. Those undertaking the technical training program had a 12% injury rate in the season studied. There was an 18% injury rate in the group following the proprioceptive program. In the subset wearing the external ankle support, the injury rate was 35%. The two players in the technical training group who sustained ankle sprains had had four or more than four prior ankle sprains in their careers, respectively. The three players who received ankle sprains in the proprioceptive program group had had three, four, or more than four ankle sprains in their careers, respectively. In the external ankle support group, of the six who sustained an ankle sprain, one had three previous ankle sprains, three had four prior ankle sprains, and a single player had received more than four previous ankle sprains in her career. The authors concluded that compressive external ankle support was only effective in players who had had fewer than four previous ankle sprains in their career. Both technical and proprioceptive training were thought to be more effective than an external ankle support for preventing ankle sprain. The limitations of this study include the obvious absence of any control group, thus making definite conclusions difficult at best. Also, as Stasinopoulos states that many players may have received the technical training before that study in some form, there may be some confusion as to what has caused the intergroup differences.

It is thought that inadequate foot posture awareness is a major risk for recurrent ankle sprain injury. Robbins *et al.* demonstrated, in a small study of 24 healthy volunteers, that ankle tapes can correct the impaired proprioception caused by athletic footwear or exercise.[57] But a study of 25 injured athletes showed no significant difference in the ability to perceive ankle joint movement between those with sprains and those with no history of injury. There was similarly no difference in movement perception between taped and untaped individuals.[58]

A cost–benefit analysis[59] across several studies showed that ankle taping was three times more expensive than bracing over the course of one competitive season. Taping is only cost-effective if used for short periods.

Conclusions

A number of problems exist with the available studies. Firstly, many papers do not make adequately clear the prior injuries of their participants. Secondly, it would be more accurate for studies to quote their findings in terms of the ankles injured rather than the players injured, as commonly occurs now. Again, there is an absence of the use of controls in many of the available studies, preventing the determination of effects due to the intervention. An effectively designed RCT would circumnavigate many of these potential weaknesses. Our review has found a paucity of research on subjects other than young healthy males in terms of prophylaxis. In order to determine the most appropriate treatment for any individual, it is of vital importance to increase the variety of our study populations.

In terms of ankle sprain treatment, early mobilization has been proven to be more comfortable, associated with less pain, and allowed a more rapid return to work than immobilization. Elastic wrap bandages have been shown to be more effective than no treatment for ankle sprains. The best evidence exists for the use of external ankle supports, suggesting that these braces are more effective than elastic bandages at getting individuals back to work and reducing subjective instability. There is currently insufficient evidence to suggest which of the many available supports provides the best outcome.

A major problem with determining the most effective intervention for ankle sprain is the widely varying methodology used in the available literature. This makes the process of meta-analysis very difficult to perform. In addition, many of the current studies have poor methodology, such as being insufficiently powered or not using controls. A large-scale, fully randomized control trial investigating the benefits of different treatments remains the ideal solution, and we await such a result with interest. It is also of note that we do not know which of the different compressive treatments are effective in which populations. Many of the current studies are conducted in young healthy males, and we must broaden the study populations in future in order to determine the most effective interventions. Finally, as mentioned earlier, most of the literature focuses on continuous compression, and it would be of interest to determine the effects of other types, such as intermittent compression, as treatment for ankle sprains.

With regard to prophylaxis, compression does appear to be at least somewhat protective against ankle sprains. In terms of the best treatment, again the evidence points to a superiority of the ankle brace over any other form of compressive treatment. The best specific type of support remains undetermined by current research. The current literature is somewhat inconclusive, but appears to suggest that compressive treatments are more effective for those who have a history of ankle sprains, and not for preventing first-time injuries.

Summary

- Ankle sprains are a common injury.
- Rest is recommended in the early stages but evidence is weak.
- Ice and elevation are routinely used.
- Compression is variably used.
- Functional treatments (including strapping, bracing, Tubigrip, and elastic bandages) significantly improved some outcomes.
- External support devices appear better than bandaging.
- Intermittent compression has not been adequately tested.
- Most studies are of poor quality, and the high-quality studies only demonstrated improvement related to returning to work.
- Prophylactic compression appears useful in preventing further injury, but those with multiple injuries in the past gain less benefit.
- There is insufficient evidence on the use of compression in other joints than the ankle to give conclusive advice.

Key messages

- External ankle braces, associated with early mobilization, are probably the most effective treatment of acute ankle sprains.
- External braces appear to help prevent further sprains, except in those with multiple previous injuries.
- Intermittent compression with continuous support may be effective in the acute phase.
- Evidence for compression in injuries other than ankle sprains is poor.

Sample examination questions

Essay questions

1. How might compression treatment help in the recovery from a ligamentous injury of the ankle?
2. What type of ankle support is best for a person who cannot weight-bear after an ankle sprain?
3. What advice would you give a rugby player who has had several ankle sprains regarding future protection of the ankle?
4. What treatments should be combined with compression treatment for ankle sprains?
5. Which people benefit from wearing an ankle support during sport?
6. Why might compression be disadvantageous in the early treatment of sprains?

7 If compression is applied to the ankle after injury, how is this best undertaken?
8 What does evidence suggest about treatment of different severities of injury?

Case study 12.1

A 26-year-old athlete with no previous ankle problems sustains an inversion injury to his right ankle. He cannot weight-bear after the injury and rapidly develops swelling and bruising over the lateral ligament. It is impossible to undertake an anterior drawer sign or talar tilt test because of the pain it induces.

Immediate action: ice is applied and his leg is elevated.

As he cannot weight-bear, he satisfies the Ottawa criteria for having a radiograph of his ankle. This shows no fracture. Elevation and ice are continued for 2 days. During this period, he is instructed on non–weight-bearing exercises. As soon as he can tolerate it, he is fitted with an ankle brace and encouraged to mobilize. He uses the brace at all times when he is weight-bearing. He continues to ice the joint and elevate when not mobilizing until all swelling has disappeared.

With a regime of increasing mobilization and joint-strengthening exercises, he is able to resume sport after 4 weeks. He is advised to continue using his ankle support during his sporting activities for several months.

He does not have any instability evident, and so does not require any further investigation.

References

1 Boyce SH, Quigley MA. A review of sports injuries presenting to an accident & emergency department. *Emerg Med Journal* 2004; **21**:704–706.
2 Watters DAK, Brooks S, Elton RA, *et al.* Sports injuries in an accident and emergency department. *Arch Emerg Med* 1984; **2**:105–111.
3 Murphy AW, Martyn C, Plunkett PK, *et al.* Sports injuries and the accident and emergency department—ten years on. *Ir Med J* 1992; **85**:30–32.
4 Colville MR, Marder RA, Boyle JJ, Zarins B. Strain measurement in lateral ankle ligaments. *Am J Sports Med* 1990; **18**:196–200.
5 Perlman M, Leveille D, DeLeonibus J, *et al.* Inversion lateral ankle trauma: differential diagnosis, review of the literature, and prospective study. *J Foot Surg* 1987; **26**:95–135.
6 Kannus P, Renström P. Treatment for acute tears of the lateral ligaments of the ankle: operation, cast, or early controlled mobilization. *J Bone Joint Surg Am* 1991; **73**:305–312.
7 Marder RA. Current methods for the evaluation of the ankle ligament injuries. *J Bone Joint Surg Am* 1994; **76**:1103–1111.
8 Hammond HK, Froelicher VF. The physiologic sequelae of chronic dynamic exercise. *Med Clin North Am* 1985; **69**:21–39.
9 Imig CJ, Randall BF, Hines HM. Effect of immobilization on muscular atrophy and blood flow. *Arch Phys Med Rehabil* 1953; **34**:296–298.
10 Akeson WH, Amiel D, Abel MF, Garfin SR, Woo SL. Effects of immobilization on joints. *Clin Orthop Relat Res* 1987; **219**:28–37.
11 Namba RS, Kabo JM, Dorey FJ, Meals RA. Continuous passive motion versus immobilization: the effect on posttraumatic joint stiffness. *Clin Orthop Relat Res* 1991; **267**:218–223.
12 Buckwalter JA. Should bone, soft-tissue and joint injuries be treated with rest or activity. *J Orthop Res* 1995; **13**:155–156.
13 Jarvinen MJ, Lehto MUK. The effects of early mobilisation on the healing process following muscle injuries. *Sports Med* 1993; **15**:78–89.
14 Knight KL. Cryotherapy in sports injury management. *Int Perspect Physiother* 1989; **4**:163–185.
15 Knight K, Londeree BR. Comparison of blood flow in the ankle of uninjured subjects during therapeutic applications of heat, cold, and exercise. *Med Sci Sport Exerc* 1980; **12**:76–80.

16 Rivenburgh DW. Physical modalities in the treatment of tendon injuries. *Clin Sports Med* 1992; **11**:645–659.
17 Swenson C, Sward L, Karlsson J. Cryotherapy in sports medicine. *Scand J Med Sci Sports* 1996; **6**:193–200.
18 McLean DA. The use of cold and superficial heat in the treatment of soft tissue injuries. *Br J Sports Med* 1989; **23**:53–54.
19 Ho SSW, Illgen RL, Meyer RW, *et al.* Comparison of various icing times in decreasing bone metabolism and blood flow in the knee. *Am J Sports Med* 1994; **23**:74–76.
20 MacAuley DC. Ice therapy: how good is the evidence? *Int J Sports Med* 2001; **22**:379–384.
21 Belitsky RB, Odam SJ, Hubley-Kozey C. Evaluation of the effectiveness of wet ice, dry ice, and cryogen packs in reducing skin temperature. *Phys Ther* 1987; **67**:1080–1084.
22 Rucinski TJ, Hooker DN, Prentice WE, Shields EW, Cote-Murray DJ. The effects of intermittant compression on oedema in post-acute ankle sprains. *J Orthop Sports Phys Ther* 1991; **14**:65–69.
23 Thorsson O, Lilja B, Nilsson P, Westlin N. Immediate external compression in the management of an acute muscle injury. *Scand J Med Sci Sports* 1997; **7**:182–190.
24 Alt W, Lohrer H, Gollhofer A. Functional properties of adhesive ankle strapping: neuromuscular and mechanical effects before and after strapping. *Foot Ankle Int* 1999; **20**:238–245.
25 Neilsen HV. Arterial pressure–blood flow relationships during limb elevation in man. *Acta Physiol Scand* 1983; **118**:405–413.
26 Baumert PW. Acute inflammation after injury. *Postgrad Med* 1995; **97**:35–49.
27 Laughman RK, Carr TA, Chao EY, Youdas JW, Sim FH. Three dimensional kinematics of the taped ankle before and after exercise. *Am J Sports Med* 1980; **8**:425–431.
28 Capasso G, Maffulli N, Testa V. Ankle taping: support given by different materials. *Br J Sports Med* 1989; **23**:239–40.
29 Viljakka T. Mechanics of knee and ankle bandages. *Acta Orthop Scand* 1986; **57**:54–8.
30 Stover CN. Air stirrup management of ankle injuries in the athlete. *Am J Sports Med* 1980; **8**:360–365.
31 Kerkhoffs GM, Rowe BH, Assendelft WJ, *et al.* Immobilisation and functional treatment for acute lateral ankle ligament injuries in adults. *Cochrane Database Syst Rev* 2002;(**3**):CD003762.
32 Brooks SC, Potter BT, Rainey JB. Treatment for partial tears of the lateral ligament of the ankle: a prospective trial. *BMJ* 1981; **282**:606–608.
33 Linde F, Hvass I, Jurgensen U, Madsen F. Compression bandage in the treatment of ankle sprains: a comparative prospective study. *Scand J Rehabil Med* 1984; **16**:177–179.
34 Tufft K, Leaman A. A better form of treatment? Comparison of wool and crepe and elasticated tubular bandage in the treatment of ankle sprains. *Prof Nurse* 1999; **9**:745–746.
35 Korkala O, Rusanen M, Jokipii P, Kytomaa J, Avikainen V. A prospective study of the treatment of severe tears of the lateral ligament of the ankle. *Int Orthop* 1987; **11**:13–17.
36 Hedges JR, Anwar RA. Management of ankle sprains. *Ann Emerg Med* 1980; **9**:298–302.
37 Dettori JR, Basmania CJ. Early ankle mobilization, part II: a one-year follow-up of acute, lateral ankle sprains (a randomized clinical trial). *Mil Med* 1994; **159**:20–24.
38 Eiff MP, Smith AT, Smith GE. Early mobilisation versus immobilization in the treatment of lateral ankle sprains. *Am J Sports Med* 1994; **22**:83–88.
39 Watts BL, Armstrong B. A randomised controlled trial to determine the effectiveness of double Tubigrip in grade 1 and 2 (mild to moderate) ankle sprains. *Emerg Med J* 2001; **18**:46–50.
40 Kerkhoffs GMMJ, Struijs PAA, Marti RK, *et al.* Different functional treatment strategies for acute lateral ankle ligament injuries in adults. *Cochrane Database Syst Rev* 2002;(**3**):CD002938.
41 Boyce SH, Quigley MA, Campbell S. Management of ankle sprains: a randomised controlled trial of the treatment of inversion injuries using an elastic support bandage or an Aircast ankle brace. *Br J Sports Med* 2005; **39**:91–96.
42 Leanderson J, Wredmark T. Treatment of acute ankle sprain: comparison of a semi-rigid ankle brace and compression bandaging in 73 patients. *Acta Orthop Scand* 1995; **66**:529–531.
43 Pope MH, Renstrom P, Donnermeyer D, Morgenstern S. A comparison of ankle taping methods. *Med Sci Sports Exerc* 1987; **19**:143–147.
44 Chartered Society of Physiotherapy. *Guidelines for the Management of Soft Tissue (Musculoskeletal) Injury with Protection, Rest, Ice, Compression and Elevation (PRICE) during the First 72 Hours.* London: Association of Chartered Physiotherapists in Sports Medicine, 1999.

45 Airaksinen O, Kolari PJ, Miettinen H. Elastic bandages and Intermittent pneumatic compression in the treatment of ankle sprains. *Arch Phys Med Rehabil* 1990; **71**:380–383.
46 Anandacoomarasamy A, Barnsley L. Long term outcomes of inversion ankle injuries. *Br J Sports Med* 2005; **39**:e14.
47 Handoll HHG, Rowe BH, Quinn KM, de Bie R. Interventions for preventing ankle ligament injuries. *Cochrane Database Syst Rev* 2001;(**3**):CD000018.
48 Thacker SB, Stroup DF, Branche CM, *et al.* The prevention of ankle sprains in sports: a systematic review of the literature. *Am J Sports Med* 1999; **27**:753–760.
49 Simon JE. Study of the comparative effectiveness of ankle taping and ankle wrapping on the prevention of ankle injuries. *J Natl Athl Trainers Assoc* 1969; **4**:6–7.
50 Ekstrand J, Gillquist J, Liljedahl SO. Prevention of soccer injuries: supervision by doctor and physiotherapist. *Am J Sports Med* 1983; **11**:116–120.
51 Surve I, Schwellnus MP, Noakes T, Lombard C. A fivefold reduction in the incidence of recurrent ankle sprains in soccer players using the Sport-Stirrup orthosis. *Am J Sports Med* 1994; **22**:601–6.
52 Sitler M, Ryan J, Wheeler B, McBride J, *et al.* The efficacy of a semirigid ankle stabilizer to reduce acute ankle injuries in basketball: a randomized clinical study at West Point. *Am J Sports Med* 1994; **22**:454–461.
53 Sharpe SR, Knapik J, Jones BH. Ankle braces effectively reduce recurrence of ankle sprains in female soccer players. *J Athl Train* 1997; **32**:21–24.
54 Amoroso PJ, Ryan JB, Bickley B, *et al.* Braced for impact: reducing military paratroopers' ankle sprains using outside-the-boot braces. *J Trauma* 1998; **45**:575–580.
55 Schumacher JT Jr, Creedon JF, Pope RW. The effectiveness of the parachutist ankle brace in reducing ankle injuries in an airborne ranger battalion. *Mil Med* 2000; **165**:944–948.
56 Stasinopoulos D. Comparison of three preventive methods in order to reduce the incidence of ankle inversion sprains among female volleyball players. *Br J Sports Med* 2004; **38**:182–185.
57 Robbins S, Waked E, Rappel R. Ankle taping improves proprioception before and after exercise in young men. *Br J Sports Med* 1995; **29**:242–247.
58 Refshauge KM, Killbreath SL, Raymond J. The effect of recurrent ankle inversion sprain and taping on proprioception at the ankle. *Med Sci Sports Exerc* 2000; **32**:10–15.
59 Olmsted LC, Vela LI, Denegar CR, Hertel J. Prophylactic ankle taping and bracing: a numbers needed to treat and cost benefit analysis. *J Athl Train* 2004; **39**:95–100.

CHAPTER 13
NSAIDs and pain management in sports

Weiya Zhang

Introduction

Nonsteroidal anti-inflammatory drugs (NSAIDs) are widely used to relieve pain due to musculoskeletal injuries.[1,2] However, NSAIDs cause significant damage to the upper gastrointestinal tract.[3–5] The risk of serious gastrointestinal ulcer complications in NSAID users is approximately 2.5 to 4.5 times that of nonusers.[6] This results in 10,000 hospitalizations and 2000 deaths per year in the UK and over 70,000 hospitalizations and 7000 deaths annually in the US.[7,8] The cost of managing gastrointestinal side effects due to NSAIDs is enormous, for example, in the UK an additional £36 million per year is spent to manage gastrointestinal bleeding and perforation due to the use of NSAIDs in the treatment of musculoskeletal conditions,[9] whereas in the US, the cost approaches up to $1.6 billion.[10]

Because of the burden of gastrointestinal side effects due to NSAIDs, safer treatment approaches have been attempted, including co-administration of gastroprotective agents (misoprostol, H_2 antagonists, and proton-pump inhibitors/PPIs), topical NSAIDs, COX-2 inhibitors, including selective COX-2 inhibitors and specific COX-2 inhibitors (coxibs). However, at present, co-administration with gastroprotective agents and the use of COX-2 inhibitors are only cost-effective for higher-risk populations,[11,12] and the latter may be associated with greater cardiovascular side effects.[13,14] Topical NSAIDs seem to be effective in acute pain due to soft-tissue injuries, strains, and sprains,[15] and appear to be safer than oral NSAIDs.[16] However, the long-term benefits of topical NSAIDs for chronic pain need further confirmation.[17]

This paper reviews the current best available evidence with regard to the risks and benefits of NSAIDs, including COX-2 inhibitors, and gastroprotective agents in the management of musculoskeletal injuries. In addition, the evidence of prophylactic effects of NSAIDs in the inhibition of bone formation after surgery was also reviewed.

Methods

Systematic literature search

A systematic search of the literature published between January 1945 and 30 April 2005 was undertaken using MEDLINE (1966–), Old MEDLINE (1950–), EMBASE (1980–), CINHAL (1980–), the Science Citation Index (1945–), and Cochrane Library databases (1996–). The search consisted of three strategies:

- Sports medicine in whatever possible terms in the databases.
- NSAIDs as a Medical Subject Heading (MeSH).

Table 13.1 Evidence hierarchy for efficacy

Ia	Meta-analysis of randomized controlled trials
Ib	Randomized controlled trial
IIa	Controlled study without randomization
IIb	Quasi-experimental study
III	Nonexperimental descriptive studies, such as comparative, correlation, and case–control studies
IV	Expert committee reports or opinion or clinical experience of respected authorities, or both

• Types of research, in the form of systematic review/meta-analysis, randomized controlled trial (RCT)/controlled trial (CT), uncontrolled trial, cohort study, case–control study, cross-sectional study and economic evaluation.

The three strategies were then combined to obtain the current available research evidence on NSAIDs in sports medicine.

The search in the Cochrane Library included a MeSH search of the Cochrane reviews, Abstracts of Quality Assessed Systematic Reviews, the Cochrane Controlled Trial Register, NHS Economic Evaluation Databases, the Health Technology Assessment Database, and the NHS Economic Evaluation Bibliography Details Only. In addition, a topics search on sport or musculoskeletal injuries was undertaken.

Inclusion/exclusion criteria

Only studies in humans with the use of NSAIDs in musculoskeletal injuries were included. Animal studies were excluded. Studies for other conditions were included only if they were associated with sport or musculoskeletal injuries, such as osteoarthritis, lateral elbow pain and patellofemoral syndrome. For efficacy, questions were answered using the best available evidence according to the level of evidence[18] (Table 13.1). For example, if a question on the effect of NSAIDs could be answered by level Ia evidence (i.e., a systematic review of RCTs) then studies of a weaker design (RCT, level Ib) were not reviewed, unless they were new studies published after the systematic review. Results of the latest systematic review including more trials were used if there was more than one systematic review for the same question. Questions on side effects, however, were answered using both RCTs and observational studies, irrespective of conditions, as RCTs are not necessarily the best method to assess adverse effects, and sport injuries may not be the target condition for which side effects of an intervention are assessed. Statistical pooling was undertaken as appropriate if there was no meta-analysis. Questions of cost-effectiveness were answered according to the outcome measure of the effectiveness. For example, if the effectiveness was measured as pain relief score or quality of life years (QALYs) gained, only studies for sports injuries or associated musculoskeletal conditions were eligible. If the effectiveness was measured as adverse events averted, any studies for the proposed interventions were included. Results of the latest economic evaluation were used if there was more than one economic evaluation for the same question.

Outcome measures

Efficacy

For treatment efficacy, effect size (ES) or weighted mean difference (WMD) compared with placebo or active control was calculated for continuous outcomes. ES is the standard mean difference—i.e., the mean difference between a treatment and a control group divided by the standard deviation of the difference. It is therefore free of units and comparable across interventions. Clinically, an ES of 0.2 is considered small, 0.5 is moderate, and greater than 0.8 is large.[19] WMD is the pooled mean difference weighted by the sampling variance. Unlike ES, WMD keeps the natural unit of outcome measure. For dichotomous data, such as the percentage of patients more than 50% pain relief, rate ratio (RR),[20] or the number needed to treat (NNT) was estimated.[21] The NNT is the estimated number of patients who need to be treated either to prevent an unwanted effect such as gastrointestinal bleeding, or to obtain a wanted outcome such as pain relief; therefore the smaller the NNT, the better the treatment effect. The 95% confidence interval (CI) of the NNT was calculated using Altman's method.[22]

Adverse effects

For adverse effects, the RR was calculated from RCTs or cohort studies for the incident risk and from cross-sectional studies for prevalent risk, whereas the odds ratio (OR) was calculated from case–control studies.[20] Both present how many times more likely (or less likely) subjects who are exposed to NSAIDs are to have adverse effects than those who are not exposed. RR or OR = 1 indicates no relationship, whereas RR or OR > 1 or < 1 indicates a positive or negative relationship.

Economic evaluation

For economic evaluation, the incremental cost-effectiveness ratio (ICER) was calculated by the different costs between the two treatments divided by their different effectiveness. When available, QALYs were used for the measurement of effectiveness, otherwise disease specific outcomes such as the reduction of pain were used. In addition, study design, comparator, perspective, time horizon, discounting, total costs, effectiveness were critically appraised.

All outcomes were presented with the point estimate (e.g., mean) and 95% CI, unless otherwise stated.

Conventional oral NSAIDs

Efficacy

Oral NSAIDs have been widely used to treat musculoskeletal pain. Four systematic reviews have been identified from the literature search, including three Cochrane reviews in acute and chronic Achilles tendonitis,[23] lateral elbow pain,[24] and patellofemoral pain symptom,[25] and one non-Cochrane review in osteoarthritis.[26] Only one RCT in each of three Cochrane reviews was relevant to the question of whether conversional oral NSAIDs are effective for the conditions studied. The results were controversial between the reviews. One review showed that oral NSAIDs were no more beneficial than placebo,[23] whereas the other two demonstrated that oral NSAIDs were beneficial for some outcomes (e.g., pain), but not for others (e.g., function)[24,25] (Table 13.2). It is difficult to interpret these results, as firstly, the reviews included different conditions; secondly, they used different outcomes; and thirdly, only one RCT was available and the sample size was small (36–128 subjects).

In contrast, a robust review of 23 RCTs with 10,845 patients in knee osteoarthritis demonstrated a superiority of oral NSAIDs over placebo in reducing pain.[26] The pooled ES

Table 13.2 Efficacy of oral nonsteroidal anti-inflammatory drugs (NSAIDs): systematic reviews of randomized and controlled trials

First author, ref.	RCTs (n)	Subjects (n)	Condition	Outcome measure	Estimate (95% CI)
NSAIDs vs. placebo					
McLauchlan 2001[23]	1	67	Achilles tendonitis	RR (return to normal activity)	0.82 (0.61 to 1.11)
			RR (symptom improved)	1.01 (0.75, 1.35)	
Green 2002[24]	1	128	Lateral elbow pain	WMD (VAS pain↓)	13.90 (4.60 to 23.32)
			WMD (VAS function↑)	3.30 (–6.53, 13.13)	
Heintjes 2004[25]	1	36	Patellofemoral pain syndrome	ES (VAS pain↓)	0.78 (0.10 to 1.46)
Bjordal 2004[26]	23	10845	Knee osteoarthritis	ES (WOMAC/ VAS pain↓)	0.32 (0.24 to 0.39)
NSAIDs vs. paracetamol					
Zhang 2004[27]	8	1622	Osteoarthritis	ES (WOMAC /VAS pain↓)	0.20 (0.10 to 0.30)

CI, confidence interval; ES, effect size (standard mean difference); NSAID, nonsteroidal anti-inflammatory drug; RCT, randomized controlled trial; RR, rate ratio; VAS, visual analogue scale; WMD, weighted mean difference; WOMAC, Western Ontario and McMaster Universities Osteoarthritis Index.

was 0.32 (95% CI, 0.24 to 0.39) (Fig. 13.1). Furthermore, another meta-analysis showed that oral NSAIDs was more effective than paracetamol.[27] The pooled ES from eight trials with 1622 patients was 0.21 (95% CI, 0.10 to 0.30). Other outcomes such as physical function and stiffness were also in favor of NSAIDs.[27] The results from these two meta-analyses clearly suggest that NSAIDs are effective agents for osteoarthritis—a common degenerative musculoskeletal condition in the elderly that may be related to sports injuries.[28]

Side effects

Although they are effective in many conditions including musculoskeletal pain, NSAIDs cause serious upper gastrointestinal damage. A systematic review scrutinized 4881 published titles and identified 16 RCTs, nine cohort studies, and 23 case–control studies.[5] The pooled OR of perforation, ulcers, and bleeds (PUB) from 16 NSAIDs versus placebo RCTs comprising 4431 patients was 5.36 (95% CI, 1.79 to 16.10). The pooled RR of PUB from nine cohort studies comprising over 750,000 person-years of exposure was 2.7 (95% CI, 2.1 to 3.5). The pooled OR of PUB from 23 case–control studies using age and gender matching, representing 25,732 patients, was 3.0 (95% CI, 2.5 to 3.7). These data support an association between the use of NSAIDs and serious upper gastrointestinal complications from different study designs. For minor gastrointestinal side effects, such as dyspepsia, a meta-analysis of 48 placebo-controlled RCTs, encompassing nearly 12,000 patients, showed that NSAIDs were associated with an increased risk of dyspepsia (OR 1.4; 95% CI,

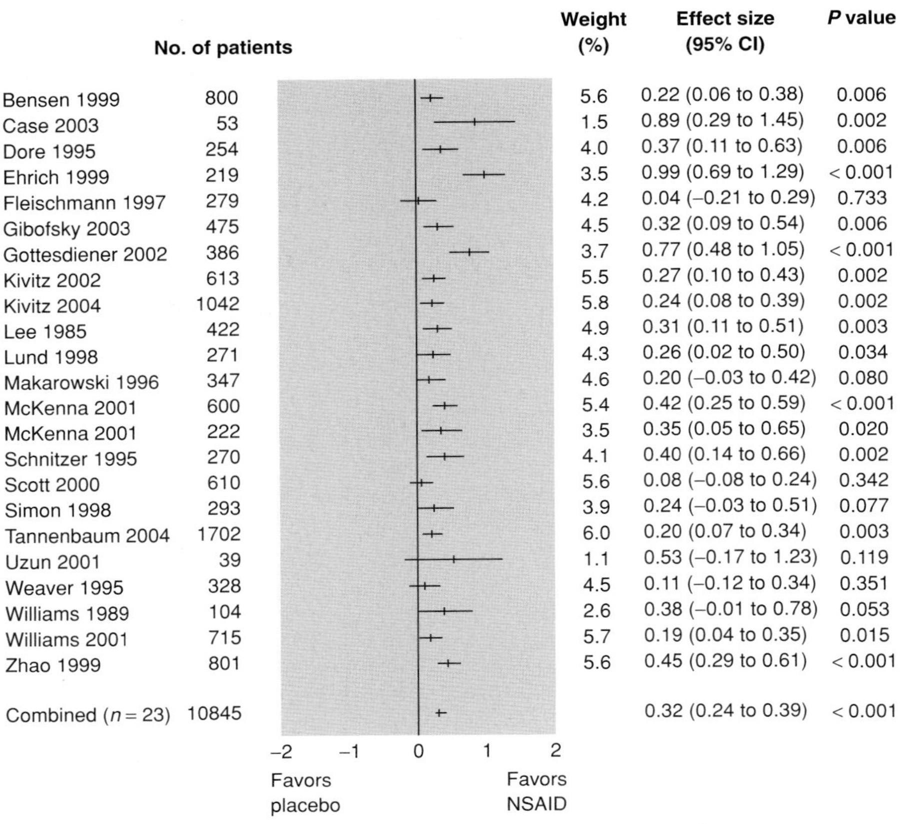

Figure 13.1 The effect size in pain reduction between nonsteroidal anti-inflammatory drugs (NSAIDs) versus a placebo in knee osteoarthritis (adapted with permission from Bjordal *et al.* 2004[26]).

1.1 to 1.8).[29] Dyspepsia was defined as any terms (including dyspepsia) relating to epigastric or upper abdominal pain/discomfort except for nausea, vomiting or heartburn in this meta-analysis. In the meantime, the reviewers also retrieved 56 case–control studies and 24 cohort studies from the literature. Unfortunately, dyspepsia was not reported to be associated with the use of NSAIDs in these study designs.[29] Individual patient meta-analysis from three case–control studies with 2472 cases of upper gastrointestinal bleeding and 5877 controls showed that ibuprofen had the lowest OR (OR 1.7; 95% CI, 1.1 to 2.5), followed by diclofenac (4.9; 95% CI, 3.3 to 7.1), indomethacin (6.0; 95% CI, 3.6 to 10.0), naproxen (9.1; 95% CI, 6.0 to 13.7), piroxicam (13.1; 95% CI, 7.9 to 21.8) and ketoprofen (34.9; 95% CI, 12.7 to 96.5) (Fig. 13.2). A dose–response relationship was seen with any NSAID.[30]

In conclusion, oral conventional NSAIDs are effective for musculoskeletal pain. However, such benefit comes at the expense of important side effects, most notably upper gastrointestinal toxicity. The efficacy differences between NSAIDs are minor, but ibuprofen seems to have least gastrointestinal toxicity among the most commonly used NSAIDs. However, the benefit–risk ratio may vary from person to person. The decision should be

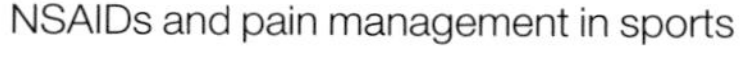

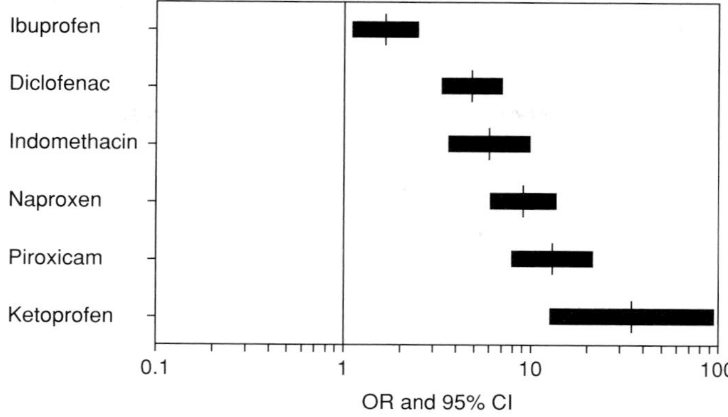

Figure 13.2 The odds ratio (OR) and 95% confidence interval (CI) of upper gastrointestinal bleeding for different types of conventional oral nonsteroidal anti-inflammatory drugs (NSAIDs).

therefore based on the individual patient response and the potential gastrointestinal risk of NSAIDs.

Cox-2 inhibitors

Efficacy

NSAIDs inhibit cyclo-oxygenase 1 (COX-1), a constitutive enzyme expressed in most tissues, including the gastrointestinal mucosa, where it maintains physiological processes. NSAIDs inhibit COX-2, an inducible proinflammatory enzyme.[31] This property makes NSAIDs act as a double-edged saw, having both anti-inflammatory effects and gastrointestinal toxicity. As a result, specific NSAIDs that selectively inhibit the COX-2 isoform have been developed. Depending on their selectivity to the COX-2 isoform, two subgroups can be identified: COX-2-selectives (such as etodolac, meloxicam, nabumetone and nimesulide), and COX-2-specifics or coxibs (celecoxib, rofecoxib, vodalecoxib, lumiracoxib, and etoricoxib). A large number of RCTs have been undertaken to examine the clinical effectiveness of these particular group of NSAIDs. In musculoskeletal injuries, for example, a head-to-head comparison showed that celecoxib was as effective as naproxen in treating acute ankle sprains, but caused significantly less dyspepsia.[32] A systematic review of RCTs comparing celecoxib with placebo or conventional NSAIDs in osteoarthritis demonstrated that celecoxib was more effective than placebo and as effective as nonselective conventional NSAIDs.[33] Three large-scale RCTs, the CLASS (n = 8059), VIGOR (n = 8076), and TARGET (n = 18,325) trials, have been undertaken to examine the gastrointestinal safety of coxibs.[34–36] The results showed that the coxibs reduced the gastrointestinal complications induced by NSAIDs by 50–70%. The results were confirmed by a systematic review of 68 RCTs, including CLASS and VIGOR, with a total of 53,742 subjects (Table 13.3).[37]

Side effects

An increased risk of myocardial infarction was observed with Vioxx (rofecoxib) in the VIGOR trial.[35] The risk has been recently confirmed by a cumulative meta-analysis, in which 18 RCTs and 11 observational studies were included.[38] The pooled RR of myocar-

Table 13.3 Efficacy of five strategies for the prevention of gastrointestinal toxicity induced by nonsteroidal anti-inflammatory drugs (NSAIDs)

Comparison	Trials (n)	Patients (n)	RR (95% CI)		
			Symptomatic ulcers	Complications	Death
COX-2-selectives vs. nonselectives	51	28178	0.41 (0.3 to 0.7)	0.61 (0.3 to 1.1)	0.68 (0.3 to 1.6)
COX-2-specifics vs. nonselectives	17	25564	0.49 (0.4 to 0.6)	0.55 (0.4 to 0.8)	1.02 (0.6 to 1.9)
Misoprostol vs. placebo	23	16945	0.36 (0.2 to 0.7)	0.57 (0.4 to 0.9)	0.89 (0.5 to 1.7)
Proton-pump inhibitor vs. placebo	6	1358	0.09 (0.0 to 0.5)	0.46 (0.1 to 2.9)	0.17 (0.0 to 4.1)
H_2-receptor antagonist vs. placebo	15	2621	1.46 (0.1 to 35.5)	0.33 (0.0 to 8.1)	3.00 (0.1 to 68.3)

CI, confidence interval; RR, relative risk.
Complications: ulcer complications including upper gastrointestinal perforation, obstruction, and bleeding (POB). COX-2-selectives include etodolac, meloxicam, nabumetone and nimesulide; COX-2-specifics include celecoxib and rofecoxib. Data obtained from Hooper *et al.* 2004.[37]

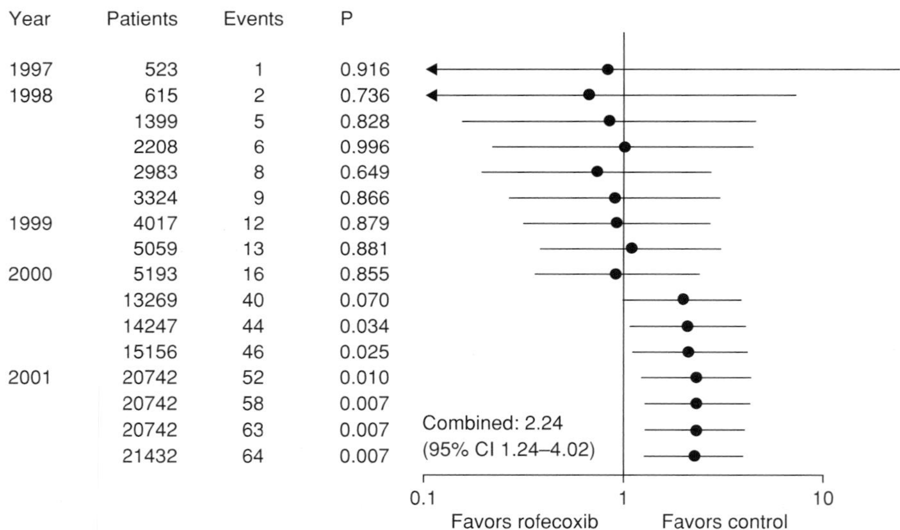

Figure 13.3 Relative risk and 95% confidence interval (CI) of myocardial infarction. A cumulative meta-analysis of randomized trials comparing rofecoxib with controls (adapted with permission from Juni *et al.* 2004[38]).

dial infarction from the RCTs was 2.24 (95% CI, 1.24 to 4.02) and it was unlikely to be caused by chance, as the estimate became stable after the year 2000 (Fig. 13.3). Meta-regression was used to examine whether the RR was affected by the dose, type of control, trial duration, etc. There was little evidence that the RR differed depending on the control group (placebo, non-naproxen NSAIDs, or naproxen; $P = 0.41$) or trial duration ($P = 0.82$).

Naproxen showed a small cardioprotective effect (RR 0.86; 95% CI, 0.75 to 0.99), which could not be explained by the findings of the VIGOR trial. As a result, rofecoxib has now been withdrawn from the market. Nevertheless, the story of the cardiovascular adverse effects of coxibs has not yet ended. On 9 December 2004, the U.S. Food and Drug Administration (FDA) issued a black-box warning for valdecoxib for life-threatening skin reactions and cardiovascular risk.[39] Just over a week later, on 17 December 2004, the National Cancer Institute (NCI) announced the premature cessation of a trial of celecoxib known as the Adenoma Prevention with Celecoxib (APC) trial, due to a significant excess of cardiovascular death, myocardial infarction, and stroke.[40] Immediately afterward, on 20 December 2004, the National Institutes of Health (NIH) suspended the Alzheimer's Disease Anti-inflammatory Prevention Trial (ADAPT), in which naproxen was found to increase cardiovascular and cerebrovascular events in comparison with a placebo.[41] More recently, a case–control study involving 8143 cases of serous coronary heart disease (CHD) and 31,496 matched controls from California suggested that not only coxibs, but also conventional oral NSAIDs, including naproxen, were associated with an elevated risk of CHD. The odds ratios were 1.14 (95% CI, 1.00 to 1.30) for naproxen, 3.00 (95% CI, 1.09 to 8.31) for rofecoxib > 25 mg/day, and 1.13 (95% CI, 1.01 to 1.27) for other NSAIDs.[42] Like the gastrointestinal adverse effects, cardiovascular toxicity of NSAIDs may be a class effect, but different extents of it cannot be excluded. It is well known that NSAIDs and coxibs increase blood pressure.[43,44] This may explain the elevated risk of congestive heart failure associated with both agents observed in a cohort study.[45] However, whether this is an independent risk factor for myocardial infarction or interacts with the inhibition of prostacyclin (PGI_2) and thromboxane (TXA_2) synthesis in the vessel wall and in platelets remains unknown. Nevertheless, what is clear is that like conventional NSAIDs, coxibs may also act as a double-edged saw, and their benefits should be carefully balanced against their risks.

Cost-effectiveness

Another problem with coxibs is that they are normally more expensive than conventional NSAIDs. The cost-effectiveness issue is therefore of great interest to society, individual patients, and third parties such as national health services and the insurance companies from which the costs are reimbursed. Two economic evaluations have been undertaken in osteoarthritis.[12,46] The results showed that both rofecoxib and celecoxib were more expensive but more effective (in terms of serious gastrointestinal events avoided) than conventional NSAIDs (Table 13.4). It would cost in average $4700 to $55,000 to avoid one serious gastrointestinal event (perforation, ulcer, and bleeding) with coxibs. The cost decreased when the patient's gastrointestinal risk increased, indicating that the use of coxibs is more cost-effective for patients with a higher risk of gastrointestinal bleeding.[12,46] Both coxibs were dominated by paracetamol—that is, coxibs are more costly and less safe than paracetamol.

In conclusion, COX-2-specific inhibitors are equally effective as conventional NSAIDs but are associated with less gastrointestinal toxicity. Coxibs are cost-effective only for the population at high gastrointestinal risk. However, COX-2 inhibitors may increase the cardiovascular risk of NSAIDs, such as hypertension, myocardial infarction, and heart failure. Although these events are rare, the agents should be used with caution in people with a high risk of cardiovascular diseases. As a result, the cost-effectiveness of COX-2 inhibitors in comparison with conventional NSAIDs needs to be reviewed with consideration of both gastrointestinal and cardiovascular safety.

Table 13.4 Cost-effectiveness of coxibs and gastroprotectors compared with conventional oral nonsteroidal anti-inflammatory drugs (NSAIDs) or paracetamol

Intervention	Comparator	Perspective	Time horizon	Discounting	Effectiveness	C1–C2	E1–E2	ICER
Rofecoxib	Ibuprofen	Institutional/payer	6 months	No	PUB averted	$471000–112000	991–980	32636
	NSAIDs	Institutional/payer	1 year	3%	PUB averted	–	–	4738
	Paracetamol	Institutional/payer	6 months	No	PUB averted	$471000–63000	991–995	Dominated
Celecoxib	Ibuprofen	Institutional/payer	6 months	No	PUB averted	$474000–112000	990–980	36200
	Paracetamol	Institutional/payer	6 months	No	PUB averted	$474000–63000	990–995	Dominated
Ibuprofen + GI protector	Ibuprofen	Institutional/payer	6 months	No	PUB averted	$556000–112000	988–980	55500
NSAIDs + misoprostol (all OA patients)	NSAIDs	Canadian Health services	3 months	No	PUB averted	$32396–25622	96–86	677
NSAIDs + misoprostol (OA patients aged ≥ 65 years)	NSAIDs	Canadian Health services	3 months	No	PUB averted	$28971–25622	91–86	670

C1, total costs with intervention; C2, total costs with comparator; E1, effect with intervention; E2, effects with comparator; ICER: incremental cost-effectiveness ratio, base case scenario; NSAID, nonsteroidal anti-inflammatory drug; OA, osteoarthritis; PUB, perforation, ulcer or bleed.

Gastrointestinal protectors

Efficacy

Hooper and colleagues undertook a systematic review of RCTs on the effectiveness of gastroprotective agents for the prevention of the gastrointestinal of NSAIDs.[37] Twenty-three studies (16,945 subjects) were included for misoprostol, six (1358 subjects) for proton-pump inhibitors (PPIs), and 15 trials (2621 subjects) for H_2-receptor antagonists. The risk of symptomatic ulcers was significantly reduced by either misoprostol or PPI. In addition, misoprostol significantly reduced the risk of the ulcer complications. However, the evidence for H_2-receptor antagonists is inconclusive (Table 13.3). Further analysis of five systematic reviews showed that all three gastroprotective agents were effective in preventing endoscopic ulcers, with RRs of 0.26 (95% CI, 0.17 to 0.39), 0.40 (95% CI, 0.32 to 0.51) and 0.44 (95% CI, 0.03 to 0.74) for misoprostol, PPIs, and double-dose H_2-receptor antagonists, respectively.[47] The standard dosage of H_2-receptor antagonists is ineffective.

Side effects

Misoprostol may cause abdominal pain and diarrhea. The RR was 1.89 (95% CI, 1.52 to 2.16).[47]

Cost-effectiveness

The co-use of gastroprotective agents obviously results in additional costs. Whether the extra benefits are worth the extra cost becomes an essential issue. Two economic evaluations have been undertaken in osteoarthritis.[11,12] Both showed that the prophylactic use of gastroprotective agents was effective in preventing the adverse gastrointestinal events caused by NSAIDs, but was more expensive (Table 13.4). The treatment was more cost-effective in a high-risk population.[11] The analyses were based on adverse effects avoided. Further studies using generic outcomes such as quality of life and years gained are still needed.

In conclusion, co-use of gastroprotective agents such as misoprostol and proton-pump inhibitors may reduce the gastrointestinal toxicity of NSAIDs. However, additional benefits have to be balanced against additional adverse effects and costs. Evidence for the co-use of H_2-receptor antagonists is less convincing; only a double dosage shows gastrointestinal protective effects.

Topical NSAIDs

Efficacy

Topical NSAIDs have been well investigated in acute pain due to musculoskeletal injuries (soft-tissue trauma, strains and sprains).[15] Thirty-seven placebo-controlled trials (3556 patients) have been systematically reviewed. The pooled RR for patient with over 50% pain reduction in 1 week was 1.7 (95% CI, 1.5 to 1.9). The NNT was four (95% CI, 3 to 4). For chronic conditions such as osteoarthritis and tendinitis, 12 placebo-controlled trials were analyzed. The pooled RR was 2.0 (95% CI, 1.5 to 2.7). The NNT was three (95% CI, 3 to 4). However, only short-term trials (2 weeks) were available. The benefits beyond 2 weeks remain uncertain.[17]

More recently, four longer-term trials (4–12 weeks) have been undertaken to compare the clinical effects of topical diclofenac with placebos (one trial including 248 patients), vehicle (dimethylsulfoxide, three trials including 790 patients), or oral diclofenac in the

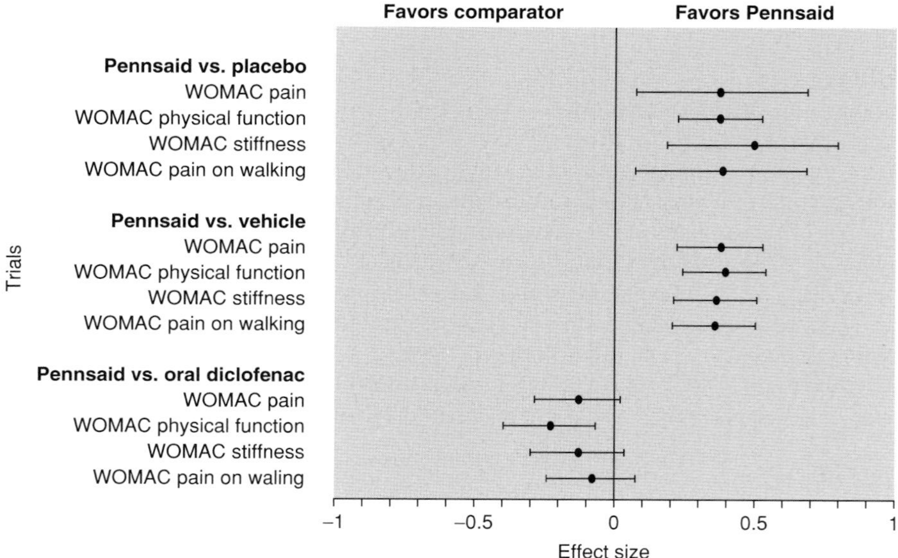

Figure 13.4 The effect size of Pennsaid (topical diclofenac 1.5% w/w diclofenac sodium in a vehicle containing dimethylsulfoxide, DMSO) in comparison with a placebo vehicle (containing the full concentration of DMSO), or oral diclofenac.

treatment of knee osteoarthritis (one trial including 622 patients).[48–51] All of the trials had double-blind parallel designs, with one trial using a double-dummy method to compare topical with oral diclofenac. A total of 1412 patients aged 40–85 years with radiographic evidence of knee osteoarthritis and at least moderate pain were involved. Two trials required patients to have a flare of pain.[48,50] Intention-to-treat (ITT) analysis was used for all studies.

The results showed that topical diclofenac was significantly superior to either placebo (ES 0.37; 95% CI, 0.07 to 0.68) or vehicle (ES 0.36; 95% CI, 0.05 to 0.67) and was equivalent to its oral formulation (ES –0.14; 95% CI, –0.29 to 0.02) in relieving pain due to knee osteoarthritis (Fig. 13.4). These effects were sustained throughout the 4–12 weeks of trial observation (Table 13.5). Similar patterns were observed for dichotomous outcomes, such as patients with more than 50% pain relief, good or very good patient global assessment, and OMERACT-OARSI responders (Fig. 13.5). The pooled NNT for patients with more than 50% pain reduction was 6 (95% CI, 4 to 10).

Side effects

Evidence from randomized controlled trials indicates that topical NSAIDs may cause some local skin side effects but are associated with fewer gastrointestinal events than oral NSAIDs.[15,27] The skin reaction is more likely to be caused by the vehicle that carries the NSAID. This was confirmed by recent trials in the treatment of knee osteoarthritis, in which topical diclofenac (including the vehicle) and the vehicle itself both led to more local skin reactions than placebo. In contrast, topical diclofenac was associated with fewer gastrointestinal events than its oral equivalent[48–51] (Table 13.6). A population-based case–control study compared previous exposure to oral or topical NSAIDs between 1101

Table 13.5 Effect size and 95% confidence intervals between topical diclofenac and vehicle control

	4 weeks	6 weeks	12 weeks	P*
WOMAC pain	0.36 (0.05 to 0.67)	0.39 (0.13 to 0.66)	0.35 (0.13 to 0.57)	0.969
WOMAC physical function	0.48 (0.16 to 0.79)	0.39 (0.12 to 0.66)	0.35 (0.13 to 0.57)	0.802
WOMAC stiffness	0.38 (0.07 to 0.69)	0.42 (0.15 to 0.69)	0.30 (0.08 to 0.52)	0.798
WOMAC pain on walking	0.47 (0.15 to 0.78)	0.33 (0.06 to 0.59)	0.31 (0.09 to 0.53)	0.714

* Chi-square test for heterogeneity.
WOMAC, Western Ontario and McMaster Universities Osteoarthritis Index.

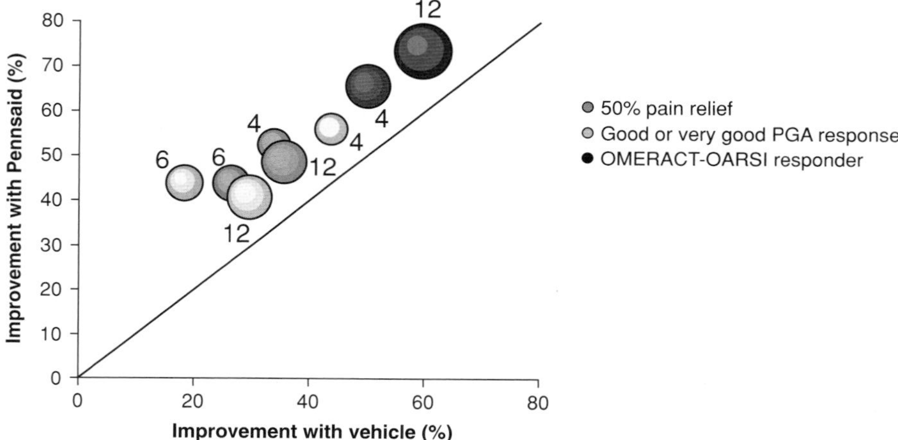

Figure 13.5 Clinical improvement (%) with topical diclofenac and vehicle control. The numbers in the bubbles indicate the weeks when the outcomes were recorded. The sizes of the bubbles reflect the sample size, ranging from 163 to 322). PGA, patient global assessment.

Table 13.6 Relative risk of skin reactions and gastrointestinal events with topical diclofenac

	RR (95% confidence interval)	
	Skin reactions*	GI events†
Placebo	1	1
Vehicle	3.25 (1.72, 6.15)	1.07 (0.44, 2.60)
Topical diclofenac + vehicle	3.66 (1.95, 6.86)	0.77 (0.31, 1.96)
Topical diclofenac + vehicle vs. vehicle	1.42 (0.71, 2.84)	0.78 (0.29, 2.06)
Topical diclofenac + vehicle vs. oral diclofenac	9.20 (5.13, 16.48)	0.57 (0.46, 0.72)

RR, relative risk.
* Skin reactions include dry skin, rash, paresthesia and pruritus. RR was calculated separately for each complaint. RRs were then pooled to present skin reactions.
† Gastrointestinal events include dyspepsia, diarrhea, nausea, and vomiting. RR was calculated separately for each complaint. RRs were pooled to present gastrointestinal events as a global outcome.

patients with upper gastrointestinal bleeding and perforation and 6593 age-matched and sex-matched controls from a community in Tayside, Scotland.[52] The gastrointestinal bleeding and perforation was significantly associated with the use of oral NSAIDs (adjusted OR 2.59; 95% CI, 2.12 to 3.16) but not with the use of topical NSAIDs (adjusted OR 1.45; 95% CI, 0.84 to 2.50).

In conclusion, topical NSAIDs are effective in the treatment of acute pain due to musculoskeletal injuries. The long-term benefits of topical NSAIDs with different vehicles need further assessment. Topical NSAIDs are equally effective as oral NSAIDs, but are associated with less gastrointestinal toxicity.

NSAIDs and bone growth

A Cochrane review has been undertaken to examine the prophylactic effects of NSAIDs in preventing heterotopic bone formation (HBF) in the soft tissues surrounding the hip joint—a common complication of hip surgery.[53] Eighteen trials (15 RCTs and 3 CTs) including 4763 patients were included. Of them, 16 trials compared NSAIDs with placebos and two compared NSAIDs with heparin. Overall, 17 trials examined the effects of medium to high dosages of NSAIDs. There was a reduced risk of developing HBF after hip surgery (RR 0.41; 95% CI, 0.36 to 0.46). In contrast, one large trial examining low-dose aspirin demonstrated no effects on the risk of HBF (RR 0.98; 98% CI 0.85 to 1.12) (Fig. 13.6). The results were not significantly altered by sensitivity analyses according to randomization, blinding, type of controls and preoperative or postoperative use of NSAIDs.

However, as for many other conditions, NSAIDs were associated with more gastrointestinal side effects than controls (RR 1.31; 95% CI, 1.00 to 1.71). When NSAIDs are used for this purpose, one should also consider the trade-off between benefits and harms.

Conclusions

NSAIDs are an effective treatment for relieving the symptoms of musculoskeletal conditions and injuries, both in the acute and chronic phases. There is little difference between types of NSAIDs in terms of efficacy, but there are some differences in terms of side effects. For example, among the conventional NSAIDs, ibuprofen appears to be equally effective as other NSAIDs but is associated with the fewest gastrointestinal events. Although coxibs can dramatically reduce the gastrointestinal toxicity of NSAIDs, they are only cost-effective in people who are at high risk of gastrointestinal bleeding. Coxibs, however, may increase the cardiovascular risk of NSAIDs. The co-use of gastroprotective agents such as misoprostol and proton-pump inhibitors, as well as double doses of H_2-blockers, may reduce the gastrointestinal side effects of NSAIDs, but also may result in additional adverse effects and costs. In contrast, topical NSAIDs may have a favorable risk–benefit ratio, provided the long-term benefits of this route for NSAIDs can be confirmed. Apart from the analgesia and anti-inflammatory effects, NSAIDs may have other effects on musculoskeletal conditions, such as the inhibition of bone formation after surgery.

Summary

- NSAIDs are beneficial in many musculoskeletal conditions, including sport injuries and bone formation.
- However, they also cause unwanted effects, such as gastrointestinal events and cardiovascular events. The potential of these unwanted events may vary from drug to drug.

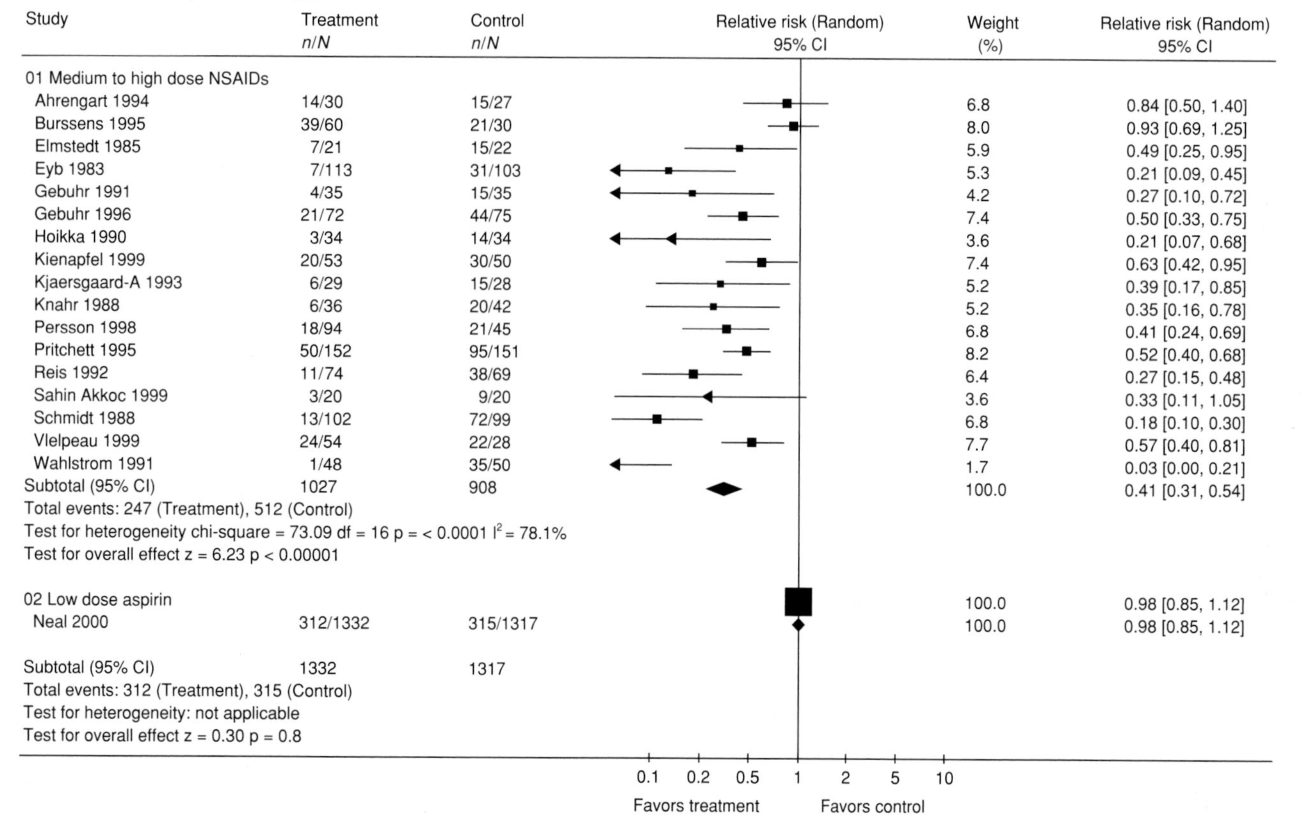

Figure 13.6 Prophylactic effects of nonsteroidal anti-inflammatory drugs (NSAIDs) in the prevention of heterotopic bone formation after hip surgery (adapted with permission from Fransen *et al.* 2003[53]).

• Co-use of gastroprotective agents may prevent the gastrointestinal side effects, but they may also induce other adverse effects and increase the treatment cost.
• The optimal use of NSAIDs should rely on a careful balance between benefits and harm/costs, as well as individual patient characteristics and preferences.

Key messages

• NSAIDs have been widely used in musculoskeletal conditions, but the optimal way of using NSAIDs has yet to be identified.
• There are robust data with regard to the benefits, side effects, and cost-effectiveness of NSAIDs in sports-related conditions, ranging from systematic reviews, large-scale randomized and controlled trials, and population-based epidemiological studies.
• Ibuprofen appears to be safer than other conventional NSAIDs. It should at least be tried in the first instance if NSAIDs are suggested.
• Topical NSAIDs are effective and safer for acute injury such as soft-tissue trauma, strains, and sprains. The long-term risk–benefit ratio of topical NSAIDs in the treatment of chronic conditions deserves further research.
• Coxibs are more useful for patients who are at high risk of gastrointestinal bleeding, but they should be used with caution in patients who are at risk of cardiovascular diseases.
• Misoprostol and proton-pump inhibitors are useful for patients who are at high risk of gastrointestinal bleeding, but possible side effects and additional costs have to be balanced.

Sample examination questions

Multiple-choice questions (answers on page 602)

1 NSAIDs are effective in relieving symptoms due to musculoskeletal injuries, but also cause:
   A Dyspepsia
   B Endoscopic or symptomatic ulcers
   C Ulcer complications such as perforation, obstruction, and bleeding (POB)
   D All of the above
2 Rare cardiovascular events have been observed with:
   A Rofecoxib
   B Celecoxib
   C Valdecoxib
   D All of the above
3 Topical NSAIDs are effective:
   A Only for acute pain
   B Only for chronic pain
   C For acute pain, and evidence for chronic pain has yet to be established
   D For both acute and chronic pain

Essay questions

1 Describe the mechanism of action for NSAIDs and the rationale of COX-2 inhibitors.
2 A male patient aged 30 with a recent ankle strain comes to your clinic. What would you like to prescribe for him to relieve his pain and swelling, and why?
3 A female patient aged 70 who has had knee pain for over 2 years comes to your clinic. What would you like to recommend to relieve her pain, and why?

Case study 13.1

John, a 25-year-old professional football player, recently stretched his knee. He consulted his doctor due to knee pain and was diagnosed as having a ligament injury. In addition to being recommended to use a brace to protect the knee and help healing of the ligament injury, he was proscribed paracetamol (1000 mg q.i.d.) to control his pain. However, after 3 days of treatment, he came back to complain that the paracetamol did not work well for his knee pain. He was then given ibuprofen (400 mg t.i.d.) for 1 week of treatment, and his knee pain was well controlled.

Case study 13.2

Joanna, a 76-year-old retired dinner lady who had been overweight since she was 45, was diagnosed as having knee osteoarthritis when she was 60. Her knee pain was a major problem for her daily activities. She had been treated with paracetamol, but it had only worked for a few months. She was then prescribed diclofenac, but it caused serious gut pain. She was then given ibuprofen and later naproxen, but both still caused her some gut pain. Misoprostol was then added, but it caused diarrhea. As she had a coronary problem, she was unable to take any coxibs. Her knee pain continued for many years until she recently joined an educational course on knee osteoarthritis and took part in once-weekly exercise sessions on the course. Her weight has fallen by 9 kg since then, and she has also been given topical diclofenac as needed.

Summarizing the evidence

Comparison/treatment strategies	Results	Level of evidence*
For pain relief		
Conventional NSAIDs versus placebo	23 RCTs, 10845 subjects, pooled ES = 0.32, 95% CI, 0.24 to 0.39	Ia
Coxibs versus conventional NSAIDs	17 RCTs, 25564 subjects, risk of GI ulcers/ complications was reduced by 50%	Ia
NSAIDs + PPI versus NSAIDs	6 RCTs, 1358 subjects, risk of GI ulcers/ complications was reduced by at least 50%	Ia
NSAIDs + misoprostol versus NSAIDs	23 RCTs, 16945 subjects, risk of GI ulcer/ complications was reduced by at least 40%	Ia
Topical NSAIDs versus placebo	37 RCTs, 3556 subjects, NNT = 4 (95% CI, 3 to 4)	Ia
Topical NSAIDs versus oral NSAIDs	1 RCT, 622 subjects, no difference between the treatments	Ib
To prevent heterotopic bone formation		
NSAIDs versus placebo	18 RCTs/CTs, 4763 subjects, risk of HBF was reduced by 60%	Ia

* See Table 13.1 for detailed definition.

CI, confidence interval; CT, controlled trial; ES, effect size; GI, gastrointestinal; HBF, heterotopic bone formation NNT, number needed to treat; NSAID, nonsteroidal anti-inflammatory drug; PPI, proton-pump inhibitors; RCT, randomized controlled trial;

References

1 Gorsline RT, Kaeding CC. The use of NSAIDs and nutritional supplements in athletes with osteoarthritis: prevalence, benefits, and consequences. *Clin Sports Med* 2005; **24**:71–82.

2 Baldwin LA. Use of nonsteroidal anti-inflammatory drugs following exercise-induced muscle injury. *Sports Med* 2003; **33**:177–185.

3 Gabriel SE, Jaakkimainen L, Bombardier C. Risk for serious gastrointestinal complications related to use of nonsteroidal anti-inflammatory drugs: a meta-analysis. *Ann Intern Med* 1991; **115**:787–796.

4 Hernandez-Diaz S, Garcia Rodriguez LA. Association between nonsteroidal anti-inflammatory drugs and upper gastrointestinal tract bleeding/perforation an overview of epidemiologic studies published in the 1990s. *Arch Intern Med* 2000; **160**:2093–2099.

5 Ofman JJ, MacLean CH, Straus WL, *et al.* A metaanalysis of severe upper gastrointestinal complications of nonsteroidal antiinflammatory drugs. *J Rheumatol* 2002; **29**:804–812.

6 Dubois RW, Melmed GY, Henning JM, Bernal M. Risk of upper gastrointestinal injury and events in patients treated with cyclooxygenase (COX)-1/COX-2 nonsteroidal antiinflammatory drugs (NSAIDs), COX-2 selective NSAIDs, and gastroprotective cotherapy: an appraisal of the literature. *J Clin Rheumatol* 2004; **10**:178–189.

7 Blower AL, Brooks A, Fenn GC, *et al.* Emergency admissions for upper gastrointestinal disease and their relation to NSAID use. *Aliment Pharmacol Ther* 1997; **11**:283–291.

8 Silverstein FE. Improving the gastrointestinal safety of NSAIDs: the development of misoprostol—from hypothesis to clinical practice. *Dig Dis Sci* 1998; **43**:447–458.

9 Hunsche E, Chancellor JV, Bruce N. The burden of arthritis and nonsteroidal anti-inflammatory treatment: a European literature review. *Pharmacoeconomics* 2001; **19**(Suppl 1):1–15.

10 Smalley WE, Griffin MR, Fought RL, Ray WA. Excess costs from gastrointestinal disease associated with nonsteroidal anti-inflammatory drugs. *J Gen Intern Med* 1996; **11**:461–469.

11 Gabriel SE, Jaakkimainen RL, Bombardier C. The cost-effectiveness of misoprostol for nonsteroidal antiinflammatory drug-associated adverse gastrointestinal events. *Arthritis Rheumatism* 1993; **36**:447–459.

12 Kamath CC, Kremers HM, Vanness DJ, *et al.* The cost-effectiveness of acetaminophen, NSAIDs, and selective COX-2 inhibitors in the treatment of symptomatic knee osteoarthritis. *Value Health Care* 2003; **6**:144–157.

13 Bresalier RS, Sandler RS, Quan H, *et al.* Cardiovascular events associated with rofecoxib in a colorectal adenoma chemoprevention trial. *N Engl J Med* 2005; **352**:1092–1102.

14 Simmons RL, Owen S, Abbott CJ, *et al.* Naproxen sodium and paracetamol/dextropropoxyphene in sports injuries: a multicentre comparative study. *Br J Sports Med* 1982; **16**:91–95.

15 Moore RA, Tramer MR, Carroll D, Wiffen PJ, McQuay HJ. Quantitative systematic review of topically applied non-steroidal anti-inflammatory drugs. *BMJ* 1998; **316**:333–338.

16 Anon. Topical analgesics: a review of reviews and a bit of perspective. *Bandolier Extra* 2005 (available at: www.ebandolier.com).

17 Lin, Zhang WJ, Jones A, Doherty M. Efficacy of topical non-steroidal anti-inflammatory drugs in the treatment of osteoarthritis: meta-analysis of randomised controlled trials. *BMJ* 2004; **329**:324–326B.

18 Shekelle PG, Woolf SH, Eccles M, Grimshaw J. Clinical guidelines: developing guidelines. *BMJ* 1999; **318**:593–596.

19 Cohen J. *Statistical Power Analysis for the Behavioral Sciences*, 2nd ed. Hillsdale, NJ: Erlbaum, 1988.

20 Kleinbaum DG, Kuppler LL, Morgenstern H. *Epidemiologic Research: Principles and Quantitative Methods.* Belmont, CA: Lifetime Learning Publications, 1982.

21 Cook RJ, Sackett DL. The number needed to treat: a clinically useful measure of treatment effect. *BMJ* 1995; **310**:452–454.

22 Altman DG. Confidence intervals for the number needed to treat. *BMJ* 1998; **317**:1309–1312.

23 McLauchlan GJ, Handoll HHG. Interventions for treating acute and chronic Achilles tendinitis. *Cochrane Database Syst Rev* 2001; (**2**):CD000232.

24 Green SE, Assendelft WJJ, Barnsley L, *et al.* Non-steroidal anti-inflammatory drugs (NSAIDs) for treating lateral elbow pain in adults. *Cochrane Database Syst Rev* 2002; (**2**):CD003686.

25 Heintjes E, Berger MY, Bierma-Zeinstra SM, *et al.* Pharmacotherapy for patellofemoral pain syndrome. *Cochrane Database Syst Rev* 2004; (**3**):CD003470.

26 Bjordal JM, Ljunggren AE, Klovning A, Slordal L. Non-steroidal anti-inflammatory drugs, including cyclo-oxygenase-2 inhibitors, in osteoarthritic knee pain: meta-analysis of randomised placebo controlled trials. *BMJ* 2004; **329**:1317.

27 Zhang W, Jones A, Doherty M. Does paracetamol (acetaminophen) reduce the pain of osteoarthritis? A meta-analysis of randomised controlled trials. *Ann Rheum Dis* 2004; **63**:901–907.

28 Kujala UM, Kettunen J, Paananen H, *et al.* Knee osteoarthritis in former runners, soccer players, weight lifters, and shooters. *Arthritis Rheum* 1995; **38**:539–546.

29 Ofman JJ, MacLean CH, Straus WL, *et al.* Meta-analysis of dyspepsia and nonsteroidal antiinflammatory drugs. *Arthritis Rheum* 2003; **49**:508–518.

30 Lewis SC, Langman MJS, Laporte JR, *et al.* Dose–response relationships between individual nonaspirin nonsteroidal anti-inflammatory drugs (NSAIDs) and serious upper gastrointestinal bleeding: a meta-analysis based on individual patient data. *Br J Clin Pharmacol* 2002; **54**:320–326.

31 Gilroy DW, Colville-Nash PR, Willis D, *et al.* Inducible cyclooxygenase may have anti-inflammatory properties. *Nature Med* 1999; **5**:698–701.

32 Petrella R, Ekman EF, Schuller R, Fort JG. Efficacy of celecoxib, a COX-2-specific inhibitor, and naproxen in the management of acute ankle sprain: results of a double-blind, randomized controlled trial. *Clin J Sport Med* 2004; **14**:225–231.

33 Deeks JJ, Smith LA, Bradley MD. Efficacy, tolerability, and upper gastrointestinal safety of celecoxib for treatment of osteoarthritis and rheumatoid arthritis: systematic review of randomised controlled trials. *BMJ* 2002; **325**:619–623.

34 Silverstein FE, Faich G, Goldstein JL, *et al.* Gastrointestinal toxicity with celecoxib vs nonsteroidal anti-inflammatory drugs for osteoarthritis and rheumatoid arthritis—the CLASS study: A randomized controlled trial. Celecoxib Long-term Arthritis Safety Study. *JAMA* 2000; **284**:1247–1255.

35 Bombardier C, Laine L, Reicin A, *et al.* Comparison of upper gastrointestinal toxicity of rofecoxib and naproxen in patients with rheumatoid arthritis. VIGOR Study Group. *N Engl J Med* 2000; **343**:1520–1528.

36 Farkouh ME, Kirshner H, Harrington RA, *et al.* Comparison of lumiracoxib with naproxen and ibuprofen in the Therapeutic Arthritis Research and Gastrointestinal Event Trial (TARGET), cardiovascular outcomes: randomised controlled trial. *Lancet* 2004; **364**:675–684.

37 Hooper L, Brown TJ, Elliott RA, *et al.* The effectiveness of five strategies for the prevention of gastrointestinal toxicity induced lay non-steroidal anti-inflammatory drugs: systematic review. *BMJ* 2004; **329**:948–952.

38 Juni P, Nartey L, Reichenbach S, *et al.* Risk of cardiovascular events and rofecoxib: cumulative meta-analysis. *Lancet* 2004; **364**:2021–2029.

39 U.S. Food and Drug Administration. Bextra label updated with boxed warning concerning severe skin reaction and warning regarding cardiovascular risk. *FDA Talk Paper* 4 A.D.; available at: http://fda.gov/bbs/topics/ANSWERS/2004/ANS01331.html. Accessed 5 May 2005.

40 U.S. Department of Health and Human Services. NIH halts use of COX-2 inhibitor in large cancer prevention trial. *NIH News* 2004; available at: http://www.nih.gov/news/pr/dec2004/od-17.htm. Accessed 5 May 2005.

41 U.S. Department of Health and Human Services. Use of non-steroidal anti-inflammatory drugs suspended in large Alzheimer's disease prevention trial. *NIH News* 2004; http://www.nih.gov/news/pr/dec2004/od-20.htm. Accessed 13 June 2005.

42 Graham DJ, Campen D, Hui R, *et al.* Risk of acute myocardial infarction and sudden cardiac death in patients treated with cyclo-oxygenase 2 selective and non-selective non-steroidal anti-inflammatory drugs: nested case–control study. *Lancet* 2005; **365**:475–481.

43 Johnson AG, Nguyen TV, Day RO. Do nonsteroidal anti-inflammatory drugs affect blood pressure? A meta-analysis. *Ann Intern Med* 1994; **121**:289–300.

44 Aw TJ, Haas SJ, Liew D, Krum H. Meta-analysis of cyclooxygenase-2 inhibitors and their effects on blood pressure. *Arch Intern Med* 2005; **165**:490–496.

45 Mamdani M, Juurlink DN, Lee DS, *et al.* Cyclo-oxygenase-2 inhibitors versus non-selective non-steroidal anti-inflammatory drugs and congestive heart failure outcomes in elderly patients: a population-based cohort study. *Lancet* 2004; **363**:1751–1756.

46 Pellissier JM, Straus WL, Watson DJ, Kong SX, Harper SE. Economic evaluation of rofecoxib versus nonselective nonsteroidal anti-inflammatory drugs for the treatment of osteoarthritis. *Clin Ther* 2001; **23**:1061–1079.

47 Zhang W, Doherty M, Arden N, *et al.* EULAR evidence based recommendations for the management of hip osteoarthritis: report of a task force of the EULAR Standing Committee for International Clinical Studies Including Therapeutics (ESCISIT). *Ann Rheum Dis* 2005; **64**:669–681.

48 Baer P, Thomas LM, Shainhouse JZ. Treatment of osteoarthritis of the knee with a topical diclofenac solution: a randomised controlled, 6-week trial [ISRCTN53366886]. *BMC Musculoskelet Disord* 2005; **6**:44.

49 Bookman AA, Williams KS, Shainhouse JZ. Effect of a topical diclofenac solution for relieving symptoms of primary osteoarthritis of the knee: a randomized controlled trial. *CMAJ* 2004; **171**:333–338.

50 Roth SH, Shainhouse JZ. Efficacy and safety of a topical diclofenac solution (Pennsaid) in the treatment of primary osteoarthritis of the knee: a randomized, double-blind, vehicle-controlled clinical trial. *Arch Intern Med* 2004; **164**:2017–2023.

51 Tugwell PS, Wells GA, Shainhouse JZ. Equivalence study of a topical diclofenac solution (Pennsaid) compared with oral diclofenac in symptomatic treatment of osteoarthritis of the knee: a randomized controlled trial. *J Rheumatol* 2004; **31**:2002–2012.

52 Evans JMM, McMahon AD, McGilchrist MM, *et al.* Topical non-steroidal anti-inflammatory drugs and admission to hospital for upper gastrointestinal bleeding and perforation: a record linkage case–control study. *BMJ* 1995; **311**:22–26.

53 Fransen M, Neal B. Non-steroidal anti-inflammatory drugs for preventing heterotopic bone formation after hip at throplasty. The Cochrane Library 2005; Oxford (1): ID CD001160.

SECTION 3
Chronic conditions

CHAPTER 14

Benefits of regular exercise in the treatment and management of bronchial asthma

Felix S.F. Ram and Joanna Picot

Introduction

Subjects with asthma have a unique response to exercise or physical activity. On the one hand, exercise can provoke an increase in airways resistance leading to exercise-induced asthma (EIA). On the other hand, regular physical activity and participation in sports are considered to be useful in the management of asthma, especially in children and adolescents,[1] but this has not been investigated in the same detail as the mechanisms of EIA.

Exercise-induced asthma can be prevented or reduced by pretreatment with a number of medicines, including beta agonists, chromones, and leukotriene antagonists. Despite this, the fear of inducing an episode of breathlessness inhibits many patients with asthma from taking part in physical activities. A low level of regular physical activity in turn leads to a low level of physical fitness, so it is not surprising that a number of studies[2,3] have found that patients with asthma have lower cardiorespiratory fitness than their peers, although not every study has reported this.[4]

Physical training programs have been designed for patients with asthma with the aim of improving physical fitness, neuromuscular coordination and self-confidence. Subjectively, many patients report that they are symptomatically better when fit, but the physiological basis of this perception has not been systematically investigated. A possible mechanism is that an increase in regular physical activity of sufficient intensity to increase aerobic fitness will raise the ventilatory threshold, thereby lowering the minute ventilation during mild and moderate exercise. Consequently, breathlessness and the likelihood of provoking exercise-induced asthma will both be reduced. Exercise training may also reduce the perception of breathlessness through other mechanisms including strengthening of the respiratory muscles.

We have conducted a systematic review to measure the effects of physical training on subjects with asthma. This review was originally published electronically[5] in 1999 on the Cochrane Library. It has since been updated to encompass a literature search up to and including July 2005. With these reviews, every effort is made to locate all published and unpublished studies (without any restriction on language) to answer the question. Explicit criteria are used to select studies for inclusion in the review and to assess their quality. If appropriate, a meta-analysis is used to produce an overall result. Meta-analysis is a statistical procedure to quantitatively summarize the results of randomized controlled trials.

Objectives

This review was undertaken to gain a better understanding of the effects of physical training on the health of subjects with asthma. The objective was to assess the evidence from randomized, controlled clinical trials (RCTs) of the effects of physical training on resting pulmonary function, aerobic fitness, clinical status and quality of life in patients with asthma.

Key message

Having asthma need not prevent you from obtaining the benefits of increased physical activity. This review shows that people with asthma who take regular exercise can improve their cardiorespiratory fitness and work capacity. It has also shown that regular exercise does not adversely affect lung function. Therefore, there should not be any restrictions in patients with asthma wanting to participate in regular physical activity. Further studies are necessary to determine if regular exercise reduces symptoms and improves the quality of life in asthma.

Methods

Types of study and participants

Only trials of subjects with asthma who were randomized to physical training or a control intervention were selected. Subjects had to be aged 8 years and older and their asthma had to be diagnosed by a physician or by the use of objective criteria—for example, bronchodilator reversibility. Subjects with any degree of asthma severity were included. To qualify for inclusion the physical training had to include whole body aerobic exercise for at least 20 minutes, two or more times a week, for a minimum of 4 weeks.

Search strategy

The following terms were used to search for studies: asthma* AND (work capacity OR physical activity OR training OR rehabilitation OR physical fitness). The Cochrane Airways Group asthma and wheeze randomized controlled clinical trials register (up to July 2005) was searched for studies. Additional searches were carried out on MEDLINE (1966–2005), EMBASE (1980–2005), SportDiscus (1949–2005), Current Contents Index (1995–2005) and Science Citation Index (1995–2005). The reference lists of all the papers that were obtained were reviewed to identify trials not captured by electronic and manual searches. Abstracts were reviewed without language restriction. When more data were required for the systematic review, the authors of the study were contacted requesting the additional information or clarification (Box 14.1).

Data collection and analysis

The following outcome measures were looked for:

- Bronchodilator usage
- Episodes of wheeze
- Symptoms (recorded in daily diary cards)
- Exercise endurance
- Work capacity

Box 14.1 The Cochrane Collaboration and the Cochrane Airways Group

• The Cochrane Collaboration is an international network of individuals and institutions that evolved to prepare systematic, periodic reviews of randomized, controlled trials. Individual trials may be too small to answer questions on the effects of health-care interventions. Systematic reviews that include all relevant studies reduce bias and increase statistical power, and make it easier to determine whether a treatment is effective or not. With the exponential growth of the medical literature (over two million articles are published annually), systematic reviews help to distill this information and make it more manageable.
• The Cochrane Collaboration is organized into more than 50 review groups. Before the reviews are published electronically in the Cochrane Library, they are peer-reviewed. Reviews are then updated at regular intervals. More information about the Cochrane Collaboration, including abstracts of the reviews, can be found at: http://www.cochrane.org. The full texts of reviews are available on subscription, either on the Internet or on CD-ROM (http://www.thecochranelibrary.com).

• Walking distance
• Measures of quality of life
• Physiological measurements—i.e., peak expiratory flow rate (PEFR), forced expiratory volume in 1 second (FEV_1), forced vital capacity (FVC), maximum oxygen consumption (Vo_{2max}), maximum expiratory flow ($V_{E\,max}$), maximum heart rate (HR_{max}), maximum voluntary ventilation.

Two reviewers assessed the trials for inclusion by only looking at the methods section of each paper without reading the results of the study or the conclusions.[6] Each reviewer independently applied written inclusion/exclusion criteria to the methods section of each study. Disagreement about inclusion of a study was resolved whenever possible by consensus and an independent person was consulted if disagreement persisted. All trials that appeared potentially relevant were assessed, and if appropriate were included in the review. If an RCT was excluded on methodological grounds, the reason for exclusion was recorded.

The methodological quality of the included trials was assessed with particular emphasis on treatment allocation concealment, which was ranked using the Cochrane Collaboration approach:

• Grade A: adequate concealment
• Grade B: uncertain
• Grade C: clearly inadequate concealment
• Grade D: not used (no attempt at concealment).

Two of the reviewers independently extracted data from the trials. The trials were combined for meta-analysis using Review Manager 4.2.8 (Cochrane Collaboration). A fixed-effect model was used. The outcomes of interest in this review were continuous data. Data from each of the continuous outcomes were analyzed as weighted mean differences with 95% confidence intervals.

Results

The electronic search yielded 1014 potential studies: 29 references were found in EMBASE, 86 in MEDLINE, 76 in SportDiscus, and 823 from the Cochrane Register, of trials. An additional 28 references were added from bibliographic searching of relevant articles. Of a total of 1042 abstracts, 101 dealt with physical training in asthma. The full text of each of the 101 papers was obtained and translated where necessary (one each from French and German). Fifty-nine studies were excluded as they were not relevant to the topic being reviewed leaving 42 studies for potential inclusion in the review. Upon closer examination of the study methodology a further 29 studies were excluded (mostly due to not being an RCT) and the remaining thirteen[7–19] were included in this systematic review (Table 14.1).

We wrote to the first authors of the included studies to clarify areas of uncertainty. Most of the trials did not describe the method of randomization and did not make any references to allocation concealment (blinding). All trials mentioned that subject allocation was carried out randomly, but only one trial[19] reported the method used. Using the Cochrane Collaboration approach for allocation concealment, the trial reporting method of allocation (using coded random numbers) was graded "A," and all other trials included in this review were allocated a grade "B," indicating that we were uncertain as to the method of treatment allocation used by the authors in their trials.

Figure 14.1 shows how the effect of physical training on Vo_{2max} was assessed. The output from the statistical software used here (RevMan 4.2.8) shows the mean and standard deviation for the experimental group (training group) and the control group for each of the seven studies where Vo_{2max} was measured. On the right-hand side of Fig. 14.1, the weighted mean difference (WMD) is shown. This is the difference between the experimental and control groups, weighted according to the precision of the study in estimating the effect (precision is calculated as the inverse of the variance). This method assumes that all of the trials have measured the outcome on the same scale and that for each study the baseline Vo_{2max} was not significantly different between control and experimental groups. Where the weighted mean difference lies to the right of the line of zero effect, it favors physical training. If the 95% confidence interval (represented by straight horizontal black lines) does not cross the line of zero effect, the result is statistically significant. The overall weighted mean difference (95% confidence interval) for the seven studies was 5.43 mL/kg/min (4.24 to 6.61), represented by the diamond at the bottom of the figure—i.e., physical training resulted in an increase Vo_{2max} of 5.43 mL/kg/min.

The chi-squared value (10.97) provides an indication of the heterogeneity of the studies. The test of heterogeneity shows whether or not the differences in the results of the five studies are greater than would be expected by chance. In this case, the chi-squared value has to be greater than 12.59 (six degrees of freedom and $\alpha = 0.05$) before the studies would be considered heterogeneous. For Vo_{2max}, it is 10.97, and therefore it can be concluded that the RCTs contributing to this particular outcome were not heterogeneous.

Table 14.2 provides a summary of the results. The overall weighted mean difference is shown for each of the outcome measures along with the 95% confidence intervals. Physical training led to a significant increase in Vo_{2max} (seven studies), VE_{max} (four studies) (Fig. 14.2), and work capacity (three studies). Episodes of wheeze were reported in only one study.[12] Although the number of episodes of wheeze was 7.5 days less in the training group, this difference was not significant ($P = 0.3$). Physical training did not change FEV_1, FVC, or PEFR (Figs. 14.3, 14.4, and 14.5, respectively).

No usable data were available for the following outcome measures: maximum voluntary ventilation, bronchodilator use, symptom diary scores, exercise endurance, walking distance or measures of quality of life. There were insufficient studies to justify subgroup analysis by gender, age, or exercise intensity.

Table 14.1 Characteristics of the studies included

First author, ref.	Method of participant selection	Description of participants and duration of physical training	Type of physical training
Ahmaidi[8]	Participants were selected after performing incremental exercise test on a cycle ergometer and the 20-m shuttle test	Children aged 12–17. Sessions were for 1 h, 3 days a week for 3 months, 36 sessions in total	Running on an outdoor track
Cochrane[9]	6-week run-in period preceded patient selection	Participants aged 16–40. Sessions lasted 30 min, 3 days a week for 3 months	Warm-ups, cycling, jogging, light-calisthenics, stretching and aerobics
Counil[17]	1 month of acclimatization to altitude (1400 m), 6 weeks without any acute episode of wheezing, 1 year without emergency department visits for acute asthma and a baseline $FEV_1 > 70\%$ of predicted	Children aged 10–16 (mean 13 years). Training group exercised three times weekly for 6 weeks, with each session lasting 45 min	Continuous cycling activity
Fitch[10]	The 1962 American Thoracic Society definition of asthma was used for selection	Children aged 10–14. Physical training period was for 3 months	Jogging, calisthenics, soccer, netball, volleyball, sprints
Girodo[11]	Media solicitation was used to obtain volunteers	Participant age was 28–33 years. Subjects trained for 1 h, 3 times a week for 16 weeks	No details provided in published paper, but the subjects were led by a person experienced in physical education
Huang[18]	A city-wide swimming program for asthmatic children in Baltimore, Maryland	Children aged 6–12. Subjects trained for 1 h, three times a week for 2 months	Swimming training program
Matsumoto[7]	Children with asthma diagnosed according to the ATS criteria who had been admitted to hospital	Children aged 9–12 participated in the study. Subjects trained for 30 min a day for 6 days per week for 6 weeks	Swimming training program

Continued

Table 14.1 *(Continued)*

First author, ref.	Method of participant selection	Description of participants and duration of physical training	Type of physical training
Sly[12]	Participants were selected from patients attending a pediatric allergy clinic at a hospital	Children aged 9–13. Sessions were for 2 h, 3 days a week, 39 sessions in total	Swimming, calisthenics, tumbling, parallel bars, rope climbing, abdominal strengthening, wall ladder and running
Swann[13]	Participants attending an asthma clinic with > 20% fall in FEV_1 were selected	Children aged 8–14. Sessions were twice a week and lasted for 3 months	Warm-ups, squat thrusts, star jumps, sit-ups and press-ups
Van Veldhoven[16]	Children were recruited from an asthma center, following an advertisement in the local paper and from a special school	Children aged 8–13 (mean age 10.6). Physical training program was done twice a week for 1 h in a gymnasium and one 20-min exercise session per week at home for a period of 3 months	Gymnastics with focus on improving and enhancing physical competence and learning asthma coping strategies in exercise situations
Varray[14]	Participants had to meet 3 of 4 criteria: clinical, allergic, immunological, and functional (> 15% increase in FEV_1)	Children, mean age 11.4 years. Sessions lasted for 1 h each, with 10 min on and 10 min off training	Indoor swimming training
Varray[15]	Participants selected if a 15% improvement in FEV_1 by inhaling a bronchodilator	Children, mean age 10.3 years (exercise) and 11.7 years (control). Sessions lasted 30 min each, were twice a week for 3 months, 30 sessions in total	Indoor swimming with individualized training intensity
Weisgerber[19]	Subjects with moderate persistent asthma according to symptoms criteria and a need for preventive daily asthma therapy were recruited from the Medical College of Georgia Pediatric Pulmonary, Allergy/Immunology and General Pediatric clinics	Children aged 7–14. Children met for physical training twice per week for 5–6 weeks for 45 min each time	Swimming lessons

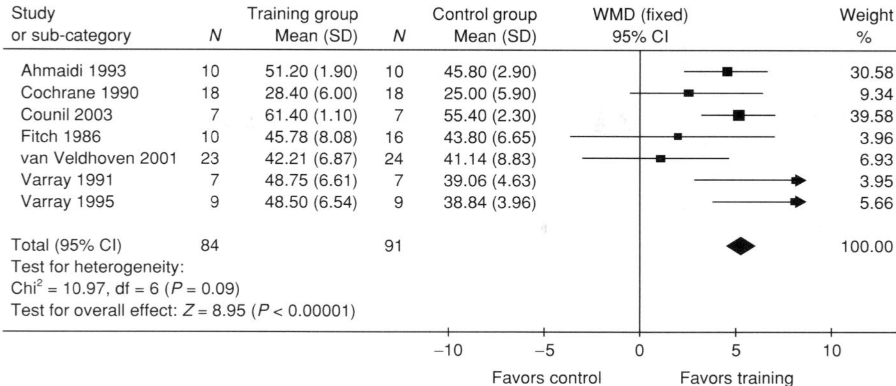

Figure 14.1 Details of the maximum oxygen consumption (Vo_{2max}; mL/kg/min) outcome. The mean value for each trial is indicated by a square box, with the line through it representing the 95% confidence interval (CI). Mean values left of the zero effect line (0) favor control, and values on the right favor physical training. The solid diamond indicates the overall mean effect that physical training has on Vo_{2max}. A percentage weighting (Weight%), which is dependent on the precision and sample size of the estimation of the mean value for each randomized controlled trial, is allocated to each study. The chi-square (χ^2, 10.97) and the degrees of freedom (df = 6) values at the bottom left give a measure of the heterogeneity of the combined results that contributed towards the overall mean result for Vo_{2max}. The Z statistic (8.95) indicates the level of significance for the overall result.

Table 14.2 Summary of mean results for each outcome

Outcome measure	Weighted mean difference	95% confidence intervals	No. of studies contributing to outcome (ref. nos.)
PEFR (L/min)	–5.47	–27.55 to 16.60	4[10,12,16,19]
FEV_1 (L)	0.01	–0.14 to 0.16	5[9,12,14,16,19]
FVC (L)	0.09	–0.12 to 0.30	4[12,14,16,19]
VE_{max} (L/min)	6.00	1.57 to 10.43	4[9,14,16,17]
Vo_{2max} (mL/kg/min)	5.43	4.24 to 6.61	7[8–10,14–17]
Work capacity (W)	14.95	11.52 to 18.38	3[7,8,16]
HR_{max} (bpm)	7.70	5.57 to 9.83	5[8,10,14,16,17]
Episodes of wheeze (days)	–7.50	–22.42 to 7.42	1[12]

FEV_1, forced expiratory volume in one second; FVC, forced vital capacity; HR_{max}, maximum heart rate; PEFR, peak expiratory flow rate; VE_{max}, maximum expiratory flow.

Discussion

The clearest finding of this meta-analysis was that aerobic power (Vo_{2max}) and maximum expiratory flow (VE_{max}) increased with physical training. This shows that the response of subjects with asthma to physical training is similar to that of healthy people,[20] and therefore presumably the benefits of an increase in cardiorespiratory fitness are also accessible to them. In addition, work capacity (i.e., maximum work output) also increased

Study or sub-category	N	Training group Mean (SD)	N	Control group Mean (SD)	WMD (fixed) 95% CI	Weight %
Cochrane 1990	18	66.00 (16.00)	18	58.00 (14.00)		20.36
Varray 1991	7	47.26 (12.80)	7	47.17 (9.73)		13.85
van Veldhoven 2001	23	62.58 (9.98)	24	60.06 (13.27)		43.82
Counil 2003	7	102.10 (7.40)	7	87.30 (10.40)		21.97
Total (95% CI)	55		56			100.00

Test for heterogeneity: $Chi^2 = 5.47$, $df = 3$ ($P = 0.14$)
Test for overall effect: $Z = 2.65$ ($P = 0.008$)

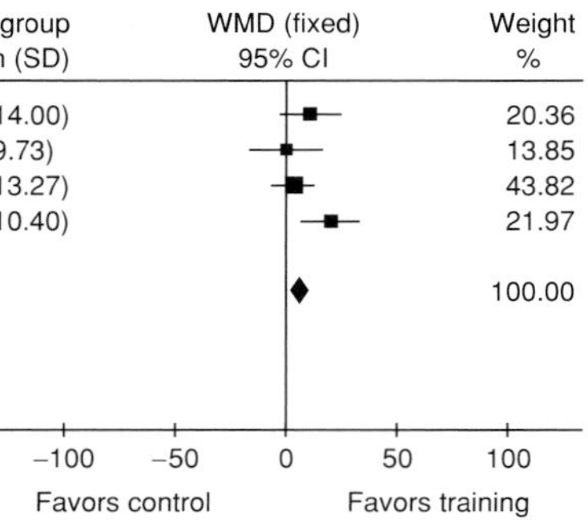

−100 −50 0 50 100
Favors control Favors training

Figure 14.2 Details of the maximum expiratory flow (VE_{max}; L/min) outcome. The solid diamond is on the right-hand side of the line of no effect (favoring training), indicating that physical training increases VE_{max}.

Study or sub-category	N	Training group Mean (SD)	N	Control group Mean (SD)	WMD (fixed) 95% CI	Weight %
Sly 1972	12	0.99 (0.45)	12	1.26 (0.55)		13.48
Cochrane 1990	18	2.97 (0.69)	18	3.13 (0.80)		9.15
Varray 1991	7	1.66 (0.25)	7	1.74 (0.42)		16.62
van Veldhoven 2001	23	2.16 (0.51)	24	2.18 (0.36)		33.96
Weisgerber 2003	5	1.52 (0.18)	3	1.22 (0.21)		26.79
Total (95% CI)	65		64			100.00

Test for heterogeneity: $Chi^2 = 6.59$, $df = 4$ ($P = 0.16$)
Test for overall effect: $Z = 0.12$ ($P = 0.90$)

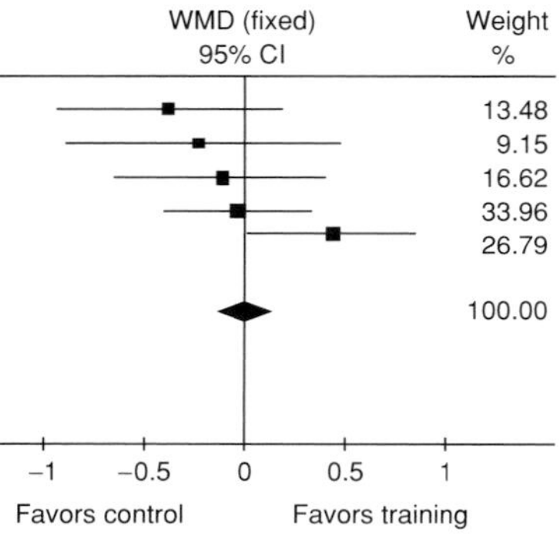

−1 −0.5 0 0.5 1
Favors control Favors training

Figure 14.3 Details of the forced expiratory volume in 1 second (FEV_1; L/min) outcome. The solid diamond crosses the line of no effect, therefore indicating that physical training does not alter FEV_1.

Study or sub-category	N	Training group Mean (SD)	N	Control group Mean (SD)	WMD (fixed) 95% CI	Weight %
Sly 1972	12	1.59 (0.68)	12	1.83 (0.74)		13.09
Varray 1991	7	2.07 (0.87)	7	2.26 (0.55)		7.28
van Veldhoven 2001	23	2.59 (0.57)	24	2.55 (0.48)		46.42
Weisgerber 2003	5	1.89 (0.16)	3	1.54 (0.29)		33.22
Total (95% CI)	47		46			100.00

Test for heterogeneity: $Chi^2 = 3.96$, $df = 3$ ($P = 0.27$)
Test for overall effect: $Z = 0.85$ ($P = 0.39$)

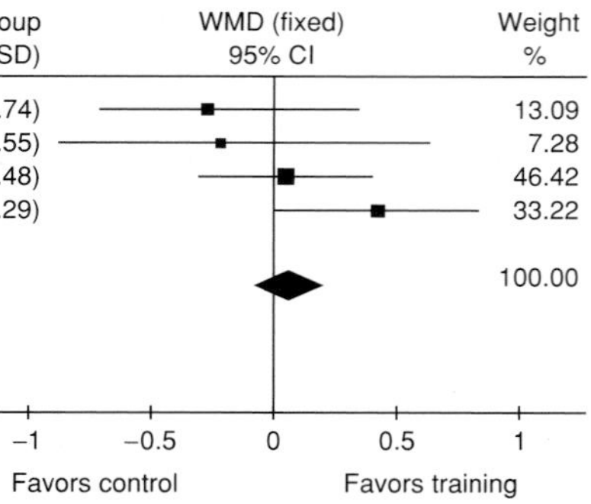

−1 −0.5 0 0.5 1
Favors control Favors training

Figure 14.4 Details of the forced vital capacity (FVC; L) outcome. The solid diamond crosses the line of no effect, therefore indicating that physical training does not alter FVC.

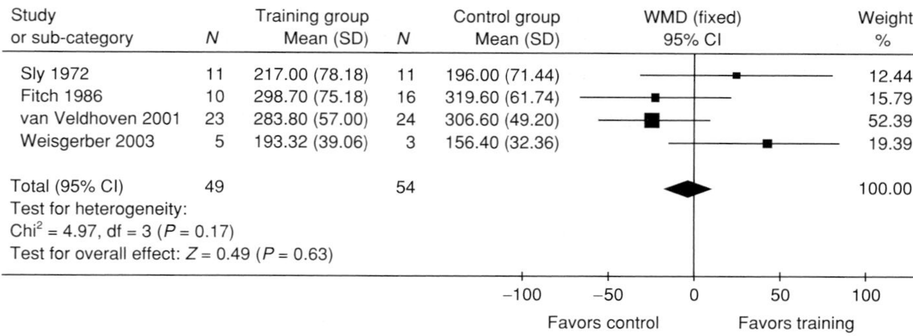

Study or sub-category	N	Training group Mean (SD)	N	Control group Mean (SD)	WMD (fixed) 95% CI	Weight %
Sly 1972	11	217.00 (78.18)	11	196.00 (71.44)		12.44
Fitch 1986	10	298.70 (75.18)	16	319.60 (61.74)		15.79
van Veldhoven 2001	23	283.80 (57.00)	24	306.60 (49.20)		52.39
Weisgerber 2003	5	193.32 (39.06)	3	156.40 (32.36)		19.39
Total (95% CI)	49		54			100.00

Test for heterogeneity: $Chi^2 = 4.97$, df = 3 ($P = 0.17$)
Test for overall effect: $Z = 0.49$ ($P = 0.63$)

Figure 14.5 Details of the peak expiratory flow rate (PEFR; L/min) outcome. The solid diamond crosses the line of no effect, indicating that physical training does not significantly alter PEFR in patients with asthma.

with physical training, which is consistent with the observation that Vo_{2max} and VE_{max} increased.

No improvement in resting lung function was shown. This is not surprising, since there is no obvious reason why regular exercise should improve PEFR, FEV_1, or FVC. It seems that any benefits of regular exercise in patients with asthma are unrelated to effects on lung function. On the other hand, evidence from this review suggests that regular exercise does not have any detrimental effect on lung function. This is reassuring for the continued promotion of exercise prescription by health professionals.[21]

Typically, physical training has no effect, or slightly reduces the maximum heart rate, whereas maximum stroke volume, and thus maximum cardiac output, are increased.[22,23] In the studies which were included in this review, maximum heart rate increased after physical training.[8,10,14,16,17] This suggests that cardiac factors did not limit the maximum exercise capacity prior to training. Breathlessness or some other noncardiac factor may have terminated the baseline tests before a true HR_{max} was achieved. The higher heart rate following physical training may reflect the ability of subjects to exercise for longer.

An alternative explanation, which is improbable, is that the medication taken to prevent EIA caused the increased HR_{max}. Inhaled beta agonists can raise heart rate above resting levels, but prophylactic medication was not changed during the study period, and there is no evidence that physical training alters the cardiac response to β-agonists. The significance of the effect of these agents on heart rate lies in their alteration of the workload–heart rate relationship and the possible consequences of this for exercise prescription based on heart rate.

Unfortunately, there were no data available on a number of outcome measures of interest for this review—i.e., exercise endurance (as distinct from Vo_{2max}), symptoms (other than frequency of wheeze), bronchodilator use, and measures of quality of life. This review has revealed an important gap in our knowledge about the effects of physical training in asthma. There is, however, evidence from one study[24] which was excluded from this review, suggesting that physical training may improve these outcomes. The study by Cambach *et al.* included subjects with asthma, but was not included in our review because they also received education about their disease and breathing retraining. This means that any benefit could not be ascribed solely to physical training. Nonetheless, the intervention resulted in significant improvements in exercise endurance time and the total score for the

Chronic Respiratory Disease Questionnaire increased by 17 points compared to the control group. In subjects with chronic obstructive pulmonary disease (COPD), pulmonary rehabilitation does not lead to an improvement in these parameters unless the subjects undertake exercise training[25] and the same may be true of asthma. A study from Brazil[26] allocated children to physical training or a control group. The study was not included in the review because the allocation of the subjects was not truly random, but it did find that physical training led to significant reductions in the use of both inhaled and oral steroids.

There are a number of pitfalls in conducting systematic reviews. Electronic searches of the literature may identify as few as 50% of the relevant studies.[27] Hand searching of journals may be useful to increase the yield, but is labor-intensive and time-intensive. The Cochrane Collaboration Randomized Controlled Trials register incorporates systematic hand searching (retrospective and prospective) of core journals in an attempt to improve the thoroughness of electronic searching. So that we did not miss any relevant papers, we used several electronic databases in addition to the Cochrane Trials register, and we checked the reference lists of all papers obtained to identify studies we had not already found. This approach will have reduced our chance of missing relevant studies.

Another source of bias can occur with the selection of relevant studies from titles and abstracts of papers. This source of bias was reduced by having written inclusion and exclusion criteria and by having two people independently review and select papers from the abstracts of the 1042 studies which were identified.

The review was restricted to randomized controlled trials. This eliminated a substantial source of data, but this approach is justified because the strength of the evidence obtained from randomized controlled trials is much greater than that of evidence obtained from other lower methodological studies. Adequate randomization technique and treatment allocation concealment have been found to be important aspects of good-quality trials. We attempted to assess the quality of randomization technique and allocation concealment in the studies that were included in the review. Unfortunately, few of the studies provided information about this, other than stating the subjects were randomized to physical training or control groups.

A potential weakness of this review is the small number of subjects included. However, the studies that measured Vo_{2max} and $\mathrm{V_E}_{max}$ were homogeneous, and all studies showed a similar effect, which was highly significant ($P < 0.00001$ and $P < 0.008$, respectively).

Conclusions

In summary, one can conclude that aerobic power and ventilation improves following regular physical training in patients with asthma. This appears to be a normal training effect and is not due to an improvement in resting lung function. It is reassuring to know that physical training does not have an adverse effect on lung function and wheeze in patients with asthma. Therefore, there is no reason why patients with asthma should not participate in regular physical activity. It is recommended that children and adolescents with asthma participate in regular physical activity. This will not only improve asthma management but also provide associated general health benefits. When recommending physical training to patients, one must also provide appropriate guidance regarding the prevention and treatment of exercise-induced asthma.

There is a need for further randomized controlled trials to assess the role of physical training in the treatment and management of bronchial asthma. In particular, it will be important to determine whether the improved exercise performance that follows physical training is translated into fewer symptoms and to an improvement in quality of life.

Summary

- Forty-two controlled trials of physical training of patients with asthma were identified in the literature covering the years 1966–2005.
- Thirteen of these trials met the inclusion criteria: objective asthma diagnosis, age (≥ 8 years), and at least 20 minutes of whole-body exercise two or more times a week for a minimum of 4 weeks.
- Outcomes of interest, resting lung function, asthma state and cardiorespiratory fitness, were subjected to a meta-analysis.

Key messages

- Physical training resulted in a significant increase in cardiorespiratory fitness as measured by increases in $\dot{V}O_{2max}$ and $\dot{V}E_{max}$.
- Work capacity also significantly increased in three of these studies.
- Physical training does not worsen lung function in patients with asthma.
- Cardiorespiratory benefits of regular exercise are available to patients with asthma as they are to nonasthmatics.
- Patients with asthma have no reason not to participate in regular physical activities.

Acknowledgments

The authors would like to thank Byzance Daglish (Aventis Pharma, Paris) for translating the French-language paper; and A. Varray, R. Sly, and J. Neder for responding to requests for further information about their trials.

Sample examination questions

Multiple-choice questions (answers on page 602)

1 In individuals with asthma, regular physical training leads to improvements in:
  A Forced expiratory volume in one second
  B Forced vital capacity
  C Peak expiratory flow rate
  D Maximal oxygen uptake
  E Bronchial hyperresponsiveness

2 For systematic reviews of clinical trials to be reliable. They should not include:
  A Unpublished studies
  B Open, uncontrolled studies
  C Non–English-language studies
  D Small studies
  E Large studies

3 In subjects with asthma, there is clear evidence that:
  A β_2 agonists should not be used before exercise
  B Physical training reduces the quality of life
  C Many types of physical training improve aerobic fitness
  D Physical training should be restricted to children under the age of 12 years
  E Only swimming improves aerobic fitness

4 Physical training of asthmatic individuals has been shown to:
   A Reduce the need for bronchodilator use
   B Reduce the frequency of exercise-induced asthma
   C Increase maximum voluntary ventilation
   D Decrease maximum exercise ventilation
   E Increase maximum work capacity
5 The Cochrane Collaboration:
   A Prepares and maintains systematic reviews of the effects of health care interventions
   B Is a collection of historical medical biographies
   C Disseminates information about nonscientific treatments for human diseases and disorders
   D Maintains a database on the epidemiology of asthma
   E Is a nonprofit organization that sponsors research into alternative therapies for asthma

Essay questions

1 Discuss the advantages and disadvantages of systematic reviews of randomized controlled trials in summarizing evidence of the effectiveness of health care interventions. Include a comparison of systematic reviews of nonrandomized controlled trials and randomized controlled trials; use examples from other health-care interventions if appropriate.
2 Write an essay on the role and benefits of physical training for patients with asthma. Compare and contrasts these benefits to nonasthmatics who undertake regular physical training.

Case study 10.1

Xavier is an 8-year-old boy who enjoys playing soccer with his class-mates on Saturday mornings during the winter season. Xavier's soccer coach, Tom, has requested his mum to take Xavier to his doctor for a check-up, as Tom believes that Xavier may not be able to continue with his soccer because of his coughing and shortness of breath during practice. Xavier comes to your clinic for a physical. You find that even with Tom's concerns, Xavier is able to ride his bike and use his skateboard throughout the year without any problems and he sleeps through the night without coughing. You also find that during soccer practice, Xavier seems to have more difficulty breathing out and does not have pain in the front of his chest or neck during these episodes. Upon further assessments, you rightly diagnose asthma and prescribe appropriate medications for Xavier's age.

Is Tom rightly concerned about Xavier's coughing and shortness of breath during practice, if so why? How will you address Xavier's mum's query about whether Xavier should be allowed to continue playing soccer, and how this may affect his asthma?

Case study 10.2

Charlotte is a 15-year-old young woman who has been doing ballet since she was 2 years old. However, over the last 6 months, she has noticed that her asthma is restricting her ability to perform with the rest of her ballet class. As a result, Charlotte often misses ballet, and her dad encourages her to stop her ballet in order to avoid being short of breath and having coughing episodes during her ballet lessons. She used to participate in sports at school, but quit because she "got too tired." Charlotte admits that she is awakened by coughing two nights a week, and more often if she visits her girlfriend's house, where there is a cat called Rusty.

Charlotte and her dad come to you for advice regarding Charlotte's asthma and her continued participation in ballet and other sports. They are particularly interested in knowing if there are any measures that Charlotte can take prior to starting her ballet lessons and if her ballet is causing her asthma. They are also interested in knowing if Rusty may be making her asthma worse.

Summarizing the evidence

Outcome measure	Results	Level of evidence*
PEFR	4 RCTs, one of moderate size and three of small size	A4
FEV_1	5 RCTs, two of moderate size and three of small size	A3
FVC	4 RCTs, one of moderate size and three of small size	A4
VE_{max}	4 RCTs, two of moderate size and two of small size	A3
VO_{2max}	7 RCTs, two of moderate size and five of small size	A3
Work capacity	3 RCTs, one of moderate size and two of small size	A4
HR_{max}	5 RCTs, one of moderate size and four of small size	A4
Episodes of wheeze	1 RCT of small size	A6

FEV_1, forced expiratory volume in 1 second; FVC, forced vital capacity; HR_{max}, maximum heart rate; PEFR, peak expiratory flow rate; VE_{max}, maximum expiratory flow; VO_{2max}, maximum oxygen consumption.

"A" grade level of evidence, from randomized controlled trials (RCTs) only, has been shown in this review, which has been graded as shown below. Arbitrarily, the following cut-off points for study size have been used; large study ≥ 60 patients per study group; moderate-sized study ≥ 15 patients per study group; small study ≤ 15 patients in each study group.

* A1: evidence from two or more large RCTs.
A2: evidence from at least one large RCT.
A3: evidence from two or more moderate-sized RCTs.
A4: evidence from at least one moderate-sized RCT.
A5: evidence from two or more small RCTs.
A6: evidence from at least one small RCT.

References

1 Orenstein DM. Asthma and sports. In: Bar-Or O, ed. *The Child and the Adolescent Athlete.* London: Blackwell, 1996: 433–454.
2 Clark CJ, Cochrane LM. Assessment of work performance in asthma for determination of cardiorespiratory fitness and training capacity. *Thorax* 1988; **43**:745–749.
3 Garfinkel S, Kesten S, Chapman K, *et al.* Physiologic and nonphysiologic determinants of aerobic fitness in mild to moderate asthma. *Am Rev Respir Dis* 1992; **145**:741–745.
4 Santuz P, Baraldi E, Filippone M, *et al.* Exercise performance in children with asthma: is it different from that of healthy controls? *Eur Respir J* 1997; **10**:1254–1260.
5 Ram FS, Robinson SM, Black PN, Picot J. Physical training for asthma. *Cochrane Database Syst Rev* 2005; (4):CD001116.
6 Oxman AD, Cook DJ and Guyatt GH. How to use an overview. *JAMA* 1994; **17**:1367–1371.
7 Matsumoto I, Araki H, Tsuda K, *et al.* Effects of swimming training on aerobic capacity and exercise induced bronchoconstriction in children with bronchial asthma. *Thorax* 1999; **54**:196–201.
8 Ahmaidi SB, Varray AL, Savy-Pacaux AM, *et al.* Cardiorespiratory fitness evaluation by the shuttle test in asthmatic subjects during aerobic training. *Chest* 1993; **104**:1135–1141.

9 Cochrane LM, Clark CJ. Benefits and problems of a physical training programme for asthmatic patients. *Thorax* 1990; **45**:345–351.
10 Fitch KD, Blitvich JD, Morton AR. The effect of running training on exercise-induced asthma. *Ann of Allergy* 1986; **57**:90–94.
11 Girodo M, Ekstrand KA, Metivier GJ. Deep diaphragmatic breathing: rehabilitation exercises for the asthmatic patient. *Arch Phys Med Rehabil* 1992; **73**:717–720.
12 Sly RM, Harper RT, Rosselot I. The effect of physical conditioning upon asthmatic children. *Ann Allergy* 1972; **30**:86–94.
13 Swann IL, Hanson CA. Double-blind prospective study of the effect of physical training on childhood asthma. In: Oseid S, Edwards A, eds. *The Asthmatic Child—in Play and Sport*. London: Pitman, 1983: 318–325.
14 Varray AL, Mercier JG, Terral CM, *et al.* Individualized aerobic and high intensity training for asthmatic children in an exercise readaptation program: is training always helpful for better adaptation to exercise? *Chest* 1991; **99**:579–586.
15 Varray AL, Mercier JG, Prefaut CG. Individualized training reduces excessive exercise hyperventilation in asthmatics. *Int Rehabil Res* 1995; **18**:297–312.
16 Van Veldhoven NHM, Vermeer A, Bogaard JM, *et al.* Children with asthma and physical exercise: effects of an exercise programme. *Clin Rehabil* 2001; **15**:360–370.
17 Counil FP, Varray A, Matecki S, *et al.* Training of aerobic and anaerobic fitness in children with asthma. *J Pediatr* 2003; **142**:179–184.
18 Huang SW, Veiga R, Sila U, *et al.* The effect of swimming in asthmatic children: participants in a swimming program in the city of Baltimore. *J Asthma* 1989; **26**:117–121.
19 Weisgerber MC, Guill M, Weisgerber JM, *et al.* Benefits of swimming in asthma: effect of a session of swimming lessons on symptoms and PFTs with review of the literature. *J Asthma* 2003; **40**:453–464.
20 Robinson DM, Egglestone DM, Hill PM, Rea HH, *et al.* Effects of a physical conditioning programme on asthmatic patients. *N Z Med J* 1992; **105**:253–256.
21 Chakravarthy MV, Joyner MJ, Booth FW. An obligation for primary care physicians to prescribe physical activity to sedentary patients to reduce the risk of chronic health conditions. *Mayo Clin Proc* 2002; **77**:165–173.
22 Haas F, Pasierski S, Levine N, *et al.* Effect of aerobic training on forced expiratory airflow in exercising asthmatic humans. *J Appl Physiol* 1987; **63**:1230–1235.
23 Brooks GA, Fahey TD, White TP. *Exercise Physiology: Human Bioenergetics and Its Applications*. Mountain View, Canada: Mayfield, 1996:295–296.
24 Cambach W, Chadwick-Straver RVM, Wagenaar RC, *et al.* The effects of community-based pulmonary rehabilitation programme on exercise tolerance and quality of life: a randomised controlled trial. *Eur Respir J* 1997; **10**:104–113.
25 Ries AL, Kaplan RM, Limberg TM, *et al.* Effects of pulmonary rehabilitation on physiologic and psychological outcomes in patients with chronic obstructive pulmonary disease. *Ann Intern Med* 1995; **122**:823–832.
26 Neder JA, Nery LE, Silva AC, *et al.* Short term effects of aerobic training in the clinical management of severe asthma in children. *Thorax* 1999; **54**:202–206.
27 Dickersin K, Scherer R, Lefebvre C. Identifying relevant studies for systematic reviews. *BMJ* 1994; **309**:1286–1291.

CHAPTER 15

What is the role of exercise in the prevention of back pain?

Joanne Dear and Martin Underwood

Low back pain is a major health and socioeconomic problem in the Western world.[1,2] Estimates of the economic burden of low back pain suggest that it is greater than that of coronary heart disease, stroke, or diabetes.[3–5] The 1998 direct, indirect, and informal health-care costs in the UK were estimated to be £1632 million, £3440 million, and £1578 million, respectively.[6] Around one-third of direct health-care costs are for the provision of services in the private sector, and it is likely that these are paid by patients or their families either directly or indirectly through health insurance. Apart from the pain, disability, and economic costs due to chronic low back pain, it can have a major impact on individual's feelings of self-worth.[7] Simple means of preventing back pain or its recurrence could have a major impact on individual patients, their families, and society overall.

Epidemiology of low back pain

Estimates suggest that the lifetime prevalence of low back pain is 49–70%, point prevalence 12–30%, and 1-month period prevalence 25–42%.[8] The South Manchester Back Pain Study collected data both from people consulting their family practitioner and the general population. Over a year, the cumulative incidence of new consulting episodes of back pain was 3% in males and 5% in females.[9] A follow-up survey 1 year later found a cumulative annual incidence of 31% in males and 32% in females.[9] Those patients with a previous history of low back pain had a higher incidence rate and, although most cases improved within a few weeks, residual symptoms and recurrences were common.[10] Occupational studies suggest that 20–44% of patients suffer a recurrence within 1 year, and that the lifetime recurrence rate is 85%.[11] Between 5% and 15% of those presenting with acute back pain subsequently develop chronic problems.[12] Some caution should be used when interpreting and using epidemiological evidence, as there appears to be little consensus on low back pain classifications. Indeed, low back pain terminology and definitions are coming under continued scrutiny.[13]

Exercise and the prevention of low back pain and disability

Lack of physical fitness and strength measured at the back and abdominal muscles have been suggested as possible risk factors for developing new and recurrent low back pain.[8] The known health benefits of physical activity suggest that lifetime physical fitness and functioning may have a role in the primary prevention of low back pain (LBP); and that continued reinforcement of the physical activity message may have some impact on low back pain occurrence and the progression towards chronicity.[14] Many other factors, such as pain, disability, job dissatisfaction, and psychosocial issues have also been linked to developing chronic LBP.[15] Thus, exercise is only one of a number of approaches that could be used in the prevention and treatment of LBP. Consideration of psychosocial factors when considering an exercise intervention might aid compliance with the recommended regimen.[16,17] Exercise therapies, either as single interventions or as part of multidisciplinary treatment programs, are commonly used for low back pain.[18–20] There are a number of systematic reviews and meta-analyses of randomized controlled trials of the effectiveness of exercise therapy.[21–24] These indicate that exercise can be beneficial for some low back pain patients. Exercise regimens for both acute and chronic LBP are included in numerous national management guidelines and more recently in the European back pain guidelines.[25,26] The focus of this chapter is on appraising the evidence for the use of exercise alone in the primary prevention of LBP and the secondary prevention of LBP disability.

Evidence-based medicine and back pain

The fashion for evidence-based health care means that we are expected to be aware of the current best evidence when recommending treatment options to our patients.[27] However, robust randomized and controlled evidence may not be available to inform treatment decisions. Randomized controlled trials are established as the "gold standard" in intervention research. However, the lack of prognostic homogeneity in study populations, the difficulty of blinding patients and therapists to the intervention, difficulty in standardizing the interventions, small sample sizes, loss to follow-up, and poor adherence to treatment may all need careful consideration when assessing trials of exercise for treatment or prevention of LBP.[28] Furthermore, there is no single clinical indicator that is regarded as a suitable outcome measure.[29] There are international guidelines for outcome measures for back pain research.[30] These suggest including back pain–specific functional outcomes (e.g., Roland Morris Questionnaire[31] or Oswestry Disability Questionnaire[32]); generic health status (e.g., SF-36[33]); Health Utility (e.g., EQ 5D[34]) pain (frequency and severity); work disability (work absenteeism), and patient satisfaction. This consensus gives little indication of clinical usefulness or whether potential benefits from treatments are meaningful to individual patients, and it is not itself evidence-based.

Applying methods derived from pharmaceutical trials of standardized preparations used for well-defined conditions with clear outcomes (e.g., death) may not be the most appropriate tool for assessing the effectiveness of exercise therapy for low back pain, a poorly defined condition with nonstandardized treatment packages for which there is a lack of clarity about how to assess the outcome. Notwithstanding these potential limitations of the evidence-based approach, critically appraising existing intervention studies can help inform the advice we give our patients.

Inclusion criteria used in back pain studies

Knowing the features of those included in trials of exercise treatment is crucial to deciding whether the findings can be applied to clinical practice. The reader must be extremely cautious as to the interpretation of the effectiveness of the intervention when comparing trials which have used different classifications of low back pain. Low back pain is usually defined as pain, muscle tension, or stiffness localized below the costal margin and above the inferior gluteal folds, with or without leg pain.[35]

A simple classification system that is gaining increased international acceptance is to triage low back pain into three categories:[27]

- Serious spinal pathology (malignancy/sepsis/osteoporotic collapse)
- Nerve root pain/ radicular pain
- Nonspecific low back pain

Nearly all low back pain is nonspecific,[8] defined as symptoms without a clear and specific cause. This diagnostic triage is a helpful first step. However, there are no generally recognized ways for further classifying these patients.

Duration is thought to be a relevant criterion when categorizing low back pain. The Quebec task force defined "acute" back pain as less than 6 weeks, "subacute" as 6 weeks to 3 months, and "chronic" as greater than 3 months.[36] For the purpose of this chapter, acute and subacute low back pain are grouped together (symptom duration 0–12 weeks), with pain lasting longer than 12 weeks considered to be chronic.[8]

What is an exercise intervention?

It is impossible to interpret the research findings without defining what is meant by an exercise intervention. Exercise regimens included within back pain intervention studies include different types of aerobic, flexibility and strengthening exercises. In addition to the mode of exercise, it is important that adequate detail is provided about the dose used. Groups such as the American College of Sports Medicine offer clear guidance on the desired dose of exercise required to affect physiological change. One recent review of the exercise evidence for chronic low back pain incorporated this helpful information into its analysis.[29] Without clear and detailed information about the exercise prescription, only limited analysis of the efficacy of the intervention can be made. The progression of the exercise prescription featured within many of the low back pain trials is governed not by the practitioner, but by the length of the intervention located within the trial design. Patients randomized to an exercise intervention will often exercise for a specified length of time, somewhere between 4 and 12 weeks, with exercise progressions determined by those guiding the trial rather than their individual needs. Practitioners would normally expect that exercise progression should be individualized to the patient; the rate of exercise progression for one LBP patient may not be similar to that of another reporting the same problems.

Exercise interventions included within trials are often characterized by a prescriptive element in their design that includes details relating to the type or mode of exercise and the dose of the prescription, a combination of frequency, intensity, and duration. In many low back pain trials, exercise is often a combination of exercise types, and seldom is one mode of exercise the focus of questions relating to its efficacy as a treatment and/or management option.

Inclusion criteria for this review

The aim of this review is to provide some guidance as to the recommended exercise interventions for both acute and chronic low back pain in primary and secondary prevention. There are a number of excellent systematic and literature reviews in this area,[21,29,37–40] but to our knowledge, none has looked solely at trials in which the exercise intervention is not part of a wider multidisciplinary program and specifically considered the constituents of the exercise programs. Studies included in this review were those in which the predominant exercise was not part of a multidisciplinary program or used in conjunction with other interventions that have been seen to be effective for low back pain patients. In this way, we have been able to summarize the effectiveness of defined exercise regimens. Studies were excluded if the exercise intervention was implemented in combination with educational programs, cognitive behavioral therapy, back schools, functional restoration programs, medical interventions, manual therapy, relaxation programs, ergonomics, and behavioral techniques. Studies included were not limited to randomized controlled trials (RCTs). A clear description of the patients was required, including duration of symptoms (acute or chronic) and diagnosis (nonspecific low back pain). All papers reviewed were in English. Every effort has been made to detail the exercise regimen used accurately to allow for future prescription.

Search strategy

The search strategy used the following search terms: exercise and back pain; exercise therapy and back pain. Searches were carried out on MEDLINE (1966–2005); AMED (1985–2005); British Nursing Index (1985–2005); CINAHL (1982–2005); SportsDiscus (1830–2005); Cochrane Collaboration; ScienceDirect and Emerald FullText. All searches were conducted in April 2005. The reference lists of all the papers obtained were reviewed for relevant articles not included in electronic searches.[41]

In contrast to previous reviews, we sought to identify and describe the specific modes of exercise evaluated for the prevention of chronic low back pain disability. The detail provided on the exercise prescriptions used in the included studies is sparse; thus, even if a clear benefit was demonstrated, replicating the results would be impossible. It is imperative that future studies clearly describe the interventions tested.

We identified 24 relevant studies, 16 RCTs and eight other studies that assessed nine different exercise regimens (Table 15.1).

Calisthenics

Calisthenics exercise can be used to develop and maintain muscular strength and endurance across all areas, including abdominals, hip flexors, gluteals and lower back. These types of exercise can be easily performed within the home if the patient has limited access to exercise facilities and equipment. Prescription and choice of exercise repertoire must be clear and the patient must be confident to exercise on his/her own if a group exercise option is not viable. Resistance is provided by body weight, and careful consideration must be given to the choice of exercise and prescription.

Prescription: two sessions per week, each session lasting 45 minutes.[42]

Leisure-time physical activity/self-exercise/sport-specific programs

This type of physical activity is often self-rated and includes nonoccupational activity quantified by hours spent engaging in physical activity. It can include sports activities, as well as the more functional leisure-time activities, including walking. This often encompasses the more general "get active—stay active" message. It is a useful regimen for all patients, particularly those with limited access to facilities or those previously considered sedentary. Of particular interest is that leisure-time physical activity often includes walking, possibly the most accessible form of activity for the majority of the population.

Table 15.1 Exercise for the primary prevention of back pain

First author, ref.	Design	Study population	Predominant exercise	Comparison/control group	Evidence for the use of exercise based on the study findings
Leisure-time physical activity/self-exercise					
Croft[10]	Prospective population-based cohort	2715 adults without current back pain	Leisure-time physical activity	Not applicable	Leisure-time physical activity is not associated with risk of back pain
Harreby[61]	Prospective cohort study	640 38-year-old adults previously surveyed at age 14	Leisure-time physical activity	Not applicable	Leisure-time physical activity over 3 h/week reduces risk of LBP
Leino[62]	Prospective cohort study	607 blue- and white-collar employees in the metal industry	Leisure-time physical activity	Not applicable	An inverse linear association between leisure-time physical activity and the 5-year change in symptoms and clinical findings of the low back was demonstrated
Multimodal exercise programs/general exercise therapy					
Gerdle[64]	RCT	97 women employed as home care service personnel. Inclusion criteria: working at least part time; employed at least 6 months; not on long-term sick leave	Exercise: 1 h of exercise, once a week for 1 year. Exercise includes warm-up, muscle strength, and aerobics (n = 46)	Control intervention: no intervention (n = 49)	Inconsistent findings for the use of general, multimodal exercise program
Gundewall[63]	Randomized prospective study	69 nurses and nurse's aides with and without back pain. 68 women. RCT with 13-month follow-up	Preventative exercise: dynamic endurance, isometric strength and functional coordination exercises during working hours, 20 min, average of six sessions a month (n = 28)	Control intervention: no intervention (n = 32)	Back strengthening and endurance exercise combined with functional coordination had a positive effect on pain, work absenteeism, and back strength.

LBP, lower back pain; RCT, randomized controlled trial.

Prescription: a benchmark of five sessions of physical activity per week, each session lasting 30 minutes, could be used.[43]

McKenzie exercises

McKenzie extension exercises are a popular approach targeting pain relief and can be prescribed as sole interventions or as part of a wider multimodal program.[20,44–46] It is an extension-oriented treatment regimen used for pain relief by "centralizing" the pain to the lower back, where the source of the pain can be treated. This exercise regimen has been used with both acute and chronic LBP patients. McKenzie exercises, like any other exercise regimen, need to be prescribed correctly, with careful consideration of type and frequency of exercise. They can be viewed as much more than simple extension, and a full range of motion is the ultimate goal. They can be used in conjunction with other modes of activity, for example strengthening and flexion exercises, as suitable progressions. Prescription ranges from three sessions per week to one session every day including a range of six exercises with ten repeats.[45,46] Liebenson provides a useful overview and exercise examples.[47,48]

Prescription: there is little consensus on the optimal prescription for the LBP patient but prescriptive elements of this exercise may need to be individualized to the patient and delivered by specially trained practitioners.

Multimodal exercise programs/general exercise therapy

Multimodal programs in most cases included aerobic, strengthening, stretching and coordination activities using bicycle ergometers, treadmills, free weights, and resistance equipment.[20,49–51] The effectiveness of this program in relation to outcome measures is very difficult to pinpoint to one mode of exercise because of the range of activities included. Although the reliance on equipment is high, the program can be adapted to suit those who wish to exercise in the home.

Prescription: dependent on the patient, their current symptoms and goals.

Spinal stabilization program/core strengthening

This is a very specific regimen designed to control pain through active segmental stabilization protecting the spine from strain and reinjury.[52] The program is based on theoretical knowledge, with clear recommendations for exercise progressions once the stabilization skill has been mastered. It involves co-contraction of transversus abdominis and multifidus, but is reliant on highly skilled exercise professionals or practitioners to teach the skill to the patient. Focused on pain relief through active segmental stabilization, progressions associated with this mode of exercise are clearly defined, especially once the skill of co-contraction has been mastered. The program advocated in the work by Sung appears advanced, particularly if the patient is advised to co-contract local musculature.[52] Both Akuthota and Nadler[53] and Richardson and Jull[54] provide useful overviews.

Prescription: this exercise program is heavily reliant on skilled practitioners to teach co-contraction of transverses abdominis and multifidus. This mode of exercise is not suitable for all patients—e.g., those who are not motivated to exercise.

Sport-specific programs

Sport-specific programs feature in a small number of studies and are included as part of wider leisure-time physical activity. Sport-specific programs utilize recognizable sports activities such as swimming and gymnastics as their chosen mode of activity.

Prescription: the prescriptive element of the program is not always detailed. The suitability of sport-specific programs for all patients is questionable and participation is often determined by the patient's personal preference.

Strengthening exercises

Strengthening exercises are the mainstay of a number of interventions, including multimodal programs.[19,20,42,49,50,55–59] Clearly, the prescription must be individualized and progressive. Progression may be achieved most easily and accurately by gradual increases in loading using resistance equipment. For patients without access to such equipment, exercises that use the patient's own body weight as resistance can be used. These exercises are included in most dynamic back and abdominal muscle programs and as an integral part of multimodal programs. Exercise progression is an important parameter of the regimen with a gradual increase in loading.

Prescription: individualized exercise program—for ease of prescription, resistance equipment can be used to quantify performance.

Whole-body vibration exercise

Vibration technology uses reflexive responses to develop muscle strength and performance. An oscillating platform produces vibration which is transferred to the body producing a stretch reflex resulting in rapid and intense muscle contractions. This type of exercise is dependent on specific equipment and is therefore limited in its applicability.

Prescription: manufacturers often provide clear guidelines regarding exercise prescription, including details relating to the type of exercise performed and the frequency and intensity.

Williams flexion exercises/lumbar flexion exercises

First developed in 1937 for chronic LBP patients in response to clinical observations, these exercises focus predominantly on pain relief through flexion exercises.[44–46,60] They have been used in studies in which a primary goal is to improve lower trunk stability. Their aim is to reduce pain and improve lower trunk stability by establishing a balance between the flexor and extensor postural musculature. Examples include posterior pelvic tilt, hip flexor stretch, abdominal curls, and standing squat. These exercises are indicated for those whose back pain is aggravated by extension. Exercise prescription needs to be tailored to the patient, with careful consideration of frequency advised. Prescription ranges from performing exercises every day to two, three or five times per week over a number of months.[45,46,60]

Prescription: little consensus has been reached regarding prescription, but individualized progressive programs should be the goal.

Role of exercise in primary prevention (Table 15.1)

The rationale for the preventative effect of physical activity is not clear, but it may be that simply improving muscle strength and gaining an overall improved level of physical fitness is enough to prevent the onset of back pain.[37,39]

Leisure-time physical activity/self-exercise/sport-specific programs

The prospective cohort study by Croft *et al.* of 2715 adults without back pain did not find that leisure-time physical activity affected the incidence of LBP.[10] However, in a cohort of

640 subjects aged 38, Harreby *et al.* found that 3 hours per week of physical activity reduced the risk of back pain measured by lifetime, 1-year, and point prevalence rates.[61] Leino[62] noted a modest inverse relationship between leisure-time physical activity and back symptoms in male metal industry employees. These observational data (level A2 evidence) need cautious interpretation, but they indicate that leisure-time physical activity, including sporting activity, does not predict the onset of back pain and that it might have a role in its prevention.

Multimodal exercise programs/general exercise therapy

Two small RCTs used a prescriptive intervention using strength and endurance modes of activity in subjects perceived to be at high risk of back pain because of their occupation.[63,64] These RCTs showed conflicting results as to preventative efficacy of prescriptive exercise (level A4 evidence).

Interpretation of these results is handicapped by lack of detail on subjects' characteristics. The included studies' sample populations could be considered asymptomatic at the time of data collection. However, they may have had symptoms associated with bouts of acute pain without progressing to chronicity. Considering that at some point during our lives most of us will suffer from low back pain, it would be extremely difficult to find a truly asymptomatic population who had never at any point had back pain.[37]

If improvements in general physical fitness can reduce rates of occurrence, then much may be said for leading a physically active life rather than looking to find the perfect exercise prescription. Those who are more physically active are often the individuals who eat a healthy diet, smoke less, and are less likely to be obese—all indicators of good physical health and reduced risk from disease. The argument for the overall benefit of physical activity is very persuasive.[65] Future studies focusing on primary prevention might further investigate the potential for leisure-time physical activity as a preventative measure. In the meantime, advising a physically active lifestyle using meaningful and functional adaptations of daily activities might help reduce the incidence of disabling back pain, as well as having other more general health benefits.

Role of exercise in secondary prevention

Secondary prevention of low back pain can be defined as the prevention of further development of pain, specifically in halting the progression to chronicity or significantly reducing recurrence rates.[37] We identified 19 relevant studies (Table 15.2). A wide range of regimens and prescriptions has been assessed. This range is particularly surprising when we consider that we have focused only on studies using exercise as the primary intervention, rather than those including it as part of a wider and often multidisciplinary therapeutic program. This may reflect uncertainty amongst practitioners with regards to what mode or modes of exercise may be best for different groups of back pain sufferers.

Calisthenics

One small RCT used a predominantly calisthenic program incorporating some flexion and abdominal strengthening exercises into the regimen. Donchin *et al.*[42] compared this regimen with a back school program and control intervention over the course of 3 months. Using performance-related outcome measures, the calisthenics group had a greater benefit on flexion and strength measures and LBP episodes in the previous month

Table 15.2 Studies of exercise for secondary prevention of back pain

First author, ref.	Design	Study population	Predominant exercise	Comparison/control group	Evidence for the use of exercise based on the study findings
Calisthenics					
Donchin[42]	RCT	142 hospital workers. Inclusion criteria: at least 3 annual episodes of low back pain	1. Exercise: calisthenics, flexion and pelvic tilt based on the Williams method, strengthening abdominal muscles, 45 min 2 x week for 3 months, groups of 10–12 (n = 46)	2. Back school: 90 min, 4 sessions, 2 weeks plus a 5th session after 2 months, groups of 10–12, instruction in body mechanics and exercises (n = 46). 3. Control intervention; waiting list controls (n = 50)	Evidence that a moderate calisthenics program is more effective than a back school and control intervention
McKenzie exercises					
Delitto[45]	RCT	24 pts with acute or subacute (< 7 weeks) with or without radiation	McKenzie extension exercises; 3 times per week; supervised; handout; advice to exercise at home (n = 14)	Williams flexion exercises; 3 times per week; supervised; handout; advice to exercise at home (n = 10)	Evidence that McKenzie extension exercises are more effective than Williams flexion exercises at improving functional status.
Descarreaux[19]	Randomized experimental study	20 pts with subacute or chronic nonspecific LBP	Exercises to increase muscle force and extensibility in the hip and trunk muscles. Details of prescription; repetitions and intensity based on preprogram assessments of force and extensibility. First 3 weeks: one set of exercises; second 3 weeks another set of exercises designed to progress training intensity. Duration 6 weeks; home-based; twice per day (n = 10)	Back school–type program: five exercises: flexion mobilization; passive extension mobilizations; stretching; abdominal reinforcement; back and hip extension. Intensity set—no progression; duration 6 weeks; home-based; twice per day (n = 10)	Lack of between-group analysis suggests conflicting evidence for the effectiveness of progressive hip and trunk muscle force and extensibility exercises

Continued

Table 15.2 *(Continued)*

First author, ref.	Design	Study population	Predominant exercise	Comparison/control group	Evidence for the use of exercise based on the study findings
Elnaggar[46]	RCT	56 pts with chronic, nonspecific LBP	McKenzie extension exercises; 30 min/day; 2 weeks; 7 sessions each week; 3 sessions supervised; 4 sessions at home; 6 types of exercise; 10 reps. each (n = 28)	Williams flexion exercises; 30 min/day; 2 weeks; 7 sessions per week; 3 sessions supervised; 4 sessions at home; 6 types of exercise; 10 reps. each (n = 28)	No significant differences in pain between groups. No evidence to suggest which type of exercise, flexion or extension is more effective
Petersen[20]	Randomized study	260 pts with subacute or chronic nonspecific LBP	McKenzie exercises: each session lasted 30 min; max of 15 sessions for 8 weeks; self-administered exercise at home or in the gym for a further 2 months (n = 132)	Multimodal group: 5–10 min stationary bike; 10 reps. low-resistance exercises for lumbopelvic muscles in flexion, extension, and rotation; dynamic back strengthening in flexion and extension. Strengthening exercises performed in sets of 10 reps. with 1-min rest between sets. Gradual progression over 8-week period; stretching; 60–90 min 2 × per week; max. of 15 sessions for 8 weeks; self-administered exercise at home or in the gym for a further 2 months (n = 128)	No evidence of effectiveness for either the McKenzie exercises or the multimodal exercise program in reducing pain and disability
Risch[59]	RCT	54 pts with chronic LBP with or without radiation	Dynamic extension program; twice a week for 4 weeks; then once a week for 6 weeks (n = 31)	Waiting list control group (n = 23)	Some evidence that extension exercises are more effective than inactive treatment, but study deemed to be of poor quality

Multimodal exercise programs/general exercise therapy					
Aure[49]	RCT with 1-y follow up	49 pts with subacute or chronic nonspecific LBP	General exercise therapy: 10 min warm-up on bike; individual 45 min programs; strengthening; stretching; mobilizing; coordination; stabilization for back, abdominal, pelvic and lower limb muscles; type, reps, sets and progressions chosen by therapist; 16 sessions over 2 months (n = 22)	Manual therapy: spinal manipulation; stretching and mobilizations; subset of 5 general exercises for spine, abdomen and lower limb; 6 specific exercises for spinal segments and pelvic girdle; 2–3 sets of 20 reps; 30 s–1 min rest between sets; each session 45 min; 16 sessions over 2 months (n = 27)	No evidence that general exercise therapy is more effective than manual therapy. Both programs affect selected outcome measures over time
Friedrich[56]	Prospective clinical randomized controlled trial	93 pts with chronic nonspecific LBP	Exercises to increase spinal mobility; trunk and lower limb muscle length; force; endurance and coordination. 10 sessions each 25 minutes; intensity and progression based on the pt; advice to exercise at home.	Exercise program + motivational program including counseling and reinforcement techniques	Between-group analysis is not clear. No evidence that exercise alone is more effective than exercise combined with a motivational program.
Gur[60]	Single-blinded randomized study	75 pts with chronic nonspecific LBP.	Lumbar flexion and extension; knee flexion; hip adduction; strengthening exercises; 2 sessions a day; 5 days a week for 4 weeks (n = 25)	Laser therapy alone—5 times a week for 4 weeks. Each session lasted 30 min (n = 25) 2. Laser therapy + exercise (n = 25)	No evidence that a multimodal exercise program is more effective than laser therapy alone or in combination with exercise.

Continued

Table 15.2 *(Continued)*

First author, ref.	Design	Study population	Predominant exercise	Comparison/control group	Evidence for the use of exercise based on the study findings
Rainville[50]	Cohort study	70 pts with chronic nonspecific low back pain	Multimodal exercise program: stretching: resistance training (machine and free weights); 10–20 reps. per exercise; weight and reps. set by a therapist; stepwise progression based on goals; endurance activities included in each session using aerobics, treadmill and bike; session lasted 2 h 3 × per week; total duration 6 weeks; following completion of program independent programs devised for each pt (stretch daily strengthening exercise 3 × per week, aerobic exercise 3 or more times per week) (n = 70)	Not applicable	Evidence to suggest that a progressive multimodal exercise program of brief duration reduces anticipated and experienced pain levels during physical activity, overall back pain and disability, back strength and flexibility
Spinal stabilization program/core strengthening					
Sung[52]	Short-term longitudinal cohort study	16 pts with subacute or chronic nonspecific LBP	Spinal stabilization exercise protocol: upper body extension; alternate arm and leg lift; alternate arm and leg extension on all fours; diagonal curl up; curl up; 5 exercises repeated daily; 3 × per week for 4 weeks (n = 16)	Not applicable	Evidence to suggest that a short-duration spinal stabilization program can reduce disability and increase back muscle endurance
Strengthening exercises					
Bentsen[55]	RCT	74 women with chronic nonspecific LBP with or without radiation	Home training + dynamic strength exercises. 3 back and abdominal strengthening exercises; 10 times a day at home; 1 y; dynamic exercises, gradually intensified; 30 min; twice per week; 3 months (n = 41)	Home training; 3 back and abdominal strength exercises; 10 times a day; 1 y (n = 33)	Conflicting evidence for the effectiveness of strengthening exercise

Hansen[57]	RCT	180 pts with chronic LBP with or without radiation	Intensive, dynamic back muscle training; 3 exercises; 5 sets of 10 reps. each; 1 h sessions; twice a week; 4 weeks (n = 60)	1. Physical therapy; 1 h sessions; twice weekly; 4 weeks (n = 59) 2. Placebo control; 1 h sessions; twice a week; 4 weeks (n = 61)	No evidence that strengthening exercise is more effective than physical therapy and placebo
Hemmila[66]	RCT	114 pts with chronic LBP with or without radiation	Bending and rotation exercises; 10 times every 15 min; 3 exercises; 10 times each; twice a day; 10 1-h sessions; 6 weeks (n = 35)	1. Bone setting; gentle mobilizations; 10 1-h sessions; 6 weeks (n = 35) 2. Physiotherapy; 10 1-h sessions; 6 weeks (n = 34)	Limited evidence that manual therapy is more effective than bending and rotation exercises at reducing disability
Johanssen[67]	RCT	40 pts with chronic nonspecific LBP with or without radiation	Dynamic back, neck and abdominal endurance exercises; supervised; up to 100 reps; 1 h sessions; twice per week; 3 months (n = 13)	Coordination and balance exercises; up to 40 reps.; twice a week; 3 months (n = 14)	No evidence to suggest which type of exercise is more effective
Ljunggren[58]	RCT	103 pts with chronic nonspecific LBP	Strengthening exercises using TerapiMaster; exercise at home for 15–30 min 3 × per week over the course of 1 y changes or modifications to the program made where necessary (n = 55)	1. Conventional physiotherapy strengthening exercises (n = 48)	No evidence that strengthening exercise is more effective than conventional physiotherapy exercises in reducing work absenteeism. Both exercise programs do reduce work absenteeism
Torstensen[51]	RCT	208 pts with chronic nonspecific LBP with or without radiation	Progressively graded exercise therapy; mobilizing and stabilizing exercises; 7–9 exercises; 1000 reps. per session; 1 h session; 3 × per week; 12 weeks (n = 71)	Self-exercise by walking; 1 h walking; 3 × per week; 12 weeks (n = 70). 2. Conventional physiotherapy; 1 h session; 3 × per week; 12 weeks (n = 67)	Evidence for the effectiveness of progressively graded exercise when compared to low intensity self exercise for a reduction in pain and functional status

Continued

Table 15.2 *(Continued)*

First author, ref.	Design	Study population	Predominant exercise	Comparison/control group	Evidence for the use of exercise based on the study findings
Whole-body vibration exercise					
Rittweger[68]	RCT	50 pts with chronic nonspecific LBP	Whole-body vibration exercise (VbX) using a Galilieo2000: platform oscillating around a resting axis between the pts feet. Amplitude adjusted by foot distance; for this group of pts: amplitude of 6 mm, vibration frequency of 18 Hz; 4 min duration for each unit; 2 min warm-up; duration increased progressively to 7 minutes; patient performed slow movements of the hips and waist, bending and rotating; increased progression to 5 kg weights applied to the shoulders; 18 exercise units in 12 weeks; first 6 weeks 2 units per week; 1 unit per week thereafter (n = 25)	Isodynamic lumbar extension exercise (LEX) using an LE Mark 1 minute warm up with lumbar extension and then 1 min rest. Repetitive contraction cycles at a constant speed at 50% of the pt baseline maximal isometric values. When able to perform LEX for longer than 105 s (11 cycles) loading progressively increased; 18 exercise units in 12 weeks; first 6 weeks 2 units per week; 1 unit per week thereafter; sit ups and leg presses performed after LEX. (n = 25)	No evidence that VbX is more effective than LEX yet both modes of exercise do increase lumbar torque, relieve pain and improve pain related limitation
Williams flexion exercises/lumbar flexion exercises					
Buswell[44]	RCT	50 pts with chronic recurrent LBP with or without radiation	Flexion exercises, 8–14 treatments (n = 25)	Extension exercises (McKenzie), 8–14 treatments (n = 25)	No evidence to suggest which type of exercise, flexion or extension is more effective

LBP, lower back pain; RCT, randomized controlled trial.

in hospital workers who reported at least three annual episodes of back pain[42] (level A4 evidence). The lack of detail provided on the description of the calisthenics prescription, including limited illustration of the exercises undertaken, makes it very difficult to assess the program used.

McKenzie exercises

Five studies used McKenzie extension exercise as the predominant regimen. Three were small RCTs, with one small and one large randomized controlled trial.[19,20,45,46,59] This regimen was used with acute and chronic patients, but the definitions of acute, subacute, and chronic low back pain were inconsistent, with three of the five studies recruiting patients who could be classified across several back pain subgroups.[19,20,45] Two RCTs found some evidence for the use of McKenzie extension exercises when compared to Williams flexion exercises and a waiting list control group in both acute and chronic patients[45,59] (level A4 evidence). Delitto *et al.*[45] used a supervised McKenzie extension program three times per week for an undisclosed period of time and compared this with a program of Williams flexion exercises. Functional status improved significantly for those patients following the McKenzie regimen in comparison with those following the Williams flexion program. Similarly, Risch *et al.*[59] found evidence for the effectiveness of a 10-week dynamic extension program when compared with a waiting list control group using pain and physical disability scores as outcome measures. A more detailed description of the prescription used was given in the three studies which found no or conflicting evidence for the use of McKenzie exercises. Elnaggar *et al.*[46] found no significant differences in pain between a group of chronic LBP patients following a 2-week, daily program of six extension exercises in comparison with an identical prescription of flexion exercises (level A4 evidence). Descarreaux *et al.*[19] used a small sample (n = 20) of subacute or chronic LBP patients randomized to either a progressive, individualized 6-week program of extension exercises or a general, nonprogressive back school program for 6 weeks. Lack of between-group analysis hampered the interpretation of the disability, pain, and muscle force and extensibility outcome measures, suggesting conflicting evidence for the use of this type of extension program (level B1 evidence). A randomized study by Petersen *et al.*[20] was the only study to recruit a large sample (n = 260) of acute or chronic LBP patients to either a McKenzie extension group (15–30-minute sessions over 8 weeks followed by self-exercise for a further 2 months) or a multimodal exercise regimen (strengthening, flexion, extension and stretching program of 60–90-minute sessions twice weekly for 8 weeks). No significant differences in pain or disability were identified in either group following intervention.

Multimodal exercise programs/general exercise therapy

Four studies looked at the use of multimodal or general exercise programs in subjects with subacute and chronic LBP. Only one cohort study found evidence of effectiveness. Aure *et al.*[49] conducted an RCT recruiting and randomizing 49 subacute or chronic LBP patients to either a general exercise therapy group (45-minute sessions, including a range of exercises in which the prescription was recommended by a therapist; 16 sessions over the course of 2 months) or a manual therapy group using the same frequency and duration of sessions but including spinal manipulation and mobilizations. Although both programs affected the selected outcome measures over time (spinal range of movement, pain intensity, disability, and general health), there was no clear evidence that general exercise therapy was more effective than manual therapy (level A4 evidence). An individualized program of general exercise for chronic patients was also used by Friedrich *et al.*,[56] focusing on improving spinal mobility, muscle length, force, endurance and coordination over 10–25-minute sessions. As a comparison, Friedrich added a motivational program to the exercise regimen measuring disability, pain and work ability at 3.5 weeks, 4 months, 12 months, and 5 years. Friedrich concluded that there was no evidence that exercise alone is more effective than exercise combined with a motivational program (level A4 evidence). A relatively short but fairly intensive program (two sessions a day, 5 days a week for 4 weeks) of general activity to include flexion, extension, and strengthening exercises was used by Gur *et al.*[60] Subjects with chronic pain were randomized to a general exercise group, a laser therapy group, or a combined exercise and laser therapy group. No significant differences were found between the groups on pain, disability, spinal range of movement or flexion following intervention (level B1 evidence). Rainville *et al.* used a cohort study to investigate the effectiveness of a multimodal program for chronic patients.[50] Seventy patients were recruited to a program including resistance, aerobic, and stretching modes of exercise conducted over a period of 6 weeks (2-hour sessions three times a week). Following intervention, there was a reduction in anticipated and experienced pain levels during activity, overall back pain and disability, back strength and flexibility (level of evidence B1).

Spinal stabilization program/core strengthening

One short-term longitudinal study included spinal stabilization as the predominant exercise regime. Sung[52] recruited 16 subacute or chronic patients to a spinal stabilization program that used a combination of five exercises repeated on a daily basis three times a week for a total of 4 weeks. Results from this study suggest that a short-duration spinal stabilization program can reduce disability and increase back muscle endurance (level B1 evidence). No further RCTs of this exercise program that used clinically relevant outcomes were found. It is important to consider the applicability of the mode of exercise for the patient, and although spinal stabilization regimens have been detailed thoroughly, this program of exercise might provide distinct adherence barriers for the patient. Spinal stabilization is a complex exercise program reliant on sound guidance from a highly-skilled exercise professional. The patient is asked to isolate and co-contract the transversus abdominis and multifidus, which requires high levels of skill and reeducation on the part of the patient. In their overview of spinal stabilization, Richardson and Jull suggest that stabilization exercises might prove difficult for those with low back pain.[54] Although this mode of specific exercise allows us to pinpoint exactly which features of the exercise tasks may be responsible for the more favorable outcomes, careful consideration should be given as to whether the patient can actually carry out the task asked of him/her. Prescribing exercises that are unachievable can have serious implications for patient self-efficacy and future adherence.

Strengthening

Six studies used strengthening exercise as their choice of intervention all focusing on chronic LBP patients. One study found evidence for the effectiveness of strengthening exercises. Torstensen conducted a small RCT comparing progressively graded exercise therapy (including mobilizing and stabilizing exercise) with both self exercise (walking) and conventional physiotherapy.[51] The duration of the programs across all arms of the study was comparable (three sessions a week for 12 weeks). However, the prescriptive exercise regime appears to have been of a greater intensity (seven to nine exercises, 1000 repeats per session). Improvements in pain and functional status were noted for those completing the progressive regime (level A4 evidence). Bentsen *et al.* found conflicting evidence for the use of a progressive home training and dynamic strength program when compared to strength exercises based in the home[55] (level A4 evidence), whilst Hansen *et al.*,[57] Hemmila *et al.*,[66] Johanssen *et al.*,[67] and Ljungren *et al.*[58] found no evidence for the effectiveness of a range of strengthening programs.

Whole-body vibration exercise

Rittweger *et al.* implemented a small RCT (n = 50) of chronic patients randomized to either a whole-body vibration exercise or an isodynamic lumbar extension exercise group.[68] Both groups completed the same number of exercise units over the same period of time, and both groups were reliant on using specialist equipment. Although both modes of exercise were seen to increase lumbar torque, relieve pain, and improve pain-related limitation, there was no evidence to suggest that whole-body vibration exercise is more effective than isodynamic lumbar extension exercise (level A4 evidence).

Williams flexion exercises/lumbar flexion exercises

One small RCT compared flexion exercises as the predominant regime. Buswell[44] recruited 50 chronic LBP patients and randomized them to either a flexion exercise or extension exercise group. The number of sessions was comparable between the groups (n = 14), but no detail was given in relation to the number, type, or progression of the prescription. There was no significant improvement in pain following the intervention, and Buswell concluded that there was no evidence of effectiveness.

What does this all mean?

Acute LBP

The Cochrane systematic review of exercise therapy for low back pain concluded that exercise interventions may not be helpful for those with acute low back pain.[21] Only two of our five studies included support the use of exercise regimens for LBP: McKenzie extension exercises[45] (level A4 evidence) and a program of spinal[52] stabilization (level B1 evidence). Both studies are of poor quality, with small sample sizes recruited and limited outcome measures used. Additionally, there are inconsistencies in the definitions of acute, subacute, and chronic low back pain in both studies.

Chronic LBP

Conflicting evidence has been found in the Cochrane systematic review on the effectiveness of exercise therapy compared to inactive treatments for chronic low back pain. Of the exercise regimens explored, extension exercises[59] (level A4 evidence), calisthenics[42] (level A4 evidence), and strengthening and progressive multimodal programs[50,51,55] (level A4 and B1 evidence) were favored. There was variable suitability of the outcome measures chosen in these studies, and so conclusions based on these studies should be approached with some caution. The evidence presented for the use of exercise interventions with chronic low pain patients is surprisingly weak. A wide range of regimens has been considered including flexion and extension, multimodal, strengthening and vibration exercise programs. None of the RCTs featured in this review was of a high quality or inclusive of large sample sizes, and the descriptions of many of the exercise regimens were simplistic.

Acute and chronic LBP

Our findings for both acute and chronic LBP are consistent with the findings of previous reviews including the 2004 European guidelines for the management of acute and chronic nonspecific low back pain.[25,27] The available data do not support the use of specific exercise regimens for people with LBP. However, the diversity of regimens evaluated means that it is inappropriate to make general statements that specific exercise regimens are ineffective. There are simply not enough data on any one approach for firm conclusions to be drawn. Neither do our data, on their own, provide evidence to support the use of general exercise regimens. However, if it is believed that enforced rest is harmful for those with back pain[69] and that promoting general physical activity has an all-round beneficial impact on general health, then advising general exercise may be appropriate. The most recent recommendations offered by the Chief Medical Officer in the UK in 2004 recommend all adults undertake a 30-minute session of moderate intensity exercise on at least five days of the week.[43] If this recommendation is used as a benchmark for low back pain patients, it will give them the best opportunity to improve not only their current pain situation but also their general physical health.

Conclusions

It is important to use the best evidence to drive practice. The research reviewed here gives little indication of which exercise regimens may or may not be effective for low back pain. Indeed, it may be that RCTs are not the right tools to investigate interventions for low back pain.[70] Indirect evidence on the potential harm from rest on back pain and on the potential general health benefits of exercise lead us to conclude that encouraging general exercise and physical fitness has a role in the primary and secondary prevention of low back pain disability. We cannot make any recommendations on specific exercise regimens.

Exercise progression may be the key in successful prescription, and every effort should be made to advise patients to exercise with gradual increases in loading. However, every patient is an individual. Thus, exercise prescriptions are essentially based on personal preference, performance, and goals, as indicated by the evidence at the disposal of the practitioner.

Summary

- There is not enough evidence to support any one exercise approach to help with low back pain.
- A careful scrutiny of the exercise prescription will inform decisions as to whether the exercise regimen is appropriate for an individual.
- Given the known health benefits of physical activity, it is possible that lifetime physical fitness and functioning may have a role in primary and secondary prevention of low back pain.

Key messages

- There is little evidence for the recommendation of specific exercise regimens for acute or chronic low back pain.

• The promotion of general activity is appropriate for improving general physical health; this may also help back pain.
• Any exercise prescription should be tailored to the individual, taking into consideration personal preference, performance, and goals.

Sample examination questions

Multiple-choice questions (answers on page 602)

1 Factors linked to the development of chronic back pain include:
  A Genetic disposition
  B Psychosocial issues
  C Smoking
  D Dietary habits
  E Hypertension
2 When considering prescribing exercise to low back pain patients, you should:
  A Not listen to your patient's preferences for mode of exercise
  B Utilize best evidence to inform your practice
  C Think carefully about exercise loading and progressions
  D Give only specific exercise regimens
  E Give the same exercise regime for every patient
3 An exercise intervention can be defined as a program that includes:
  A A mode of exercise
  B Information relating to the duration of exercise
  C No information about how often the exercise(s) should be performed
  D No information about intensity of exercise
  E Clear detail on expected exercise progressions

Essay questions

1 Discuss the evidence for the prescription of specific exercise regimens for both acute and chronic low back pain patients.
2 Devise and design an exercise regimen for a chronic low back pain patient, giving a rationale for all aspects of your prescription.
3 Provide a detailed overview of the rationale for some of the mode of exercise featured within low back pain literature.

Case study 15.1

Mr. Jones, a 45-year-old office worker, presents with nonspecific low back pain which he says has been a problem for the last 2 months. Mr. Jones has sought help previously and has been utilizing nonsteroidal anti-inflammatories when in severe pain. Mr. Jones is currently sedentary, but suggests that he has been previously active, reporting time spent swimming and at the gym. In discussion, Mr. Jones states that he would like to be more active and that perhaps his lack of activity is not helping his current episode of low back pain. Consider the exercise prescription appropriate for Mr. Jones.

Case study 15.2

Ms. Smith is a 24-year-old elite gymnast presenting with acute low back pain as a result of a training injury. Ms. Smith reports that she has been unable to train at her normal intensity for the past week and is concerned as she has an important international competition in 4 weeks' time. She is keen to resume normal training and activity as soon as possible and seeks your advice on what should be her best course of action.

Summarizing the evidence for the use of exercise regimens

Exercise Regimen	Results	Level of evidence*
Primary prevention		
Leisure-time physical activity	3 cohort studies; both large study size; conflicting evidence[10,61,62]	A2
Multimodal program including aerobic, strengthening and functional components	1 RCT and 1 prospective cohort study, none of moderate size, conflicting evidence[63,64]	A4
Secondary prevention (acute–subacute)		
McKenzie extension vs. Williams flexion	1 RCT not of moderate size, results in favor of McKenzie extension exercises[45]	A4
Muscle force and extensibility exercise vs. back school	1 cohort study not of moderate size, conflicting evidence[19]	B1
McKenzie extension vs. multimodal program including strengthening and stretching	1 randomized study of large study size, no evidence of effectiveness[20]	A2
Spinal stabilization program	1 cohort study, not of moderate size, in favor of spinal stabilization programs[52]	B1
Multimodal program including strengthening, stretching, mobilization coordination and stabilization vs. program of manual therapy	1 RCT not of moderate size, no evidence of effectiveness[49]	A4
Secondary prevention (chronic)		
Home training and dynamic strength exercise (progressive) vs. home training and back/abdominal exercise (no progression)	1 RCT not of moderate size, conflicting evidence[55]	A4
Flexion exercises vs. McKenzie extension	2 RCTs, none of moderate size, no evidence of effectiveness[44,46]	A4
Intensive dynamic back muscle training vs. control (conventional physiotherapy exercise; physical therapy; placebo control)	2 RCTs, none of moderate size, no evidence of effectiveness[57,58]	A4
Bending and rotation exercise vs. gentle mobilizations vs. physiotherapy	1 RCT, not of moderate size, no evidence of effectiveness[66]	A4
Dynamic back, neck and abdominal endurance exercise vs. coordination and balance exercise	1 RCT, not of moderate size, no evidence of effectiveness[67]	A4

Summarizing the evidence for the use of exercise regimens *(Continued)*

Exercise Regimen	Results	Level of evidence*
Dynamic extension exercises vs. waiting list control	1 RCT, not of moderate size, limited evidence of the effectiveness of dynamic extension exercises[59]	A4
Progressively graded exercise therapy vs. self-exercise	1 RCT, not of moderate size, evidence of the effectiveness of progressively graded exercise therapy[51]	A4
General exercise program vs. exercise program with motivational program	1 RCT, not of moderate size, no evidence of effectiveness[56]	A4
Calisthenics vs. back school vs. waiting list control	1 RCT, not of moderate size, evidence for the use of a moderate calisthenics program[42]	A4
Lumbar flexion and extension vs. laser therapy vs. laser therapy and exercise	1 randomized study, not of moderate size, no evidence of effectiveness[60]	B1
Multimodal exercise program	1 cohort study, not of moderate size, evidence for the use of progressive multimodal exercise program[50]	B1
Whole-body vibration exercise vs. isodynamic lumbar extension	1 RCT, not of moderate size, no evidence of effectiveness[68]	A4

A1: evidence from large randomized controlled trials (RCTs) or systematic review (including meta-analysis).
A2: evidence from at least one high-quality cohort.
A3: evidence from at least one moderate-sized RCT or systematic review.
A4: evidence from at least one RCT.
B: evidence from at least one high-quality study of nonrandomized cohorts.
B1: evidence from at least one cohort study.
C: expert opinions.
N.b.: moderate size is deemed to be a sample size of over 100 in each intervention and comparison group.

References

1 Andersson G. The epidemiology of spinal disorders. In: Frymoyer J, ed. *The Adult Spine: Principles and Practice.* Philadelphia: Lippincott-Raven, 1997: 93–141.
2 Waddell G. *Models of Disability. Using Low Back Pain as an Example.* London: The Royal Society of Medicine, 2002.
3 Maniadakis N, Rayner M. *Coronary Heart Disease Statistics: Economics Supplement.* London: British Heart Foundation, 1988.
4 Dale S. *Stroke.* London: Office of Health Economics, 1989.
5 Gray A, Fenn P, McGuire AJ. The cost of insulin-dependent diabetes mellitus in England and Wales. *Diabet Med* 1995; 12:1068–1076.

6 Maniadakis N, Gray A. The economic burden of back pain in the UK. *Pain* 2000; **84**:95–103.
7 Harding G, Parsons S, Rahman A, Underwood M. "It struck me that they didn't understand pain": The specialist pain clinic experience of patients with chronic musculoskeletal pain. *Arthritis Rheum* 2005; **53**:691–696.
8 Van Tulder M, Koes B, Bombardier C. Low back pain. *Best Pract Res Clin Rheumatol* 2002; **16**:761–775.
9 Papageorgiou AC, Croft PR, Thomas E. Influence of previous pain experience on the episode incidence of low back pain: results from the South Manchester Back Pain Study. *Pain* 1996; **66**:181–185.
10 Croft PR, Papageorgiou AC, Thomas E, Macfarlane GJ, Silman AJ. Short-term physical risk factors for new episodes of low back pain: prospective evidence from the South Manchester Back Study. *Spine* 1999; **24**:1556–1561.
11 Andersson G. Epidemiological features of chronic low back pain. *Lancet* 1999; **354**:581–585.
12 Quittan M. Management of back pain: review. *Disabil Rehabil* 2002; **24**:423–434.
13 McCarthy C, Arnall FA, Strimpakos N, Freemont A, Oldham JA. The biopsychosocial classification of nonspecific low back pain: a systematic review. *Phys Ther Rev* 2004; **9**:17–30.
14 Underwood M. Exercise and the prevention of back pain disability. *Br J Sports Med* 2000; **34**:5.
15 Pincus T, Burton AK, Vogel S, Field AP. A systematic review of psychological factors as predictors of chronicity/disability in prospective cohorts. *Spine* 2002; **27**:E109–E120.
16 Cats-Baril WL, Frymoyer JW. Identifying patients at risk of becoming disabled because of low back pain: the Vermont Rehabilitation Engineering Center predictive model. *Spine* 1991; **16**:605–607.
17 Gatchel RJ. The dominant role of psychosocial risk factors in the development of chronic low back pain disability. *Spine* 1995; **20**:2702–2709.
18 UK BEAM Trial Team. United Kingdom Back Pain Exercise and Manipulation (UK BEAM) randomised trial: effectiveness of physical treatments for back pain in primary care. *BMJ* 2004; **329**:1377.
19 Descarreaux M, Normand MC, Laurencelle L, Dugas C. Evaluation of a specific home exercise program for low back pain. *J Manip Physiol Ther* 2002; **25**:497–503.
20 Petersen T, Kryger P, Ekdahl C, Olsen S. The effect of McKenzie therapy as compared with that of intensive strengthening training for the treatment of patients with subacute or chronic low back pain. *Spine* 2002; **27**:1702–1709.
21 Van Tulder MW, Malmivaara A, Esmail R, Koes B. Exercise therapy for low back pain: a systematic review within the framework of the Cochrane Collaboration Back Review Group. *Spine* 2000; **25**:2784–2796.
22 Kool J, De Bie R, Oesch P, Knusel O, van den Brandt P, Bachmann S. Exercise reduces sick leave in patients with nonacute nonspecific low back pain: a meta-analysis. *J Rehabil Med* 2004; **36**:49–62.
23 Hayden JA, van Tulder M, and Tomlinson G. Systematic review: strategies for using exercise therapy to improve outcomes in chronic low back pain. *Ann Intern Med* 2005; **142**:776–785.
24 Hayden JA, van Tulder M, Malmivaara A, Koes B. Meta-analysis: exercise therapy for nonspecific low back pain. *Ann Intern Med* 2005; **142**(9):765–775.
25 Airaksinen O, Hildebrandt J, Mannion A, *et al.* European guidelines for the management of chronic nonspecific low back pain. 2004. Available at: http://www.backpaineurope.org/web/files/WG2_Guidelines.pdf (accessed 7 September 2006).
26 Van Tulder M, Becker A, Bekkering T, *et al.* European guidelines for the management of acute nonspecific low back pain in primary care. 2004. Available at: http://www.backpaineurope.org/web/files/WG1_Guidelines.pdf (accessed 7 September 2006).
27 European Commission COST B13 Management Committee. European guidelines for the management of low back pain. *Acta Orthop Scand Suppl* 2002; **73** (305):20–25.
28 Koes BW. How to evaluate manual therapy: value and pitfalls of randomized clinical trials. *Man Ther* 2004; **9**:183–184.
29 Liddle SD, Baxter GD, and Gracey JH. Exercise and chronic low back pain: what works? *Pain* 2004; **107**:176–190.
30 Battie M, Beurskens AJ, Bombardier C, Croft PR, Koes B. Outcome measures for low back pain research: a proposal for standardized use. *Spine* 1998; **23**:2003–2013.
31 Roland M, Morris R. A study of the natural history of back pain. Part I: development of a reliable and sensitive measure of disability in low back pain. *Spine* 1983; **8**:141–144.
32 Fairbank JC, Couper J, Davies JB, O'Brien JP. The Oswestry low back pain disability questionnaire. *Physiotherapy* 1980; **66**:271–273.

33 Ware JEJ, Sherbourne CD. The MOS 36-item short-form health survey (SF-36). Conceptual framework and item selection. *Med Care* 1992; **30**:473–483.

34 EuroQol Group. EuroQol: a new facility for the measurement of health-related quality of life. *Health Policy* 1990; **16**:199–208.

35 Van Tulder M, Koes B. Low back pain (acute). *Clin Evid* 2004; **12**:1643–1658.

36 Spitzer WO, Leblanc FE. Scientific approach to the assessment and management of activity-related spinal disorders: a monograph for clinicians. Report of the Quebec Task Force on Spinal Disorders. *Spine* 1987; **12** (7 Suppl):S1–59.

37 Linton SJ, van Tulder MW. Preventative interventions for back and neck pain problems: what is the evidence? *Spine* 2001; **26**:778–787.

38 Vuori IM. Dose–response of physical activity and low back pain, osteoarthritis, and osteoporosis. *Med Sci Sports Exerc* 2001; **33**(6 Suppl):S551–S586.

39 Lahad A, Malter AD, Berg AO, Deyo RA. The effectiveness of four interventions for the prevention of low back pain. *JAMA* 1994; **272**:1286–1291.

40 Rainville J, Hartigan C, Martinez E, *et al.* Exercise as a treatment for chronic low back pain. *Spine J* 2004; **4**:106–115.

41 Van Tulder M, Assendelft WJ, Koes BW, Bouter LM. Method guidelines for systematic reviews in the Cochrane Collaboration Back Review Group for Spinal Disorders. *Spine* 1997; **22**:2323–2330.

42 Donchin M, Woolf O, Kaplan L, Floman Y. Secondary prevention of low back pain: a clinical trial. *Spine* 1990; **15**:1317–1320.

43 Department of Health. *At Least Five a Week: Evidence on the Impact of Physical Activity and its Relationship to Health.* London: TSO, 2004.

44 Buswell J. Low back pain: a comparison of two treatment programmes. *N Z J Physiother* 1982; **10**:13–17.

45 Delitto A, Cibulka MI, Erhard RE, *et al.* Evidence for the use of an extension–mobilization category in acute low back syndrome: a prescriptive validation pilot study. *Phys Ther* 1993; **73**:216–222.

46 Elnaggar IM, Nordin M, Sheikhzadeh A, Parnianpour M, Kahanovitz N. Effects of spinal flexion and extension exercises on low back pain and spinal mobility in chronic mechanical low back pain patients. *Spine* 1991; **16**:967–972.

47 Liebenson C. Self-treatment advice and the McKenzie approach for back trouble. *J Bodyw Mov Ther* 2005; **9**:35–39.

48 Liebenson C. McKenzie self-treatments for sciatica. *J Bodyw Mov Ther* 2005; **9**:40–42.

49 Aure AF, Nilsen JH, Vasseljen O. Manual therapy and exercise therapy in patients with chronic low back pain. *Spine* 2003; **28**:525–532.

50 Rainville J, Hartigan C, Jouve C, Martinez E. The influence of intense exercise-based physical therapy program on back pain anticipated before and induced by physical activities. *Spine J* 2004; **4**:176–183.

51 Torstensen TA, Ljunggren AE, Meen HD, *et al.* Efficiency and costs of medical exercise therapy, conventional physiotherapy, and self-exercise in patients with chronic low back pain: a pragmatic, randomized, single-blinded, controlled trial with 1 year follow up. *Spine* 1998; **23**:2616–2624.

52 Sung PS. Multifidi muscles median frequency before and after spinal stabilization exercises. *Arch Phys Med Rehabil* 2003; **84**:1313–1318.

53 Akuthota V, Nadler SF. Core strengthening. *Arch Phys Med Rehabil* 2004; **85**(Suppl 1):S86–S92.

54 Richardson CA, Jull GA. Muscle control–pain control. What exercises would you prescribe? *Man Ther* 1995; **1**:2–10.

55 Bentsen H, Lindgarde F, Manthorpe R. The effect of dynamic strength back exercise and/or home training programme in 57-year-old women with chronic low back pain: results of a prospective randomized study with a 3-year follow-up period. *Spine* 1997; **22**:1494–1500.

56 Friedrich M, Gittler G, Arendasy M, Friedrich KM. Long-term effect of a combined exercise and motivational program on the level of disability of patients with chronic low back pain. *Spine* 2005; **30**:995–1000.

57 Hansen FR, Bendix T, Skov P, *et al.* Intensive, dynamic back-muscle exercises, conventional physiotherapy, or placebo control treatment of low back pain. *Spine* 1993; **18**:98–107.

58 Ljunggren AE, Weber H, Kogstad O, Thom E, Kirkesola G. Effect of exercise on sick leave due to low back pain: a randomized, comparative, long-term study. *Spine* 1997; **22**:1610–1617.

59 Risch SV, Norvell NK, Pollock MK, *et al.* Lumbar strengthening in chronic low back pain patients. *Spine* 1993; **18**:232–238.

60 Gur A, Karakoc M, Cevik R, *et al.* Efficacy of low power laser therapy and exercise on pain and functions in chronic low back pain. *Lasers Surg Med* 2003; **32**:233–238.
61 Harreby M, Hesslesoe G, Kjer J, Neergaard K. Low back pain and physical exercise in leisure time in 38-year-old men and women: a 25-year prospective cohort study of 640 school children. *Eur Spine J* 1997; **6**:181–186.
62 Leino PI. Does leisure time physical activity prevent low back disorders? a prospective study of metal industry employees. *Spine* 1993; **18**:863–871.
63 Gundewall B, Liljeqvist M, Hansson T. Primary prevention of back symptoms and absence from work. *Spine* 1993; **18**:587–594.
64 Gerdle B, Brulin C, Elert J, *et al.* Effect of a general fitness program on musculoskeletal symptoms, clinical status, physiological capacity, and perceived work environment among home care service personnel. *J Occup Rehabil* 1995; **5**:1–16.
65 Department of Health. *Choosing Health: Making Healthier Choices Easier.* London: TSO, 2004.
66 Hemmila HM, Keinanen-Kiukaanniemi SM, Levoska S, Puska P. Long-term effectiveness of bone setting, light exercise therapy, and physiotherapy for prolonged back pain: a randomized controlled trial. *J Manip Physiol Ther* 2002; **25**:99–104.
67 Johanssen F, Remvig L, Kryger P, *et al.* Exercises for chronic low back pain: a clinical trial. *J Orthop Sports Phys Ther* 1995; **22**:52–59.
68 Rittweger J, Just K, Kautzsch K, Reeg P, Felsenberg D. Treatment of chronic lower back pain with lumbar extension and whole body vibration exercise: a randomized controlled trial. *Spine* 2002; **27**:1829–1834.
69 Waddell G. *The Back Pain Revolution.* Edinburgh: Churchill–Livingstone, 1998.
70 Wyatt M, Underwood M, Cassidy J, Nagel P, Scheel I. Health policy research and back pain: what, why, how, who and when? *Spine* 2004; **29**:E468–475.

CHAPTER 16

How should you treat spondylolysis in the athlete?

Christopher J. Standaert and Stanley A. Herring

Introduction

The diagnosis and management of spondylolysis in adolescent athletes is a controversial topic in the medical literature. Despite the frequency with which symptomatic spondylolysis occurs in this population, there are no controlled trials on the treatment of these athletes, and a number of diagnostic and treatment strategies have been proposed. In the classification of Wiltse *et al.*,[1] the term "isthmic spondylolysis" is used to identify those patients who have sustained a lesion in the pars interarticularis of the vertebral arch. Establishing the clinical diagnosis of symptomatic spondylolysis is contingent upon radiographic demonstration of such a lesion. However, there is a relatively high prevalence of asymptomatic pars lesions in the general population, and likely an even higher rate in adolescent athletes. Often, multiple radiological studies may be required to adequately assess an athlete with a suspected pars lesion. In the absence of any controlled trials, optimal treatment needs to be based upon a thorough understanding of the available information, despite its limitations. This chapter will review the current medical literature in order to allow for the derivation of a rational diagnostic and treatment strategy for adolescent athletes with spondylolysis.

Methods

Computer-based searches of multiple databases were performed. MEDLINE (PubMed, 1966–November 2005) was searched for the following terms, either individually or in multiple combinations: spondylolysis, pars interarticularis, adolescents, low back pain, and sports medicine. The Cochrane Library and Current Controlled Trials were also searched for "spondylolysis." Searches for controlled trials on spondylolysis in the above databases, along with Proquest Health and Medical Complete and the Web of Science, yielded no articles. Additional references were obtained from a review of multiple textbooks felt likely to contain information on spondylolysis, the authors' personal collections of related articles, and a review of references in all articles identified by the above methods. Over 200 publications were ultimately reviewed fully. Publications were selected for inclusion in this chapter on the basis of perceived scientific and historical merit, particularly as felt relevant to providing a thorough understanding of the available knowledge about spondylolysis. As no controlled clinical trials were identified, this could not be used as an inclusion criterion.

Epidemiology and natural history

The incidence of spondylolysis for the Caucasian population generally has been reported to be about 3–6%.[2–4] Roche and Rowe[4] studied 4200 cadaveric spines and found an overall incidence of 4.2%. This number varied within subgroups of the population, however, with rates of 6.4% for Caucasian males, 2.8% for African–American males, 2.3% for Caucasian females, and 1.1% for African–American females. There was no significant change in these rates with increasing age from 20 to 80 years old. Other authors have similarly noted males being affected two to three times as frequently as females.[2,3] The vast majority of spondylitic defects occur at L5 (80–95%), with L4 being the next most commonly affected level (5–15%). More proximal lumbar levels are affected much less frequently.[2–10] Multiple studies have shown a strong association between pars defects and the presence of spina bifida occulta (Fig. 16.1).[3,4,10–12] It is the general agreement of multiple authors that the majority of cases likely occur in the early school-age years.[1,3,13–15] The overwhelming majority of cases occurring in children of this age are asymptomatic.[3] Interestingly, Rosenburg *et al.*[16] studied 143 adults who had never walked and found that none of them had a pars defect on plain radiographs, although the views obtained were limited in some patients. The rate of spondylolisthesis occurring with spondylolysis has varied widely in different reports in the literature, but generally seems to range between 30% and 50%.[3,8,17–19]

Spondylolysis seems to occur much more frequently in the young athletic population than in the general population. In a review of radiographs from 4234 elite adolescent athletes suffering from low back pain, Rossi and Dragoni[8] found that 13.9% of these athletes had spondylolysis present on plain radiographs. Divers, weight lifters, wrestlers, gymnasts, track and field athletes, and soccer players were among those groups that had disproportionately higher rates of spondylolysis identified. In a review of 3152 elite

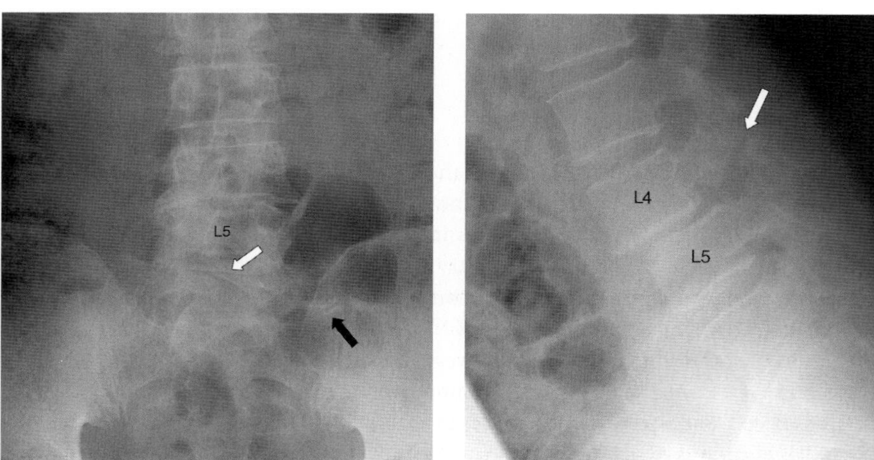

Figure 16.1 (**a**) Radiograph showing a transitional vertebral segment, representing a partially lumbarized S1 vertebra, with spina bifida occulta (white arrow) and an anomalous lumbosacral articulation on the left (black arrow). (**b**) Lateral radiograph of the same individual, showing a spondylolisthesis at L4–5 with pars defects in L4 (arrow).

Spanish athletes, Soler and Calderon[9] found a slightly lower overall rate of spondylolysis at 8.02% for the group as a whole. The athletes in this study were being seen for medical check-ups and did not necessarily have low back complaints; the prevalence in this group, therefore, may be closer to the true prevalence in asymptomatic athletes. Soler and Calderon also noted higher rates of spondylolysis in gymnasts and weightlifters, with throwing track and field athletes and rowers additionally showing particularly high prevalence rates. Other authors have similarly noted increased rates of spondylolysis in gymnasts,[20] football players,[21,22] cricketers,[21,22] and other athletes.[13,24–27]

The natural history of spondylolysis has been studied in a variety of manners. In the only study group of its kind in the literature, Fredrickson *et al.*[3] prospectively studied 500 first-grade students with plain radiographs and Beutler *et al.*[28] subsequently provided 45-year follow-up data on this population. The initial study found an overall incidence of spondylolysis of 4.4% at age six. This number increased to 5.2% by age 12 and 6% by adulthood. Family members of affected individuals had a much higher rate of spondylolysis noted than did the population as a whole, a finding similar to that reported by other researchers.[3,29] In the follow-up study of the initial group of patients identified with spondylolysis, Beutler *et al.*[28] noted that, after 45 years of follow-up, these individuals seemed to have a clinical course similar to that of the general population. No individuals with unilateral pars defects developed a slip, and progression of spondylolisthesis slowed every decade. There was no association between slip progression and pain.

Two of the most frequently mentioned concerns in the extended natural history of adolescents with spondylolysis are the risks of progressive spondylolisthesis and of disk degeneration. Overall, the risk of progression of spondylolysis with or without low-grade spondylolisthesis to a more significant slip is small. However, the literature in this regard is somewhat problematic, as there is no standard used to define what degree of slip progression is significant. Frennered *et al.*[30] followed 47 patients ≤ 16 years old with symptomatic spondylolysis or low-grade spondylolisthesis for a mean of 7 years. The initial degree of slip was 9–14%. Only two of their patients (4%) progressed ≥ 20% over the follow-up period. They found no radiographic or clinical correlates to the risk of slip progression. Similar numbers have been reported by other authors, with significant slip progression being uncommon in individuals presenting with slips of less than 20–30%.[11,19,31–33]

Muschik *et al.*[34] specifically assessed the risk of slip progression in child and adolescent athletes. They found similar numbers to those reported for the general population, with 12% of their patients showing a slip progression of > 10% over an average follow-up of 4.8 years. Only one of their 86 patients progressed > 20%, and 9% of their patients actually showed a partial reversal of displacement on follow-up. They found no significant relationship between the presence of spina bifida occulta and progression, but they did note an increased tendency to progress during the early growth spurt of puberty. All of their athletes remained asymptomatic during the follow-up period, and they felt that there was no increased risk for progression with active sports participation for athletes with a low-grade slip. Frennered *et al.*[30] also noted no correlation between athletic training and slip, progression of slip, or pain.

There are very few studies on disk degeneration developing in association with spondylolysis. In general, there is reported to be an increase in the frequency with which disk degeneration occurs over time at the level subjacent to a spondylitic lesion when individuals with low back pain and spondylolysis with or without spondylolisthesis are compared to unaffected controls.[35,36] The increase in disk degeneration was particularly noted in older patients. Overall, the studies reported on this topic have been small, and it is not clear if there are differences between those patients with unilateral or bilateral lesions or those with or without associated spondylolisthesis.

Pathophysiology

The lesion of the pars interarticularis in spondylolysis is generally considered to result from mechanical stress to that portion of the neural arch.[15,26,37–42] Wiltse *et al.*[15] suggested that most cases of isthmic spondylolysis should be considered fatigue fractures due to repetitive load and stress, rather than being caused by a single traumatic event, although a single traumatic event may result in completion of the fracture already developing. Several authors have looked at the effects of mechanical loading on the pars interarticularis. In a modeling experiment, Dietrich and Kurowski[40] found that the greatest loads with flexion/extension movements occur at L5/S1 and that the highest mechanical stresses occur at the region of the pars interarticularis. Chousa *et al.*[37] modeled the L4–5 motion segment and found that the stress in the pars was greatest under extension and rotational loads, suggesting that repetitive loading of this nature may be a significant risk factor for the development of spondylolysis. Green *et al.*[43] found that activities involving repetitive flexion and extension subject the pars to significant stress due to relative motion of the inferior articular process associated with these movements. Based on their studies of cadaveric vertebrae, Cyron and Hutton felt that the genetic predisposition for spondylolysis may be related to a possible genetic tendency for relatively lower cortical bone density at the pars.[44]

Clinical presentation

Given the frequency with which spondylolysis occurs in adolescent athletes, the diagnosis needs to be considered in essentially any young athlete presenting with a complaint of low back pain. The clinical presentation of symptomatic spondylolysis is described by many authors as a complaint of focal low back with radiation of pain into the buttock or proximal lower extremities noted occasionally.[13,14,24,38,45,46] The onset of pain can be gradual or start after an acute injury, and mild symptoms can be present for some time with an acute worsening after a particular event.[13,15] Some authors feel that activities involving lumbar spinal extension or rotation may particularly increase symptoms, and, as noted previously, athletes participating in these sports may be at increased risk for the development of pars lesions.[9,15,45,47] Physical examination is often felt to show a hyperlordotic posture with tight hamstrings, although there is no formal study on these somewhat subjective findings.[45,48] The only possible pathognomonic sign noted in the literature is reproduction of pain by performing the one-legged hyperextension maneuver (the patient stands on one leg and leans backwards), with unilateral lesions frequently resulting in pain when standing on the ipsilateral leg.[15,38,45,48] This maneuver may clearly stress spinal structures other than the pars, and, as with any clinical examination finding, the results of this maneuver should be assessed in the context of the overall clinical picture. Neurologic examination in isolated spondylolysis should generally be normal, with radicular findings suggestive of alternative or additional pathology. Additional diagnostic considerations in this population of patients with low back pain include discogenic pain, facet-mediated pain, a seronegative spondyloarthropathy or other rheumatologic disorders, and other bony injuries (e.g., transverse process, vertebral body, or sacral fractures).[45]

Diagnostic imaging

Clearly, the diagnosis of symptomatic spondylolysis cannot be made without demonstrating a lesion in the pars radiographically. Traditionally, plain radiography has been used in the identification or pars lesions, but there are significant limitations to the information that can be gained through the isolated use of radiographs. These limitations also affect the utility of much of the clinical information in the medical literature, as many older studies relied entirely upon plain radiography for the evaluation of patients studied. Literature utilizing computed tomography (CT), nuclear imaging, and magnetic resonance imaging (MRI) has clearly shown the increased sensitivity of these modalities when compared to plain radiography and has provided additional insights on the pathology and treatment of pars lesions. The literature remains problematic, however, in that there is no universally accepted algorithm for imaging of these patients, nor agreement on the optimal technical parameters for CT and MRI. The different imaging choices available have their own individual benefits and limitations, and the best approach to imaging currently involves the use of multiple imaging modalities.

Plain radiographs generally show the defect in isthmic spondylolysis as a lucency in the region of the pars interarticularis (Fig.16.1). The lesion is commonly described as having the appearance of a collar or a broken neck on the "Scotty dog" seen in lateral oblique radiographs (Fig. 16.2). Visualizing a defect in the pars on plain radiographs can be difficult, however, and frequently requires multiple views of the lumbosacral spine. Using anterior/posterior, lateral, and lateral oblique views, both Libson *et al.*[17]and Amato *et al.*[2] found that roughly 19% of the pars defects identified were seen only on the lateral oblique views. The single most sensitive view in the study of Amato *et al.*[2] was the lateral spot view of the lumbosacral junction, which revealed the lesion in 84% of their cases.

Multiple studies utilizing radionuclide imaging have shown that bone scan and, particularly, single photon emission computed tomography (SPECT) offer many advantages over isolated plain radiographs in the diagnosis of spondylolysis (Figs. 16.3, 16.4). Initial studies by Jackson *et al.*[49] and Elliot *et al.*[50] found that planar bone scan identified pars lesions in a significant number of patients in whom plain radiographs were negative. Subsequent studies have consistently shown that SPECT is significantly more sensitive than either plain films or planar bone scan in the identification of pars lesions.[51–56] For

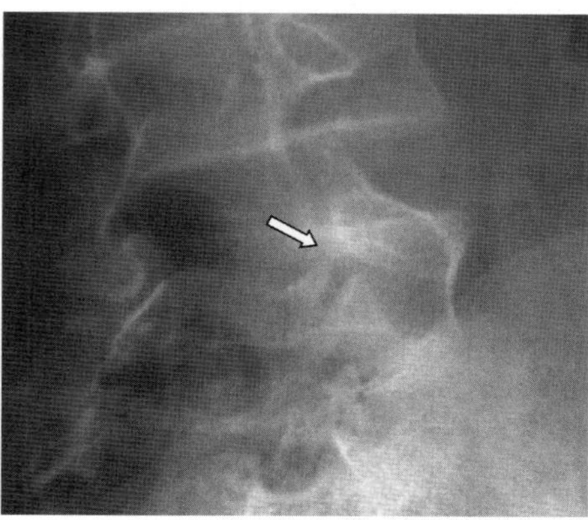

Figure 16.2 Oblique radiograph showing an elongated, thinned pars interarticularis with a subtle fracture line (arrow).

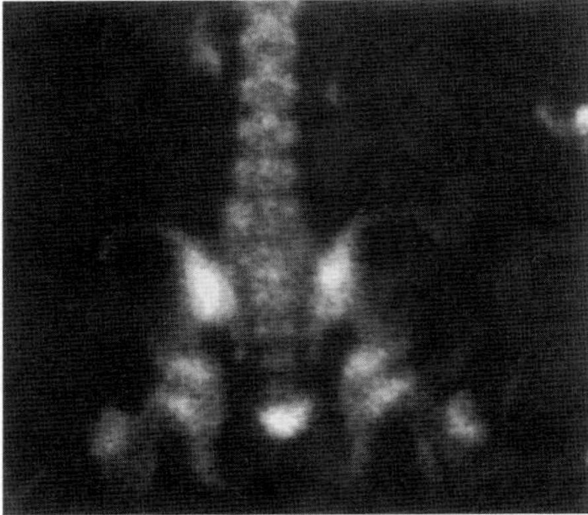

Figure 16.3 Planar bone scan, posterior view, showing a mild increase in uptake posteriorly on the left at L5.

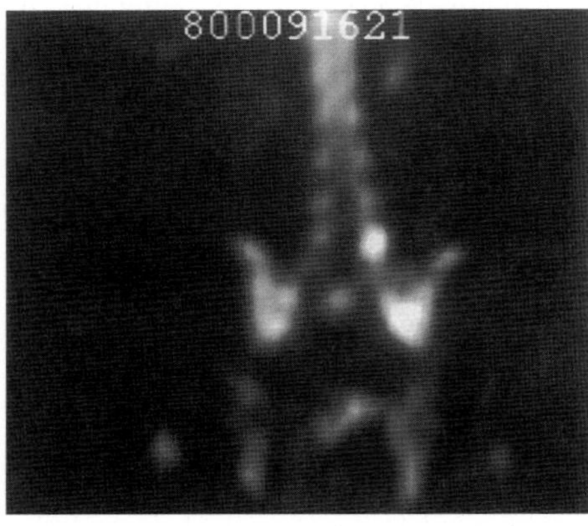

Figure 16.4 Single photon emission computed tomography (SPECT) imaging, anterior view, of the patient in Fig. 16.3, showing a clear increase in uptake in the left posterior neural arch of L5.

example, Anderson *et al.*[51] found that, compared with SPECT, plain radiography failed to demonstrate the pars lesion in 53% of their patients and planar bone scan in 19%.

In addition to simply being more sensitive in the identification of pars lesions than plain radiography, several studies have shown that bone scan or SPECT may be helpful with the crucial task of identifying symptomatic lesions. Studies by Elliot *et al.*[50] and Lowe *et al.*[57] both suggested that a positive bone scan correlates with a symptomatic lesion. Studies on SPECT provide additional support for this concept. Collier *et al.*,[58] Itoh *et al.*,[59] Lusins *et al.*,[60] and Raby and Matthews,[61] all using different lines of research, similarly concluded that a positive SPECT scan correlated strongly with a symptomatic lesion.

An important issue to consider in the use of radionuclide imaging is that, while it is seemingly quite sensitive in the identification of pars lesions, the specificity of this type of imaging is limited. It has been noted by several authors that not all abnormalities seen in the posterior elements on SPECT or bone scan represent pars lesions, a finding consistent with our clinical experience as well.[52,62–65] Potential abnormalities that may result in an abnormal SPECT that would otherwise be consistent with spondylolysis include facet arthropathy or fracture, infection and osteoid osteoma. Additional imaging, particularly with CT, is generally required to clarify the bony abnormality in a patient with a positive SPECT study.

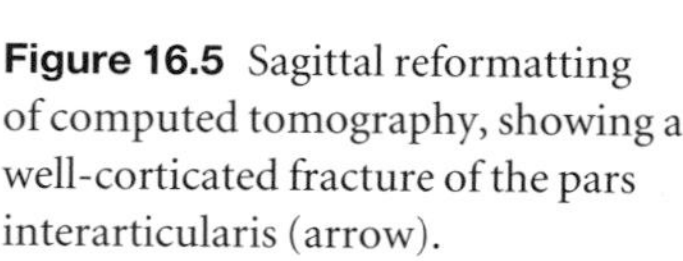
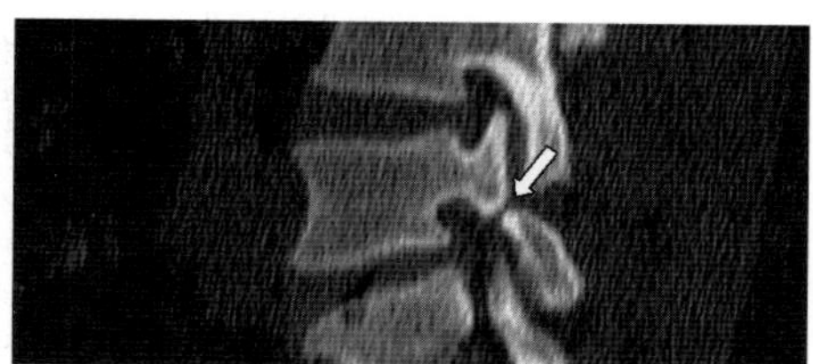

Figure 16.5 Sagittal reformatting of computed tomography, showing a well-corticated fracture of the pars interarticularis (arrow).

Like radionuclide imaging, CT has been shown to be more sensitive than plain radiography in revealing pars lesions, although it may be less sensitive than SPECT (Fig. 16.5).[54,56,62,64,66,67] Congeni *et al.*[62] compared CT to plain films and radionuclide imaging in 40 young athletes with lower back pain, negative plain films, and a presumptive diagnosis of spondylolysis based on a positive bone scan or SPECT. They found pars lesions on CT in 34 of these patients, while six patients had no clear fracture on CT, including several with stress reactions and one with an avulsion fracture of an apophyseal joint. Other authors have similarly identified a number of patients in whom there is increased activity in the area of the pars on SPECT but either an incomplete fracture or no fracture noted on CT.[23,54,55,63] While Congeni *et al.*[62] interpreted their finding of six patients with negative CT and positive radionuclide imaging as showing a 15% false-positive rate for radionuclide imaging, it could also be that these cases represented false-negatives for CT. Gregory *et al.*[63] interpreted the findings of an abnormal SPECT with a negative CT as indicating a bone stress response, rather than as a falsely positive SPECT scan.

CT may additionally play a significant role in staging pars defects to allow for better treatment stratification. CT can distinguish between well-corticated fracture margins, termed "chronic" lesions or "nonunions" by various authors, and differing stages of more recent or incomplete fractures.[54,55,63,64,68] (Fig. 16.6) The appearance of the pars on CT has been classified into different categories by multiple authors, and these findings have been found to be associated with the potential for bony healing.[55,68]

There are some limitations to the studies using CT, as there are no standard imaging parameters. Some authors prefer the use of reverse-angle gantry axial images in order to have the scan plane perpendicular to the presumed fracture line.[62–64,66] Various studies also describe significantly different slice thicknesses and skip intervals being utilized, while many authors do not mention these variables at all.[54,56,61–64,66,67,69,70] Comparison studies looking at standard versus reverse-angle gantry images and different slice thicknesses certainly would be helpful in defining imaging standards for CT.

Although less well studied than CT and radionuclide imaging, MRI may also play a role in the diagnosis of spondylolysis (Fig. 16.7). Its efficacy in visualizing the pars appeared somewhat problematic in early studies, but more recent work with improved technical approaches has proven more useful.[64,71,72] MRI clearly offers advantages over SPECT and CT in terms of revealing other types of pathology present in the lumbar spine, and the lack of ionizing radiation with MRI may also contribute to this being a particularly desirable modality in studying pars lesions,[64] especially in the female adolescent population. Yamane *et al.*[73] studied MRI in comparison with CT and found that MRI may be useful in identifying lesions in the pars before they are noted on CT, and thus may have the potential to identify stress lesions early in their clinical course. There was no comparison with SPECT included in this study, however, nor any data on clinical correlation to the findings

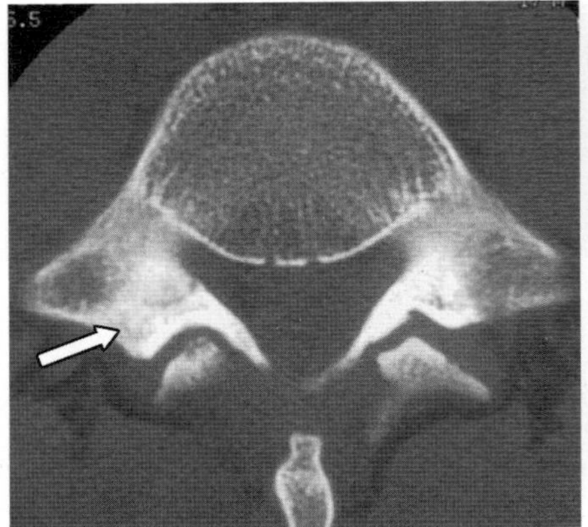

(a)

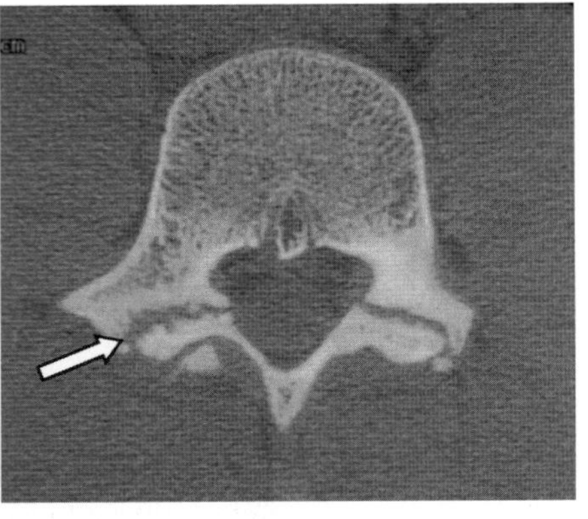

(b)

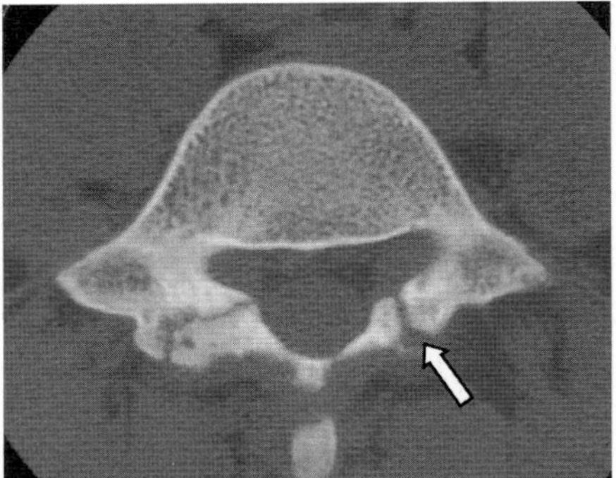

(c)

Figure 16.6 (**a**) Computed tomography (CT) scan, showing an early-stage pars lesion (arrow) associated with sclerosis and an incomplete fracture line, but no significant separation, cortication, or cystic change. (**b**) CT scan, showing a progressive-stage pars lesion (arrow) associated with sclerosis, fracture with minimal separation, and cyst formation. There is no cortication of the fracture margins. (**c**) CT scan, showing a terminal-stage pars lesion (arrow) with separation and clearly defined, corticated margins. (Reproduced with permission from Standaert CJ, *Oper Tech Sports Med* 2005; **13**:101–107.)

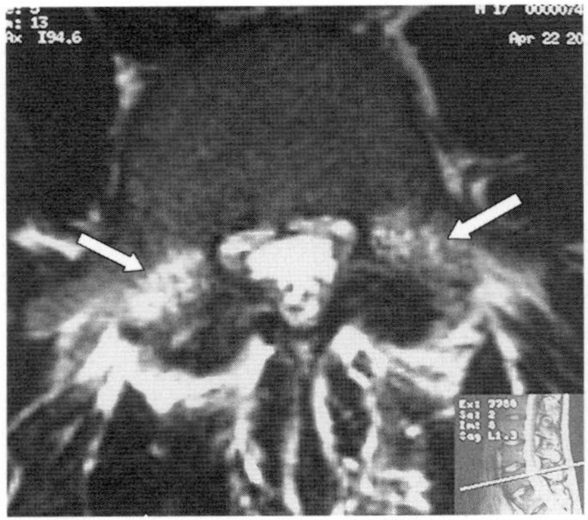

(a)

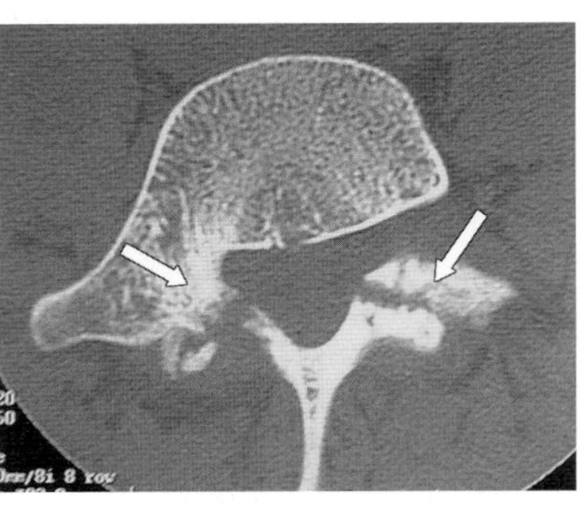

(b)

Figure 16.7 (**a**) Magnetic resonance imaging (MRI) scan, T2-weighted axial sequence, showing a hyperintense signal in the pedicles bilaterally (arrows), associated with bilateral pars fractures. (**b**) The corresponding computed tomography (CT) scan of the same patient as in Fig. 16.2a, showing bilateral pars fractures (arrows) that correlate to the areas of abnormality on the MRI. Note that the actual fractures are appreciated far better on the CT. (Reproduced with permission from Standaert CJ, *Oper Tech Sports Med* 2005; **13**:101–107.)

on MRI. Hollenberg *et al.*[74] presented a classification system for MRI findings in the pars interarticularis based upon the appearance of the pars and graded on a 0–4 scale, with defined criteria for each grade thought to correspond with varying types of injuries or pathological states of the pars. Although the authors did feel that their classification system was reliable, the clinical utility of this system is unclear. Unfortunately, there was no comparison of MRI to either SPECT or CT, no clinical data on outcome, no clear means of establishing pathological correlates to the findings, and no discussion of the prevalence of these findings in a normal control group.

There has been one published article comparing the use of CT, SPECT, and MRI in the diagnosis of spondylolysis in adolescents with low back pain.[75] In this study, the authors assessed 72 patients (8–26 years old) with a recent onset or exacerbation of extension-related low back pain with SPECT, CT, and MRI. Using CT and SPECT as the "gold standard" for diagnosis, there were 40 pars defects identified in these individuals, 25 of which were chronic and only 15 felt to be "acute or active lesions" with a positive SPECT study. Twenty-nine of these 40 total lesions were correctly graded by MRI, although 39 of the 40 had some degree of abnormality on MRI. However, there were also two pars with abnormal SPECT activity and no evidence of edema on MRI and seven pars identified as having marrow edema on MRI with normal SPECT imaging, an issue the authors had difficulty reconciling. The greatest discrepancy between MRI and SPECT occurred in cases of stress reaction without a pars defect and for the grading of incomplete defects, which are frequently the more clinically relevant lesions. This study contains no information on clinical outcome, treatment, or the degree of sports participation among the subjects. It is also extremely important to realize that this study utilized nonstandard MRI imaging techniques, including oblique sagittal images and reverse-angle oblique axial images. It is doubtful that standard MRI sequences would yield similar results. Despite the authors' enthusiasm in the use of MRI as a "first-line" imaging modality in the diagnosis of spondylolysis, in our estimation the role of MRI is still unclear in this setting, and more clinical data are needed.

Treatment

Treatment for spondylolysis has been studied using a variety of diagnostic standards, therapeutic interventions, and outcome measures. The lack of consensus on these issues and the lack of any large scale, controlled clinical trials on the diagnosis and management of spondylolysis make it difficult to define an optimal treatment algorithm. Advances in imaging technology also limit the practical utility of older studies that were based upon plain radiography for diagnosis and follow-up. Studies that stratify patients based upon the radiographic appearance of the pars lesion suggest that there are likely clinical subgroups that should be managed differently. Although the comprehensive answers to questions on the treatment of spondylolysis await further study, some of the currently available studies on treatment are discussed below.

In a widely referenced study, Steiner and Micheli[76] assessed bony healing and clinical outcome in 67 patients with spondylolysis or low-grade spondylolisthesis who were treated with an antilordotic modified Boston brace. All of their patients were diagnosed and followed using plain radiography, and 25 of them underwent a planar bone scan. Their patients followed a treatment regimen of brace use for 23 hours per day for 6 months followed by a 6-month weaning period, physical therapy, and allowance for athletic participation in the brace provided that the patient was asymptomatic. Twelve of their patients showed evidence of bony healing, with the earliest changes appearing at four months, and 78% of their patients had good to excellent clinical results including full return to activity and no brace use. The overall rate of healing was 25% when patients with only spondylolysis were considered. This study is significantly limited by the relatively small size, lack of controls, and the reliance upon plain radiography for assessment of healing. Several other relatively small, noncontrolled studies are hampered by similar methodological issues and use varying treatment protocols. Despite the different treatment methods utilized, however, these studies show similar results in terms of functional outcome (Table 16.1).[5,6,56,69]

Morita *et al.*[70] and Fujii *et al.*[68] attempted to assess the relationship between bony healing and the radiographic stage of the pars lesion. The authors classified the pars lesions into early, progressive, and terminal stages based upon either plain radiography (Fig. 16.1) or CT. Morita *et al.*[70] studied 185 adolescents with spondylolysis. Plain radiography or CT was used for diagnosis and follow-up, and treatment consisted of activity restriction, bracing with a nonspecified "conventional lumbar corset" for 3–6 weeks, followed by the use of an extension limiting corset for 3–6 months, and rehabilitation once healing occurred. Healing was noted in 73% of the early stage, 38.5% of the progressive stage, and none of the terminal defects. Fujii *et al.*[68] studied 134 patients ≤ 18 years old with CT pre- and post-treatment. Treatment consisted of relative rest and the use of a corset. Healing was noted in 62% of the early-stage defects while none of the terminal defects healed. Clinical outcome was not reported for these studies. Overall, multiple studies have noted that unilateral fractures have a much higher rate of healing than bilateral fractures.[5,54,56,68,70]

The use of bracing in the treatment of spondylolysis has been controversial. There are many authors who advocate the routine use of a rigid brace,[5,27,56,69,76] and there are reports by others who do not routinely use a rigid brace in the management of these patients.[49,62,68,70] Bony healing has been shown to occur with the use of either a rigid brace,[5,76] a soft brace,[70] or no brace.[49] Excellent clinical outcomes are frequently achieved in the absence of bony healing and there has been no association noted between the stage of the fracture and clinical outcome, with the exception that bilateral defects may develop an associated spondylolisthesis with time.[5,6,54,56,76] Biomechanical studies show that intervertebral motion at the lumbosacral junction can be increased by the use of a brace and that the greatest effect of a lumbosacral brace is to limit gross body motion rather than intervertebral motion.[77–79] It may be that the role of a brace in a patient with spondylolysis is to limit gross motion and hence overall physical activity, rather than to limit intervertebral motion in an effort to achieve bony healing.

There are limited reports on other modes of treatment, including external bone stimulators and oxygen–ozone treatment.[80–82] A recent review on the use of external electrical stimulation for the treatment of spondylolysis concluded that the data is too limited to conclude whether or not it can be used for this condition.[83] As with other aspects of care for athletes with spondylolysis, these issues warrant further study.

Surgical treatment for spondylolysis has generally been reserved for patients in whom conservative care fails. Surgery is reported to be necessary in about 9–15% of cases with spondylolysis and/or low-grade spondylolisthesis.[5,76] Potential indications for surgical intervention include progressive slip, intractable pain, the development of neurologic deficits, and segmental instability associated with pain.[14,38] Surgery is generally not required to control pain and should likely be used rarely in the management of isolated spondylolysis.[49]

Table 16.1 Outcomes of treatment for spondylolysis

Study	Design	Diagnosis	N	Mean age	Diagnostic imaging	Treatment summary	Radiographic outcome	Clinical outcome
Turner, Bianco 1971[10]	Retrospective case series	Spondylolysis and/or spondylolisthesis (spondylolysis only subgroup addressed in this table)	59	<19 years	Not reported, plain radiograph presumed	24 of 59 (41%) with minimal symptoms were not treated 20 of 59 (34%) treated with activity modification, "supportive garments," and exercises 15 of 59 (17%) fused surgically	Not reported	One of non-operatively treated patients underwent surgery, others that were available for follow-up with minimal to no complaints
Jackson, *et al.* 1981[49]	Prospective cohort	Low back pain and history suggestive of spondylolysis	37	15.5 years	Limited plain radiograph and bone scan	Activity restriction only	Bone scans normal or >75% improved in 14 of 15 patients with pars lesions No change on plain radiographs Follow-up on others not reported	12 of 15 (80%) returned to sports, including all with positive bone scans and radiographs either negative or with only unilateral defects in the pars
Pizzutillo, Hummer 1989[80]	Retrospective case series	Spondylolysis and/or spondylolisthesis, all had to have interfering pain and only conservative treatment	82	14.3 years	Plain radiograph assumed but not clearly specified	Mixed, including exercise, casting, bracing and rest to differing degrees	Not reported	48 of 70 (62%) of patients with up to a 50% spondylo-listhesis had significant pain relief. 1 of 12 (8%) with greater than 50% slip had significant pain relief.
Steiner, Micheli 1985[76]	Retrospective case series	Spondylolysis and/or <25% spondylo-listhesis	67	16.0 years	Plain radiograph Planar bone scan in 25	Anti-lordotic modified Boston brace 23 hours/day × 6 months, 6 month wean, physical therapy	Osseous healing in 12 of 67 patients, 11 of 44 (25%) with only spondylolysis	57% Excellent 21% Good 13% Fair 9% Poor
Blanda, *et al.* 1993[5]	Retrospective case series	Spondylolysis with or without spondylo-listhesis	82	14.9 years	Plain radiograph with or without planar bone scan	Rigid lordotic brace, physical therapy, wean from brace when pain free, surgery in 9 of 62 with spondylolysis	Osseous healing in 23 of 62 (37%) with only spondylolysis	84% Excellent 12% Good 3% Fair
Daniel, *et al.* 1995[85]	Retrospective case series	Spondylolysis, low back pain of discrete onset	29	21 years	Plain radiograph with planar bone scan if inconclusive	All had >4 months care before study, then treated with activity modification, bracing (usually thoraco-lumbar orthosis)	Osseous healing in 2 of 29 (6.8%) by plain radiograph at 3 months	6.8% treated successfully, all others failed non-operative treatment

Continued

Table 16.1 *(Continued)*

Study	Design	Diagnosis	N	Mean age	Diagnostic imaging	Treatment summary	Radiographic outcome	Clinical outcome
Morita, *et al.* 1995[70]	Retrospective case series	Spondylolysis	185	13.9 years	Plain radiograph, staged as early, progressive, or terminal. CT in some	Rest from sports, conventional corset for 3–6 months, physical therapy with extension limiting corset	Osseous healing in: Early lesions: 73% Progressive: 38.5% Terminal: 0%	Not reported
Congeni, *et al.* 1997[62]	Prospective cohort	Spondylolysis Restricted to positive bone scan/SPECT with negative plain radiographs	40	14.6 years	Planar bone scan or SPECT with negative radiographs	Initial activity modification, rigid anti-lordotic brace if pain persisted after 2–4 weeks (2 of 40), physical therapy	Not reported, but CT obtained 10 weeks after diagnosis by nuclear imaging, graded by CT appearance	73% maintained very high activity level
Sys 2001[56]	Cohort	Spondylolysis with "subtle fractures": negative radiographs, positive SPECT	34	17.2	Plain X-ray, planar bone scan and SPECT, CT	Rigid brace (Boston Overlap Brace) with thigh extension 23° per day until follow-up scintigraphy negative or 6 months (average 15.9 weeks)	100% of unilateral fractures healed, 5 of 17 bilateral fractures healed fully (7 additionally showed unilateral healing)	92.9% "excellent" or "good" outcome, 89.3% returned to prior level of competition at average of 5.5 months, 1 had surgery
D'Hemecourt 2002[69]	Retrospective case series	Spondylolysis by radiographs or CT, 4 of 73 patients with spondylolisthesis	73	15.7	Plain X-ray, SPECT, CT	Rigid brace antilordotic Boston Overlap Brace) 23%/day for 6 months, then weaned, physical therapy with flexion bias	Not reported	77% "excellent" or "good" outcome
Stretch 2003[55]	Prospective cohort	Fast bowlers with spondylolysis, all with positive SPECT	10	15–22	Plain X-ray, SPECT, CT	Activity restriction, for 3 months (no bowling or tasks with lumbar extension or rotation) and active rehabilitation program	80% healed at 1 year (2 of 10 that did not heal had "old bilateral fractures")	Not reported
Fujii, *et al.* 2004 (68)	Retrospective cohort	Spondylolysis with or without low-grade spondylolisthesis	134	13.8	Plain X-ray CT	Discontinuation of sports, Damen corset for 3 months, isometric then isotonic trunk exercises	62% of early defects, 9% of progressive defects, and 0% of terminal defects healed	Not reported
Miller 2004[54]	Longitudinal cohort	Spondylolysis, negative radiographs with positive bone scan or SPECT	40	12–20	Plain X-ray, bone scan/SPECT, CT 8–12 weeks after diagnosis	Activity restriction, nonrigid bracing, active rehabilitation after 2–4 weeks, rigid brace if not better at 4 weeks (2/40, 5%)	7–11 year follow-up imaging on 11/40 patients. No bilateral defects healed and 38 developed grade I slip, all unilateral defects healed	7–11 year follow-up in 32/40 patients, 91% "good or excellent" function, 100% active in sports
Iwamoto 2004[6]	Prospective cohort	Spondylolysis on plain radiographs	40	20.7	Plain X-ray	Activity restriction, rigid antilordotic brace until symptoms reduced	Not specified	87.5% returned to sports at mean of 5.4 months

Current management

The preceding review of the literature on spondylolysis still leaves the primary question of this chapter unanswered; namely, how should you treat the adolescent athlete with spondylolysis? Our approach to this question follows and is based on our understanding of the natural history, pathophysiology, diagnostic assessment, and treatment options discussed above, along with our own clinical experience. The goals of our approach are to accurately identify symptomatic lesions of the pars where present, to provide appropriate treatment to reduce pain and allow for any potential healing of the lesion when possible, and, ultimately, to optimize the athlete's functional outcome, both short-term and long-term. We are fully aware that other practitioners may approach the problem quite differently, but we have found the approach described here to be very effective for our patients.

In an adolescent athlete in whom the diagnosis of spondylolysis is suspected, we will initially obtain standing anteroposterior and lateral plain radiographs of the lumbar spine. Oblique and coned-down views of the lumbosacral junction are not obtained routinely. The primary purpose of obtaining the plain films is to identify spondylolisthesis or any other readily apparent bony anomalies. Assuming the plain films do not indicate the presence of another pathologic process, a bone scan with SPECT imaging of the lumbosacral spine is obtained to identify any metabolically active bony lesions, including a symptomatic lesion of the pars. If the SPECT shows an area of increased radionuclide uptake consistent with a pars lesion, a thin-cut CT scan (with 1.0-mm axial, stacked images) is obtained through the region of the spine in which the abnormality is identified on SPECT. This is done in order to both fully define the nature of the bony abnormality and to stage the lesion by radiographic appearance. The initial step in treatment of patients with an identified symptomatic pars lesion is rest, including avoidance of all sports activities and any physical activity not required for basic daily function. Significant activity limitation is used in order to reduce the stress applied to the pars by motion. If the patient's pain is not dramatically improved after 2–3 weeks of rest, the patient is fitted for a lumbosacral brace to be used for additional activity restriction until the patient is asymptomatic. If the patient's CT scan showed an early or progressive stage lesion without significant cortication and separation, rest is continued for three full months, the minimum time required to obtain bony healing.[73] At that point, if asymptomatic and with a full, pain-free range of motion in the lumbar spine, the athlete is started in a rehabilitation program and can return to sport when he or she has regained significant aerobic conditioning and can participate in sports-specific retraining without any symptoms. This rehabilitation period usually takes an additional 2–4 months to complete. If the pars lesion is a late-stage, well-corticated fracture, physical restoration for return to sport is begun once the patient is asymptomatic, usually after about 4–6 weeks of rest. Prolonged rest is not used in these patients as the likelihood of obtaining bony healing is extremely low.

If, at any point in the treatment program, an athlete is not progressing as expected, further investigation is performed in order to identify any additional physical or psychosocial factors that may be playing a role in the patient's condition. Radiographic follow-up is not routinely obtained in patients without spondylolisthesis if they are progressing well clinically. Patients with spondylolisthesis frequently do require routine follow-up with radiographs, but the comprehensive management of spondylolisthesis is beyond the scope of this chapter.

Conclusions

Spondylolysis is a relatively common radiographic finding that predominantly develops during early childhood without any associated symptoms but may be a significant cause of pain in certain individuals, particularly adolescent athletes involved in sports with repetitive spinal motions. The pars lesion likely represents a fatigue fracture due to the effects of repetitive stress imposed by physical activity. Although the pars defect can frequently be identified by plain radiography, radionuclide imaging (particularly SPECT), CT, and possibly MRI may be needed to identify and stage a pars lesion or to exclude other spinal pathology that may be present. The vast majority of patients have excellent clinical outcomes with conservative care, although there is limited long-term follow-up reported of athletes suffering pars lesions in adolescence. Actual healing of the pars lesion seems more likely to occur in unilateral defects and in lesions with earlier appearing radiologic characteristics.[5,54,56,68,70] The varied approaches and outcomes described in the literature make it difficult to clearly define the role of bracing, and rigid bracing does not seem to be mandatory for the appropriate management of adolescent athletes with symptomatic spondylolysis. One common thread to the majority of treatment approaches in spondylolysis is relative rest and the avoidance of activities that are associated with increased pain. This may well be the central aspect of treatment, with the primary goal of early-stage treatment being minimization of the biomechanical forces responsible for the propagation of the stress reaction in the pars. Clearly, further clinical study of spondylolysis is needed, particularly longitudinal studies to enhance our understanding of the natural history of this disorder and controlled clinical trials to study the type and extent of treatment necessary to optimize patient outcomes. It is our current opinion that treatment should proceed on an individual basis after a careful assessment of the patient's overall status and identification of concrete treatment goals.

Summary

- Isthmic spondylolysis is found in roughly 4–6% of the general population.
- The vast majority of radiographically evident pars defects develop during early childhood without symptoms.
- The prevalence of spondylolysis is higher in adolescent athletes, ranging from 8% to 15% in studies of large groups of athletes.
- Spondylolysis is a frequent source of low back pain in adolescent athletes.
- Approximately 20% of pars defects seen on plain radiography are identified on lateral oblique views only.
- SPECT and CT have been shown to be more sensitive at identifying pars lesions than plain radiography.
- Studies indicate that a positive SPECT scan correlates with a symptomatic lesion.
- MRI may potentially offer significant advantages over some other imaging modalities, but there is insufficient data on its use in the management of athletes with spondylolysis.
- The vast majority of patients with symptomatic spondylolysis do well with conservative care.
- Early-stage, unilateral pars defects have a relatively high chance of healing, but later stage defects with more extensive cortication and separation have a much lower rate of healing.

• Osseous healing is not necessary to achieve an excellent clinical outcome with full return to activities, although this would seem desirable to achieve where possible.
• There are no published controlled trials on treatment for spondylolysis.

Clinical implications

• Spondylolysis is a very common cause of low back pain in adolescent athletes, particularly those involved in sports with repetitive spinal motions.
• SPECT scanning represents the best radiographic screening tool currently, although its specificity is limited.
• Radiographic staging of the lesion by CT may allow for better patient stratification.
• MRI may be of some utility, but data on the clinical application of MRI findings is lacking and optimal imaging sequences are not well-defined.
• Relative rest is essential in treatment and should continue for at least 3 months after the resolution of symptoms in earlier-stage lesions with potential for healing.

Sample examination questions

Multiple-choice questions (answers on page 602)

1 The prevalence of spondylitic defects identified on plain radiographs in asymptomatic, elite-level adolescent athletes is closest to which of the following?
   A Less than 1%.
   B 3–5%.
   C 8–15%
   D 15–20%
   E Greater than 20%.

2 In an adolescent athlete with a suspected symptomatic pars lesion in whom SPECT imaging is consistent with such a lesion in the lower lumber spine, which of the following is true about the role of CT?
   A A CT of the lumbar spine is not necessary, as all such cases are noted to have a clear pars fracture on CT.
   B A CT scan can help determine the radiographic stage of the pars lesion, which has been shown to correlate to the potential for obtaining bony healing.
   C A CT scan can identify the extent of marrow edema and thus may potentially identify a stress reaction in the bone occurring in the absence of an overt fracture.
   D A CT scan of the lumbar spine is not necessary, as there is no chance it will change the management approach for this patient.
   E A CT scan of the lumbar spine is not necessary, as MRI has clearly been shown to provide superior information for the clinical management of patients with spondylolysis.

3 Which of the following is true of the published studies on the management of adolescent athletes with symptomatic spondylolysis?
   A All studies use the same imaging protocols.
   B Studies utilizing a rigid antilordotic lumbosacral orthosis report a significantly higher rate of bony union than studies in which such a brace has not been used.
   C It is clearly important to continue high-level sports participation during the initial phase of treatment.

D There are no published randomized, controlled trials on the treatment of these athletes.
E The literature on the biomechanics of lumbar orthoses consistently shows that these devices limit intervertebral motion at the lumbosacral junction.

Essay questions

1 What is the underlying prevalence of pars defects on plain radiographs in an asymptomatic population and how does this affect the interpretation of diagnostic studies for an adolescent athlete with low back pain?
2 What are the advantages and limitations of each of the currently available imaging modalities in the assessment of an adolescent athlete with suspected spondylolysis?
3 In the absence of any randomized trials, how can a clinician best use the medical literature to arrive at an optimal treatment strategy for spondylolysis in an adolescent athlete?

Case study 16.1

A 14 year-old female presents with a primary complaint of low back pain. The patient has been playing competitive volleyball for the previous 2 years and has been performing ballet since age 9. She first noticed low back pain 2 months prior to presentation while playing volleyball. The pain was not particularly severe, initially, and she continued her competitive season. Near the end of her season, she had an acute increase in her pain as she extended her spine while jumping to block a shot during a volleyball game. She has since discontinued all competitive and recreational sports and takes two or three tablets of a codeine-based pain medication daily for her pain. She predominantly complains of midline low back pain that increases with activity or bending forward or backward. She has some vague radiating discomfort into her lateral hips, but no paresthesias or pain radiating past her knees. She notes no neurological changes. Her pain has diminished somewhat since discontinuing her sports activities.

Her past medical history is limited to significant problems with gastroesophageal reflux at age 10. This is currently well managed. She takes no medications on a regular basis. Her family history is notable for multiple family members having back problems.

On physical examination, she is a pleasant, healthy-appearing girl in no acute distress. Her lumbar spine is nontender to palpation. Forward flexion at the waist is to 90°, with slight tightness in her low back but no overt pain. Lumbar extension is more uncomfortable for her, in general, with more guarded motion in this direction. She is neurologically intact with no decrements to range-of-motion in her lower extremities.

Imaging studies obtained before presentation consist of plain radiographs of her lumbar spine and a lumbar spine MRI. The radiographs show hemisacralization of the L5 vertebra on the left. No spondylolisthesis or spondylolysis is evident on the plain films, although oblique views had not been obtained. The MRI is interpreted as showing evidence of a transitional lumbar vertebra, as noted on the radiographs, and a small focal midline disk protrusion at L4–5, with no displacement of the nerve roots or thecal sac. The patient subsequently underwent a bone scan with SPECT imaging of her lumbar spine, which revealed increased radiotracer uptake in the posterior elements of L4 and L5 on the right. A limited CT scan of the lower lumbar spine was then obtained which showed sclerosis of the right L4 pars interarticularis with a faint lucency in the pars, consistent with a subtle fracture. Reevaluation of the lumbar MRI revealed no findings consistent with edema in the area of the right L4 pars.

On the basis of her presentation and imaging, the patient was diagnosed with spondylolysis on the right at L4. She was treated with a program of relative rest, including the avoidance of all sporting activities. Her narcotic analgesics were discontinued. After 3 months of rest, she was initiated in a physical therapy program. At that time, she noted her only functional limitation was her ability to perform aggressive sporting tasks. At the completion of her physical therapy care, about 4.5 months after presentation, she started low-level recreation sports and progressed with no discomfort. By 8 months from presentation, her only discomfort occurred with lifting heavy objects with suboptimal motion patterns. Over the next few years, she was able to participate in ballet and competitive track and field events, both middle-distance running and jumping, without any discomfort.

Summarizing the evidence

Comparison/treatment strategies	Results	Level of evidence*
Brace versus rest	No RCTs or other comparative studies, 1 or more case-series on each, no substantial benefit shown for one over the other	Level 3
Rigid brace versus soft brace	No RCTs or other comparative studies, 1 or more case-series on each, no substantial benefit shown for one over the other	Level 3
3 months versus 6 months of brace use or rest	No RCTs or other comparative studies, no substantial benefit shown for one or the other	Level 3

RCT, randomized controlled trial.*
U.S. Preventive Services Task Force:
Level I: Evidence obtained from at least one properly designed randomized controlled trial.
Level II-1: Evidence obtained from well-designed controlled trials without randomization.
Level II-2: Evidence obtained from well-designed cohort or case-control analytic studies, preferably from more than one center or research group.
Level II-3: Evidence obtained from multiple time series with or without the intervention. Dramatic results in uncontrolled trials might also be regarded as this type of evidence.
Level III: Opinions of respected authorities, based on clinical experience, descriptive studies, or reports of expert committees.

References

1 Wiltse LL, Newman PH, Macnab I. Classification of spondylolysis and spondylolisthesis. *Clin Orthop Rel Res* 1976; **117**:23–29.
2 Amato ME, Totty WG, Gilula LA. Spondylolysis of the lumbar spine: demonstration of defects and laminal fragmentation. *Radiology* 1984; **153**:627–629.
3 Fredrickson BE, Baker D, McHolick WJ, Yuan HA, Lubicky JP. The natural history of spondylolysis and spondylolisthesis. *J Bone Joint Surg Am* 1984; **66**:699–707.
4 Roche MA, Rowe GG. The incidence of separate neural arch and coincident bone variations: a survey of 4,200 skeletons. *Anat Rec* 1951; **109**:233–252.
5 Blanda J, Bethem D, Moats W, Lew M. Defects of pars interarticularis in athletes: a protocol for non-operative treatment. *J Spinal Disord* 1993; **6**:406–411.
6 Iwamoto J, Takeda T, Wakano K. Returning athletes with severe low back pain and spondylolysis to original sporting activities with conservative treatment. *Can J Med Sci Sports* 2004; **14**:346–351.
7 Rossi F. Spondylolysis, spondylolisthesis and sports. *J Sports Med Phys Fitness* 1978; **18**:317–340.

8 Rossi F, Dragoni S. The prevalence of spondylolysis and spondylolisthesis in symptomatic elite athletes: radiographic findings. *Radiography* 2001; 7:37–42.

9 Soler T, Calderon C. The prevalence of spondylolysis in the Spanish elite athlete. *Am J Sports Med* 2000; **28**:57–62.

10 Turner RH, Bianco AJ. Spondylolysis and spondylolisthesis in children and teen-agers. *J Bone Joint Surg Am* 1971; **53**:1298–1306.

11 Danielson BI, Frennered AK, Irstam LK. Radiologic progression of isthmic lumbar spondylolisthesis in young patients. *Spine* 1991; **16**:422–425.

12 Jackson DW, Wiltse LL, Cirincione RJ. Spondylolysis in the female gymnast. *Clin Orthop Rel Res* 1976; **117**:658–673.

13 Hambly MF, Wiltse LL, Peek RD. Spondylolisthesis. In: Watkins RG, Williams L, Lin P, Elrod B, eds. *The Spine in Sports.* St. Louis: Mosby, 1996: 157–163.

14 Shook JE. Spondylolysis and spondylolisthesis. *Spine State Art Rev* 1990; **4**:185–197.

15 Wiltse LL, Widell EH, Jackson DW. Fatigue fracture: the basic lesion in isthmic spondylolisthesis. *J Bone Joint Surg Am* 1975; **57**:17–22.

16 Rosenberg NJ, Bargar WL, Friedman B. The incidence of spondylolysis and spondylolisthesis in nonambulatory patients. *Spine* 1981; **6**:35–38.

17 Libson E, Bloom RA, Dinari G. Symptomatic and asymptomatic spondylolysis and spondylolisthesis in young adults. *Int Orthop* 1982; **6**:259–261.

18 Lonstein JE. Spondylolisthesis in children: cause, natural history, and management. *Spine* 1999; **24**:2640–2648.

19 Saraste H. Long-term clinical and radiological follow-up of spondylolysis and spondylolisthesis. *J Pediatr Orthop* 1987; **7**:631–638.

20 Goldstein JD, Berger PE, Windler GE, Jackson DW. Spine injuries in gymnasts and swimmers: an epidemiologic investigation. *Am J Sports Med* 1991; **19**:463–468.

21 McCarroll JR, Miller JM, Ritter MA. Lumbar spondylolysis and spondylolisthesis in college football players: a prospective study. *Am J Sports Med* 1986; **14**:404–406.

22 Semon RL, Spengler D. Significance of lumbar spondylolysis in college football players. *Spine* 1981; **6**:172–174.

23 Gregory PL, Batt ME, Kerslake RW. Comparing spondylolysis in cricketers and soccer players. *Br J Sports Med* 2004; **38**:737–742.

24 Comstock CP, Carragee EJ, O'Sullivan GS. Spondylolisthesis in the young athlete. *Phys Sportsmed* 1994; **22**:39–46.

25 Gerbino PG, Micheli LJ. Back injuries in the young athlete. *Clin Sports Med* 1995; **14**:571–590.

26 Letts M, Smallman T, Afanasiev R, Gouw G. Fracture of the pars interarticularis in adolescent athletes: a clinical–biomechanical analysis. *J Ped Orthop* 1986; **6**:40–46.

27 Letts M, MacDonald P. Sports injuries to the pediatric spine. *Spine State Art Rev* 1990; **4**:49–83.

28 Beutler WJ, Fredrickson BE, Murthlan A, *et al.* The natural history of spondylolysis and spondylolisthesis: 45-year follow-up evaluation. *Spine* 2003; **28**:1027–1035.

29 Wynne-Davies R, Scott JHS. Inheritance and spondylolisthesis: a radiographic family survey. *J Bone Joint Surg Br* 1979; **61**:301–305.

30 Frennered AK, Danielson BI, Nachemson AL. Natural history of symptomatic isthmic low-grade spondylolisthesis in children and adolescents: a seven year follow-up study. *J Ped Orthop* 1991; **11**:209–213.

31 Blackburne JS, Velikas EP. Spondylolisthesis in children and adolescents. *J Bone Joint Surg Br* 1977; **59**:490–494.

32 Lindholm TS, Ragni P, Ylikoski M, Poussa M. Lumbar isthmic spondylolisthesis in children and adolescents: radiologic evaluation and results or operative treatment. *Spine* 1990; **15**:1350–1355.

33 Seitsalo S, Osterman K, Hyvarinen H, *et al.* Progression of spondylolisthesis in children and adolescents: a long-term follow-up of 272 patients. *Spine* 1991; **16**:417–421.

34 Muschik M, Hahnel H, Robinson PN, Perka C, Muschik C. Competitive sports and the progression of spondylolisthesis. *J Pediatr Orthop* 1996; **16**:364–369.

35 Dai L. Disc degeneration in patients with lumbar spondylolysis. *J Spinal Disord* 2000; **13**:478–486.

36 Szypryt EP, Twining P, Mulholland RC, Worthington BS. The prevalence of disc degeneration associated with neural arch defects of the lumbar spine assessed by magnetic resonance imaging. *Spine* 1989; **14**:977–981.

37 Chousa E, Totoribe K, Tajima N. A biomechanical study of lumbar spondylolysis based on a three-dimensional finite element method. *J Orthop Res* 2004; **22**:158–163.

38 Ciullo JV, Jackson DW. Pars interarticularis stress reaction, spondylolysis, and spondylolisthesis in gymnasts. *Clin Sports Med* 1985; **4**:95–110.

39 Cyron BM, Hutton WC. The fatigue strength of the lumbar neural arch in spondylolysis. *J Bone Joint Surg Br* 1978; **60**:234–238.

40 Dietrich M, Kurowski P. The importance of mechanical factors in the etiology of spondylolysis: a model analysis of loads and stresses in human lumbar spine. *Spine* 1985; **10**:532–542.

41 Farfan HF, Osteris V, Lamy C. The mechanical etiology of spondylolysis and spondylolisthesis. *Clin Orthop Rel Res* 1976; **17**:40–55.

42 O'Neill DB, Micheli LJ. Postoperative radiographic evidence for fatigue fracture as the etiology in spondylolysis. *Spine* 1989; **14**:1342–1355.

43 Green TP, Allvey JC, Adams MA. Spondylolysis: bending of inferior articular processes of lumbar vertebrae during simulated spinal movements. *Spine* 1994; **19**:2683–2691.

44 Cyron BM, Hutton WC. Variations in the amount and distribution of cortical bone across the partes interarticulares of L5: a predisposing factor in spondylolysis? *Spine* 1979; **4**:163–167.

45 Anderson SJ. Assessment and management of the pediatric and adolescent patient with low back pain. *Phys Med Rehabil Clin North Am* 1991; **2**:157–185.

46 Micheli LJ, Wood R. Back pain in young athletes: significant differences from adults in causes and patterns. *Arch Pediatr Adolesc Med* 1995; **149**:15–18.

47 Stinson JT. Spondylolysis and spondylolisthesis in the athlete. *Clin Sports Med* 1993; **12**:517–528.

48 Micheli LJ. Back injuries in gymnastics. *Clin Sports Med* 1985; **4**:85–93.

49 Jackson DW, Wiltse LL, Dingeman RD, Hayes M. Stress reactions involving the pars interarticularis in young athletes. *Am J Sports Med* 1981; **9**:304–312.

50 Elliott S, Hutson MA, Wastie ML. Bone scintigraphy in the assessment of spondylolysis in patients attending a sports injury clinic. *Clin Radiol* 1988; **39**:269–272.

51 Anderson K, Sarwark JF, Conway JJ, Logue ES, Schafer MF. Quantitative assessment with SPECT imaging of stress injuries of the pars interarticularis and response to bracing. *J Ped Orthop* 2000; **20**:28–33.

52 Bellah RD, Summerville DA, Treves ST, Micheli LJ. Low back pain in adolescent athletes: detection of stress injury to the pars interarticularis with SPECT. *Radiology* 1991; **180**:509–512.

53 Bodner RJ, Heyman S, Drummond DS, Gregg JR. The use of single photon emission computed tomography (SPECT) in the diagnosis of low back pain in young patients. *Spine* 1988; **13**:1155–1160.

54 Miller SF, Congeni J, Swanson K. Long-term functional and anatomical follow-up of early detected spondylolysis in young athletes. *Am J Sports Med* 2004; **32**:928–933.

55 Stretch RA, Botha T, Chandler S, Pretorius P. Back injuries in young fast bowlers: a radiologic investigation of the healing of spondylolysis and pedicle sclerosis. *S Afr Med J* 2003; **93**:611–616.

56 Sys J, Michielsen J, Bracke P, Martens M, Verstreken J. Nonoperative treatment of active spondylolysis in elite athletes with normal X-ray findings: literature review and results of conservative treatment. *Eur Spine J* 2001; **10**:498–504.

57 Lowe J, Schachner E, Hirschberg E, Shapiro Y, Libson E. Significance of bone scintigraphy in symptomatic spondylolysis. *Spine* 1984; **9**:653–655.

58 Collier BD, Johnson RP, Carrera GF, *et al.* Painful spondylolysis or spondylolisthesis studied by radiography and single photon emission computed tomography. *Radiology* 1985; **154**:207–211.

59 Itoh K, Hashimoto T, Shigenobu K, Yamane S, Tamaki N. Bone SPECT of symptomatic lumbar spondylolysis. *Nucl Med Comm* 1996; **17**:389–396.

60 Lusins JO, Elting JJ, Cicoria AD, Goldsmith SJ. SPECT evaluation of lumbar spondylolysis and spondylolisthesis. *Spine* 1994; **19**:608–612.

61 Raby N, Mathews S. Symptomatic spondylolysis: correlation of CT and SPECT with clinical outcome. *Clin Radiol* 1993; **48**:97–99.

62 Congeni J, McCulloch J, Swanson K. Lumbar spondylolysis: a study of natural progression in athletes. *Am J Sports Med* 1997; **25**:2148–2153.

63 Gregory PL, Batt ME, Kerslake RW, Scammell BE, Webb JF. The value of combining single photon emission computerised tomography and computerised tomography in the investigation of spondylolysis. *Eur Spine J* 2004; **13**:503–509.

64 Harvey CJ, Richenberg JL, Saifuddin A, Wolman RL. The radiological investigation of lumbar spondylolysis. *Clin Radiol* 1998; **53**:723–728.

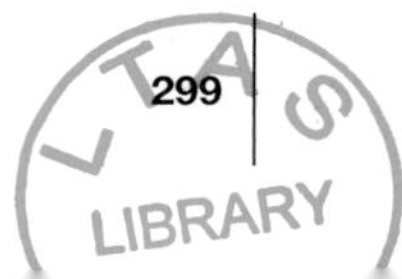

65 Mannor DA, Lindenfeld TN. Spinal process apophysitis mimics spondylolysis: case reports. *Am J Sports Med* 2000; **28**:257–260.
66 Saifuddin A, White J, Tucker S, Taylor BA. Orientation of lumbar pars defects: Implications for radiological detection and surgical management. *J Bone Joint Surg Br* 1998; **80**:208–211.
67 Teplick JG, Laffey PA, Berman A. Diagnosis and evaluation of spondylolisthesis and/or spondylolysis on axial CT. *Am J Neuroradiol* 1986; 7:479–491.
68 Fujii K, Katoh S, Sairyo K, Ikata T, Yasui N. Union of defects in the pars interarticularis of the lumbar spine in children and adolescents: the radiologic outcome after conservative treatment. *J Bone Joint Surg Br* 2004; **86**:225–231.
69 D'Hemecourt PA, Zurakowski D, Kriemler S, Micheli LJ. Spondylolysis: returning the athlete to sports participation with brace treatment. *Orthopedics* 2002; **23**:653–657.
70 Morita T, Ikata T, Katoh S, Miyake R. Lumbar spondylolysis in children and adolescents. *J Bone Joint Surg Br* 1995; 77:620–625.
71 Campbell RSD, Grainger AJ. Optimization of MRI pulse sequences to visualize the normal pars interarticularis. *Clin Radiol* 1999; **54**:63–68.
72 Udeshi UL, Reeves D. Routine thin slice MRI effectively demonstrates the lumbar pars interarticularis. *Clin Radiol* 1999; **54**:615–619.
73 Yamane T, Yoshida T, Mimatsu K. Early diagnosis of lumbar spondylolysis by MRI. *J Bone Joint Surg Br* 1993; 75:764–768.
74 Hollenberg GM, Beattie PF, Meyers SP, Weinberg EP, Adams MJ. Stress reactions of the lumbar pars interarticularis: the development of a new MRI classification system. *Spine* 2002; **27**:181–186.
75 Campbell RSD, Grainger AJ, Hide IG, Papastefanou S, Greenough CG. Juvenile spondylolysis: a comparative analysis of CT, SPECT, and MRI. *Skelet Radiol* 2005; **34**:63–73.
76 Steiner ME, Micheli LJ. Treatment of symptomatic spondylolysis and spondylolisthesis with the modified Boston brace. *Spine* 1985; **10**:937–943.
77 Axelsson P, Johnsson R, Stromqvist B. Effect of lumbar orthosis on intervertebral mobility. *Spine* 1992; 17:678–681.
78 Calmels P, Fayolle-Minon I. An update on orthotic devices for the lumbar spine based on a review of the literature. *Rev Rheum Engl Ed* 1996; **63**:285–291.
79 Lantz SA, Schultz AB. Lumbar spine orthosis wearing I: restriction of gross body motions. *Spine* 1986; 11:834–837.
80 Bonetti M, Fontana A, Albertini F. CT-guided oxygen-ozone treatment for first degree spondylolisthesis and spondylolysis. *Acta Neurochir Suppl* 2005; **92**:87–92.
81 Fellander-Tsai L, Micheli LJ. Treatment of spondylolysis with external stimulation and bracing in adolescent athletes: a report of two cases. *Clin J Sport Med* 1998; **8**:232–234.
82 Maharam LG, Sharkey I. Electrical stimulation of acute spondylolysis: 3 cases. *Med Sci Sports Exerc* 1992; **24** (Suppl):538.
83 Stasinopoulos D. Treatment of spondylolysis with external electrical stimulation in young athletes: a critical literature review. *Br J Sports Med* 2004; **38**:352–354.
84 Pizzutillo PD, Hummer CD. Nonoperative treatment for painful adolescent spondylolysis or spondylolisthesis. *J Pediatr Orthop* 1989; **9**(5):538–40.
85 Daniel JN, Polly DW, van Dam BE. A study of the efficacy of nonoperative treatment of presumed traumatic spondylolysis in a young patient population. *Mil Med* 1995; **160**(ii):553–5.

SECTION 4
Injuries to the upper limb

CHAPTER 17

How evidence-based is our examination of the shoulder?

Anastasia M. Fischer and William W. Dexter

Introduction

Acute and chronic injuries of the shoulder are common problems presenting to primary-care physicians and orthopedic surgeons. As the joint is inherently large and unstable, with a complicated bony joint and numerous soft-tissue structures to support it, the physician is faced with many possible causes of pain. While the patient's history will often point to the diagnosis—e.g., age greater than 60 with night pain, indicating a probable rotator cuff tear—shoulder symptoms are often nonspecific. Complicating the situation further, the treatment of each may vary, ranging from rest to specific exercises, to surgical intervention. Therefore, the physician must use various diagnostic techniques in an attempt to determine the precise nature of the problem and prescribe treatment accordingly. Methods range from physical examination, to imaging studies, to arthroscopic visualization. After a thorough history, the physical examination should include: inspection, palpation, range of motion, strength, and special tests. This chapter is intended to discuss and provide evidence for the special tests used to determine the need for and type of treatment prescribed for shoulder pain.

Special tests for the rotator cuff

Impingement syndrome

To investigate specific tests used to evaluate impingement syndrome of the shoulder, the PubMed database was searched using the keywords "shoulder AND impingement AND Neer OR Hawkins." From this search, we identified 428 articles. Of these, six specifically addressed either the original description of the test, or compared the test to a gold standard and reported sensitivities and specificities.

Neer first described the "impingement sign" that now commonly bears his name in 1972.[1] More fully explained in 1983,[2] the test is performed "with the patient seated and the examiner standing. Scapular rotation is prevented by one hand as the other raises the arm in forced forward elevation (somewhere between flexion and abduction), causing the greater tuberosity to impinge against the acromion." A positive test was described as "pain at the anterior edge of the acromion," and was intended to reveal patients with impingement lesions of all stages, as well as stiffness, instability, arthritis, calcium deposits, and bone lesions. In order to differentiate pain due to impingement from pain due to other processes, it was suggested that an injection of 10 mL of 1.0% Xylocaine beneath the anterior acromion could be used, which could usually eliminate or markedly reduce the pain from impingement.

Hawkins and Kennedy described the impingement test that now bears the common name of the "Hawkins test" in 1980.[3] In this test, the patient's humerus is forward-flexed to 90° and forcibly internally rotated at the shoulder. This maneuver was thought to drive the greater tuberosity farther under the coracoacromial ligament and reproduce impingement pain. Interestingly, the authors stated that this technique was not as reliable as the Neer's sign.

McFarland *et al.*[4] investigated positive results of the Neer and Hawkins impingement test versus bursitis and cuff abnormalities seen during arthroscopy. It was found that there was no significant difference in the rate of impingement seen surgically in a positive Neer versus a positive Hawkins test.

Calis *et al.*[5] tested the Neer test, Hawkins test, horizontal adduction test, the painful arc (pain with active abduction of the shoulder between 60° and 120°), the drop-arm test (inability to hold the shoulder at 90° of flexion in the scapular plane with the elbow extended if pressure is applied), the Yergason test, and Speed's test (both discussed in biceps tendon pathology) in patients with shoulder pain. These patients were then given anterior subacromial injections of 10 mL of 1% lidocaine and observed for 30 min for the resolution of pain. Those with relief were diagnosed with subacromial impingement, those without were said to have pain of other etiologies. Patients then had radiographs and standard magnetic resonance imaging (MRI) of the shoulder done as the gold standard for comparison. The results are listed in Table 17.1.[5–8] The study also evaluated the combination of tests and found that as the number of positive tests increased, the specificity of the combined tests increased, but the sensitivity decreased. The positive predictive value appears to remain fairly constant at around 80%, regardless of how many tests are positive. Although this study does not compare the results with surgical findings, it does bear merit as a "first-response" type of study, in that most physicians believing the patient has subacromial impingement syndrome will first attempt conservative measures for treatment, possibly even before other diagnostic tests are done. However, one shortcoming of the study is that the sensitivity and specificity of MRI with or without arthrogram is limited in comparison with arthroscopy in assessing shoulder pathology.

The diagnostic accuracy of the Neer and Hawkins impingement signs for predicting subacromial bursitis or rotator cuff pathology, using arthroscopy as a gold standard, was tested by MacDonald *et al.* in 2000.[6] In their evaluation, the study did not attempt to differentiate pain caused by subacromial impingement from other causes of potential pain with an injection of anesthetic, as was originally described. The findings are described in Table 17.1. Although both tests are seen to be rather sensitive, they are not adequately specific and have a poor positive predictive value. This might be expected due to the aforementioned lack of use of anesthesia in the patients, but it does reflect the common use of the tests. The tests do not appear to complement each other in the diagnosis of bursitis or rotator cuff tear.

Further investigation of the impingement sign (Neer test) was done by Litaker *et al.* in 2000.[7] In this study, the Neer test was evaluated and compared with four other physical examination findings (infraspinatus and supraspinatus atrophy, weakness with either elevation or external rotation, and arc of pain) with respect to its ability to predict a rotator cuff tear. The results are seen in Table 17.1. This study will be revisited in the chapter section on rotator cuff tears.

Table 17.1 Comparison of special tests for evaluating shoulder impingement

Test studied	First author, ref.	Study design	Patients (n)	Diagnosis researched	Gold standard	Sensitivity (%)	Specificity (%)	PPV	NPV
Neer test	MacDonald (2000)[6]	Prospective	85	Subacromial bursitis	Arthroscopy	75	48	36	83
Neer test	Calis (1999)[5]	Prospective	120 (125 shoulders)	Subacromial impingement syndrome	MRI	89	31	76	52
Neer test	MacDonald (2000)[6]	Prospective	85	Rotator cuff tear	Arthroscopy	83	51	40	89
Neer test	Litaker (2000)[7]	Retrospective	448	Rotator cuff tear	Arthroscopy	97	9	67	63
Hawkins test	MacDonald (2000)[6]	Prospective	85	Subacromial bursitis	Arthroscopy	92	44	39	93
Hawkins test	Calis (1999)[5]	Prospective	120 (125 shoulders)	Subacromial impingement syndrome	MRI	92	25	75	56
Hawkins test	MacDonald (2000)[6]	Prospective	85	Rotator cuff tear	Arthroscopy	88	43	38	90
Neer *and* Hawkins	MacDonald (2000)[6]	Prospective	85	Subacromial bursitis	Arthroscopy	71	51	36	82
Neer *and* Hawkins	MacDonald (2000)[6]	Prospective	85	Rotator cuff tear	Arthroscopy	83	56	43	56
Neer *or* Hawkins	MacDonald (2000)[6]	Prospective	85	Subacromial bursitis	Arthroscopy	96	41	39	96
Neer *or* Hawkins	MacDonald (2000)[6]	Prospective	85	Rotator cuff tear	Arthroscopy	88	38	36	89
Horizontal adduction test	Calis (1999)[5]	Prospective	120 (125 shoulders)	Subacromial impingement syndrome	MRI	82	28	74	38
Speed's test	Calis (1999)[5]	Prospective	120 (125 shoulders)	Subacromial impingement syndrome	MRI	69	56	79	42
Yergason's test	Calis (1999)[5]	Prospective	120 (125 shoulders)	Subacromial impingement syndrome	MRI	37	86	87	36
Painful arc test	Calis (1999)[5]	Prospective	120 (125 shoulders)	Subacromial impingement syndrome	MRI	33	81	81	33
Drop-arm test	Calis (1999)[5]	Prospective	120 (125 shoulders)	Subacromial impingement syndrome	MRI	8	97	88	30
IRRST	Zaslav (2001)[8]	Prospective	110 with + Neer	Subacromial outlet impingement	Arthroscopy	88	96	88	96

IRRST, internal rotation resistance stress test; MRI, magnetic resonance imaging; NPV, negative predictive value; PPV, positive predictive value.

Zaslav introduced a test called the internal rotation resistance stress test (IRRST) in 2001 to attempt to differentiate between outlet impingement syndrome and nonoutlet (intra-articular) causes of shoulder pain in patients with a positive Neer test.[8] The test is "performed in the standing position with the examiner positioned behind the patient. The arm is positioned in 90° abduction in the coronal plane and approximately 80° of external rotation. A manual isometric muscle test is performed for external rotation and then compared with one for internal rotation in the same position. If a patient with a positive impingement sign has good strength in external rotation in this position and apparent weakness in internal rotation, the IRRST result is considered positive." A positive test indicated an intra-articular source of pain, such as a superior labrum anterior–posterior (SLAP) lesion (discussed later in this text). The test was compared to findings in arthroscopy, and the results are shown in Table 17.1. It is interesting to note that in this study, those with a positive IRRST were on average 50 years of age or younger, while those with a negative test were on average 50 years of age or older. On the basis of this one study, the test appears to help differentiate between outlet and nonoutlet causes of pain; however, this might be related to the age of the patient.

On the basis of our evaluation of the literature regarding tests to evaluate impingement syndrome in the shoulder, we recommend using the Neer and Hawkins tests to assist the physician in diagnosis and prescription of treatment. Although these tests are lacking in specificity, they appear to have a reasonable negative predictive value when used alone or together. Another test that may show promise is the IRRST described by Zaslav *et al.*,[8] but as this test has only been evaluated by the creators and authors of the original study, it will be more helpful if other authors are able to repeat their results.

Rotator cuff tears

To investigate specific tests used to evaluate the rotator cuff, the PubMed database was searched using the keywords "shoulder AND Jobe" to search for the Jobe's sign, "shoulder AND lift off" to search for the lift-off test, "shoulder AND lag" to search for the lag signs, "shoulder AND empty can" to search for the empty can test, and "shoulder AND rotator cuff tear AND exam" to try to catch any tests that had been missed. From this search, we identified 96 articles for Jobe's test, two of which described the original test; 15 articles for the lift-off sign, two of which described and studied the test; 25 articles for the lag sign, one of which described and studied the test; 11 articles for the empty can test, one of which described and studied both the full can and empty can tests, and 174 articles describing examinations of the shoulder to predict rotator cuff tears, two of which described and studied several tests.

Pathology of the rotator cuff muscles should be evident by pain with active motion, weakness, instability, or a combination of these symptoms produced by each muscle.[9,10] As such, various methods for testing the individual muscles of the rotator cuff have been suggested.

Jobe and Jobe described the "supraspinatus test" in 1983 as a means of testing for supraspinatus weakness or insufficiency.[11] The patient's arm is placed in 90° abduction with 30° forward horizontal angulation with the thumb pointing at the floor. In this position, muscle testing against resistance can reproduce pain or weakness suggestive of impingement or tear. This method, also called the "empty can test," was not evaluated in comparison with surgical or radiographic findings.

Yocum described a test similar to Jobe's test for supraspinatus strength, with the arm in 90° abduction, 30° forward flexion, and maximal internal rotation.[12] This test was said to have demonstrated a selective way to test the supraspinatus via measurement of electromyographic (EMG) activity in studies conducted at the Centinela Hospital Medical Center biomechanics laboratory. Also mentioned in the article is a test for the subscapularis, in which the patient sits with the arm adducted to the side and the elbow flexed to 90° and resists internal rotation. There are no supporting data or references for either test.

Gerber *et al.* developed a test called the "lift-off test" in 1991 to diagnose tears of the subscapularis tendon.[13] The test consists of placing the arm in full extension and internal rotation, and then asking the patient to lift the dorsum of the hand off the back. If the patient is unable to do so, the test is noted to be positive. To validate the test, they tested nine patients with a subscapularis tear proven surgically in comparison with 100 healthy shoulders. A statistical analysis was not calculated by the authors of the study, but a post-hoc analysis was done by the author of this chapter (AMF) to assess predictive values, and these results are seen in Table 17.2.[13] While the validation numbers are low, given the data presented by Gerber, the lift-off test would appear to be a good test for assessing the integrity of the subscapularis musculotendinous unit.

Gerber *et al.* furthered their study in 1996 by studying 16 men with subscapularis tears, without comparing them with healthy controls.[14] The results are shown in Table 17.3.[14] In this study, the definition of a pathologic lift-off test was different from that in the previous study—the test was considered positive when the patient was unable to maintain maximum internal rotation after having been placed in that position passively. The authors also presented a few new conclusions: that a lift-off lag sign was specific for a small or incomplete tear, that patients who could not reach behind their back due to pain could perform a "belly-press" test (although data on this are not given in the study), and that increased passive external rotation with a feeling of apprehension could improve the accuracy of the diagnosis preoperatively. As this study had no controls, it is difficult to assess its validity.

Greis *et al.*[15] studied Gerber's lift-off test in five patients. Placing the patient's arm in different positions behind the back, they found that muscle activity of the subscapularis (determined electromyographically) was highest when the hand was placed further up the back, as opposed to at the level of the buttock (a maneuver that provides further internal rotation of the humerus).

Kelly *et al.*[16] used electromyographic techniques to attempt to standardize the manual muscle examination on the nondominant shoulder in 11 male subjects. The subjects were asked to perform isometric contractions in 29 different positions while EMG measurements were taken from the supraspinatus muscle, infraspinatus muscle, and subscapularis. Although studies were not done to establish the relevance to rotator cuff muscle pathology seen either on imaging or arthroscopically, the results in Table 17.4 show the positions that produced the greatest activation of muscle units. It should be noted that the "full can test" was compared with the "empty can test" (or Jobe's test), and although the results were not significantly different with regard to activation of the supraspinatus muscle, the "full can test" resulted in less activation of the infraspinatus and better isolation of the supraspinatus. It is not known if this would therefore better predict location of pathology.

The above techniques for isolating the individual muscles of the rotator cuff may assist the physician in locating pathology within the shoulder joint. Although one can assume that pain and/or weakness with a movement specific to a certain muscle points to pathology within that muscle, this is an area that would greatly benefit from further research.

Table 17.2 Special test for evaluating subscapularis rupture

Test studied	First author, ref.	Study design	Patients (n)	Diagnosis researched	Gold standard	Sensitivity (%)	Specificity (%)	PPV	NPV
Lift-off test	Gerber (1991)[13]	Retrospective	162	Subscapularis tendon rupture	Arthroscopy	89	100	100	99

NPV, negative predictive value; PPV, positive predictive value.

Table 17.3 Special tests for evaluating subscapularis rupture

Test studied	First author, ref.	Study design	Patients (n)	Diagnosis researched	Gold standard	Patients with positive test/patients tested
Lift-off test	Gerber (1996)[14]	Nonrandomized retrospective	16	Subscapularis tendon rupture	Arthroscopy	13/16
Increased passive external rotation	Gerber (1996)[14]	Nonrandomized retrospective	16	Subscapularis tendon rupture	Arthroscopy	10/16
Weak lift off test	Gerber (1996)[14]	Nonrandomized retrospective	16	Subscapularis tendon rupture	Arthroscopy	3/16

Table 17.4 Special tests for evaluating rotator cuff strength

Muscle evaluated	Position producing greatest EMG response
Supraspinatus muscle	"Full can test": 90° scapular elevation with 45° humeral rotation
Infraspinatus muscle	External rotation at 0° with −45° humeral rotation
Subscapularis muscle	"Gerber push with force test": full combined internal rotation with resistance

EMG, electromyography.

In 1996, Hertel *et al.* introduced three new signs to evaluate for rotator cuff tears in the supraspinatus, infraspinatus, and subscapularis tendons.[17] The first, called the "external rotation lag sign," is performed with the patient seated with his or her back to the physician. The elbow is "passively flexed to 90° and the shoulder is held at 20° elevation (in the scapular plane) and near maximal external rotation by the physician. The patient is then asked to actively maintain the position of external rotation in elevation as the physician releases the wrist while maintaining support of the limb at the elbow. The sign is positive when a lag, or angular drop, occurs." The second test, called the "drop sign," is performed with the patient in the same position. The physician "holds the affected arm at 90° of elevation (in the scapular plane) and at almost full external rotation, with the elbow flexed at 90°. The patient is asked to actively maintain this position as the physician releases the wrist while supporting the elbow. The sign is positive if a lag or 'drop' occurs." The third and final test described is the "internal rotation lag sign," again performed with the patient seated with his or her back to the physician. "The affected arm is held by the physician at almost maximal internal rotation. The elbow is flexed to 90°, and the shoulder is held at 20° elevation and 20° extension. The dorsum of the hand is passively lifted away from the lumbar region until almost full internal rotation is reached. The patient is then asked to actively maintain this position as the physician releases the wrist while maintaining support at the elbow. The sign is positive when a lag occurs."

Hertel *et al.*[17] then compared the preoperative physical examination with diagnoses found at surgery. Grouping the findings into two categories—posterosuperior cuff tear (supraspinatus and infraspinatus disease) and subscapularis tear—they compared the three new lag signs with two previously documented tests, Jobe's sign (the empty can test), and the drop sign. Table 17.5[17,18] lists the results. The tests all have excellent positive predictive values (meaning that a positive test is a good indicator of disease); however, all but the internal rotation lag sign have a relatively poor negative predictive value (meaning that a negative test is not a good indicator for ruling out the disease).

Itoi *et al.*[18] asked "which is more useful, the 'full can test' or the 'empty can test,' in detecting the torn supraspinatus tendon?" A total of 143 consecutive shoulders were evaluated with the tests, and a positive test was recorded when the patient experienced pain, muscle weakness, or both. The physical examination was compared versus a 1.5-T MRI without arthrography. The results are shown in Table 17.5. The authors concluded that although the tests were statistically similar, the full can test was preferable as it caused less pain, although the difference was not statistically significant.

A very large retrospective study was conducted by Litaker *et al.* in 2000 to investigate signs and symptoms of rotator cuff tears in comparison with arthroscopic findings.[7] The results are shown in Table 17.6.[7] Logistic regression analysis showed that the three factors

Table 17.5 Special tests for evaluating rotator cuff tears

Test studied	First author, ref.	Study design	Patients (n)	Diagnosis researched	Gold standard	Sensitivity (%)	Specificity (%)	PPV	NPV
External rotation lag sign	Hertel (1996)[17]	Prospective	100	Posterosuperior cuff tear	Open or arthroscopic visualization	70	100	100	56
Drop sign	Hertel (1996)[17]	Prospective	100	Posterosuperior cuff tear	Open or arthroscopic visualization	21	100	100	32
Internal rotation lag sign	Hertel (1996)[17]	Prospective	100	Subscapularis tear	Open or arthroscopic visualization	97	96	97	96
Lift-off sign	Hertel (1996)[17]	Prospective	100	Subscapularis tear	Open or arthroscopic visualization	62	100	100	69
Jobe's sign (empty can test)	Hertel (1996)[17]	Prospective	100	Posterosuperior cuff tear	Open or arthroscopic visualization	84	58	84	58
Jobe's sign (empty can test)	Itoi (1999)[18]	Prospective	143	Supraspinatus tear	MRI	89	50	36	93
Full can test	Itoi (1999)[18]	Prospective	143	Supraspinatus tear	MRI	86	57	39	93

MRI, magnetic resonance imaging; NPV, negative predictive value; PPV, positive predictive value.

Table 17.6 Special tests for evaluating rotator cuff tears

Test studied	First author, ref.	Study design	Patients (n)	Diagnosis researched	Gold standard	Sensitivity (%)	Specificity (%)	PPV	NPV
History of trauma	Litaker (2000)[7]	Retrospective	448	Rotator cuff tear	Arthroscopy	36	73	72	37
Night pain	Litaker (2000)[7]	Retrospective	448	Rotator cuff tear	Arthroscopy	88	20	70	43
Supraspinatus atrophy	Litaker (2000)[7]	Retrospective	448	Rotator cuff tear	Arthroscopy	56	73	81	44
Infraspinatus atrophy	Litaker (2000)[7]	Retrospective	448	Rotator cuff tear	Arthroscopy	56	73	81	43
Elevation < 170°	Litaker (2000)[7]	Retrospective	448	Rotator cuff tear	Arthroscopy	30	78	74	36
External rotation < 70°	Litaker (2000)[7]	Retrospective	448	Rotator cuff tear	Arthroscopy	19	84	70	34
Neer's test	Litaker (2000)[7]	Retrospective	448	Rotator cuff tear	Arthroscopy	97	9	67	63
Weakness with elevation	Litaker (2000)[7]	Retrospective	448	Rotator cuff tear	Arthroscopy	64	65	78	48
Weakness with external rotation	Litaker (2000)[7]	Retrospective	448	Rotator cuff tear	Arthroscopy	76	57	79	54
Arc of pain	Litaker (2000)[7]	Retrospective	448	Rotator cuff tear	Arthroscopy	98	10	67	69
Expert diagnosis	Litaker (2000)[7]	Retrospective	448	Rotator cuff tear	Arthroscopy	90	53	80	78

NPV, negative predictive value; PPV, positive predictive value.

best able to statistically predict a rotator cuff tear were: weakness on external rotation, age > 65 years, and the presence of night pain.

The authors of this chapter recommend a holistic approach to diagnosing tears of the rotator cuff. While many of the tests described either have poor statistical value for predicting pathology or are not well supported by research, they can still be used to assist the physician in diagnosis. We would use the patient's history, strength testing of the rotator cuff musculature (supported by an external or internal rotation lag sign), and a lack of response to treatment including physical therapy to guide the physician towards the time and placement of surgical intervention.

Labral tears

To investigate specific tests used to evaluate the glenoid labrum, the PubMed database was searched using the keywords "shoulder AND labral tear", "shoulder AND glenoid labral tear", and "shoulder AND SLAP". From this search, we identified 102 articles describing labral tears, five of which described and studied specific tests; 57 articles describing glenoid labral tears, four of which were appropriate for this chapter; and 101 articles describing SLAP lesions, four of which were appropriate for this chapter. Subsequent to this step, the reference section of the aforementioned articles was reviewed to find any articles that might have been missed by our search. In this way, an additional four articles were found that were described and studied specific tests.

Glenoid labral tears constitute another conundrum for diagnosis. Ideally, surgeons would prefer to be able to diagnose these lesions prior to surgery so that the patient can provide consent for a repair procedure, to ensure that the appropriate equipment is available at the time of surgery, and to ensure that a surgeon skilled in the repair of these lesions is present at the time of surgery.[19] Although tears of the glenoid labrum can occur anywhere around the circumference, the SLAP lesion is perhaps the most notorious. An acronym for a tear in the *s*uperior *l*abrum, extending from *a*nterior to *p*osterior, the lesion was first described by Snyder *et al.*[20] in 1990. At that time, the authors claimed that SLAP lesions could only be diagnosed surgically. However, two diagnostic tests were introduced—the "biceps tension test" (resisted shoulder flexion with the elbow extended and forearm supinated) and the "joint compression–rotation test" (the supine patient's shoulder is abducted 90°, the elbow flexed to 90°, and a compressive force is applied longitudinally through the humerus while rotating it, attempting to catch the torn portion of labrum between the humeral head and the glenoid rim). Both were intended to cause pain or clicking to suggest a labral tear. Although the lesions were visualized surgically, no statistical analysis of the physical examination findings was done.

Liu *et al.*[21] conducted a study published in 1996 that evaluated the use of the apprehension test, relocation test, crank test, or shift and load test to predict labral tears in comparison with MRI (with and without saline arthrography). A positive test was considered a feeling of instability or clicking with any one or more of the four tests. Both special tests and MRI were compared with the arthroscopic findings. The results are shown in Table 17.7;[21] the study combined tests used for both instability and labral tears (which can certainly coexist), but did not distinguish between them.

To narrow their results and formally introduce the "crank test," Liu *et al.* published a follow-up study later in 1996.[22] In this study, 62 patients with a history of shoulder pain underwent the crank test to evaluate prediction of glenoid labral tears versus arthroscopic findings. Patients with physical examination findings suggestive of a rotator cuff tear were

Table 17.7 Special tests for evaluating labral tears versus magnetic resonance imaging

Test studied	First author, ref.	Study design	Patients (n)	Diagnosis researched	Gold standard	Sensitivity (%)	Specificity (%)	PPV	NPV
Apprehension, relocation, load and shift, *or* crank test	Liu (1996)[21]	Retrospective	54	Labral tear	Arthroscopy	90	85	95	73
MRI	Liu (1996)[21]	Retrospective	54	Labral tear	Arthroscopy	59	85	92	39

NPV, negative predictive value; PPV, positive predictive value.

eliminated from the study. The crank test was now described with the "patient in the standing position with the arm elevated to 160° in the scapular plane. A joint load was applied along the axis of the humerus with one hand while the other performed humeral rotation. A positive test was determined either by 1) pain during the maneuver with or without a click or 2) reproduction of the symptoms, usually pain or catching felt by the patient during athletic or work activities." The results are shown in Table 17.8.[19,22–31]

Although the sensitivity and specificity of this test for predicting labral tears are very high, it must be remembered that patients with shoulder pain of perhaps another etiology were eliminated from this study. It is possible that including them would have decreased the accuracy of the test.

O'Brien *et al.* introduced the "active compression test" (now often called the O'Brien test) in 1998.[29] The original description stated: "The standing patient forward flexed the arm to 90° with the elbow in full extension and then adducted the arm 10° to 15° medial to the sagittal plane of the body and internally rotated it so that the thumb pointed downward. The examiner, standing behind the patient, applied a uniform downward force to the arm. With the arm in the same position, the palm was then fully supinated and the maneuver was repeated. The test was considered positive if pain was elicited during the first maneuver, and was reduced or eliminated with the second. Pain localized to the acromioclavicular joint or 'on top' was diagnostic of acromioclavicular joint abnormality, whereas pain or painful clicking described as 'inside' the shoulder was considered indicative of labral abnormality." The results are shown in Table 17.8. Physical examination findings for lesions suspected of being labral tears were compared with the surgical findings. Postoperative repeat studies were not carried out to report the resolution of pain with the examination.

The anterior slide test was introduced by Kibler *et al.* in 1995.[24] In this test, "the patient is examined either standing or sitting, with their hands on the hips with thumbs pointing posteriorly. One of the examiner's hands is placed across the top of the shoulder from the posterior direction, with the last segment of the index finger extending over the anterior aspect of the acromion at the glenohumeral joint. The examiner's other hand is placed behind the elbow and a forward and slightly superiorly directed force is applied to the elbow and upper arm. The patient is asked to push back against this force. Pain localized to the front of the shoulder under the examiner's hand, and/or a pop or click in the same area, was considered to be a positive test." The results are shown in Table 17.8.

The biceps load test was introduced by Kim *et al.* in 1999, to evaluate the integrity of the superior glenoid labrum in shoulders with recurrent anterior dislocations.[25] The test was described with the patient in a supine position and the shoulder abducted to 90° with the forearm supinated. The shoulder was then externally rotated to the position of pain (standard apprehension test) and stopped. Active flexion of the elbow against resistance followed, and if the discomfort was increased or stayed the same, the test was considered positive for a SLAP lesion. The results are shown in Table 17.9.[32] Statistically, this is a very good test, but it should be noted that it was only used in patients with documented recurrent anterior shoulder dislocations, all of whom had Bankart lesions. To remedy this problem, Kim *et al.*[26] introduced the biceps load test II to examine painful shoulders for isolated SLAP lesions. This test is similar to the test described above, except that the arm is abducted to 120° instead of 90°, and the test is only considered positive if the amount of pain in the shoulder increases (it was positive in the previous test if pain remained the same). The results are shown in Table 17.8. Neither of these tests has been studied by other authors.

Table 17.8 Special tests for evaluating labral pathologies

Test studied	First author, ref.	Study design	Patients (n)	Diagnosis researched	Gold standard	Sensitivity (%)	Specificity (%)	PPV	NPV
Crank test	Liu (1996)[22]	Prospective	62	Labral tear	Arthroscopy	91	93	94	90
Crank test	Guanche (2000)[23]	Prospective	46	SLAP lesion	Arthroscopy	45	69		
Crank test	Guanche (2000)[23]	Prospective	46	Non-SLAP labral lesion	Arthroscopy	47	68		
Crank test	Guanche (2000)[23]	Prospective	46	Any labral lesion	Arthroscopy	42	77		
Crank test	Stetson (2002)[31]	Nonrandomized prospective study	65	Labral tear	Arthroscopy	46	56	41	61
Crank test	Parentis (2002)[30]	Prospective	132	Type I or II SLAP lesion	Arthroscopy	13	83		
Crank test	Guanche (2003)[19]	Prospective	60	Labral tear (including SLAP lesions)	Arthroscopy	40	73	82	29
Crank test	Guanche (2003)[19]	Prospective	60	SLAP lesion	Arthroscopy	39	67	59	47
O'Brien test	O'Brien (1998)[29]	Prospective	318	Labral tear	Arthroscopy	100	98.5	88.7	100
O'Brien test	Morgan (1998)[28]	Retrospective	102	SLAP lesion II	Arthroscopy	85	41		
O'Brien test	Guanche (2000)[23]	Prospective	46	SLAP lesion	Arthroscopy	50	50		
O'Brien test	Guanche (2000)[23]	Prospective	46	Non-SLAP labral lesion	Arthroscopy	87	68		
O'Brien test	Guanche (2000)[23]	Prospective	46	Labral lesion	Arthroscopy	64	85		
O'Brien test	Parentis (2002)[30]	Prospective	132	Type I or II SLAP lesion	Arthroscopy	63	50		
O'Brien test	Stetson (2002)[31]	Nonrandomized prospective study	65	Labral tear	Arthroscopy	54	31	34	50
O'Brien test	McFarland (2002)[27]	Retrospective consecutive case series	426	SLAP lesions II–IV	Arthroscopy	47	55	10	91
O'Brien test	Guanche (2003)[19]	Prospective	60	Labral tear (including SLAP)	Arthroscopy	63	73	87	40
O'Brien test	Guanche (2003)[19]	Prospective	60	SLAP lesion	Arthroscopy	54	47	57	45
Jobe relocation test	Morgan (1998)[28]	Retrospective	102	SLAP lesion II	Arthroscopy	59	54		
Relocation test	Parentis (2002)[30]	Prospective	132	Type I or II SLAP lesion	Arthroscopy	50	53		
Jobe relocation test	Guanche (2003)[19]	Prospective	60	Labral tear (including SLAP)	Arthroscopy	44	87	91	34
Jobe relocation test	Guanche (2003)[19]	Prospective	60	SLAP lesion	Arthroscopy	36	63	55	45

Continued

Table 17.8 *(Continued)*

Test studied	First author, ref.	Study design	Patients (n)	Diagnosis researched	Gold standard	Sensitivity (%)	Specificity (%)	PPV	NPV
Anterior apprehension test	Guanche (2003)[19]	Prospective	60	Labral tear (including SLAP)	Arthroscopy	40	87	90	33
Anterior apprehension test	Guanche (2003)[19]	Prospective	60	SLAP lesion	Arthroscopy	30	63	50	43
O'Brien test *or* crank test	Guanche (2000)[23]	Prospective	46	SLAP lesion	Arthroscopy	65	38		
O'Brien test *or* crank test	Guanche (2000)[23]	Prospective	46	Non-SLAP labral lesion	Arthroscopy	93	52		
O'Brien test *or* crank test	Guanche (2000)[23]	Prospective	46	Labral lesion	Arthroscopy	76	69		
Jobe *or* O'Brien *or* apprehension test	Guanche (2003)[19]	Prospective	60	Labral tear (including SLAP)	Arthroscopy	72	73	88	47
Anterior slide	Kibler (1995)[24]	Retrospective	226	Superior glenoid labral tear	Arthroscopy	78	92		
Anterior slide	McFarland (2002)[27]	Retrospective consecutive case series	419	SLAP lesions II–IV	Arthroscopy	8	84	5	90
Anterior slide	Parentis (2002)[30]	Prospective	132	Type I or II SLAP lesion	Arthroscopy	10	82		
Compression–rotation	McFarland (2002)[27]	Retrospective consecutive case series	426	SLAP lesions II–IV	Arthroscopy	24	76	9	90
Speed's test	Morgan (1998)[28]	Retrospective	102	SLAP lesion II	Arthroscopy	78	37		
Speed's test	Parentis (2002)[30]	Prospective	132	Type I or II SLAP lesion	Arthroscopy	40	67		
Speed's test	Guanche (2003)[19]	Prospective	60	Labral tear (including SLAP)	Arthroscopy	18	87	80	26
Speed's test	Guanche (2003)[19]	Prospective	60	SLAP lesion	Arthroscopy	9	74	30	40
Biceps load test I	Kim (1999)[25]	Prospective nonrandomized double-blind	75	SLAP lesion	Arthroscopy	90.9	96.9	83	98
Biceps load test II	Kim (2001)[26]	Prospective double-blind	127	SLAP lesion	Arthroscopy	89.7	96.9	92.1	95.5

NPV, negative predictive value; PPV, positive predictive value; SLAP, superior labrum anterior–posterior (lesion).

Table 17.9 Special test for evaluating biceps tendon or labral pathology

Test studied	First author, ref.	Study design	Patients (n)	Diagnosis researched	Gold standard	Sensitivity (%)	Specificity (%)	PPV	NPV
Speed's test	Bennett (1998)[32]	Prospective	46	Biceps/labral pathology	Arthroscopy	90	14	23	83

NPV, negative predictive value; PPV, positive predictive value.

Morgan *et al.* compared O'Brien's test, Jobe's relocation test (discussed in instability), and Speed's test (discussed in biceps tendon pathology) to surgical findings in 102 patients with type II SLAP lesions.[28] The results are shown in Table 17.8. The authors determined that Speed's and O'Brien's tests were useful in predicting anterior SLAP lesions, whereas the Jobe relocation test was useful in predicting posterior SLAP lesions.

Guanche and Quick compared O'Brien's test and the crank test with arthroscopic findings in 2000.[23] The results are shown in Table 17.8. The authors concluded that neither test definitively identifies labral lesions and that the combination of tests does not increase the reliability of the diagnosis.

Stetson and colleagues conducted a study to compare the crank test and O'Brien test with arthroscopic findings.[31] The results are shown in Table 17.8. The authors found that a great number of positive crank tests and O'Brien tests did not reveal a labral tear, but instead identified bursitis or rotator cuff tears. However, the study included an older patient population as well as patients with suspected rotator cuff tears, which may have substantially affected the results.

McFarland *et al.* conducted a study to compare the O'Brien test, the anterior slide test, and the compression rotation test (Snyder's joint compression test) with arthroscopic findings.[27] The control group consisted of patients who retrospectively had either no SLAP lesion on arthroscopy, or a type I SLAP lesion, in comparison with the study group, who had types II, III, or IV SLAP lesions (77% of whom had other coexistent intra-articular pathology). The physical examination of the patients was done before they were diagnosed surgically, but only 69% of the patients received all three tests. The results are shown in Table 17.8. It is interesting to note that none of the patients had positive results on all three tests in the SLAP lesion group, but that 5% of patients in the control group did. Also, there was no significant difference between groups for patients who had zero, one, or two tests with positive results. McFarland *et al.* also concluded that a pop, click, or clunk appreciated with the test was of no diagnostic significance.

Parentis *et al.*[30] conducted a study to compare the active compression test (O'Brien's test), anterior slide test, pain provocation test, crank test, relocation test, Hawkins' test, Neer's test, Speed's test, and Yergason's test with arthroscopic findings of type I and II SLAP lesions. The results are shown in Table 17.8. None of the tests studied had sensitivities high enough to be used diagnostically, although the specificities could be useful in helping to rule out pathology.

Guanche and Jones conducted a study to examine several tests in comparison with arthroscopy.[19] Sixty patients in whom shoulder surgery was planned were examined with Speed's test, the anterior apprehension test, Yergason's test, O'Brien's test, Jobe's relocation test (see the section on instability below for a description), the crank test, and a test for tenderness of the bicipital groove. The results are shown in Table 17.8. The authors concluded that O'Brien's test and the Jobe relocation test were statistically correlated with labral tears found surgically, and that the apprehension test approached statistical significance. The other tests were not found to be useful in diagnosing labral tears, and none of the tests performed provided statistically significant results for identifying SLAP lesions in particular.

Although none of the tests to evaluate for glenoid labral tears individually exhibit a repeatedly high sensitivity or specificity sufficient for diagnosis, it appears that using multiple tests can help guide the physician in diagnosis. The studies conducted by Guanche *et al.* in 2000 and 2003 reveal that the sensitivity can be improved with only a small decrease in the specificity if the O'Brien test, crank test, and Jobe test are conducted together, with any positive result predictive of a tear.[19,23] The biceps load tests also appear to have promise in diagnosis, but it would be helpful if other investigators could repeat the results of the originators of the technique. As none of these tests is particularly time-consuming, the authors of this chapter suggest that physicians use all four tests in their evaluation of the glenoid labrum when prompted by patient history, perhaps in conjunction with a lack of response to physical therapy, to guide their decision to pursue additional imaging or surgical intervention.

Biceps tendon pathology

To investigate specific tests used to evaluate the biceps tendon, the PubMed database was searched using the keywords "shoulder AND biceps tendon AND test." From this search, we identified 37 articles, one of which described and studied the test. The reference for Yergason's sign was found by searching the reference section of a review article describing the test.[9] The authors of this study were unable to find this reference in the database used for this chapter.

Yergason's sign was introduced in 1931.[33] In this test, "if the elbow is flexed to 90°, the forearm being pronated; and the examining surgeon holds the patient's wrist so as to resist supination, and then directs that active supination be made against his resistance; pain, very definitely localized in the bicipital groove, indicates a condition of wear and tear of the long head of the biceps, or synovitis of its tendon sheath."

Speed's test (never described by Dr. Speed himself) was originally developed to examine for bicipital tendonitis, SLAP lesions, and/or biceps avulsions. Dr. Speed had found that when he elevated his arm with elbow extension, he had pain in the proximal shoulder area. He was later diagnosed with bicipital tendonitis. Bennett was the first to compare the test results with arthroscopic findings of intra-articular biceps tendon/labral injury or macroscopic bicipital groove injury, and/or biceps tendon inflammation at the level of the groove.[32] The results are shown in Table 17.9. It was suggested that the poor specificity of the test was because the test causes pain with subacromial bursitis, instability, a tight posterior capsule, a coracoacromial ligament spur, a subscapularis or supraspinatus injury, or a Bankart lesion. One patient with a fully avulsed biceps tendon had a negative test, presumably because the tendon was retracted from the groove. Although this test is sensitive, it does not appear to be helpful in narrowing the etiology of shoulder pain. The authors of this chapter therefore suggest that this test should be used with caution.

Laxity

To investigate specific tests used to evaluate shoulder laxity and instability, the PubMed database was searched using the keywords "shoulder AND instability". This search produced 1528 articles, three of which described and studied specific tests. The reference sections of these articles were then searched for descriptions or studies of tests that were missed by the initial search. This provided an additional three articles that were appropriate for this chapter.

The sulcus sign was first referenced by Neer and Foster in 1980,[34] and more fully described in 1993 by Silliman and Hawkins.[35] In this test, downward traction is applied to the humerus, and if the examiner observes dimpling beneath the acromion, the test is said to be positive.

In 1984, Gerber and Ganz introduced two tests for shoulder laxity: the anterior and posterior drawer tests, said to be comparable to testing for ligamentous laxity in the knee.[36]

In the anterior drawer test, the patient is supine, and "the examiner stands facing the affected shoulder. He fixes the patient's hand in his own (opposite) axilla by adducting his own humerus. The patient should not grasp the surgeon's axilla but should be completely relaxed. The affected shoulder is held in 80° to 120° of abduction, 0° to 20° of forward flexion, and 0° to 30° of lateral rotation." The examiner then stabilizes the scapula with one hand, while drawing the humeral head anteriorly with the other to determine the grade of movement and therefore, laxity of the joint. The posterior drawer test is also done with the patient supine, but the shoulder is placed in 80–120° abduction and 20–30° of forward flexion, with the elbow at 120° of flexion. The examiner then slightly rotates the humerus medially while flexing the shoulder to 60–80° in an attempt to sublux the humeral head posteriorly. A positive test is described with appreciable posterior subluxation and is often associated with a feeling of apprehension by the patient. Although no statistical analysis was done, the authors state that the anterior drawer test was positive in all of their patients with recurrent anterior dislocations except for two. There is no mention of the incidence of positive posterior drawer tests.

Silliman and Hawkins described the load and shift test in 1993.[35] This test, designed to evaluate glenohumeral translation anteriorly and posteriorly, is performed with the patient sitting. The examiner stands behind the patient and stabilizes the scapula with one hand, while grasping the humeral head with the other. As the head is "loaded" concentrically into the glenoid fossa, both anterior and posterior stresses are applied, and the amount of translation is noted.

The loose shoulder may or may not be more prone to instability than a tighter shoulder. Although there are several tests designed to evaluate the laxity of the shoulder, it is important to understand that findings do not necessarily imply instability or even a predisposition to instability.

Instability

The apprehension test was first described in 1981 by Rowe and Zarins, in a study evaluating treatment of patients with chronic repetitive shoulder subluxation.[37] With the patient in either a seated or standing position, the shoulder is passively moved into "maximum external rotation in abduction and forward pressure is applied to the posterior aspect of the humeral head." A positive test is noted when the patient becomes apprehensive and complains of pain in the shoulder. Although a statistical analysis was not performed, all of the subluxing patients in this study (n = 58) had a positive apprehension test.

The apprehension–relocation test was described by Jobe and Kvitne in 1989.[38] In this test, the patient is supine and the apprehension test is performed. When apprehension is experienced, a posteriorly directed force is applied to the humeral head. "Patients with primary impingement will generally have no change in their pain, whereas patients with instability (subluxation) and secondary impingement will have pain relief and will tolerate maximal external rotation with the humeral head maintained in a reduced position." No statistical analysis was done to compare the physical examination findings with a gold standard.

Speer *et al.* studied the apprehension–relocation test in 1994.[39] A total of 100 patients undergoing shoulder surgery were tested with and without an anterior force being applied, and with pain and apprehension being separate primary end points. The results are shown in Table 17.10.[39] The authors concluded that the test best predicted instability with apprehension as the primary end point, instead of pain, and noted that the test was not

Table 17.10 Special tests for evaluating shoulder laxity

Test studied	First author, ref.	Study design	Patients (n)	Diagnosis researched	Gold standard	Sensitivity (%)	Specificity (%)	PPV	NPV
Shoulder pain test @ 90/90 with a positive relocation test	Speer (1994)[39]	Prospective nonrandomized	100	Anterior instability	Arthroscopy	30	58	38	49
Shoulder pain test @ 90/90 with an anterior force and positive relocation test	Speer (1994)[39]	Prospective nonrandomized	100	Anterior instability	Arthroscopy	54	44	45	53
Shoulder apprehension test @ 90/90 with a positive relocation test	Speer (1994)[39]	Prospective nonrandomized	100	Anterior instability	Arthroscopy	57	100	100	73
Shoulder apprehension test @ 90/90 with an anterior force and positive relocation test	Speer (1994)[39]	Prospective nonrandomized	100	Anterior instability	Arthroscopy	68	100	100	78

NPV, negative predictive value; PPV, positive predictive value.

significantly different if an anterior force was applied to the humerus or not. "In all probability, if a patient acknowledges apprehension in the position of 90/90 or 90/90ANT, there is anterior instability and any further pursuit of the relocation test is moot."

In a paper presented in 2000, Tzannes *et al.* conducted a study of 100 symptomatic shoulders and examined them for laxity, among other physical examination tests.[40] All patients underwent arthroscopic surgery to determine the cause of their symptoms. Unstable shoulders had a greater degree of internal rotation and a higher incidence of laxity than those shoulders determined to be stable or have SLAP lesions. They were also found to have a lower incidence of decreased strength, positive impingements tests, as well as positive O'Brien's tests. The predictive values of laxity or instability testing was not reported.

The authors of this chapter suggest using the shoulder relocation test with apprehension as a positive end point to evaluate for shoulder instability.

Conclusions

Special tests used to evaluate the shoulder for various conditions are fraught with uncertainty. As seen in the tables presented in this chapter, research done by various authors has documented widely ranging sensitivities and specificities for any one test. In many cases, the special tests introduced by authors had excellent positive predictive value in diagnosis, but other investigators were unable to repeat the results seen in the original studies. There has been some effort to combine various special tests in an attempt to increase the accuracy, but the combinations researched to date have not been able to do so. This is an area that deserves further research.

It becomes obvious, then, that prediction of injuries necessitating surgical repair is difficult when special tests alone are used. Physicians have a responsibility to the patient to acquire a detailed history of the injury, its progress, and response to physical therapy if applicable. They must also exercise appropriate use of physical examination skills and imaging acquisition and interpretation when considering a surgical referral for shoulder pathology.

Summary

• There are very few special tests of the shoulder that can reliably predict internal derangement.
• The examiner should gain a level of expertise with several maneuvers for each entity and consider combining these to form a diagnosis based on physical examination of the painful shoulder.
• Further studies should continue to explore physical examination techniques as a reliable means of diagnosis.
• The patient's history and response to conservative treatment may better guide the practitioner towards surgical repair than physical examination techniques.

Key messages

• Shoulder impingement syndrome may best be predicted by the Hawkins and Neer tests, although these tests may also be positive in other shoulder pathologies.
• Rotator cuff tears are difficult to predict on the basis of a physical examination alone, but the lift-off and lag signs can be helpful in assessing the integrity of the rotator cuff.

• Labral tears are difficult to predict on the basis of a physical examination alone; a combination of tests may give the examiner more confidence in diagnosing SLAP lesions.
• The apprehension and apprehension–relocation tests better predict shoulder instability than shoulder pain with these tests.

Sample examination questions

Multiple-choice questions (answers on page 602)

1 Although lacking in specificity, the combination of tests (with good negative predictive value) best suited to evaluate impingement syndrome in the shoulder is:
   A Neer and Hawkins tests
   B O'Brien's and internal rotation stress tests
   C Speed's and Yergason's tests
   D Painful arc and internal rotation stress tests
   E Horizontal abduction and Hawkins tests
2 The following statements about rotator cuff tests are relatively well supported by the literature:
   A The full can test seems to be a better indicator of supraspinatus pathology (tears) than the empty can sign
   B Lag signs (IRLS, ERLS) have reasonable sensitivity and positive predictive value for diagnosing rotator cuff tears
   C EMG data suggest that the infraspinatus muscle is most fully activated with full internal rotation against resistance
   D A and B
   E All of the above
3 SLAP (superior labrum anterior–posterior) tears of the glenoid labrum are reliably diagnosed by the following test:
   A O'Brien's test
   B Anterior slide test
   C Crank test
   D Biceps load test
   E No single test has either high sensitivity or specificity for labral injury

Essay questions

1 Describe the tests that will give the best assessment of outlet impingement of the shoulder (Neer, Hawkins, and internal rotation stress test).
2 What are "lag signs" and how are they utilized in diagnosing pathology of the shoulder?
3 Describe three tests that might be used to assess the integrity of the glenoid labrum and discuss their diagnostic accuracy and optimal utilization.

Case study 17.1

A swimmer presents to the clinic with complaints of bilateral shoulder pain of about 3 months' duration. The onset was insidious and correlated with a rapid increase in swimming distance. The pain is worse when swimming (all strokes hurt, but breast stroke less so). There are no associated symptoms in this otherwise healthy athlete. The resident is interested in learning examination maneuvers to confirm the presumptive diagnosis.

Case study 17.2

A tennis player presents 3 weeks after an acute injury to the dominant shoulder. The injury was sustained while completing an overhead shot. The athlete felt something pop, which was painful deep in the shoulder, and now notes a nagging pain and complains of a sense of instability and a clunking sensation with overhead shots and serves. The athlete is wondering whether surgery is needed. MRI scanning is not possible, and a clinical diagnosis is therefore necessary to direct care.

Case study 17.3

A 50-year-old weekend warrior presents to the clinic with complaints of increasing shoulder pain. There was no specific inciting injury. The athlete now complains of pain that limits sleep and an inability to throw and notes a sense of weakness with most resisted activities. Application of various focused physical examinations maneuvers led to a diagnosis.

Summarizing the evidence

Physical examination Test	Results	Level of evidence*
Impingement		
Neer test	2 RCTs, one of large size, good sensitivity	A3
Hawkins test	2 RCT, one of large size, very good sensitivity, conflicting negative predictive value	A3
Neer *or* Hawkins test	1 RCT, moderate size, good negative predictive value	A3
Rotator cuff tears		
Lift-off test	3 non-RCTs, one of large size, excellent sensitivity and specificity	B
Empty can test	2 RCTs, both of large size, poor specificity with conflicting positive predictive value	A3
Internal rotation lag sign	1 RCT, large size, excellent positive predictive value	A3
External rotation lag sign	1 RCT, large size, excellent positive predictive value	A3
Labral tears		
Crank test	5 RCTs, one of large size, conflicting results	A3
O'Brien test	7 RCTs, 4 of large size, conflicting results	A4
O'Brien test *or* crank test	1 RCT, of small size, fair sensitivity and specificity	A4
Shoulder laxity		
Shoulder apprehension test with a positive relocation test	1 RCT, large size, excellent specificity and positive predictive value	A3

* A1: evidence from large randomized controlled trials (RCTs) or systematic reviews (including meta-analysis).†

A2: evidence from at least one high-quality cohort.
A3: evidence from at least one moderate-sized RCT or systematic review.[†]
A4: evidence from at least one RCT.
B: evidence from at least one high-quality study of nonrandomized cohorts.
C: expert opinions.
† Arbitrarily, the following cut-off points have been used; large study size: ≥ 100 patients per intervention group; moderate study size: ≥ 50 patients per intervention group.

References

1 Neer CS II. Anterior acromioplasty for the chronic impingement syndrome in the shoulder: a preliminary report. *J Bone Joint Surg Am* 1972; **54**:41–50.
2 Neer CS II. Impingement lesions. *Clin Orthop* 1983; **173**:70–77.
3 Hawkins RJ, Kennedy JC. Impingement syndrome in athletes. *Am J Sports Med* 1980; **8**:151–158.
4 McFarland EG, Hsu CY, Neira C, O'Neil O. Internal impingement of the shoulder: a clinical and arthroscopic analysis. *J Shoulder Elbow Surg* 1999; **8**:458–460.
5 Calis M, Akgun K, Birtane M, *et al.* Diagnostic values of clinical diagnostic tests in subacromial impingement syndrome. *Ann Rheum Dis* 2000; **59**:44–47.
6 MacDonald PB, Clark P, Sutherland K. An analysis of the diagnostic accuracy of the Hawkins and Neer subacromial impingement signs. *J Shoulder Elbow Surg* 2000; **9**:299–301.
7 Litaker D, Pioro M, El Bilbeisi H, Brems J. Returning to the bedside: using the history and physical exam to identify rotator cuff tears. *J Am Geriatr Soc* 2000; **48**:1633–1637.
8 Zaslav KR. Internal rotation resistance strength test: a new diagnostic test to differentiate intra-articular pathology from outlet (Neer) impingement syndrome in the shoulder. *J Shoulder Elbow Surg* 2001; **10**:23–27.
9 Tennent TD, Beach WR, Meyers JF. A review of the special tests associated with shoulder examination. Part I: the rotator cuff tests. *Am J Sports Med* 2003; **31**:154–160.
10 Tennent TD, Beach WR, Meyers JF. A review of the special tests associated with shoulder examination. Part II: laxity, instability, and superior labral anterior and posterior (SLAP) lesions. *Am J Sports Med* 2003; **31**:301–307.
11 Jobe FW, Jobe CM. Painful athletic injuries of the shoulder. *Clin Orthop* 1983; **173**:117–124.
12 Yocum LA. Assessing the shoulder: history, physical examination, differential diagnosis, and special tests used. *Clin Sports Med* 1983; **2**:281–289.
13 Gerber C, Krushell RJ. Isolated rupture of the tendon of the subscapularis muscle: clinical features in 16 cases. *J Bone Joint Surg Br* 1991; **73**:389 – 394.
14 Gerber C, Hersche O, Farron A. Isolated rupture of the subscapularis tendon. *J Bone Joint Surg Am* 1996; **78**:1015–1023.
15 Greis PE, Kuhn JE, Schultheis J, Hintermeister R, Hawkins R. Validation of the lift-off test and analysis of subscapularis activity during maximal internal rotation. *Am J Sports Med* 1996; **24**:589–593.
16 Kelly BT, Kadrmas WR, Speer KP. The manual muscle examination for rotator cuff strength: an electromyographic investigation. *Am J Sports Med* 1996; **24**:581–588.
17 Hertel R, Ballmer FT, Lambert SM, Gerber S. Lag signs in the diagnosis of rotator cuff rupture. *J Shoulder Elbow Surg* 1996; **5**:307–313.
18 Itoi E, Kido T, Sano A, Urayama M, Sato K. Which is more useful, the "full can test" or the "empty can test," in detecting the torn supraspinatus tendon? *Am J Sports Med* 1999; **27**:65–68.
19 Guanche CA, Jones DC. Clinical testing for tears of the glenoid labrum. *Arthroscopy* 2003; **19**:517–523.
20 Snyder SJ, Karzel RP, Del Pizzo W, *et al.* SLAP lesions of the shoulder. *Arthroscopy* 1990; **6**:274–279.
21 Liu SH, Henry MH, Nuccion S, Shapiro MS, Dorey F. Diagnosis of glenoid labral tears: a comparison between magnetic resonance imaging and clinical examinations. *Am J Sports Med* 1996; **24**:149–154.
22 Liu SH, Henry MH, Nuccion SL. A prospective evaluation of a new physical examination in predicting glenoid labral tears. *Am J Sports Med* 1996; **24**:721–725.
23 Guanche CA, Quick DC. Prospective correlation of clinical examination with arthroscopy in the diagnosis of glenoid labral tears [abstract]. *Arthroscopy* 2000; **16**:432–433.
24 Kibler WB. Specificity and sensitivity of the anterior slide test in throwing athletes with superior glenoid labral tears. *Arthroscopy* 1995; **11**:296–300.

25 Kim S, Ha K, Han K. Biceps load test: a clinical test for superior labrum anterior and posterior lesions in shoulders with recurrent anterior dislocations. *Am J Sports Med* 1999; **27**:300–303.

26 Kim S, Ha KI, Ahn JH, Kim SH, Choi HJ. Biceps load test II: a clinical test for SLAP lesions of the shoulder. *Arthroscopy* 2001; **17**:160–164.

27 McFarland EG, Kim TK, Savino RM. Clinical assessment of three common tests for superior labral anterior–posterior lesions. *Am J Sports Med* 2002; **30**:810–815.

28 Morgan CD, Burkhart SS, Palmeri M, *et al.* Type II SLAP lesions: three subtypes and their relationships to superior instability and rotator cuff tears. *Arthroscopy* 1998; **14**:553–565.

29 O'Brien SJ, Pagnani MJ, Fealy S, McGlynn SR, Wilson JB. The active compression test: a new and effective test for diagnosing labral tears and acromioclavicular joint abnormality. *Am J Sports Med* 1998; **26**:610–613.

30 Parentis MA, Mohr KJ, El Attrache NS. Disorders of the superior labrum: review and treatment guidelines. *Clin Orthop Relat Res* 2002; (**400**):77–87.

31 Stetson WB, Templin T. The crank test, the O'Brien test, and routine magnetic resonance imaging scans in the diagnosis of labral tears. *Am J Sports Med* 2002; **30**:806–809.

32 Bennett WF. Specificity of the Speed's test: arthroscopic technique for evaluating the biceps tendon at the level of the bicipital groove. *Arthroscopy* 1998; **14**:789–796.

33 Yergason RM. Supination sign. *J Bone Joint Surg* 1931; **13**:160.

34 Neer CS II, Foster CR. Inferior capsular shift for involuntary inferior and multidirectional instability of the shoulder: a preliminary report. *J Bone Joint Surg Am* 1980; **62**:897–908.

35 Silliman JF, Hawkins RJ. Classification and physical diagnosis of instability of the shoulder. *Clin Orthop Relat Res* 1993; (**291**): 7–19.

36 Gerber C, Ganz R. Clinical assessment of instability of the shoulder, with special reference to anterior and posterior drawer tests. *J Bone Joint Surg Br* 1984; **66**:551–556.

37 Rowe CR, Zarins B. Recurrent transient subluxation of the shoulder. *J Bone Joint Surg Am* 1981; **63**:863–87.

38 Jobe FW, Kvitne RS. Shoulder pain in the overhand or throwing athlete: the relationship of anterior instability and rotator cuff impingement. *Orthop Rev* 1989; **18**:963–975.

39 Speer KP, Hannafin JA, Altchek DW, Warren RF. An evaluation of the shoulder relocation test. *Am J Sports Med* 1994; **22**:177–183.

40 Tzannes A, Walton J, Murrell G. The validity of 23 clinical tests in determining shoulder instability. [Paper presented at the 2000 Pre-Olympic Congress on Sports Medicine and Physical Education International Congress on Sport Science, 7–13 September, Brisbane, Australia 2000.]

CHAPTER 18

How effective are diagnostic tests for the assessment of rotator cuff disease of the shoulder?

Jeremy Lewis and Duncan Tennent

Introduction

Musculoskeletal disorders of the shoulder are extremely common, with one in three people experiencing shoulder pain at some stage of their lives.[1] After lumbar and cervical pathology, shoulder disorders are the most common musculoskeletal condition treated in primary care, with between 1.1% and 1.6% of the population attending their family practitioner annually because of shoulder pain and dysfunction.[2–5] The incidence of shoulder pain substantially increases with age, rising to approximately 20% in individuals aged over 70 years.[1] In addition to the high incidence, shoulder dysfunction is often persistent and recurrent, and associated with substantial morbidity,[6] with 54% of sufferers reporting on-going symptoms after 3 years.[7]

Uhthoff and Sarkar[8] have stated that the majority of shoulder pain arises as a result of the peri-articular soft tissues, especially the rotator cuff. This assertion is supported by the findings of primary-care studies which have reported that the most frequent shoulder diagnosis is that of rotator cuff tendinitis, accounting for approximately one-third of all shoulder diagnoses made by family practitioners.[2,9] The incidence of rotator cuff disease, as a percentage of shoulder pathology presenting to primary care, ranges from 30% to 70%.[1,6]

The spectrum of rotator cuff (RC) and bursal pathologies is extensive and includes: RC tendinosis, RC tendinitis, partial (joint-side, bursal-side, intrasubstance) tears, full-thickness tears, acute bursitis, chronic bursitis, and bursal reaction.[10–19] In addition to this, the hypothesized mechanisms of pathology are broad and have been attributed to; extrinsic causes (acromial impingement, coracoid impingement, internal impingement), intrinsic overload and degeneration, oxidative stress, dietary deficiencies, abnormalities of posture, scapular dyskinesis, evolution, and glenohumeral instability.[19–27] The common clinical classifications of RC disease, such as RC tendinitis and subacromial bursitis are supported by equivocal research findings. Fukuda *et al.*[28] reported no infiltrations or aggregates of neutrophils, lymphocytes or plasma cells, the cells classically associated with acute and chronic inflammation, in rotator cuff tendon specimens taken from 12 subjects with rotator cuff disease during surgery. Uhthoff and Sano[16] stated that the terms "supraspinatus tendinitis" or "rotator cuff tendinitis" appear to be clinical diagnostic terms rather than ones supported by histological or biochemical evidence. This shift in the interpretation of tendon pathology has been supported by a number of authorities.[29–33]

However, Mathews *et al.*[34] reported that biopsies taken at the time of surgery from small and large rotator cuff tears (n = 40) and compared to rotator cuff tissue taken from control subjects (patients undergoing surgery for traumatic instability, n = 4) suggest a different pattern of pathology. The findings revealed an increase in blood vessels, leukocytes and fibroblasts associated with the small tears, and a decrease in blood vessels, leukocytes and fibroblasts, together with increased degeneration, edema, amyloid deposition and chondroid metaplasia associated with the larger tears. No inflammatory cells were identified in the larger tears. There was no correlation between the size of the tears and, age or duration of symptoms. These findings have important implications for management, as the absence of inflammatory cells and the extent of the degeneration in larger tears suggest that they may never heal.

Current understanding of the disease process is lacking, and there is a distinct need for histological and biochemical research across the stages (acute through chronic), as well as the causes (traumatic and nontraumatic), in all the clinical, imaging, and observational interpretations of RC and bursal pathology.

A number of conflicting theories have been proposed to describe the mechanisms causing, and the pathology associated with, rotator cuff disease. Neer[10] proposed that the main mechanism of rotator cuff disease occurred as a result of irritation to the rotator cuff tendons from the overlying acromion during elevation of the arm leading to tendon tissue irritation and inflammation, hence the term tendinitis. In this model, the site of the irritation is hypothesized to be on the superior or bursal surface of the tendon, which is the aspect of the tendon adjacent to the acromion. Although the acromial irritation theory is appealing and has been widely embraced, the evidence to support it is inadequate and largely equivocal. Findings from cadaver studies have demonstrated that rotator cuff tendon pathology occurs more commonly within the internal substance of the tendon (intrasubstance) or on the undersurface (articular or joint side) of the tendon. These are regions of the tendon not coming in contact with the acromion and to a large extent these findings refute the acromial theory.[13,35]

Most anatomical textbooks describe the rotator cuff tendons as distinct structures,[36–38] but Clark and Harryman[39] described a layered structure of the rotator cuff and capsule and reported that all four tendons fuse to form a common insertion into the humeral tuberosities. In the deepest layers of the rotator cuff, the fibers of subscapularis and infraspinatus combine with those of the supraspinatus. Fibers from supraspinatus and subscapularis tendons join to form the floor of the sheath of the biceps tendon, and a slip from the supraspinatus tendon forms a roof over the biceps tendon. The anatomical structure of the rotator cuff and capsule has profound clinical implications. Muscle testing procedures have been proposed that aim at identifying tendon pathology that is associated with weakness and pain. The structural overlap between the tendon fibers and capsule suggests that no test can selectively challenge any one of the rotator cuff tendons, and any response from muscle testing may implicate a number of structures.

An understanding of the nature of rotator cuff pathology is further complicated as a result of the lack of correlation between macroscopic tendon failure, including partial and full-thickness tears, observed in imaging techniques, such as; radiographs, diagnostic ultrasound and magnetic resonance imaging, and symptoms.[40–42] Recent research attention has been directed towards the potential role of oxidative stress[25,43] and biochemical mediation of the symptoms, including the cytokines; vascular endothelial growth factor, interleukin-Iβ (IL-Iβ), and tumor necrosis factor-α (TNFα), and the positively charged neuropeptide, substance P,[44–47] as potential factors involved in tendon pathology and pain. A greater understanding of these biochemical factors may provide opportunities for future management of rotator cuff disease as the extent to which structural pathology correlates with symptoms and functional loss remains uncertain.

Recommendations regarding the diagnosis of rotator cuff disease include; clinical investigations and diagnostic imaging. The clinical investigations involve: history-taking, observation, palpation, range of movement testing, assessment of strength and special tests, and, diagnostic imaging including; radiographs, ultrasound, arthrography, magnetic resonance imaging (MRI) and magnetic resonance arthrography (MRA), and arthroscopy.

The aim of this chapter is to review the literature on clinical testing and diagnostic imaging relating to rotator cuff disease in order to make recommendations to inform clinical practice.

Summary

- Rotator cuff lesions are considered to be the most common musculoskeletal pathology affecting the shoulder.
- Conflicting theories have been proposed to describe the mechanisms leading to the pathology.
- Equivocal findings have been reported from histological research investigating the pathology associated with rotator cuff lesions.

Methods: search strategy

Literature was identified through the MEDLINE, PubMed, EMBASE, CINAHL, AMED and Cochrane databases. Manual searches were also performed. Due to financial and time constraints, only English-language publications were reviewed. Search terms included: shoulder, glenohumeral, subacromial, rotator cuff, tendinitis, tendinosis, tendinopathy, bursa, bursitis, palpation, injection, assessment, tests, imaging, ultrasound, radiograph, magnetic resonance imaging, arthroscope, and outcome measures.

Results

Outcome measures

The benefits of using patient-based functional outcome assessments include: inclusion of the patient's perception of the problem, simplicity, ease of administration, and correlation with overall patient satisfaction.[48–51] The Oxford Shoulder Scale was demonstrated to be more sensitive to change than the SF-36, and more stable over time than the Constant score in patients with and without cuff tears undergoing surgery for impingement.[52] The Oxford Shoulder Scale and the Shoulder Pain and Disability Index demonstrated good and comparable reliability in subjects with subacromial impingement.[53]

Clinical investigation

History

Limited research pertaining to the patient's history was identified following the literature search. The presence of rotator cuff tears identified by arthrography were compared with information taken from the patient's history and physical examination.[54] Although arthrography is not considered to be the "gold standard" for identifying a rotator cuff tear, Litaker *et al.*[54] reported that night pain predicted the presence of a rotator cuff tear. The presence of night pain was reported to have a sensitivity of 87.7%, and a specificity of 19.7%. The associated positive and negative likelihood ratios were: 1.1 and 0.6, respectively. Although the sensitivity is acceptable, the low specificity suggests that conditions, other than RC tears, will also present with a history of night pain.

Observation

Observed muscle wasting in the supra and/or infrascapular fossa was found to be statistically associated ($P < 0.001$) with the presence of a rotator cuff tear.[54] However, the sensitivity (55.6%), specificity (72.9%), the positive likelihood ratio (2.1), and the negative likelihood ratio (0.6) of this observation lack sufficient clinical accuracy to predict a tear.

Posture and muscle imbalance is thought to lead to an alteration in scapular position which in turn may lead to subacromial impingement and rotator cuff pathology.[55–58] Equivocal findings have been reported regarding the relationship between posture and function and presently there is no certainty that an ideal posture exists[27,59] or that it follows the patterns established in the literature.[27,60–63] As such, clinical conclusions relating posture to function and pathology should presently only be considered as speculative. Kibler[20,22] proposed that a positive lateral scapular slide test (LSST) would indicate inadequate scapular stabilization, which may result in subacromial impingement. The test involves measuring the distance between the inferior angle of the scapula and the corresponding thoracic spinous process in three positions. A positive LSST is associated with a side-to-side difference of greater than 1 cm[20] to 1.5 cm[22] in two or more positions. The reliability, sensitivity, and specificity of this test have been challenged,[64,65] and there is no certainty that any observed asymmetry in scapular position equates with impairment occurring as a result of the scapular stabilizing muscles. In addition to this, attempts to classify scapular position and movement patterns from observation into four defined categories currently lack both intra- and interrater reliability.[66]

Palpation

Tendon palpation is recommended as a clinical test to identify tendon pathology. Cook *et al.*[67] reported that although palpation of the patella tendon was a valuable screening test in a symptomatic population and was sufficiently sensitive it lacked specificity. Based on the findings from 24 shoulders (n = 12 cadavers), the positions described in the literature[68,69] to palpate the tendons of the rotator cuff may not be optimal.[70] Table 18.1 is a summary of the findings and recommended positions to palpate the rotator cuff tendons.

No evidence is available for the reliability of palpating the rotator cuff tendons in these positions, or others, or how palpation correlates with symptoms, or its efficacy in predicting outcome.

Transdeltoid palpation (the rent test) requires the patient to relax. Standing behind the patient, the examiner performs palpation through the deltoid anterior to the anterior margin of the acromion.[71] With the elbow flexed, the examiner supports the patient's forearm. The shoulder is positioned in extension and the arm is passively internally and externally rotated. In the presence of a tear both an eminence (the greater tuberosity) and rent are palpable. The sensitivity, specificity, positive and negative likelihood ratios are presented in Table 18.3 (See pp. 337–42 below).

Table 18.1 Recommended positions for rotator cuff tendon palpation

Tendon	Optimal position	Comments
Supraspinatus	Shoulder adduction (10°), internal rotation (85°) and maximal hyperextension (35°) exposed tendon slightly, just in front of acromion adjacent to lateral end of clavicle	Forearm behind back did not expose tendon. Forearm on abdomen did not expose tendon. Exposure is predominantly dependent on hyperextension. This would normally be unacceptable clinically due to patient's pain levels
Infraspinatus and teres minor	Shoulder flexion (90°), shoulder adduction (10°) and external rotation (20°), exposed tendon deep to deltoid at posterior aspect of acromial angle. The teres minor tendon is in ferior to that of infraspinatus	Shoulder hyperextension and forearm behind back do not expose the infraspinatus tendon
Subscapularis	Shoulder adducted to thorax (0°), neutral (no flexion or extension, no internal/ external rotation). Tendon best palpated in deltopectoral triangle between long and short heads of biceps	Shoulder adduction and internal rotation places a substantial portion of the tendon under the short head of biceps and coracobrachialis. Shoulder extension and lateral rotation places the lesser tuberosity and tendon attachment deep to the deltoid muscle
Long head of biceps brachii	Shoulder adduction (0°), internal rotation (20°) ("hands-on-lap position") exposes tendon maximally in deltopectoral triangle (bonded by clavicle superiorly, medial border of deltoid and pectoralis major)	Shoulder external rotation places the tendon under the lateral aspect of the deltoid. Shoulder neutral rotation places the tendon under the anterior aspect of the deltoid muscle

Measuring range of movement

Range of movement is frequently limited in patients with rotator cuff disease,[26,27,72,73] and appropriate clinical methods for assessing movement are therefore required. Recommendations for the clinical measurement of shoulder range of movement include: visual estimation, goniometry, inclinometry, digital devices, photography, and tape measurements.[74–80] Positions for measuring shoulder range also vary and include: seated in a chair with support,[81] seated in a chair without support,[82,83] supine with hips flexed,[83] and standing.[77,78] In addition, both active and passive ranges of movement have been recommended, as well as movement to the end of available range, as well as the first onset of pain. Table 18.2 details the findings of reliability studies that have investigated measuring shoulder range of movement.[74,79,80,84–86] A summary of the findings suggests that no measurement protocol (patient position, measuring equipment, or method of measurement (active or passive range) has demonstrated acceptable reliability to be accredited as the clinical method of choice when assessing range of shoulder movement. The implications of this are that shoulder range of movement assessment and reassessment, are likely to be inaccurate, and determining any change in range post intervention must be done so with caution.

Table 18.2 Measuring range of movement

First author, ref.	Measurement	Subjects	Method	Position	Intrarater reliability	Interrater reliability	Clinical comment
Riddle 1987[74]	Flexion—passive*	S	Short goniometer	Variable	ICC (1,1) 0.98	ICC (1,1) 0.87	SEM and 95% CI not reported
Riddle 1987[74]	Flexion—passive*	S	Long goniometer	Variable	ICC (1,1) 0.98	ICC (1,1) 0.89	SEM and 95% CI not reported
Green 1998[79]	Flexion—active to P1	S	Inclinometer	Sitting	ICC 0.49	ICC 0.72	SEM and 95% CI not reported
Sabari 1998[84]	Flexion—passive	AS +?S	Goniometer	Supine	ICC (2) 0.94		SEM and 95% CI not reported
Sabari 1998[84]	Flexion—active	AS +?S	Goniometer	Supine	ICC (2) 0.95		SEM and 95% CI not reported
Sabari 1998[84]	Flexion—passive	AS +?S	Goniometer	Sitting	ICC (2) 0.95		SEM and 95% CI not reported
Sabari 1998[84]	Flexion—active	AS +?S	Goniometer	Sitting	ICC (2) 0.97		SEM and 95% CI not reported
Hayes 2001[80]	Flexion—passive to end ROM	S	Visual	Sitting	ICC (2,1) 0.59, SEM 13°, 95% CI ± 26°	ICC (2,1) 0.70, SEM 19°, 95% CI ± 38°	Not reliable
Hayes 2001[80]	Flexion—active to end ROM	S	Goniometer	Sitting	ICC (2,1) 0.53, SEM 17°, 95% CI ± 34°	ICC (2,1) 0.69, SEM 25°, 95% CI ± 50°	Not reliable
Riddle 1987[74]	Abduction—passive*	S	Short goniometer	Variable	ICC (1,1) 0.98	ICC (1,1) 0.84	SEM and 95% CI not reported
Riddle 1987[74]	Abduction—passive*	S	Long goniometer	Variable	ICC (1,1) 0.98	ICC (1,1) 0.87	SEM and 95% CI not reported
Croft 1994[85]	Abduction—passive to P1	S	Diagram	Not stated		ICC 0.84	SEM and 95% CI not reported
Croft 1994[85]	Abduction—passive end ROM	S	Diagram	Not stated		ICC 0.95	SEM and 95% CI not reported
Croft 1994[85]	Abduction—preselected range	Not stated	Visual—ROP	Not stated		ICC 0.99	SEM and 95% CI not reported
Green 1998[79]	Abduction—active to P1	S	Inclinometer	Sitting	ICC 0.38	ICC 0.77	SEM and 95% CI not reported
Sabari 1998[84]	Abduction—passive	AS +?S	Goniometer	Supine	ICC (2) 0.98		SEM and 95% CI not reported
Sabari 1998[84]	Abduction—active	AS +?S	Goniometer	Supine	ICC (2) 0.99		SEM and 95% CI not reported
Sabari 1998[84]	Abduction—passive	AS +?S	Goniometer	Sitting	ICC (2) 0.95		SEM and 95% CI not reported
Sabari 1998[84]	Abduction—active	AS +?S	Goniometer	Sitting	ICC (2) 0.97		SEM and 95% CI not reported
Hayes 2001[80]	Abduction—passive to end ROM	S	Visual	Sitting	ICC (2,1) 0.60, SEM 21°, 95% CI ± 42°	ICC (2,1) 0.66, SEM 19°, 95% CI ± 38°	Not reliable

Hayes 2001[84]	Abduction—active to end ROM	S	Goniometer	Sitting	ICC (2,1) 0.58, SEM 23°, 95% CI ± 46°	ICC (2,1) 0.69, SEM 21°, 95% CI ± 38°	Not reliable
Riddle 1987[74]	ER—passive*	S	Short goniometer	Variable	ICC (1,1) 0.98	ICC (1,1) 0.90	SEM and 95% CI not reported
Riddle 1987[74]	ER—passive*	S	Long goniometer	Variable	ICC (1,1) 0.99	ICC (1,1) 0.88	SEM and 95% CI not reported
Croft 1994[85]	ER—passive to end ROM	S	Diagram	Not stated		ICC 0.43	Not reliable
Croft 1994[85]	ER—preselected range	Not stated	Visual—ROP	Not stated		ICC 0.37	Not reliable
Green 1998[79]	ER in neutral—active to P1	S	Inclinometer	Supine	ICC 0.85	ICC 0.88	SEM and 95% CI not reported
Green 1998[79]	ER in abduction—active to P1	S	Inclinometer	Supine	ICC 0.75	ICC 0.65	SEM and 95% CI not reported
Hayes 2001[80]	ER—passive to end ROM	S	Visual	Sitting	ICC (2,1) 0.67, SEM 11°, 95% CI ± 22°	ICC (2,1) 0.57, SEM 14°, 95% CI ± 28°	Not reliable
Hayes 2001[80]	ER—active to end ROM	S	Goniometer	Sitting	ICC (2,1) 0.65, SEM 14°, 95% CI ± 28°	ICC (2,1) 0.57, SEM 14°, 95% CI ± 28°	Not reliable
Riddle 1987[74]	IR—passive*	S	Short goniometer	Variable	ICC (1,1) 0.93	ICC (1,1) 0.43	SEM and 95% CI not reported
Riddle 1987[74]	IR—passive*	S	Long goniometer	Variable	ICC (1,1) 0.94	ICC (1,1) 0.55	SEM and 95% CI not reported
Green 1998[79]	IR in abduction—active to P1	S	Inclinometer	Supine	ICC 0.82	ICC 0.44	SEM and 95% CI not reported
Green 1998[79]	HBB to P1	S	Visual	Standing	ICC 0.84	ICC 0.73	SEM and 95% CI not reported
Hayes 2001[80]	HBB—active to end ROM	S	Tape measure	Standing	ICC (2,1) 0.39, SEM 6 cm, ± 95% CI ± 12 cm	ICC (2,1) 0.39, SEM 6 cm, 95% CI ± 12 cm	Not reliable
Hayes 2001[80]	HBB—passive to end ROM	S	Tape measure	Sitting	ICC (2,1) 0.14, SEM 2SL, 95% CI ± 4SL	ICC (2,1) 0.26, SEM 2SL, 95% CI ± 4SL	Not reliable
Edwards 2002[86]	HBB—preselected level SEM and 95% CI not reported	AS	Visual	Not stated	ICC 0.44, 1–2 SL error from actual level	ICC 0.21 1–2 SL error from actual level	

*, end of range or point of pain not stated; AS, a symptomatic; CI, confidence interval; ER, external rotation; HBB, hand behind back; ICC, intraclass correlation coefficient; ROM, range of movement; ROP, recorded on paper; S, symptomatic; SEM, standard error of measurement; SL, spinal levels.

Measuring strength

Rotator cuff pathology is associated with shoulder weakness.[87–90] The intrarater and interrater reliability of assessing strength of four shoulder movements using a hand-held dynamometer, a spring-scale dynamometer and manual muscle testing was investigated. Shoulder elevation, external rotation, internal rotation and hand behind back lift-off strength were investigated with the hand-held dynamometer and manual testing. Shoulder elevation, external rotation, internal rotation and adduction strength were investigated with the spring-scale dynamometer. The intrarater study involved nine subjects (10 shoulders), eight of whom were symptomatic and within 36 months post rotator cuff repair, and the interrater study involved eight symptomatic subjects (six following RC repair, one with frozen shoulder, and one subject 17 months following scapulothoracic fusion).[90] Although standard error of measurement results were not presented, the intraclass correlation coefficient (ICC) results suggested good to excellent reliability for measuring strength with both the hand-held and spring-scale dynamometers for all the measurements of interest for both intra and interrater reliability. The reliability of manual muscle tests was found to be less reliable than the two measuring devices. These findings were also reflected in the 95% confidence interval results.

The extent to which weakness is attributable to muscle pathology (size and location of tears) is uncertain. Shoulder strength tests were performed with a hand held dynamometer in sixty-one subjects diagnosed with unilateral rotator cuff tears and/or impingement who were scheduled for arthroscopic surgery, at which point tear size was determined by two surgeons blinded to the clinical data. In comparison with the asymptomatic contralateral side, there was no significant relationship between tear size and strength, when strength was tested at 90° of shoulder abduction in the plane of the scapula, external rotation at 90° abduction, or during the "full can test." The only significant finding was that weakness of greater than 50% relative to the asymptomatic side was associated with a large or massive RC tear, when tested at 10° of shoulder abduction.[91] The reliability of the clinical measurements as well as the intraoperative observation of RC tears was not reported.

Perceived weakness during clinical testing may be better explained as occurring as a result of pain inhibition.[87–89] Immediate and significant increases in maximal isometric abduction strength were reported following subacromial local anaesthetic injection in 10 subjects with RC tendinosis.[88] This finding suggests pain inhibition may contribute substantially to a finding of muscle weakness in patients with shoulder pain during clinical tests of strength. This finding is supported by Ben-Yishay *et al.*[87] who reported significant increases in range of movement and strength in 14 patients with impingement syndrome (nine with full-thickness RC tears) following a subacromial injection. This finding was not influenced by the presence of the tear.

At present, no guidance is available to determine whether muscle strength testing should be performed as an isometric contraction or a through-range contraction.

Special clinical tests

Injections

The response to an analgesic injection into the anterior subacromial space (Neer test) is advocated to clinically determine the source of shoulder symptoms.[11] A reduction in pain and increase in range of movement during the Neer sign, Hawkins and Kennedy test, active shoulder elevation, painful arc, following the injection, implicates subacromial tissues as a source of symptoms.[11,92,93] Although this test is in common use, a search of the literature failed to identify any study that has validated it, including the exact mechanism of its action. Appropriately trained physiotherapists are as accurate (67%) as consultant orthopedic surgeons (67%) in therapeutic subacromial injection placement, and both groups are more accurate than registrars (48%), which suggests a learning effect.[94] However, there is concern relating to the ability to accurately locate the subacromial space without imaging guidance.[95–97] Of interest, improvement in shoulder score was obtained in 70% of patients with accurate injections, and in 59% of patients with inaccurate placement, which suggests a generalized "field" effect within the shoulder.[94]

Clinical tests

Recommendations for the clinical evaluation of the integrity of the rotator cuff and the structures within the subacromial space include: shoulder active range of movement tests, shoulder passive range of movement tests, passive tests, resisted movement tests (hypothesized to test muscle strength), passive–active tests, and palpation. The reliability of the clinical examination of rotator cuff pathology has been the subject of investigation in a number of studies.

De Winter *et al.*[98] reported that reliability (Cohen's kappa) was moderate ($\kappa = 0.5$, 95% CI, −0.1 to 1.0) between two physiotherapists for the clinical diagnosis of acute bursitis. The reliability of diagnosing subacromial pathology was moderate ($\kappa = 0.56$, 95% CI, 0.45 to 0.68). Overall the weakest agreement occurred in subjects with chronic complaints, bilateral involvement, and, a high degree of pain. Ostor *et al.*[99] investigated the interrater reliability of a series of clinical tests in 136 patients with shoulder pain ($n = 159$ painful shoulders in total), between a consultant rheumatologist, a specialist registrar and a nurse. Agreement between the clinicians (Cohen's kappa) for a diagnosis of rotator cuff pathology (undifferentiated) ranged between 0.38 (specialist registrar/nurse) to 0.46 (consultant/specialist registrar) suggesting fair to moderate reliability. The 95% confidence interval results were not presented. Agreement between the clinicians for the presence of impingement syndrome ranged from 0.16 (consultant/nurse) to 0.43 (specialist registrar/nurse) suggesting slight to fair reliability. Using the Cyriax assessment approach,[100,101] four clinicians completed a series of clinical tests in 53 patients with a range of shoulder conditions.[102] They reported that on the basis of the findings, the interrater reliability (Cohen's kappa coefficient) results for the diagnosis of subacromial bursitis ranged from 0.35 (expert assessor and assessor 1, 95% CI, −0.03 to 0.73), to 0.58 (expert assessor and assessor 2, 95% CI, 0.29 to 0.87), suggesting fair reliability. For the diagnosis of a rotator cuff lesion, the interrater kappa results ranged from 0.71 (expert assessor and assessor 1, and expert assessor and assessor 3, 95% CI, 0.49 to 0.93) to 0.79 (expert assessor and assessor 2, 95% CI, 0.61 to 0.96), suggesting moderate reliability.

Most clinical tests have two possible outcomes. A positive result implies the condition is present, and a negative result implies the condition is not present. Sensitivity is the "true-positive rate"—true-positive/(true-positive + false-negative)—for a test, and is the percentage of subjects with the diagnosis (condition) who are correctly identified (by the test) as positive. For a sensitive test, a positive result will rule in the condition and a negative result will rule out the presence of that condition. Specificity is the "true-negative rate"—true-negative/(true-negative + false-positive)—for a test, and is the percentage of subjects without the diagnosis (condition) who are correctly identified (by the test) as negative. For a specific test, a negative result will rule out the condition and a positive result will rule in the presence of that condition. An ideal clinical test will have a sensitivity of 100% and a specificity of 100%. Likelihood ratios provide an additional method to describe the accuracy of a clinical test. A positive likelihood ratio (sensitivity/[1-specificity]), or the ratio of the true-positive rate to the false-positive rate, provides an indication of how much more likely a positive test finding is in people with the condition than those without, and a negative likelihood ratio ([1-sensitivity]/specificity), or the ratio of the false-positive rate to the true-negative rate, provides an indication of how much more likely a negative test finding is for patients who have the condition than for those who do not. In clinical practice, positive likelihood ratios with values greater than 3 suggest the test is useful, and values greater than 10 suggest the test is very useful. The smallest negative likelihood ratio possible is zero; tests with values less than 0.33 (one-third) are useful and values less than 0.1 (one-tenth) are very useful. Table 18.3 presents the results of the sensitivity, specificity, and positive and negative likelihood ratios for clinical tests designed to detect rotator cuff pathology against a defined reference test (diagnostic ultrasound, MRI, arthroscopy). Detailed descriptions of the clinical tests included in this review are available.[54,71,93,99,103–108]

Combinations of tests

Calis *et al.*[93] reported that a negative finding in all seven tests they investigated indicated with a high probability that the diagnosis was not impingement syndrome. A positive Hawkins test together with a positive drop-arm sign indicated that the patient had Zlatkin stage 3 impingement (complete disruption of the supraspinatus tendon identified on MRI). Zlatkin stage 2 impingement (increased signal intensity with irregularity and thinning of the tendon) was best identified with a combination of the Neer sign and the horizontal adduction test.

Litaker *et al.*[54] reported that weakness in external rotation and night pain in patients aged 65 years or older strongly supported a diagnosis of RC tear (observed on arthrogram). The sensitivity decreased (70.8%) and the specificity increased (50.8%) for the clinical assessment of bursitis when the Neer impingement sign and Hawkins test were combined. The specificity increased (55.7%) and the sensitivity remained constant (83.3%) for the clinical assessment of RC pathology when the Hawkins test and Neer sign were combined. The specificity marginally increased (50.8%) and the sensitivity decreased (70.8%) when these two tests were combined to assess bursitis.[105] These findings suggest that separately or in combination, the Neer sign and Hawkins test, are sensitive tests for the pathology observed arthroscopically suggestive of subacromial bursitis or partial or full-thickness RC tears. However these tests individually or in combination lack sufficient specificity.

When the "full cans" and "empty cans" tests are compared, it appears that muscle weakness is a stronger predictor of full-thickness RC tears observed in MRI than the presence of pain, and both tests are equivalent in terms of diagnostic accuracy. The presence of pain during the "full cans" test is a better predictor of a full-thickness RC tear than the "empty cans" test.[106]

Murrell and Walton[109] compared the diagnostic value of 23 clinical tests with the status of the rotator cuff observed arthroscopically in 400 patients. They reported that an individual had a 98% chance of having a rotator cuff tear if the combination of three clinical tests (supraspinatus weakness, weakness in external rotation and the presence of impingement) was present. If two of these tests were positive and the patient was aged 60 years or older, there was also a 98% chance of having a rotator cuff tear.

Table 18.3 Clinical tests designed to detect rotator cuff pathology against defined reference tests

First author, ref.	Comments	Sensitivity (%)	Specificity (%)	LR+	LR–	Reference test(s)
Active tests						
Test: painful arc (Kessel and Watson 1977)						
Calis (2000)[93]	Neer impingement test performed on 120 patients with shoulder pain. Following injection, 84 patients (85 shoulders) were considered to have SIS/RC pathology	32.5	80.5	1.6	0.8	Neer test (10 mL 1% lignocaine anterior approach). MRI (Zlatkin *et al.* 1989 SIS stages)
Litaker (2000)[54]	448 patients with suspected RC tear undergoing arthrography. 301 patients (67.2%) had evidence of a complete or partial RC tear	97.5	9.9	1.1	0.3	Presence of partial or complete RC tear on shoulder arthrogram
Park (2005)[104]	Series of clinical tests performed in 913 patients with shoulder conditions. All tests performed with the subjects standing. 361 excluded and final study involved assessment of 552. Study population divided into 2 groups: nonimpingement (n = 193) and impingement (n = 359). Impingement group subdivided into impingement with no tear (bursitis) (n = 72), partial-thickness tear (n = 72), and full-thickness tear (n = 215).					Shoulder arthroscopic
	Bursitis	70.6	46.9	1.3	0.6	
	Partial-thickness RC tear	67.4	47.0	1.3	0.7	
	Full-thickness RC tear	75.8	61.8	1.9	0.4	
	All categories combined	73.5	81.1	3.9	0.3	
Shoulder passive range of movement tests						
Test: passive elevation						
Litaker (2000)[54]	See above. Patient supine, examiner elevates shoulder to maximal range, defined as ≥ 170°	30.2	78.1	1.4	0.9	See above
Test: passive external rotation						
Litaker (2000)[54]	See above. Patient supine, elbow flexed to 90°. Examiner externally rotates shoulder to maximal range, defined as ≥ 70°	19.0	83.6	1.2	0.9	See above

Continued

Table 18.3 *(Continued)*

First author, ref.	Comments	Sensitivity (%)	Specificity (%)	LR+	LR–	Reference test(s)
Shoulder passive tests						
Test: Neer impingement sign (Neer 1972, 1983)						
Calis (2000)[93]	See above (patient upright)	88.7	30.5	1.3	0.4	See above
Litaker (2000)[54]	See above (patient supine)	97.4	9.0	1.2	0.3	See above
MacDonald (2000)[105]	85 consecutive subjects assessed with the Neer sign. The results were then compared with the appearance of the shoulder at arthroscopy					Shoulder arthroscopy
	Appearance suggestive of bursitis (24/85)	75.0	47.5	1.4	0.5	
	Appearance suggestive of RC tear (24/85)	83.5	50.8	1.7	0.3	
	Bursitis and RC tear	77.0	62.5	2.1	0.4	
Park (2005)[104]	See above					See above
	Bursitis	85.7	42.9	1.7	0.3	
	Partial-thickness RC tear	75.4	47.5	1.4	0.5	
	Full-thickness RC tear	59.3	47.2	1.1	0.9	
	All categories combined	68.0	68.7	2.2	0.5	
Test: Hawkins test (Hawkins and Kennedy 1980)						
Calis (2000)[93]	See above	92.1	25.0	1.2	0.3	See above
MacDonald (2000)[105]	85 consecutive subjects clinical assessed with the Hawkins test. The results were then compared with the appearance of the shoulder at arthroscopy					See above
	Appearance suggestive of bursitis (24/85)	91.7	44.3	1.7	0.2	
	Appearance suggestive of RC tear (24/85)	87.5	42.6	1.5	0.3	
	Bursitis and RC tear	88.9	60.0	2.2	0.2	
Park (2005)[104]	See above					See above
	Bursitis	75.7	44.5	1.4	0.6	
	Partial-thickness RC tear	75.4	44.4	1.4	0.6	
	Full-thickness RC tear	68.7	48.3	1.3	0.7	
	All categories combined	71.5	66.3	2.1	0.4	

Test: horizontal adduction "cross body test" (McLaughlin 1951)						
Calis (2000)[93]	Arm is passively horizontally adducted across the body with elbow flexed. Pain indicates positive test	82.0	27.7	1.1	0.7	See above
Park (2005)[104]	See above					See above
	Bursitis	25.4	79.7	1.3	0.9	
	Partial-thickness RC tear	16.7	78.5	0.8	1.1	
	Full-thickness RC tear	23.4	80.8	1.2	0.9	
	All categories combined	22.5	82.0	1.3	0.9	
Resisted movement tests						
Test: "full can test" (Kelly *et al.* 1996)						
Itoi (1999)[106]	Clinical assessment of the "full can test" in 136 consecutive patients (n = 143 shoulders). Test interpreted as positive in the presence of pain, weakness, or, pain and weakness					MRI. 35 shoulders with RC FTT. Ss FTT, 19 tears; Ss +Is FTT, 11 tears; Ss + Is + Subs FTT, 5 tears
	Pain	66.0 (23/35)	64.0 (69/108)	1.8	0.5	
	Muscle weakness	77.0 (27/35)	74.0 (80/108)	2.9	0.3	
	Pain, muscle weakness, or both	86.0 (30/35)	57.0 (62/108)	2.1	0.2	
Test: "empty can test" (Jobe and Moynes 1982)						
Itoi (1999)[106]	See above. Clinical assessment of the "empty can test"					See above
	Pain	63.0 (22/35)	55.0 (59/108)	1.4	0.7	
	Muscle weakness	77.0 (27/35)	68.0 (73/108)	2.4	0.3	
	Pain, muscle weakness, or both	89.0 (31/35)	50.0 (54/108)	1.8	0.2	
Park (2005)[104]	See above					See above
	Bursitis	25.0	66.9	0.8	1.1	
	Partial-thickness RC tear	32.1	67.8	1.0	1.0	
	Full-thickness RC tear	52.6	82.4	3.0	0.6	
	All categories combined	44.1	89.5	4.2	0.6	
Test: Speed (Gilcreest and Albi 1939)						
Calis (2000)[93]	Shoulder flexed to 60°, elbow extended, forearm supinated. Humeral elevation resisted. Pain in the bicipital groove indicates biceps tendon pathology	68.5	55.5	1.5	0.6	See above

Continued

Table 18.3 *(Continued)*

First author, ref.	Comments	Sensitivity (%)	Specificity (%)	LR+	LR–	Reference test(s)
Park (2005)[104]	See above					See above
	Bursitis	33.3	69.8	1.1	0.9	
	Partial-thickness RC tear	33.3	70.6	1.1	0.9	
	Full-thickness RC tear	39.9	75.3	1.6	0.8	
	All categories combined	38.3	83.3	2.3	0.7	
Test: external rotation (Leroux *et al.* 1995)						
Park (2005)[104]	See above					See above
	Bursitis	25.0	68.9	0.8	1.1	
	Partial-thickness RC tear	19.4	69.1	0.6	1.2	
	Full-thickness RC tear	50.5	84.0	3.2	0.6	
	All categories combined	41.6	90.1	4.2	0.7	
Test: Yerganson Test						
Calis (2000)[93]	Elbow flexed to 90°, forearm pronated. Patient actively supinated forearm against resistance. Pain localized to the bicipital grove indicates disorder of long head of biceps	37.9	86.1	2.7	0.73	See above
Test: internal rotation resistance strength test (Zaslav 2001)						
Zaslav (2001)[107]	Shoulder in 90° abduction and 80° to 85° of external rotation. Patient is then requested to maximally resist first external and then internal rotation. Purpose to guide choice of surgery. Prospective findings from 110 patients with positive impingement sign who had failed conservative treatment (injection and exercise therapy). Weakness of internal rotation (n = 26) hypothesized to differentiate intra-articular pathology or secondary impingement (due to microinstability) versus weakness in external rotation (n = 84) hypothesized to detect subacromial impingement. Postoperative results not reported	88	96	22	0.1	Arthroscopic findings

Shoulder passive–active tests						
Test: drop sign (Hertel *et al.* 1996)						
Hertel (1996)[108]	100 consecutive patients with impingement syndrome. Patient seated, shoulder 90° abduction and full external rotation. Examiner releases arm and if observed to "drop" indicates loss of integrity of infraspinatus	44.4	98.3	26.1	0.6	Presence of no tear, partial-thickness tear, or full-thickness tear at operation. 24: no structural lesion; 19: PTT supraspinatus; 17: FTT supraspinatus; 11: rupture supra- and infraspinatus; 5: PTT subscapularis; 8: FTT subscapularis; 16: PTT or FTT of supra- and infraspinatus and subscapularis
Test: drop-arm sign (Codman 1934)						
Calis (2000)[93]	See above. Patient is requested to control lowering of the arm (adduction) from 90° abduction. Inability to do this is suggestive of an RC tear	7.8	97.2	2.8	0.9	See above
Park (2005)[104]	See above					See above
	Bursitis	13.6	77.3	0.6	1.1	
	Partial-thickness RC tear	14.3	77.5	0.6	1.1	
	Full-thickness RC tear	34.9	87.5	2.8	0.7	
	All categories combined	26.9	88.4	2.3	0.8	
Test: external rotation lag sign						
Hertel (1996)[108]	See above. Patient seated. Elbow passively flexed to 90°, shoulder elevated 20° (in scapular plane) and held 5° off maximal external rotation. The patient is then requested to maintain the position actively when the examiner releases the wrist while maintaining support through the elbow. Designed to test the integrity of the supraspinatus and infraspinatus tendons	68.3	100	34.8	0.3	See above

Continued

Table 18.3 *(Continued)*

First author, ref.	Comments	Sensitivity (%)	Specificity (%)	LR+	LR−	Reference test(s)
Test: internal rotation lag sign						
Hertel (1996)[108]	See above. Patient is seated with the arm of the hand of the painful shoulder placed at the lumbar region (hand behind back). The hand is passively lifted from the lumbar spine until almost full internal rotation is reached. The patient is then asked to actively maintain the position. A lag is positive. Designed to test the integrity of the subscapularis tendon	62	100	31	0.4	Presence of no tear, partial-thickness tear, or full-thickness tear at operation
Palpation						
Test: transdeltoid palpation (the rent test)						
Wolf (2001)[71]	The rent test is performed by palpating through the anterior deltoid, anterior to the anterior margin of the acromion and is used to diagnose a full-thickness rotator cuff tear. For a full description refer to Codman 1934, and, Wolf and Agrawal 2001. The test was performed on 109 patients prior to surgery. 46/109 had a full-thickness tear identified at surgery. 44/109 had a positive rent test for a full-thickness tear of the rotator cuff. 61/63 who had a negative rent test were reported to have impingement, partial-thickness tear or acromioclavicular pathology					Shoulder arthroscopy in 109 patients, MRI in 71 of 109 patients
	Palpation versus arthroscope (n = 109)	95.7	96.8	29.9	0.04	
	Palpation versus MRI (n = 71)	90.9	89.5	8.7	0.10	

FTT, full-thickness tear; Is, infraspinatus; LR–, negative likelihood ratio; LR+, positive likelihood ratio; MRI, magnetic resonance imaging; RC, rotator cuff; SIS, shoulder impingement syndrome; Ss, supraspinatus; Subs, subscapularis.

A positive Hawkins test together with the presence of a painful arc and weakness in external rotation was found to provide the best combination for the clinical diagnosis of impingement syndrome. The combination of a positive painful arc, positive drop-arm sign and weakness in external rotation provides the best diagnosis of a full-thickness rotator cuff tear.[104]

Summary

• The majority of clinical tests used to identify rotator cuff pathology lack sufficient sensitivity and specificity to accurately predict a rotator cuff lesion.
• Currently, no assessment protocol has demonstrated sufficient clinical reliability for measuring shoulder range of movement or strength.
• Perceived deficiencies in strength during clinical testing may be attributable more to pain inhibition than true muscle weakness.
• Although the mechanism of action is unknown, analgesic injection into the anterior subacromial space may inform the clinical decision-making process regarding the region of symptoms.
• Combinations of clinical tests may be more useful in the clinical reasoning process than the results of individual tests.

Imaging investigations

The use of imaging

Imaging procedures are frequently requested and interpretations of findings are based on the premise that observable structural failure is associated with pain and functional limitation. To assist in the diagnosis of rotator cuff pathology a number of imaging modalities are available. These include radiographs, ultrasound, and MRI. Studies have been conducted to ascertain their efficacy, and comparisons have been made between their ability to distinguish full-thickness and partial-thickness tears, and, in some cases tendinopathy.

However, the assumption that a correlation exists between structural pathology, symptoms, and functional loss has not been demonstrated, and findings from imaging studies in subjects without a history of shoulder pain or loss of function have suggested that normal pain-free function may continue in the presence of substantial structural pathology.

MRI scanning of the dominant asymptomatic shoulder was performed in 96 subjects.[41] Questionnaires were administered to exclude a history of shoulder symptoms. Between the ages of 40 to 60 years, one in three subjects were found to have an RC tear (4% full-thickness tear, 24% partial-thickness tear). Structural pathology was demonstrated in one in two asymptomatic subjects aged 60 years or more (28% full-thickness tear, 26% partial-thickness tear). Milgrom *et al.*[40] reported a 55% incidence of asymptomatic full-thickness RC tears, and that the presence of pathology was equal for the dominant and nondominant shoulders. Frost *et al.*[42] matched 42 subjects with impingement syndrome with 31 asymptomatic controls. They reported that 55% of the symptomatic group and 52% of the asymptomatic group had supraspinatus pathology observed in MRI. Of note, in the 31–39-year-old age group, tears were more prevalent in subjects without symptoms (43%) than those with (20%). In the 40–49-year-old group, an equal number of tears (48%) were present. The percentage of those with tears increased to 78%, but continued to remain equal between the subjects with and without symptoms in the older group (50–59 years). Miniaci *et al.*[110] reported that in an MRI study of 14 asymptomatic professional baseball pitchers (mean age 20.1 years) that 79% had RC changes in the supraspinatus and infraspinatus of the throwing arm, and 86% had changes in RC of the nonthrowing arm. Of note, glenoid labrum abnormalities were noted in 76% of subjects in the dominant shoulder and 76% in the nondominant shoulder. Two subjects were found to have asymptomatic SLAP (superior labrum anterior to posterior) lesions. Schibany *et al.*[111] reported that a complete rupture of the RC was identified by ultrasound in 6% of 212 individuals without symptoms aged between 56 and 83 years. This was confirmed in MRI in 90% of subjects.

Three distinct shapes of the acromion have been described: type I, flat; type II, curved; and type III, hooked. It was proposed that these shapes represent morphological variations that are identifiable radiologically[12,112] and that individuals with the type II or type III morphological variation are more susceptible to impingement syndrome and RC pathology. However, the concept of morphological variations in the shape of the acromion has been challenged and these changes have been described as degenerative changes and the hook associated with the Bigliani type III acromion represents a degenerative osteophytic spur growing within the coracoacromial ligament due to tension on the ligament.[35,113–116] Furthermore, Worland *et al.*[116] reported findings following a study correlating age, rotator cuff tearing, and acromial morphology in 59 asymptomatic individuals and concluded that clinicians should interpret the radiological presence of curved or hooked acromions, as well as RC tears with caution, due to the high incidence in people without symptoms.

The conclusions of these imaging studies in asymptomatic individuals were that structural RC pathology is related to age and do not correlate with painful shoulder dysfunction, and, treatment should be based on clinical and not on imaging findings.

Although there is no evidence to suggest that any imaging modality has the sensitivity to detect painful and symptomatic rotator cuff lesions associated with a functional loss, the following analysis is undertaken to review research evidence for the efficacy of imaging modalities to identify RC structural pathology. To determine the usefulness of these modalities, they need to be compared against an appropriate reference test. Arthroscopy is an invasive procedure where a fiberoptic endoscope is introduced into the shoulder to allow direct visualization of the shoulder structures. Arthroscopy allows for visualization of both sides of the RC and may be better than arthrography at detecting partial-thickness tears.[117]

Diagnostic ultrasound

Ultrasound uses linear transducers with frequencies usually in the range of 5–13 MHz to generate a pulse to record reflected waves of a sound beam in two dimensions and is used primarily to generate images of soft tissue.[117] Zehetgruber *et al.*[118] retrospectively compared ultrasound findings in a group of 332 consecutive patients undergoing shoulder surgery (arthroscopic n = 205, open n = 96). They did not differentiate between full and partial-thickness tears and reported 98% sensitivity and 93% specificity for either a complete nonvisualization of the cuff tendons or localized absence and focal discontinuity. Size and location of the tear was correctly identified in 69/96 cases (72%). The surgeons were aware of the ultrasound findings at the time of surgery. They concluded that ultrasound was of limited value for evaluation of the small RC tears. Prickett *et al.*[119] reported a sensitivity of 91% and specificity of 86% for the pooled results of partial and full-thickness RC tears in a retrospective analysis of ultrasound results compared with arthroscopic findings in 44 subjects undergoing revision surgery. Again, the surgeons were aware of the ultrasound findings. Teefey *et al.*[120] prospectively compared ultrasound and MRI in 124 consecutive patients, of whom 71 (55%) underwent arthroscopy. The ultrasound findings for full and partial-thickness tears were pooled as tears, and the findings for partial-thickness tears and no tears were pooled as no tears. The sensitivity and specificity of ultrasound compared with arthroscopic findings to detect a tear was 97% and 67%, respectively. They also reported that ultrasound correctly identified 45/46 (98%) full-thickness tears and 13/19 (68%) partial-thickness tears. Iannotti *et al.*[121] reported that in comparison to surgical findings (open and arthroscopic) a correct diagnosis was made using ultrasound in 37/42 (88%) full-thickness tears and 70% (20/37) partial-thickness tears, and 16/20 (80%) of normal tendons. They also reported that there was no significant difference between ultrasound and MRI in the detection of full-thickness tears.

From a surgical management perspective, the distinction between partial and full-thickness tears is important and it is essential that any diagnostic tool be able to distinguish between the two. Studies not making this distinction have not been included in the following review. Although arthroscopy has certain limitations, it is considered to be the gold standard reference test due to its ability to directly visualize the rotator cuff and distinguish between partial and full-thickness tears. As such, this review will only consider imaging modalities referenced against arthroscopy.[117] Table 18.4 depicts studies that have compared the sensitivity and specificity of ultrasound compared with arthroscopic findings.[122–133]

Magnetic resonance imaging

MRI allows multiplanar imaging. Patients lie in a magnetic field which causes certain nuclei to align in the direction of the field. Radiofrequency pulses are then generated which produce an image.[117] Teefey *et al.*[120] reported that MRI correctly identified 46/46 (100%) full-thickness tears and 12/19 (63%) partial-thickness tears. The sensitivity and specificity of MRI compared with arthroscopic findings to detect a tear (pooled results of full and partial-thickness tears) was 100% and 67%, respectively. MRI led to a correct diagnosis in 95% (40/42) full-thickness tears, 73% (27/37) partial-thickness tears, and 75% (15/20) normal tendons, in comparison with surgical findings.[121] Zlatkin *et al.*[134] reported that in 130 patients undergoing surgery (arthroscopy n = 103, open n = 57) for RC tears, the sensitivity and specificity of MRI for pooled partial-thickness (n = 34) and full-thickness tears (n = 96) was 90% and 93%, respectively.

In the following analysis, for the reasons outlined earlier, only MRI findings that have attempted to differentiate partial and full-thickness tears, and compared with arthroscopy will be presented.[117] These findings are presented in Table 18.5.[122,130,132,135–140]

The results suggest that both MRI and ultrasound are relatively accurate modalities for the diagnosis of rotator cuff pathology when referenced against arthroscopy. Both are less accurate in the diagnosis of partial-thickness tears. In all papers included in this review, the specificity of the two imaging modalities is higher than the sensitivity in relation to diagnosing a partial-thickness tear. This indicates that these modalities are more accurate for ruling out a partial structural lesion than ruling one in. As all the subjects in these studies underwent arthroscopic or open shoulder surgery in secondary-care institutions, it is most probable that they represent a more extreme spectrum of rotator cuff and subacromial pathology than that encountered in primary care and the patient group not requiring specialist attention. The sensitivity, accuracy, and therefore usefulness of the modalities to diagnose pathology in a less advanced stage of a condition potentially will be lower. The

Table 18.4 The use of diagnostic ultrasound to identify rotator cuff pathology

First author, ref. (patients)	Any tear		Full-thickness tear		Partial-thickness tear		Prevalence	Comments
	Sensitivity (95% CI)	Specificity (95% CI)	Sensitivity (95% CI)	Specificity (95% CI)	Sensitivity (95% CI)	Specificity (95% CI)		
Nelson 1991 (n = 19)[122]			60 (23–88)	93 (69–99)	36 (15–65)	75 (41–93)	FTT 37%, PTT 57%	Preoperative assessment Prospective
Brenneke 1992 (n = 120)[123]	78 (67–87)	82 (70–90)	95 (83–97)	93 (85–97)	41 (25–59)	91 (84–96)	AT 54%, FTT 32%, PTT 23%	Subjects had both US and MRI
Wiener 1993 (n = 225)[124]	95 (90–97)	94 (86–98)	93 (86–97)	99 (96–100)	94 (86–98)	97 (93–99)	AT 70%, FTT 40%, PTT 30%	Preoperative assessment. Surgeon unaware of US findings
Van Holsbeeck 1995 (n = 52)[125]	98 (98–100)	83 (61–94)	100 (90–100)	100 (90–100)	93 (70–99)	94 (84–98)	AT 73%, FTT 51%, PTT 22%	Preoperative assessment. Interpretation not blinded to surgical findings
Van Moppes 1995 (n = 41)[126]	80 (58–92)	95 (77–99)	100 (57–100)	100 (90–100)	73 (48–89)	96 (81–99)	AT 49%, FTT 12%, PTT 37%	Symptoms suggestive of RC pathology. Not all subjects underwent surgery

Takagishi 1996 (n = 122)[127]	72 (60–82)	89 (79–95)	76 (61–87)	100 (96–100)	50 (30–70)	90 (83–95)	AT 48%, FTT 31%, PTT 16%	Preoperative assessment
Sonnabend 1997 (n = 110)[128]	70 (58–79)	95 (84–99)	84 (71–92)	92 (83–97)	25 (12–45)	99 (94–100)	AT 48%, FTT 31%, PTT 16%	Preoperative assessment. Consecutive patients
Read 1998 (n = 42)[129]	79 (63–90)	88 (53–98)	100 (72–100)	97 (84–99)	46 (23–71)	97 (83–99)	AT 81%, FTT 24%, PTT 31%	Preoperative assessment. Prospective. Surgeon aware of US findings
Swen 1999 (n = 21)[130]			69 (42–87)	88 (53–98)			FTT 62%	Failed conservative treatment. No comment on PTT
Teefey 2000 (n = 100)[131]	90 (81–95)	85 (64–95)	100 (94–100)	91 (78–97)	47 (25–70)	93 (85–97)	AT 80%, FTT 65%, PTT 15%	Preoperative assessment. Retrospective. Surgeon aware of US findings
Martin-Hervas 2001 (n = 61)[132]	71 (54–83)	67 (48–81)	58 (39–74)	100 (90–100)	13 (2–47)	68 (55–79)	AT 56%, FTT 43%, PTT 13%	Subjects had both US and MRI
Roberts 2001 (n = 24)[133]	76 (53–90)	100 (65–100)	80 (49–94)	100 (78–100)	71 (36–92)	100 (82–100)	AT 71%, FTT 42%, PTT 29%	Prospective. Surgeon aware of US findings

AT, any tear; CI, confidence interval; FTT, full-thickness tear; MRI, magnetic resonance imaging; PTT, partial-thickness tear; RC, rotator cuff; US, ultrasonography.

Table 18.5 The use of magnetic resonance imaging to identify rotator cuff pathology

First author, ref. (patiects)	Any tear		Full-thickness tear		Partial-thickness tear		Prevalence	Comments
	Sensitivity (95% CI)	Specificity (95% CI)	Sensitivity (95% CI)	Specificity (95% CI)	Sensitivity (95% CI)	Specificity (95% CI)		
Nelson 1991 (n = 21)[122]	88 (53–98)	77 (50–92)	86 (49–97)	93 (69–99)	67 (39–86)	89 (56–98)	FTT 33%, PTT 57%	Preoperative assessment Prospective compared MRI and US
Hodler 1992 (n = 36)[135]	41 (22–64)	79 (57–91)	100 (51–100)	88 (72–95)	80 (10–33)	91 (73–98)	AT 57%, FTT 11%, PTT 47%	Arthroscopy from notes
Traughber 1992 (n = 28)[136]	71 (45–88)	93 (69–99)	100 (57–100)	100 (86–100)	56 (27–81)	95 (75–99)	AT 50%, FTT 18%, PTT 32%	Failed conservative treatment Retrospective
Quinn 1995 (n = 100)[137]	84 (67–93)	97 (90–99)	85 (64–95)	99 (93–100)	82 (52–95)	99 (94–100)	AT 31%, FTT 20%, PTT 11%	Failed conservative treatment Retrospective from surgical notes
Tuite 1995 (n = 100)[138]	93 (83–97)	75 (61–85)	91 (72–97)	95 (87–98)	74 (55–87)	87 (76–93)	AT 56%, FTT 25%, PTT 31%	Consecutive patients who had both MRI and arthroscopy. MRI known at surgery

Balich 1997 (n = 222)[139]	76.0 (65–84)	94 (89–97)	96 (85–99)	97 (93–98)	42 (26–61)	97 (93–99)	AT 30%, FTT 20%, PTT 18%	Failed conservative treatment. Results for most experienced MRI reader 5 radiologists reported pre- and postarthroscopy
Wnorowski 1997 (n = 39)[140]	86a (60–96)	52a (33–70)	56a (27–81)	73a (56–86)	33a (60–79)	100a (91–100)	AT 37%, FTT 23%, PTT 13%	Compared nonspecialist radiographers (a) to specialist radiologists (b)
	71b (45–88)	71b (51–85)	78b (45–94)	83b (65–92)	0b (0–43)	68b (51–81)		
Swen 1999 (n = 21)[130]			85 (58–96)	88 (53–98)			FTT 57%	Conservative treatment failed No comment on PTT
Martin-Hervas 2001 (n = 61)[132]	91 (77–97)	74 (55–87)	81 (62–91)	97 (85–99)	50 (22–78)	75 (62–85)	AT 56%, FTT 43%, PTT 13%	Preoperative patients Subjects had both US and MRI

AT, any tear; CI, confidence interval; FTT, full-thickness tear; MRI, magnetic resonance imaging; PTT, partial-thickness tear; US, ultrasonography.

results of the reported studies may have been influenced by the prior knowledge the majority of surgeons had regarding the imaging findings in the intraoperative setting and this prior knowledge had the very real potential of biasing the findings. The fact that different models and generations of ultrasound and MRI equipment, together with different imaging protocols, would also have introduced other confounding factors into the study findings. The findings of some studies were difficult to interpret, as different RC structural pathologies were pooled by some authors, with full-thickness tears and partial-thickness tears being grouped together as tears, or partial-thickness tears and no tears being classified as no tears.

In conclusion, there is good evidence that both ultrasound and MRI are accurate at identifying full-thickness tears in the rotator cuff and to a lesser extent diagnosing partial-thickness tears. However, the significance of these findings is open to interpretation, as neither of the imaging modalities is capable of detecting a symptomatic tear from a tear not associated with pain or functional loss.

Summary

• The incidence of rotator cuff tears observed in imaging studies appears to be equal in symptomatic populations and in people without shoulder symptoms.

• No correlation between positive imaging findings and symptoms has been demonstrated.

• Clinicians are advised to interpret radiological, ultrasound, and MRI findings of rotator cuff pathology with caution.

• Both MRI and ultrasound are accurate modalities for the diagnosis of rotator pathology when referenced against arthroscopy.

• Both modalities are more accurate at identifying full-thickness tears and less accurate at identifying partial-thickness tears.

• Bias in the reported studies, together with study design, may have influenced the reported findings.

• Limited research is available to determine the diagnostic accuracy of MRI and ultrasound for patients in the early or less severe stages of rotator cuff pathology.

Conclusions

Within the spectrum of musculoskeletal disorders of the shoulder, pathologies involving the rotator cuff and subacromial bursa are the most common. Our understanding of factors leading to rotator cuff disease and the disease process itself is limited and based more upon clinical theory than conclusive evidence. The incidence of structural rotator cuff pathology increases with advancing age. Degenerative, partial and full thickness tears of the rotator cuff occur in people without shoulder symptoms and the radiological and imaging evidence suggests that the incidence of rotator cuff pathology appears to equal and in some cases exceeds that of patients with symptoms. The relatively poor correlation between imaging findings and symptoms has an impact on clinical decision making.

A myriad of clinical tests have been proposed to selectively compress, stretch, contract or relax the tissues of the rotator cuff and subacromial bursa, which aim at differentiating the involved structure or structures. The findings of this review suggest that there is an insufficient number of studies that have evaluated the spectrum of clinical tests in the same manner, using the same reference tests to draw definitive conclusions to guide practice regarding the clinical assessment of the rotator cuff and subacromial bursa. Clinical tests require a reference test to be compared against in order to determine the diagnostic accuracy of the test. No reference test has emerged that may be considered as the one gold standard. This is because the reference tests identify structural pathology, and there is no evidence for the correlation of structural pathology and symptoms. Arthroscopy appears to be the gold standard in identifying both partial-thickness and full-thickness rotator cuff tears. Studies that have used arthroscopy as a reference test will possibly have included patients with more severe pathology, which introduces a selection bias, and generalizing the results of these studies to patients with less severe presentations of shoulder pathology may not be appropriate.

Pain appears to be a major factor influencing the ability to generate muscle strength, and research investigating the potential biochemical mediation of tendon and bursal pathology and degeneration may change our understanding of the pathological process and provide new directions for management of the disease process.

Information from the patient's history, observational findings, and a collection of symptoms may increase the likelihood that a disorder of the rotator cuff and bursa exists. One conclusion based on this review suggests a definitive understanding of the pathology and a definitive diagnosis is currently beyond our ability. This view is supported by Smidt and Green,[141] who acknowledge that the reproducibility and validity of the diagnosis and classification system for shoulder complaints are inadequate. There is a distinct need for continuing research in this area.

Key messages

- Pathologies involving the rotator cuff are considered to be the most common musculoskeletal pathology involving the shoulder.
- People without shoulder symptoms and without loss of function appear to have a similar incidence of RC tears as symptomatic populations.
- There does not appear to be a correlation between positive imaging findings and painful shoulder dysfunction.
- There is no certainty as to what constitutes rotator cuff disease that correlates with loss of function and/or pain.
- There does not appear to be a gold standard reference test to determine the accuracy of clinical assessment procedures designed to diagnose rotator cuff disease.
- A definitive understanding of rotator cuff pathology has not yet been achieved.
- A method for the definitive diagnosis of rotator cuff disease is not currently available.

Sample examination questions

Multiple-choice questions (answers on page 602)

1 Rotator cuff pathology is the most common musculoskeletal disorder of the shoulder, and:

A Accounts for approximately one-third of all shoulder diagnoses made by family practitioners
B Is always associated with signs of inflammation
C Is thought to be caused exclusively by irritation from a type II or type III acromion
D Is identified by the presence of a painful arc
E Is best diagnosed with MRI

2 The reference test(s) that best correlate(s) the findings of clinical tests and structural pathology is/are:
   A Arthroscopy
   B MRI
   C Direct visualization during open surgery
   D A combination of ultrasound and MRI
   E All of the above
3 Strength testing of the rotator cuff:
   A Should be performed as an isometric contraction
   B Implicates the muscle tendon unit involved in the pathology
   C Correlates with observed imaging findings
   D May be influenced more by pain than actual weakness
   E Is of no use in the clinical examination

Essay questions

1 Evaluate the structural, histological, and biomechanical changes associated with rotator cuff tendon and subacromial bursal disease, and contrast these findings with people without symptoms or with other shoulder pathologies.
2 Design a study to investigate the accuracy of clinical tests to identify rotator cuff and subacromial bursal pathology.
3 Critically discuss why current clinical tests and imaging techniques cannot provide a definitive diagnosis relating to the patient's symptoms.

Case study 18.1

Ms. S.F., a 63-year-old Australian retired businesswoman, presented to a consultant shoulder physiotherapist clinic in a secondary-care orthopedic outpatient clinic 6 weeks after the onset of right dominant shoulder pain. Onset of symptoms was sudden and occurred when trying to force a carry-on suitcase into an overhead luggage rack at the start of a 2-hour train journey. There was an immediate sharp pain, and by the end of the journey Ms. S.F. was unable to elevate her arm. Prior to this, there was no history of any shoulder symptoms, and the medical history was remarkably uneventful, with no report of any previous surgery, serious illness, or current comorbidity. Ms. S.F. had attended circuit training in a local gym two or three times each week (for over 5 years) before the onset of the shoulder pain. As a result of the current injury, she was unable to continue with this program. Prior to attending the clinic, Ms. S.F. had been referred privately for a diagnostic ultrasound, which had revealed a full-thickness tear of the right supraspinatus and infraspinatus. An image of the left shoulder was not available. Ms. S.F. reported that she was unable to sleep on her right shoulder and was limited in all functional activities, including dressing, carrying, lifting, and attending to personal hygiene. The Oxford Shoulder Score at the time of the initial consultation was 53 out of a possible 60. (The Oxford Shoulder Score ranges from 12 to 60, where 60 is maximum disability and 12 is the best possible result). Clinically, no wasting was observed around the shoulder. Cervical movements were full-range and pain-free, and no local tenderness was provoked during palpation in the cervical and upper thoracic regions. Shoulder movements were measured with a 360° inclinometer. Left active shoulder flexion was limited to 20° by severe pain—9/10 on a visual analogue scale (VAS; passive range 100°), abduction 20° (9/10 VAS; passive 90°), and external rotation (measured with the elbow by the side and flexed to 90° with a tape measure from the umbilicus to the ulnar styloid process, with the forearm supinated) was 22 cm (8/10 VAS). The corresponding measurements for left active shoulder movement were 160° flexion, 160° abduction, and 43 cm external rotation. With the thumb extended, the left hand behind back reached the spinal level corresponding with the inferior angle of the scapula. The right side was recorded as reaching the level of the right iliac crest laterally (9/10 VAS). The following tests were positive for the right shoulder: Neer sign, Hawkins test, and drop-arm sign. The resisted tests of abduction (tested at 10°), external rotation (with elbow by the side) were tested manually and were weak in comparison with the contralateral side and painful (both 8–9/10). Due to pain, no further evaluation was possible, and following the investigation the clinical diagnosis was rotator cuff pathology possibly involving a symptomatic structural lesion and/or pain inhibition. Management options were discussed with Ms. S.F., and following consent, the following treatments were implemented: advice, subacromial analgesic injection (administered by the consultant physiotherapist), shoulder taping, manual therapy, and a graduated supervised exercise program. Eight months after the initial presentation, the range of movement for the right shoulder was recorded as equaling the left for all movements tested. Strength had improved and appeared equal to that of the left side. The Oxford Shoulder Score had decreased to 15, and Ms. S.F. reported a full return to function and was again attending the gym (with occasional discomfort in some overhead activities). Although it was within the consultant physiotherapist's scope of practice to directly request MRI and diagnostic ultrasound, this was not ordered at the end of treatment, although this would have been of interest in an attempt to determine if the improvement was due to structural change or some other mechanism.

Summarizing the evidence

Comparison	Result	Level of evidence*
Painful arc versus Neer test + MRI/arthrogram/arthroscope	3 CTs—2 large, 1 moderate-sized Sp, Se, +LH, –LH results suggest presence of painful arc may not confirm or refute the presence of RC disease	B
Passive elevation versus arthrogram	1 CT–large Sp, Se, +LH, –LH results suggest the passive elevation test may not confirm or refute the presence of RC disease	B
Passive external rotation versus arthrogram	1 CT—large Sp, Se, +LH, –LH results suggest the passive external rotation test may not confirm or refute the presence of RC disease	B
Neer impingement sign versus Neer test + MRI/arthrogram /arthroscope	4 CTs–2 large, 2 moderate-sized Sp, Se, +LH, –LH results suggest the Neer impingement sign may not confirm or refute the presence of RC disease	B
Hawkins test versus Neer test + MRI/arthroscope	3 CTs—1 large, 2 moderate-sized Sp, Se, +LH, –LH results suggest the Hawkin's test may not confirm or refute the presence of RC disease	B

Continued

Summarizing the evidence (*Continued*)

Comparison	Result	Level of evidence*
Horizontal adduction test versus Neer test + MRI/arthroscope	2 CTs—1 large, 1 moderate-sized Sp, Se, +LH, –LH results suggest the horizontal adduction test may not confirm or refute the presence of RC disease	B
"Full cans" test versus MRI	1 CT—1 moderate-sized Sp, Se, +LH, –LH results suggest the "full cans" test may not confirm or refute the presence of RC disease	B
"Empty cans" test versus MRI/arthroscope	2 CTs—1 large, 1 moderate-sized Sp, Se, +LH, –LH results suggest the "empty cans" test may not confirm or refute the presence of RC disease	B
Speed test versus Neer test + MRI/arthroscope	2 CTs—1 large, 1 moderate-sized Sp, Se, +LH, –LH results suggest the Speed test may not confirm or refute the presence of RC disease	B
Resisted external rotation versus arthroscope	1 CT—large Sp, Se, +LH, –LH results suggest the resisted external rotation test may not confirm or refute the presence of RC disease	B
Yerganson test versus Neer test + MRI	1 CT—moderate-sized Sp, Se, +LH, –LH results suggest the Yerganson test may not confirm or refute the presence of RC disease	B
IRRST versus arthroscope	1 CT— large Sp, Se, +LH, –LH results suggest the IRRST may confirm or refute the presence of RC disease due to "impingement" versus intraarticular pathology or pathology due to "secondary impingement," postoperative results not reported	B
Drop sign versus operative findings	1 CT— large Sp, Se, +LH, –LH results suggest the drop sign may not confirm or refute the presence of RC disease	B
Drop-arm sign versus Neer test + MRI/arthroscope	2 CTs—1 large, 1 moderate-sized Sp, Se, +LH, –LH results suggest the drop-arm sign may not confirm or refute the presence of RC disease	B
External rotation lag sign versus operative findings	1 CT— large Sp, Se, +LH, –LH results suggest the external rotation lag sign may not confirm or refute the presence of RC disease	B

Summarizing the evidence (*Continued*)

Comparison	Result	Level of evidence*
Internal rotation lag sign versus operative findings	1 CT— large Sp, Se, +LH, –LH results suggest the internal rotation lag sign may not confirm or refute the presence of RC disease	B
Rent test versus arthroscope/MRI	1 CT— large (arthroscope n = 109), moderate-sized (MRI n = 71) Sp, Se, +LH, –LH results suggest the rent test may confirm or refute the presence of RC disease	B

CT, controlled trial; IRRST, internal rotation resistance strength test; +LH, positive likelihood ratio; –LH, negative likelihood ratio; MRI, magnetic resonance imaging; RC, rotator cuff; Sp, specificity; Se, sensitivity.

* A1: evidence from large randomized controlled trials (RCTs) or systematic reviews (including meta-analysis).†

A2: evidence from at least one high-quality cohort.

A3: evidence from at least one moderate-sized RCT or systematic review.†

A4: evidence from at least one RCT.

B: evidence from at least one high-quality study of nonrandomized cohorts.

C: expert opinions.

† Arbitrarily, the following cut-off points have been used; large study size: ≥ 100 patients per intervention group; moderate study size: ≥ 50 patients per intervention group.

References

1 Chard MD, Hazleman R, Hazleman BL, King RH, Reiss BB. Shoulder disorders in the elderly: a community survey. *Arthritis Rheum* 1991; **34**:766–769.

2 Van der Windt DA, Koes BW, de Jong BA, Bouter LM. Shoulder disorders in general practice: incidence, patient characteristics, and management. *Ann Rheum Dis* 1995; **54**:959–964.

3 Van der Heijden GJ. Shoulder disorders: a state-of-the-art review. *Baillière's Clin Rheumatol* 1999; **13**:287–309.

4 Luime JJ, Koes BW, Hendriksen IJ, *et al.* Prevalence and incidence of shoulder pain in the general population; a systematic review. *Scand J Rheumatol* 2004; **33**:73–81.

5 Bot SD, van der Waal JM, Terwee CB, *et al.* Incidence and prevalence of complaints of the neck and upper extremity in general practice. *Ann Rheum Dis* 2005; **64**:118–123.

6 Van der Windt DA, Koes BW, Boeke AJ, *et al.* Shoulder disorders in general practice: prognostic indicators of outcome. *Br J Gen Pract* 1996; **46**:519–523.

7 Macfarlane GJ, Hunt IM, Silman AJ. Predictors of chronic shoulder pain: a population based prospective study. *J Rheumatol* 1998; **25**:1612–1615.

8 Uhthoff HK, Sarkar K. An algorithm for shoulder pain caused by soft-tissue disorders. *Clin Orthop Relat Res* 1990; (**254**):121–127.

9 Silverstein B, Welp E, Nelson N, Kalat J. Claims incidence of work-related disorders of the upper extremities: Washington state, 1987 through 1995. *Am J Public Health* 1998; **88**:1827–1833.

10 Neer CS 2nd. Anterior acromioplasty for the chronic impingement syndrome in the shoulder: a preliminary report. *J Bone Joint Surg Am* 1972; **54**:41–50.

11 Neer CS 2nd. Impingement lesions. *Clin Orthop Relat Res* 1983; (**173**):70–77.

12 Bigliani LU, Morrison DS, April EW. The morphology of the acromion and its relationship to rotator cuff tears. *Orthop Trans* 1986; **10**:228.

13 Ozaki J, Fujimoto S, Nakagawa Y, Masuhara K, Tamai S. Tears of the rotator cuff of the shoulder associated with pathological changes in the acromion: a study in cadavers. *J Bone Joint Surg Am* 1988; **70**:1224–1230.

14 Meister K, Andrews JR. Classification and treatment of rotator cuff injuries in the overhand athlete. *J Orthop Sports Phys Ther* 1993; **18**:413–421.

15 Soslowsky LJ, An CH, Johnston SP, Carpenter JE. Geometric and mechanical properties of the coracoacromial ligament and their relationship to rotator cuff disease. *Clin Orthop Relat Res* 1994; (**304**):10–17.

16 Uhthoff HK, Sano H. Pathology of failure of the rotator cuff tendon. *Orthop Clin North Am* 1997; **28**:31–41.

17 Budoff JE, Nirschl RP, Guidi EJ. Debridement of partial-thickness tears of the rotator cuff without acromioplasty: long-term follow-up and review of the literature. *J Bone Joint Surg Am* 1998; **80**:733–748.

18 Sano H, Ishii H, Trudel G, Uhthoff HK. Histologic evidence of degeneration at the insertion of 3 rotator cuff tendons: a comparative study with human cadaveric shoulders. *J Shoulder Elbow Surg* 1999; **8**:574–579.

19 Lewis J, Green A, Dekel S. The aetiology of subacromial impingement syndrome. *Physiotherapy* 2001; **87**:458–469.

20 Kibler W. Role of the scapula in the overhead throwing motion. *Contemp Orthop* 1991; **22**:525–532.

21 Warner JJ, Micheli LJ, Arslanian LE, Kennedy J, Kennedy R. Scapulothoracic motion in normal shoulders and shoulders with glenohumeral instability and impingement syndrome: a study using Moire topographic analysis. *Clin Orthop Relat Res* 1992;(**285**):191–199.

22 Kibler WB. The role of the scapula in athletic shoulder function. *Am J Sports Med* 1998; **26**:325–337.

23 Edelson G, Teitz C. Internal impingement in the shoulder. *J Shoulder Elbow Surg* 2000; **9**:308–315.

24 Lewis J, Green A, Yizhat Z, Pennington D. Subacromial impingement syndrome: has evolution failed us? *Physiotherapy* 2001; **87**:191–198.

25 Mavrogenis S, Johannessen E, Jensen P, Sindberg C. The effect of essential fatty acids and antioxidants combined with physiotherapy treatment in recreational athletes with chronic tendon disorders: a randomised, double-blind, placebo-controlled study. *Phys Ther Sport* 2004; **5**:194–199.

26 Lewis JS, Wright C, Green A. Subacromial impingement syndrome: the effect of changing posture on shoulder range of movement. *J Orthop Sports Phys Ther* 2005; **35**:72–87.

27 Lewis JS, Green A, Wright C. Subacromial impingement syndrome: the role of posture and muscle imbalance. *J Shoulder Elbow Surg* 2005; **14**:385–392.

28 Fukuda H, Hamada K, Yamanaka K. Pathology and pathogenesis of bursal-side rotator cuff tears viewed from en bloc histologic sections. *Clin Orthop Relat Res* 1990; (**254**):75–80.

29 Khan KM, Cook JL, Bonar F, Harcourt P, Astrom M. Histopathology of common tendinopathies. Update and implications for clinical management. *Sports Med* 1999; **27**:393–408.

30 Khan KM, Cook JL, Maffulli N, Kannus P. Where is the pain coming from in tendinopathy? It may be biochemical, not only structural, in origin. *Br J Sports Med* 2000; **34**:81–83.

31 Maffulli N, Khan KM, Puddu G. Overuse tendon conditions: time to change a confusing terminology. *Arthroscopy* 1998; **14**:840–843.

32 Maffulli N, Wong J, Almekinders LC. Types and epidemiology of tendinopathy. *Clin Sports Med* 2003; **22**:675–692.

33 Perry SM, McIlhenny SE, Hoffman MC, Soslowsky LJ. Inflammatory and angiogenic mRNA levels are altered in a supraspinatus tendon overuse animal model. *J Shoulder Elbow Surg* 2005; **14**(1 Suppl S):79S–83S.

34 British Elbow and Shoulder Society. British Elbow and Shoulder Society 16th Annual Scientific Meeting, 6–8 July 2005; Cambridge.

35 Ogata S, Uhthoff HK. Acromial enthesopathy and rotator cuff tear: a radiologic and histologic postmortem investigation of the coracoacromial arch. *Clin Orthop Relat Res* 1990; (**254**):39–48.

36 Basmajian JV. *Grant's Method of Anatomy*, 9th ed. Baltimore: Williams and Wilkins, 1975.

37 Romanes G. *Cunningham's Manual of Practical Anatomy*, 14th ed. London: Oxford University Press, 1976.

38 Williams P, Bannister L, Berry M, *et al. Gray's Anatomy*, 38th ed. Edinburgh: Churchill Livingstone, 1995.

39 Clark JM, Harryman DT 2nd. Tendons, ligaments, and capsule of the rotator cuff: gross and microscopic anatomy. *J Bone Joint Surg Am* 1992; **74**:713–725.

40 Milgrom C, Schaffler M, Gilbert S, van Holsbeeck M. Rotator-cuff changes in asymptomatic adults: the effect of age, hand dominance and gender. *J Bone Joint Surg Br* 1995; 77:296–298.

41 Sher JS, Uribe JW, Posada A, Murphy BJ, Zlatkin MB. Abnormal findings on magnetic resonance images of asymptomatic shoulders. *J Bone Joint Surg Am* 1995; 77:10–15.

42 Frost P, Andersen JH, Lundorf E. Is supraspinatus pathology as defined by magnetic resonance imaging associated with clinical sign of shoulder impingement? *J Shoulder Elbow Surg* 1999; **8**:565–568.

43 Radak Z, Naito H, Kaneko T, *et al.* Exercise training decreases DNA damage and increases DNA repair and resistance against oxidative stress of proteins in aged rat skeletal muscle. *Pflugers Arch* 2002; **445**:273–278.

44 Gotoh M, Hamada K, Yamakawa H, Inoue A, Fukuda H. Increased substance P in subacromial bursa and shoulder pain in rotator cuff diseases. *J Orthop Res* 1998; **16**:618–621.

45 Gotoh M, Hamada K, Yamakawa H, *et al.* Interleukin-1-induced subacromial synovitis and shoulder pain in rotator cuff diseases. *Rheumatology (Oxford)* 2001; **40**:995–1001.

46 Sakai H, Fujita K, Sakai Y, Mizuno K. Immunolocalization of cytokines and growth factors in subacromial bursa of rotator cuff tear patients. *Kobe J Med Sci* 2001; **47**:25–34.

47 Gotoh M, Hamada K, Yamakawa H, *et al.* Interleukin-1-induced glenohumeral synovitis and shoulder pain in rotator cuff diseases. *J Orthop Res* 2002; **20**:1365–1371.

48 Williams JW Jr, Holleman DR Jr, Simel DL. Measuring shoulder function with the Shoulder Pain and Disability Index. *J Rheumatol* 1995; **22**:727–732.

49 Dawson J, Fitzpatrick R, Murray D, Carr A. The problem of "noise" in monitoring patient-based outcomes: generic, disease-specific and site-specific instruments for total hip replacement. *J Health Serv Res Policy* 1996; **1**:224–231.

50 Dawson J, Fitzpatrick R, Carr A. A self-administered questionnaire for assessment of symptoms and function of the shoulder. *J Bone Joint Surg Am* 1998; **80**:766–767.

51 Dawson J, Hill G, Fitzpatrick R, Carr A. The benefits of using patient-based methods of assessment: medium-term results of an observational study of shoulder surgery. *J Bone Joint Surg Br* 2001; **83**:877–882.

52 Dawson J, Hill G, Fitzpatrick R, Carr A. Comparison of clinical and patient-based measures to assess medium-term outcomes following shoulder surgery for disorders of the rotator cuff. *Arthritis Rheum* 2002; **47**:513–519.

53 Cloke DJ, Lynn SE, Watson H, *et al.* A comparison of functional, patient-based scores in subacromial impingement. *J Shoulder Elbow Surg* 2005; **14**:380–384.

54 Litaker D, Pioro M, El Bilbeisi H, Brems J. Returning to the bedside: using the history and physical examination to identify rotator cuff tears. *J Am Geriatr Soc* 2000; **48**:1633–1637.

55 Ayub E. Posture and the upper quarter. In: Donatelli R, ed. *Physical Therapy of the Shoulder*, 2nd ed. Melbourne: Churchill Livingstone, 1991;81–90.

56 Kendall F, McCreary E, Provance P. *Muscle Testing and Function*, 4th ed. Baltimore: Williams and Wilkins, 1993.

57 Grimsby O, Gray J. Interrelation of the spine to the shoulder girdle. In: Donatelli R, ed. *Physical Therapy of the Shoulder*, 3rd ed. New York: Churchill Livingstone, 1997:95–129.

58 Sahrmann S. *Diagnosis and Treatment of Movement Impairment Syndromes.* London: Mosby, 2002.

59 Grimmer K. An investigation of poor cervical resting posture. *Aust J Physiother* 1997; **43**:7–16.

60 DiVeta J, Walker ML, Skibinski B. Relationship between performance of selected scapular muscles and scapular abduction in standing subjects. *Phys Ther* 1990; **70**:470–476; discussion 476–479.

61 Greenfield B, Catlin PA, Coats PW, *et al.* Posture in patients with shoulder overuse injuries and healthy individuals. *J Orthop Sports Phys Ther* 1995; **21**:287–295.

62 Raine S, Twomey LT. Head and shoulder posture variations in 160 asymptomatic women and men. *Arch Phys Med Rehabil* 1997; **78**:1215–1223.

63 Lewis J. Posture and subacromial impingement syndrome: does a relationship exist? *J OCPPP* 2004; **108** (autumn):8–17.

64 Odom CJ, Taylor AB, Hurd CE, Denegar CR. Measurement of scapular asymmetry and assessment of shoulder dysfunction using the lateral scapular slide test: a reliability and validity study. *Phys Ther* 2001; **81**:799–809.

65 Koslow PA, Prosser LA, Strony GA, Suchecki SL, Mattingly GE. Specificity of the lateral scapular slide test in asymptomatic competitive athletes. *J Orthop Sports Phys Ther* 2003; **33**:331–336.

66 Kibler WB, Uhl TL, Maddux JW, *et al.* Qualitative clinical evaluation of scapular dysfunction: a reliability study. *J Shoulder Elbow Surg* 2002; **11**:550–556.
67 Cook JL, Khan KM, Kiss ZS, Purdam CR, Griffiths L. Reproducibility and clinical utility of tendon palpation to detect patellar tendinopathy in young basketball players. Victorian Institute of Sport Tendon Study Group. *Br J Sports Med* 2001; **35**:65–69.
68 Hoppenfeld S. *Physical Examination of the Spine and Extremities.* New York: Appleton-Century-Crofts, 1976.
69 Magee D. *Orthopedic Physical Assessment.* Philadelphia: Saunders, 1987.
70 Mattingly GE, Mackarey PJ. Optimal methods for shoulder tendon palpation: a cadaver study. *Phys Ther* 1996; **76**:166–173.
71 Wolf EM, Agrawal V. Transdeltoid palpation (the rent test) in the diagnosis of rotator cuff tears. *J Shoulder Elbow Surg* 2001; **10**:470–473.
72 Lukasiewicz AC, McClure P, Michener L, Pratt N, Sennett B. Comparison of 3-dimensional scapular position and orientation between subjects with and without shoulder impingement. *J Orthop Sports Phys Ther* 1999; **29**:574–583; discussion 584–586.
73 Ludewig PM, Cook TM. Alterations in shoulder kinematics and associated muscle activity in people with symptoms of shoulder impingement. *Phys Ther* 2000; **80**:276–291.
74 Riddle DL, Rothstein JM, Lamb RL. Goniometric reliability in a clinical setting. Shoulder measurements. *Phys Ther* 1987; **67**:668–673.
75 Williams J, Callaghan M. Comparison of visual estimation and goniometry in determination of a shoulder joint angle. *Physiotherapy* 1990; **76**:655–657.
76 Croft P, Pope D, Boswell R, Rigby A, Silman A. Observer variability in measuring elevation and external rotation of the shoulder. Primary Care Rheumatology Society Shoulder Study Group. *Br J Rheumatol* 1994; **33**:942–946.
77 Kumar VP, Satku SK. Documenting rotation at the glenohumeral joint: a technical note. *Acta Orthop Scand* 1994; **65**:483–484.
78 Youdas JW, Carey JR, Garrett TR, Suman VJ. Reliability of goniometric measurements of active arm elevation in the scapular plane obtained in a clinical setting. *Arch Phys Med Rehabil* 1994; **75**:1137–1144.
79 Green S, Buchbinder R, Forbes A, Bellamy N. A standardized protocol for measurement of range of movement of the shoulder using the Plurimeter-V inclinometer and assessment of its intrarater and interrater reliability. *Arthritis Care Res* 1998; **11**:43–52.
80 Hayes K, Walton JR, Szomor ZR, Murrell GA. Reliability of five methods for assessing shoulder range of motion. *Aust J Physiother* 2001; **47**:289–294.
81 Trombly C. *Occupational Therapy for Physical Dysfunction*, 4th ed. Baltimore: Williams and Wilkins, 1995.
82 Clarkson H, Gilewich G. *Musculoskeletal Assessment: Joint Range of Motion and Manual Muscle Strength.* Baltimore: Williams and Wilkins, 1989.
83 Palmer M, Epler M. *Clinical Assessment Procedures in Physical Therapy.* Philadelphia: Lippincott, 1990.
84 Sabari JS, Maltzev I, Lubarsky D, Liszkay E, Homel P. Goniometric assessment of shoulder range of motion: comparison of testing in supine and sitting positions. *Arch Phys Med Rehabil* 1998; **79**:647–651.
85 Croft P, Pope D, Zonca M, O'Neill T, Silman A. Measurement of shoulder related disability: results of a validation study. *Ann Rheum Dis* 1994; **53**:525–528.
86 Edwards TB, Bostick RD, Greene CC, Baratta RV, Drez D. Interobserver and intraobserver reliability of the measurement of shoulder internal rotation by vertebral level. *J Shoulder Elbow Surg* 2002; **11**:40–42.
87 Ben-Yishay A, Zuckerman JD, Gallagher M, Cuomo F. Pain inhibition of shoulder strength in patients with impingement syndrome. *Orthopedics* 1994; **17**:685–688.
88 Brox JI, Roe C, Saugen E, Vollestad NK. Isometric abduction muscle activation in patients with rotator tendinosis of the shoulder. *Arch Phys Med Rehabil* 1997; **78**:1260–1267.
89 Bryant L, Shnier R, Bryant C, Murrell GA. A comparison of clinical estimation, ultrasonography, magnetic resonance imaging, and arthroscopy in determining the size of rotator cuff tears. *J Shoulder Elbow Surg* 2002; **11**:219–224.
90 Hayes K, Walton JR, Szomor ZL, Murrell GA. Reliability of 3 methods for assessing shoulder strength. *J Shoulder Elbow Surg* 2002; **11**(1):33–39.
91 McCabe RA, Nicholas SJ, Montgomery KD, Finneran JJ, McHugh MP. The effect of rotator cuff tear size on shoulder strength and range of motion. *J Orthop Sports Phys Ther* 2005; **35**:130–135.

92 Birtane M, Calis M, Akgun K. The diagnostic value of magnetic resonance imaging in subacromial impingement syndrome. *Yonsei Med J* 2001; **42**:418–424.

93 Calis M, Akgun K, Birtane M, Karacan I, Calis H, Tuzun F. Diagnostic values of clinical diagnostic tests in subacromial impingement syndrome. *Ann Rheum Dis* 2000; **59**:44–47.

94 Chambers I, Hide G, Bayliss N. An audit of accuracy and efficacy of injections for subacromial impingement comparing consultant, registrar and physiotherapist. *J Bone Joint Surg Br* 2004; **87** (Suppl II Orthop Proc):160.

95 Eustace JA, Brophy DP, Gibney RP, Bresnihan B, FitzGerald O. Comparison of the accuracy of steroid placement with clinical outcome in patients with shoulder symptoms. *Ann Rheum Dis* 1997; **56**(1):59–63.

96 Partington PF, Broome GH. Diagnostic injection around the shoulder: hit and miss? A cadaveric study of injection accuracy. *J Shoulder Elbow Surg* 1998; **7**:147–150.

97 Yamakado K. The targeting accuracy of subacromial injection to the shoulder: an arthrographic evaluation. *Arthroscopy* 2002; **18**:887–891.

98 De Winter AF, Jans MP, Scholten RJ, *et al.* Diagnostic classification of shoulder disorders: interobserver agreement and determinants of disagreement. *Ann Rheum Dis* 1999; **58**:272–277.

99 Ostor AJ, Richards CA, Prevost AT, Hazleman BL, Speed CA. Interrater reproducibility of clinical tests for rotator cuff lesions. *Ann Rheum Dis* 2004; **63**(10):1288–1292.

100 Cyriax J, Cyriax P. *Diagnosis of Soft Tissue Lesions*, 8th ed. London: Baillière Tindall, 1982.

101 Cyriax J. *Illustrated Manual of Orthopaedic Medicine*, 2nd ed. Oxford: Butterworth Heinemann, 1993.

102 Hanchard NC, Howe TE, Gilbert MM. Diagnosis of shoulder pain by history and selective tissue tension: agreement between assessors. *J Orthop Sports Phys Ther* 2005; **35**:147–153.

103 Tennent TD, Beach WR, Meyers JF. A review of the special tests associated with shoulder examination. Part I: the rotator cuff tests. *Am J Sports Med* 2003; **31**:154–160.

104 Park HB, Yokota A, Gill HS, El Rassi G, McFarland EG. Diagnostic accuracy of clinical tests for the different degrees of subacromial impingement syndrome. *J Bone Joint Surg Am* 2005; **87**:1446–1455.

105 MacDonald PB, Clark P, Sutherland K. An analysis of the diagnostic accuracy of the Hawkins and Neer subacromial impingement signs. *J Shoulder Elbow Surg* 2000; **9**:299–301.

106 Itoi E, Kido T, Sano A, Urayama M, Sato K. Which is more useful, the "full can test" or the "empty can test," in detecting the torn supraspinatus tendon? *Am J Sports Med* 1999; **27**:65–68.

107 Zaslav KR. Internal rotation resistance strength test: a new diagnostic test to differentiate intra-articular pathology from outlet (Neer) impingement syndrome in the shoulder. *J Shoulder Elbow Surg* 2001; **10**:23–27.

108 Hertel R, Ballmer FT, Lombert SM, Gerber C. Lag signs in the diagnosis of rotator cuff rupture. *J Shoulder Elbow Surg* 1996; **5**:307–313.

109 Murrell GA, Walton JR. Diagnosis of rotator cuff tears. *Lancet* 2001; **357**:769–770.

110 Miniaci A, Mascia AT, Salonen DC, Becker EJ. Magnetic resonance imaging of the shoulder in asymptomatic professional baseball pitchers. *Am J Sports Med* 2002; **30**:66–73.

111 Schibany N, Zehetgruber H, Kainberger F, *et al.* Rotator cuff tears in asymptomatic individuals: a clinical and ultrasonographic screening study. *Eur J Radiol* 2004; **51**:263–268.

112 Morrison DS, Bigliani LU. The clinical significance of variations in acromial morphology. *Orthop Trans* 1987; **11**:234.

113 Edelson JG, Taitz C. Anatomy of the coraco-acromial arch: relation to degeneration of the acromion. *J Bone Joint Surg Br* 1992; **74**:589–594.

114 Prescher A. Anatomical basics, variations, and degenerative changes of the shoulder joint and shoulder girdle. *Eur J Radiol* 2000; **35**:88–102.

115 Gill TJ, McIrvin E, Kocher MS, *et al.* The relative importance of acromial morphology and age with respect to rotator cuff pathology. *J Shoulder Elbow Surg* 2002; **11**:327–330.

116 Worland RL, Lee D, Orozco CG, SozaRex F, Keenan J. Correlation of age, acromial morphology, and rotator cuff tear pathology diagnosed by ultrasound in asymptomatic patients. *J South Orthop Assoc* 2003; **12**:23–26.

117 Dinnes J, Loveman E, McIntyre L, Waugh N. The effectiveness of diagnostic tests for the assessment of shoulder pain due to soft tissue disorders: a systematic review. *Health Technol Assess* 2003; **7**:iii, 1–166.

118 Zehetgruber H, Lang T, Wurnig C. Distinction between supraspinatus, infraspinatus and subscapularis tendon tears with ultrasound in 332 surgically confirmed cases. *Ultrasound Med Biol* 2002; **28**:711–717.

119 Prickett WD, Teefey SA, Galatz LM, *et al.* Accuracy of ultrasound imaging of the rotator cuff in shoulders that are painful postoperatively. *J Bone Joint Surg Am* 2003; **85**:1084–1089.

120 Teefey SA, Middleton WD, Payne WT, Yamaguchi K. Detection and measurement of rotator cuff tears with sonography: analysis of diagnostic errors. *AJR Am J Roentgenol* 2005; **184**:1768–1773.

121 Iannotti JP, Ciccone J, Buss DD, *et al.* Accuracy of office-based ultrasonography of the shoulder for the diagnosis of rotator cuff tears. *J Bone Joint Surg Am* 2005; **87**:1305–1311.

122 Nelson MC, Leather GP, Nirschl RP, Pettrone FA, Freedman MT. Evaluation of the painful shoulder: a prospective comparison of magnetic resonance imaging, computerized tomographic arthrography, ultrasonography, and operative findings. *J Bone Joint Surg Am* 1991; **73**:707–716.

123 Brenneke SL, Morgan CJ. Evaluation of ultrasonography as a diagnostic technique in the assessment of rotator cuff tendon tears. *Am J Sports Med* 1992; **20**:287–289.

124 Wiener SN, Seitz WH, Jr. Sonography of the shoulder in patients with tears of the rotator cuff: accuracy and value for selecting surgical options. *AJR Am J Roentgenol* 1993; **160**:103–107; discussion 109–110.

125 Van Holsbeeck MT, Kolowich PA, Eyler WR, *et al.* US depiction of partial-thickness tear of the rotator cuff. Radiology 1995; **197**:443–446.

126 Van Moppes FI, Veldkamp O, Roorda J. Role of shoulder ultrasonography in the evaluation of the painful shoulder. *Eur J Radiol* 1995; **19**:142–146.

127 Takagishi K, Makino K, Takahira N, *et al.* Ultrasonography for diagnosis of rotator cuff tear. *Skeletal Radiol* 1996; **25**:221–224.

128 Sonnabend DH, Hughes JS, Giuffre BM, Farrell R. The clinical role of shoulder ultrasound. *Aust N Z J Surg* 1997; **67**:630–633.

129 Read JW, Perko M. Shoulder ultrasound: diagnostic accuracy for impingement syndrome, rotator cuff tear, and biceps tendon pathology. *J Shoulder Elbow Surg* 1998; **7**:264–271.

130 Swen WA, Jacobs JW, Algra PR, *et al.* Sonography and magnetic resonance imaging equivalent for the assessment of full-thickness rotator cuff tears. *Arthritis Rheum* 1999; **42**:2231–2238.

131 Teefey SA, Hasan SA, Middleton WD, *et al.* Ultrasonography of the rotator cuff: a comparison of ultrasonographic and arthroscopic findings in one hundred consecutive cases. *J Bone Joint Surg Am* 2000; **82**:498–504.

132 Martin-Hervas C, Romero J, Navas-Acien A, Reboiras JJ, Munuera L. Ultrasonographic and magnetic resonance images of rotator cuff lesions compared with arthroscopy or open surgery findings. *J Shoulder Elbow Surg* 2001; **10**:410–415.

133 Roberts CS, Walker JA 2nd, Seligson D. Diagnostic capabilities of shoulder ultrasonography in the detection of complete and partial rotator cuff tears. *Am J Orthop* 2001; **30**:159–162.

134 Zlatkin MB, Hoffman C, Shellock FG. Assessment of the rotator cuff and glenoid labrum using an extremity MR system: MR results compared to surgical findings from a multi-center study. *J Magn Reson Imaging* 2004; **19**:623–631.

135 Hodler J, Kursunoglu-Brahme S, Snyder SJ, *et al.* Rotator cuff disease: assessment with MR arthrography versus standard MR imaging in 36 patients with arthroscopic confirmation. *Radiology* 1992; **182**:431–436.

136 Traughber PD, Goodwin TE. Shoulder MRI: arthroscopic correlation with emphasis on partial tears. *J Comput Assist Tomogr* 1992; **16**:129–133.

137 Quinn SF, Sheley RC, Demlow TA, Szumowski J. Rotator cuff tendon tears: evaluation with fat-suppressed MR imaging with arthroscopic correlation in 100 patients. *Radiology* 1995; **195**:497–500.

138 Tuite MJ, Yandow DR, DeSmet AA, Orwin JF, Quintana FA. Diagnosis of partial and complete rotator cuff tears using combined gradient echo and spin echo imaging. *Skeletal Radiol* 1994; **23**:541–545.

139 Balich SM, Sheley RC, Brown TR, Sauser DD, Quinn SF. MR imaging of the rotator cuff tendon: interobserver agreement and analysis of interpretive errors. *Radiology* 1997; **204**:191–194.

140 Wnorowski DC, Levinsohn EM, Chamberlain BC, McAndrew DL. Magnetic resonance imaging assessment of the rotator cuff: is it really accurate? *Arthroscopy* 1997; **13**:710–719.

141 Smidt N, Green S. Is the diagnosis important for the treatment of patients with shoulder complaints? *Lancet* 2003; **362**:1867–1868.

CHAPTER 19

How should you treat an athlete with a first-time dislocation of the shoulder?

Marc R. Safran, Fredrick J. Dorey, and Duncan Hodge

Introduction

The glenohumeral joint is the most commonly dislocated major joint in the body.[1] The shoulder most frequently dislocates anteriorly, representing approximately 97% of all shoulder dislocations.[2] Hovelius found a 1.7% prevalence of anterior shoulder dislocations in a randomized population of 2092 Swedish people aged 18–70.[3] Many investigators have suggested the incidence to be even greater in athletes. Supporting this notion, Hovelius studied Swedish ice hockey players and reported an incidence of 7% of players with a shoulder dislocation.[4]

While recurrence of shoulder dislocation has been reported in between 20% and 50% in general populations,[5–9] recurrence rates have been reported to be much higher in young patients, ranging from 47% (48 of 102) to 100% (21 of 21).[2,6,8,10–15] In athletes who are young, the recurrence rate is reported to be even higher, ranging between 80 and 94%.[4,9,10,15]

Management of the patient with a first-time shoulder dislocation has been a matter of controversy since 1982.[11] Henry and Genung advocated primary surgical reconstruction at the time of first dislocation in the young athlete, due to the purported high risk of recurring instability.[11] However, this approach did not attract much enthusiasm for nearly a decade. Surgical intervention after a first-time shoulder dislocation has gained more support with better surgical techniques, particularly because current techniques have demonstrated greater reliability and the good results are reproducible. Now, with the advent of newer, less traumatic, and possibly safer arthroscopic techniques, many more surgeons are recommending early surgical stabilization for patients with shoulder dislocations, particularly for athletes soon after their first shoulder dislocation.

To determine the best treatment regimen for the athlete with a first-time shoulder dislocation, having large, prospective randomized trials with long-term follow-up is of paramount importance. It is also helpful to know the natural history of first-time shoulder dislocations, designate consistent criteria for determining what constitutes failure of nonoperative management and then determine if an intervention, surgical or not, will alter the natural history. This is, of course, only if the natural history results in a poor or unacceptable outcome.

A critical question when analyzing studies of the natural history or treatment of shoulder dislocations is to know what definition of failure was used. One outcome used to judge the natural history is recurrence of shoulder dislocation. Some studies of the natural history describe recurrence as re-dislocation, some as subluxation, some as the need for surgery (or re-operation). Some studies are based on subjective and/or objective rating scales, such as the Rowe, the Western Ontario Shoulder Instability (WOSI) Index,[16] the Constant score, or apprehension, crank, or fulcrum tests. Not knowing the evaluation or outcome criteria utilized in the study being reviewed can lead to confusion of apparently conflicting results.

Knowing the goals of intervention is crucial in determining the best method to treat the young athlete with the first-time shoulder dislocation. Is the goal to alter the rate of recurrent dislocation or the need for surgery? Clinicians and researchers need to determine how much improvement is needed before implementing a treatment method. Furthermore, if surgery is recommended for the treatment of all first-time shoulder dislocators, even within a defined subpopulation, where does the risk of surgery on patients who may not need the surgery outweigh the benefit?

Any valid clinical study designed to compare different treatment options properly for initial or recurrent dislocation of the shoulder would have to meet several criteria. First, several outcomes would have to be evaluated: a) the need for re-operation, b) the number of subsequent dislocations or instability episodes, c) some measure of the functional ability and limitation of the patients, d) some quality-of-life evaluation, including some measures of the patients' real functional ability (i.e., the ability to perform those items that are desired). In addition, these outcomes must be evaluated in a way that their effect on the age categories under 20, 20–30, and over 30 can be determined. The comparisons should of course be prospective and randomized, with a blinded evaluation of the patients as far as possible. In cases where one of the treatments involves surgery and the other involves nonsurgery, a double-blinded evaluation will be difficult, if not impossible. Finally, other possible covariates such as the cause of dislocation, severity of trauma, dominant side versus involved side, occupational status and athletic involvement should be available for a multivariate statistical analysis of the results. Only then can sufficient knowledge of the potential benefits of one treatment over another be determined so that a cost benefit analysis may be considered.

Unfortunately, none of the reports in the existing literature on this subject meets the above criteria, so that decisions about treatment approaches must be made based on incomplete data. The existing studies fail to use randomized trials of sufficient sample size, to present the data in a way that comparisons can be evaluated in different age subgroups, to include functional ability or quality-of-life evaluations. These studies also use highly specialized patient populations.

In this chapter, with the limitations in the lack of good studies from which to base our decisions, the authors will review existing literature to determine, using the principles of evidence based medicine where possible, if adequate information exists to answer the question of how to treat an athlete with a first-time shoulder dislocation. There has been very little new information published in the literature since the first edition of this chapter, thus, further statistical analysis of the data available with the addition of the few new papers is presented. Still, prospective, randomized clinical trials with controls, studied in a double-blinded fashion, provide the best available scientific evidence from which to base treatment strategies. However, knowledge of the natural history of the first-time shoulder dislocation also must be understood to help bring the treatment options in better perspective.

Methods

We identified citations from the reference sections of more than 38 textbooks of sports medicine, orthopedics, and shoulder surgery. We searched electronic databases (MEDLINE 1978–2006, Current Contents 1996–2006) in the English language using the subject term "shoulder dislocation." We then limited the search using the terms "treatment" and "first-time shoulder dislocation." We then further limited the search using the terms, "clinical trial" and "randomized controlled trial." We attempted to identify further citations from the reference sections of the research papers retrieved, contacted experts in the field (including first authors of prospective randomized controlled studies addressing the management of first-time shoulder dislocations), and searched the Cochrane Collaboration (an international network of experts who conduct synthetic searches for relevant citations).[17–19] Papers were excluded that did not provide primary research data, that only addressed methods of reduction or that provided previously published data. All articles were screened by two reviewers (M.R.S., D.H.). From 3282 citations identified in our search of papers on shoulder dislocations, we identified 2343 articles that reported on the treatment of shoulder dislocations and 67 papers on the treatment of first-time shoulder dislocations. Of these manuscripts, six published papers prospectively compared alternative methods of treatment of patients with first-time shoulder dislocations in a randomized fashion.[18–25] These six papers report the results of three separate study groups by three different institutions.

Two additional abstracts were identified that initially appeared to meet the inclusion criteria, but were excluded. One abstract was excluded because surgical treatment consisted of primary open repair.[26] The other abstract involved combined data from two different investigators at two different centers, and was found not to meet controlled randomization standards after the lead author had been contacted for further information.[27–29]

Additionally, three published manuscripts following the same cohort of patients with first-time shoulder dislocations were identified as the only published prospective natural history study.[5,6,30] However, we have included the presented but as yet unpublished data from one author of this chapter (R.S.) who has been performing the first prospective natural history study of first-time shoulder instability in North America.[31] Papers reporting the results of five large retrospective natural history series were identified,[2,7–9,12,14,32,33] as was one prevalence study[34] and three published articles of prospective, nonrandomized comparison trials of first-time shoulder dislocations performed by two groups.[10,15,35]

Assessment of study quality

Two authors (M.S. and D.H.) assessed the methodological quality of each study using the PEDro scale with respect to randomization; blinding of patients, clinicians, and those assessing outcomes; and proportion of patients lost to follow-up.[36] The 10-point study-quality assessment scale provides a quantitative rating for each study (Table 19.1).

Data extraction

Data extraction from the studies in this review was not blinded. The very limited number of randomized, controlled studies precluded effective blinding. Studies have found that such masking of identifying data in meta-analyses "imposes substantial burdens without significantly altering the results of a review."[37]

Table 19.1 Methodological quality scores of prospective, randomized studies in systematic review

	Wintzell *et al.* (1999)[22]	Kirkley *et al.* (1998)[16]	Bottoni *et al.* (2002)[25]
1 Eligibility criteria were specified	+	+	+
2 Subjects were randomly allocated to groups	+	+	+
3 Allocation was concealed	+	+	+
4 Groups were similar at baseline	+	+	+
5 Subjects were blinded	0	0	0
6 Surgeons who administered treatment were blinded	0	0	0
7 Assessors were blinded	0	+	0
8 Measures of key outcomes were obtained from > 85% of pts	+	+	+
9 Data were analyzed by intention to treat	+	0	0
10 Statistical comparisons between groups were conducted	+	+	+
11 Patient measures and measures of variability were provided	+	+	+
Total score	7/10	7/10	5/10

The total score is determined by counting the number of criteria that are satisfied, except that scale item 1 is not used to generate the total score, so total scores are out of 10.
+ indicates that the criterion was clearly satisfied; – indicates that it was not; ? indicates that it is not clear if the criterion was satisfied.

Natural history

General population

To make an informed decision on the appropriate management of the first-time shoulder dislocator, one must know the natural history of this problem. In orthopedic surgery, there are few entities for which the natural history has been studied as well as that of the first-time shoulder dislocation. Several retrospective studies suggest that age at the time of initial dislocation is the most important factor, and often the only variable, that can provide the prognosis for recurrent shoulder dislocation.[2,7–9,14,38] An increased recurrence rate of shoulder dislocation has been identified in younger patients (Table 19.2).[2,7–9,14,38] Patients with greater-tuberosity fractures have a better prognosis and a lower recurrence rate in comparison with patients with no fracture.[2,5,6,8,9,12,39]

Another important issue to consider is the consequence of shoulder dislocations with regard to the potential of other shoulder problems, particularly rotator cuff tears and shoulder degenerative arthritis. Retrospective studies have shown that while a first-time shoulder dislocation in a patient in the over 40-year-old age group may be associated with

Table 19.2 Retrospective natural history studies relating age to recurrence

First author, ref.	Patients (n)	Young age group and recurrence	Middle age group and recurrence	Older age group and recurrence
McLaughlin (1950)[7]	101	< 20 y/o = 90%	20–40 y/o = 60%	> 40 y/o = 10%
Rowe (1956)[8]	308	< 20 y/o = 83%	20–40 y/o = 63%	> 40 y/o = 16%
Rowe (1961)[2]	324	< 20 y/o = 94%	20–40 y/o = 74%	> 40 y/o = 14%
Simonet (1984)[9]	116	< 20 y/o = 66%	20–40 y/o = 40%	> 40 y/o = 0%
Lill (1998)[38]	175	< 30 y/o = 86%		> 30 y/o = 21%

a rotator cuff tear, the same has not been shown for those under the age of 40.[40,41] Recurrent dislocations in subjects has not been shown to be associated with rupture or tearing of the rotator cuff tendons either. Additionally, the rate of glenohumeral joint degenerative arthritis is not greater in patients who have had a single dislocation when compared with those with recurrent dislocations.[5] It is likely that the trauma sustained at the time of the first dislocation is the causative factor for those with dislocation arthropathy, and not recurrent dislocations. Thus, there does not appear to be any documented evidence of adverse consequences of recurrent dislocations other than recurrence itself.

Young population

Natural history studies on young patients have been performed and are important to help determine the prognosis of shoulder instability, to serve as a guide to treatment and to determine which patients, if any, need surgery. Several retrospective studies on young patients have reported a recurrence rate of up to 100% of first-time shoulder dislocations.[12–14,33] Hovelius *et al.* published their landmark prospective natural history study of first-time shoulder dislocations in young patients at 2 years, 5 years, and 10 years.[5,6,30] The authors began the study with 257 patients and reported a 10-year follow-up in 245 patients aged 12–40. They found that 44% of patients under 40 had at least two recurrent dislocations and 4% had only one recurrence in 10 years. Their findings on recurrence, listed by age and time of follow-up are shown in Table 19.3. An ongoing prospective natural history study of shoulder instability in a general population is currently being performed in the United States by one of the present authors (R.S.).[31] A total of 131 patients (of an initial total 139 patients) with a first-time shoulder instability (dislocation or subluxation) episode were evaluated every 6 months for an average follow-up period of

Table 19.3 Summary of the 10-year data for recurrence and surgery for first-time shoulder dislocations in young patients presented by Hovelius *et al.*[5,6,30]

Age at first dislocation	Recurrence at 2 years (%)	Recurrences at 5 years (%)	Recurrences at 10 years (%)	Surgery by 10 years (%)
All subjects (12–40)	32	44	52	23
12–22	47	64	66	34
23–29	28	48	56	28
30–40	13	19	23	9

4 years (2–7 years). Instability was uncommon over the age of 40 (one recurrence out of 41 patients over 40). There were 90 patients under the age of 40. This group was considered to be at risk for recurrent instability and was evaluated separately. Fifty-one of these 90 patients (57%) remained stable during the follow-up period, while 39 of the 90 (43%) suffered recurrent dislocations. Eighteen of the 39 unstable patients (46%) eventually had surgery, while one of the 51 stable patients (2%) had surgery for a rotator cuff repair. Several factors were evaluated for those having recurrence of instability. Specifically, the following demographic data did *not* differ between the groups: gender, dominant arm, percent of injuries to dominant versus nondominant arm, family history of instability, patient history of previous instability in other joints, type or degree of trauma causing the shoulder dislocation, amount of time the shoulder was dislocated, method of reduction, place of reduction, and time in sling. On physical examination, the two groups showed no difference in initial range of motion, strength, hyperlaxity signs, or radiographic findings. Total sports hours did not differ in the recurrence group in comparison with the nonrecurrence group, though hours spent in contact and collision sports were highly correlated with recurrence and request for surgery. Patients who used their arm at or above chest level in their occupation were more likely to have an instability event and to have instability surgery.[31] Te Slaa *et al.* also found, in their prospective study of 31 patients with first-time shoulder dislocations aged under 40 (range 16–39 years), that 55% sustained a recurrence at a follow-up of 5 years.[42] For those aged under 18 years, 71% (five of seven) had a recurrence of instability, and the authors found that age was the only predictor of recurrence.

Athletic population

Athletics has long been felt to be a risk factor for recurrent shoulder instability. While Hovelius noted recurrence of dislocation in a general population of 20%,[3] he noted recurrent shoulder instability in 90% of ice hockey players younger than 20 and 65% of players aged 20–25 at the time of their first dislocation.[4] Simonet *et al.*, in their retrospective natural history study, reported that 82% of young athletes had recurrent shoulder dislocations, while only 30% of nonathletic patients in a similar age category had recurrent instability.[9] Others have reported, in studies without comparison groups, that recurrent shoulder instability is much higher in athletes, ranging between 80% and 94% in comparison with historical controls.[10,15] Some authors have therefore recommended surgical reconstruction for young athletes with a first-time shoulder dislocation, due to the purported high risk of recurrence in this subpopulation.[11,43]

However, not all retrospective studies have confirmed this increased risk in athletes.[12] Unfortunately, the prospective natural history studies are of no help in solving this issue. Hovelius reported in his natural history study that the long-term prognosis concerning recurrent dislocation was the same for similarly aged patients who had a high level of activity in comparison with those who were sedentary.[39,44] Sachs *et al.*, in a natural history study of first-time dislocations in the United States with a minimum 2-year follow-up, did find associations between type of sports and amount of participation with recurrence in young patients with first-time dislocation of the shoulder.[31] They found that while total sports hours did not correlate with recurrence of instability, those participating in contact and collision sports had more instability and requested surgery more frequently than those not participating in contact and collision sports.[31] Sixty-five percent of young athletes involved in overhead and collision sports sustained a recurrent dislocation.[31]

With these apparently conflicting results, we attempted to evaluate this critical subgroup of patients to determine if there is a difference in the natural history of athletes with regard to recurrence in the first-time shoulder dislocation. We combined the natural history studies where the data for athletic patients is presented separately from those prospective studies where athletic control groups existed and have the data presented. Although some studies have suggested that there is little difference between athletic and nonathletic populations, we feel that the best available data should be based on information involving athletic or highly active patients only. Ten studies were identified that reported details on either highly active (military academy where collision sports are mandatory[35]) or athletic populations (Table 19.4) who did not receive any surgical intervention. Three of the studies represent subsets of the controls involved in randomized studies, and the remaining studies were based on populations in which patients elected not to have surgical intervention or to whom surgery was not offered.[20–25] There were a total of 277 patients involved, with 160 having a subsequent re-dislocation or subsequent instability for an estimated unstable incidence of 57.8% over a 2–4-year period. The 95% confidence intervals are 51.7% to 63.6%. Thus, for patients treated without surgery, we can expect between 52% and 64% to become unstable within a period of a few years. In most of the studies, the incidences of instability in athletes occurred within the first 2 years following the index incident. In the Wintzell randomized study of 30 patients, 47% of the nonsurgical patients re-dislocated within 6 months, 53% within the first year, and only 7% re-dislocated between the first and second year.[22–24]

Factors to consider, as brought to light by Sachs *et al.*, are the amount of sporting activity with regard to collision/contact sports (versus low-demand sports such as running, cycling, etc.).[31] These have generally not been addressed by other investigators. Hovelius did attempt to separate young athletes on the basis of groupings of sport and found no difference between the types of sport and recurrence.[39,44] His inability to find a difference may have been due to his groupings of sports, not having enough athletes in each group to show a difference, or because the amount of time spent by the athletes in the sports concerned may not have been sufficient (e.g., as a result of infrequently playing certain high-risk sports). These factors may account for the apparent difference between studies. The subjects in the series from West Point and the United States military are involved in rigorous, high-contact and collision sports nearly every day, which may account for their very high rate of recurrence.[10,15,25]

Need for surgery

When evaluating the best approach to the management of the patient with a first-time shoulder dislocation, one must know the likelihood that the patient will need surgery. As noted earlier, the end point of some natural history studies and the definition for failure of nonoperative treatment varies with each study. The need for surgery as a determinant for failure of nonoperative treatment is subjective as well and may vary in relation to surgeon and patient preferences.

Henry and Genung, in a retrospective study of first-time and recurrent dislocations in young athletes, reported that 75% of these athletes required surgery to participate in sports activities.[11] Simonet *et al.* noted that 33% of all first-time shoulder dislocators in a general population studied retrospectively had recurrent dislocations and that 21% of the entire group required surgery at an average of 1.9 years from the date of injury.[9] When one evaluates Simonet's data more closely, it is found that 63% of those with recurrent shoulder

Table 19.4 Natural history of first-time shoulder dislocations in young athletes. The data are from studies of highly active or athletic populations, including controls in randomized trials and where possible, natural history studies in which the data for young athletes are presented individually

First author, ref.	Population	Follow-up period	Average age	Participants (n)	Recurrences (n)	Recurrences (%)	Surgery (n)	% of all surgery	% of recurrence surgery
Aronen (1984)[46]	Navy midshipmen	3 y	19	20	5	25	4	20	80
Bottoni (2002)[25]	Military	37 months	23	12	9	75	6	50	67
Arciero (1994)[10]	West Point	23 months	19.5	15	12	80	7	47	58
Wheeler (1989)[15]	West Point	> 14 months	19	38	35	92	n/a	n/a	n/a
Simonet (1984)[9]	General athletic	4.6 y	All < 30	33	27	82%	n/a	n/a	n/a
Kirkley (2005)[21]	General athletic	6.5 y	23 y	15	9	60%	7	47	77
Wintzell (1999)[22]	Participant sports	1 y	24	23	11	48%	n/a	n/a	n/a
Sachs (2005)[31]	General population	4 y	< 40	90	39	43%	18	20%	46%
Sachs, subset	Collision/overhead sports	4 y	< 40			65		32.3%	
Sachs, subset	No collision/overhead sports	4 y						9.3%	
Hovelius (1999)[39]	Athletic	2 y	< 23	39	21	54%	n/a	n/a	n/a
Hovelius (1999)[39]	Athletic	2 y	< 30	53	24	45%	n/a	n/a	n/a
Hovelius (1999)[39]	Recreational	2 y	< 23	35	14	40%	n/a	n/a	n/a
Hovelius (1999)[39]	Recreational	2 y	< 30	57	20	35%	n/a	n/a	n/a
Te Slaa (2003)[42]	Recreational	5 y	24	31	17	55%	3	10%	18%

N/a, data not available.

dislocations required surgery and that 67% of the 21 patients under 20 years of age who had a recurrence underwent shoulder stabilization surgery.[9]

Milgrom performed a prevalence study on the basis of the Israeli Defense Forces Medical Corps Computer Database.[34] This database allows monitoring of citizens with recurrent shoulder dislocations before the individuals are eligible for military induction, during the years of regular military service (ages 18–21 years for men, 18–19.5 years for women) and during the time of eligibility for reserve army service.[34] Between the years of 1978 and 1995, the prevalence rate of subjects with recurrent shoulder dislocations 21 years and younger was found to be 19.7 per 10,000 for men and 5.01 per 10,000 for women. The prevalence rate for men between the ages of 22 and 33 with a history of shoulder dislocation was 42.4 per 10,000. The authors found that 44% of subjects were deemed sufficiently unstable enough to warrant surgery, but only 55% of these young adults actually underwent surgery.

Te Slaa *et al.* followed 31 active individuals under the age of 40 (16–39, average age 24) at the time of their first shoulder dislocation for 5 years.[42] Although 17 subjects (55%) had recurrences, only three had requested surgery by the time of the final follow-up (18% of those with recurrences).

In the prospective study by Hovelius *et al.* the authors found that only 23% of the young patients studied (under 40 years of age) underwent surgery within 10 years from the time of their initial dislocation.[5] The group that underwent surgery is about half of all subjects with two or more recurrent dislocations and less than half of all subjects with at least one dislocation.[5,44] Sachs *et al.* found that 22% of individuals under the age of 40 underwent surgery and that 22% of those over the age of forty came to surgery in the 2–7 years following their initial dislocation.[31] In those under the age of 40, most underwent shoulder stabilization surgery, while those over 40 almost always underwent rotator cuff repair surgery.[31] Interestingly, Sachs *et al.* noted that the need for immediate surgery was not predictable with any accuracy in their population. Even in their high-risk subgroup of young collision athletes, they could not, in retrospect, have predicted who would eventually ask for surgery.

Reviewing other prospective, but not randomized, comparison studies of shoulder instability in which recurrences were observed in the nonoperative group or failed treatment group, significant information can be gleaned (Table 19.5). The rates of surgery for those patients in whom early surgical intervention for first-time dislocations fails range from 0% to 100%.[10,15,20–23,24,25,35] Wintzell's study of 30 patients treated with arthroscopic lavage and followed for 1 year revealed no further surgery in this group, including the three who had recurrent instability at 1 year.[22] However, at 2 years, only one subject of the three who redislocated in the initial group of 15 patients underwent a re-operation (a re-operation rate of 33%).[23] Also, among the patients who underwent surgery in Bottoni's study, the procedure only failed in one patient, and that patient elected to have a second operation, leading to the 100% total.[25]

More interesting are the rates of surgery for patients in whom nonoperative treatment failed (Table 19.5). For those considered high-risk—i.e., young patients—only 10–50% of the young subjects treated nonoperatively requested surgery.[9,10,20–23,24,25,42] In the three studies in which the rate of surgery was greatest for the nonoperatively treated "control groups," each study used military groups with young, active, and homogeneous populations.[10,25,35]

Since, unfortunately, most of the reports in the existing literature do not comment on the need for surgery in a young, athletic population, we performed a meta-analysis. Of the

Table 19.5 First-time shoulder dislocation—recurrence rates with surgical and nonsurgical management. Evaluation of studies looking at: 1, the rates of surgery for failed surgery for first-time shoulder dislocations; and 2, rates of surgery for failed nonoperative treatment of first-time shoulder dislocations, divided into those in whom nonoperative treatment failed and all those treated nonoperatively. The last series shows rates for the different age groups as described by Simonet *et al.*

Author	Surgery failed (%)	Repeat surgery failed (%)	Nonoperative treatment failed (%)	% of nonoperative patients with failure requesting surgery	% of all nonoperative patients requesting surgery
Kirkley (1999)[20]	26	60	56	64	37
Kirkley (2005)[21]	38	50	73	64	47
Wintzell (1999)[22]	13	0	43	23	10
Wintzell (1999)[23]	20	66	60	66	40
Bottoni (2002)[25]	11	100	75	66	50
DeBerardino (2001)[35]	12	50	66	75	50
Arciero (1994)[10]	14	33	80	58	47
Wheeler (1989)[15]	22	100	92		
Milgrom (1998)[34]			44	55	
Simonet (1984)[9]					
All subjects			33	63	21
Age < 20			66%	67%	44% of all < 20
Age 20–40			40%	59%	23% of all 20–40

93 patients reported, 32 (34%) required subsequent surgery. The 95% confidence intervals are 25% to 45%. Thus, the best available data indicates that for the young highly active patient not treated with surgery initially, we can expect that between 25% and 45% of patients will require subsequent surgery.

Many factors affect an individual's choice of whether to have surgery for recurrent dislocations. Some athletes are more committed to their sport and/or sports participation than others. This motivation to return to the same sports at the same level will vary with different individuals. Some athletes simply must get back to their sport, while others, having suffered a significant injury, would rather switch to a less risky sport or play their sport less often or at a lower level. This may potentially account, at least in part, for some of the athletes with recurrences not requesting surgery. In addition, not all re-dislocations episodes are alike. Some patients' shoulders dislocate weekly, while others dislocate every 5 years. Some patients' shoulders dislocate with significant trauma and pain, while some slip in and out with very little discomfort or trauma to the patient. Some patients are disabled by their re-dislocations, while some patients are minimally inconvenienced by the recurrence.

Although the published data is not as detailed or extensive, it can be surmised that the percentage of subsequent instability will drop substantially for patients whose age is over 25 at the time of the original dislocation. For example, Hovelius reported an incidence of instability of 54% (21/39) of athletic patients under 23 years of age at the index dislocation, but only 21% (3/14) in patients aged 23 to under 30.[39] Finally, there is some existing data on the more general population that suggests that the incidence of re-dislocation/instability may be considerably lower in the less active, nonathletic population, although this has not been universally observed.

Treatment

Immobilization

Treatment of shoulder instability has traditionally consisted of various types of immobilization in adduction and internal rotation for varying amounts of time. Some studies report a benefit from 3 weeks of immobilization in comparison with shorter periods of immobilization[2,45] and a benefit from withholding patients from athletic participation for more than 6 weeks in comparison with allowing them return to sports earlier.[9] Aronen and Regan reported a recurrence rate of only 25% in U.S. Naval Academy midshipmen with a closely supervised postimmobilization rehabilitation program,[46] a finding that has been supported by a study by Yoneda *et al.* (17.3% recurrence).[47] However, many other authors have studied the effect of immobilization on recurrence after a first-time shoulder dislocation, and no benefit has been identified.[2,5,8,11–13,38] The studies that have not found a benefit of immobilization are larger ones, and some are retrospective.

The lack of benefit from immobilization may be explained by the fact that in shoulders with anterior dislocation, the anteroinferior aspect of the labrum is often inverted and shifted medially.[48,49] The pathology in first-time shoulder dislocations includes a Bankart lesion (anteroinferior labral detachment from the glenoid rim) in over 90% of cases.[10,20,25,50–52] Holding the arm in adduction and internal rotation, such as in a sling, may not provide adequate coaptation of the labrum to the glenoid rim, since the anterior soft-tissue structures are not on tension.[48,49,53] As a result, the labrum may not be held in adequate apposition for healing, and thus we may not be immobilizing patients correctly. In 2003, Itoi *et al.* published the results of a prospective randomized controlled study comparing methods of postreduction immobilization after shoulder dislocation.[54] He compared immobilization in external rotation (essentially, the arm was orientated outwards with the forearm away from the chest) with immobilization in internal rotation (where the arm could rest against the chest). In this study of 40 participants with a mean age of 39 years and 15 months of follow-up, the investigators found recurrent instability in six subjects (30%) treated in internal rotation and in none of those treated with external rotation.[54] The difference in the recurrence rate was even greater among those who were aged under 30 (45% in the internal rotation group and 0% in the external rotation group). Of note was that a similar number of participants in the two groups removed their immobilizer before 1 week had passed.[54]

Changing the position of arm immobilization still may not produce a benefit. It should be noted that there have been no prospective, randomized studies with controls evaluating the effect of immobilization, and therefore no definitive conclusions may be made regarding this form of treatment to alter the natural history of first-time shoulder dislocation.[19]

Furthermore, other studies have not reported a benefit from exercises on the rate of recurrence.[9] The lack of benefit of therapeutic exercise to reduce the rate of recurrent dislocation has been shown to be particularly true for traumatic shoulder dislocations.[55] Controlled, prospective, randomized clinical trials on the effect of immobilization and on the effect of rehabilitation exercises (with or without immobilization) are needed to conclude whether these interventions are beneficial.

Surgery

The data involving comparisons of surgery with nonsurgical intervention in the athletic population are also not very satisfying. There are only three available randomized studies (involving about 60 patients in each group) and four nonrandomized studies that provide the best evidence for evaluation of the efficacy of surgical intervention versus nonsurgical intervention.

Starting our review with the studies that provide the lowest confidence level in research—i.e., single-treatment group studies with no controls or case series studies—Boszotta and Helperstorfer reported on 67 patients with an average age of 27 (range 19–39) who were treated with arthroscopic suture repair for first-time shoulder dislocation.[56] These patients were followed for 5 years and one and a half years. The authors reported that 85% of the patients returned to sports with a 7% recurrent dislocation rate (in patients with an average age of 20 years). Salmon and Bell reported a retrospective evaluation of 17 athletic patients treated with arthroscopic stabilization after their first dislocation with an average age of 21.6 years.[57] They noted one patient with a recurrent dislocation (6%) and no patients with recurrent subluxation. Interestingly, only 10 of the subjects returned to contact sports at the same or a higher level. Five patients reported a lack of confidence in their shoulder, although none had any indication of shoulder subluxation or dislocation. Three of the five with a lack of confidence in their shoulder gave this reason for why they did not return to sports at the same level.[57] Uribe and Hechtman reported on a prospective evaluation of 11 young patients treated with arthroscopic stabilization following their first shoulder dislocation.[58] At an average of 2 years, these young patients (averaging 20 years old) had only one subluxation and no re-operations. Fabbriciani *et al.* noted no recurrence of shoulder dislocations and similar Constant scores in a prospective randomized trial comparing open and arthroscopic stabilization in the treatment of shoulder dislocation after 2 years' follow-up.[59]

A higher level of confidence in research findings are nonrandomized clinical trials with contemporaneous controls (Table 19.6), such as the study by Wheeler *et al.*[15] Wheeler *et al.* published the first prospective series comparing arthroscopic treatment for patients with first-time shoulder dislocations with nonoperative controls enrolled in the United States Military Academy at West Point.[15] Nine patients underwent arthroscopy—six had staple capsulorraphy and three just had abrasion of the glenoid rim. This group was compared with 38 patients who were treated nonoperatively, some concurrently and some retrospectively. There were two failures in the surgery (total failure rate of 22%) group, one with staple stabilization and one with glenoid abrasion. Both of these patients had open revision stabilization surgery. In the "control" group, 35 of the 38 subjects treated nonoperatively had recurrent instability—four subluxations, 14 dislocations, and 17 dislocations with subluxations—giving a failure rate of 92%.

A prospective, nonrandomized study provides a higher level of confidence in the results of treatment. Arciero *et al.* published such a study where the patients could choose their treatment.[10] This study, also performed on subjects enrolled in the United States Military Academy at West Point, compared 36 subjects who had first-time dislocations of the shoulder requiring reduction. These patients are a homogeneous group of subjects with an average age of 20 (18–24) and all very active in sports, as required by the United States Military Academy. Fifteen of these patients were treated with immobilization for four weeks, and 12 (80%) had a recurrent dislocation within the 23-month average follow-up period. Seven of the patients with recurrent instability chose surgical stabilization of their

Table 19.6 Studies of non-randomized comparisons of surgical and nonsurgical active/athletic patients. Both studies, the only ones in the literature, are from the United States Military Academy at West Point, New York. All subjects are young, within a tight age range, and are highly active in sports, particularly collision and contact sports.

First author, ref.	Population	Group	Average follow-up (months)	Average age	n	Unstable		Surgery (n)	% Surgery after redislocation	% Surgery, total
						n	%			
Arciero (1994)[10]	Whole group	Bankart	32	20.5	21	3	14	1	33	5
		Control	23	19.5	15	12	80	7	58	47
Arciero (1994)[10]	Varsity athletes	Bankart	32		8	1	13	1	100	13
		Control	23		10	8	80	7	88	70
DeBerardino (2001)[35]	Whole group	Bankart	37	20	49	6	12	3	50	6
		Control	17	20	6	4	66	3	75	50
Wheeler (1989)[15]	All athletes	Bankart	> 14	19	9	2	22	n/a	n/a	n/a
		Control	> 14	18.5	38	35	92	n/a	n/a	n/a

N/a, data not available.

shoulders. The seven patients who eventually had a shoulder-stabilizing procedure represented 58% of those who had recurrent instability who were originally treated nonoperatively and 47% of all those treated nonoperatively. Using the Rowe scale of shoulder instability as a measurement tool, only two patients' shoulders were rated as excellent in this group, one good, and 12 poor. Of the 21 patients who elected to have their initial dislocation treated surgically using arthroscopic suture stabilization, only three had recurrent instability (14%) at the average 32-month follow-up. One patient sustained a single subluxation and did not experience any further instability episodes or require any other treatment, while a second patient re-dislocated their shoulder and gave up contact sports. Only one of the three with recurrent instability eventually had a revision stabilization for multiple subluxation episodes after the initial surgery. The ratings using the Rowe scale indicated 16 patients with excellent results, two good results and three poor results. Evaluating the subgroup of varsity athletes, Arciero and co-authors found that 80% of athletes treated nonoperatively experienced recurrent instability, while one in eight varsity athletes treated with surgery had a recurrence (13%).[10] These data parallel their results for the whole group.

This group recently published a similar study using newer arthroscopic stabilization techniques.[35] The authors noted difficulty in recruiting more military subjects to select the nonoperative arm of their study.[35] Of the 54 patients with 55 acute initial dislocations, only six cadets wished to be treated nonoperatively for their first shoulder dislocation. Of these six, four redislocated at an average 17 months after the initial dislocation. Three of the four went on to have surgical stabilization. Forty-eight patients with 49 dislocations were treated with arthroscopic stabilization with an absorbable tack. These 45 men and three women, with an average age of 20, were followed for 37 months. Six had recurrent instability episodes, and three of them underwent revision stabilization. They were evaluated with Rowe scores (average 92). More importantly, the authors also used quality-of-life indices for evaluation of their subjects, rather than just the Rowe scores, recurrence of instability, and surgery. The authors used the Single Assessment Numeric Evaluation (SANE)[60] (average 95.5) and the validated quality-of-life measure SF-36 (average 99 for the stable shoulders).

DeBerardino *et al.* also attempted to determine risk factors for recurrent dislocations in those treated with early stabilization.[35] They found that a history of bilateral shoulder instability had a positive predictive value of 75% and a negative predictive value of 93.3% in a small group treated nonoperatively. On physical examination under anesthesia, a 2+ sulcus sign had a positive predictive value for recurrent instability of 100% and a negative predictive value of 91.5%. Lastly, the authors stated that the finding of poor-quality capsulolabral tissue at the time of surgery had a positive predictive value of 44.4% and a negative predictive value of 95%. Unfortunately, the authors did not apply this methodology to evaluating the predictive values for determining which subjects treated nonoperatively would eventually require surgery.

Certainly, the best information on decision-making is based on prospective, randomized trials. Three study groups have been identified in the English-language literature (Table 19.6). Kirkley *et al.* conducted a prospective, randomized, double-blind study on patients under 30 years of age with first-time shoulder dislocations.[20] The 40 patients, with an average age of 22, were randomized into an immobilization group for 3 weeks, followed by physical therapy, and a surgery group in which arthroscopic suture stabilization was performed. All patients were followed for a minimum of 24 months. Nineteen of the original 21 patients treated with immobilization followed by physical therapy were evaluated. Nine patients sustained recurrent dislocations, while two more patients experienced subluxations (11/21 = 56% recurrent instability). Three of the 19 patients treated with primary arthroscopic shoulder stabilization developed recurrent dislocations, and two other patients had subluxation episodes as well (5/19 = 26% instability). With a longer-term follow-up of 79 months, Kirkley *et al.* were able to locate 16 of the surgically treated patients and 15 of the nonsurgically treated patients.[21] At 83 months' follow-up, six of the 16 subjects treated with primary surgical stabilization had recurrent instability (38%), of whom three patients underwent revision surgery for apprehension, dislocation, and/or subluxation. Additionally, one had recurrent instability treated nonoperatively and two had persistent subluxation, although there were no cases of new recurrent dislocation after 24 months. Of the 15 subjects treated with initial sling immobilization, 11 had recurrent instability at a 75-month follow-up. Of those with recurrence of instability treated in the conservatively treated group, seven eventually underwent shoulder stabilization surgery (one patient twice). Additionally, two had recurrence of instability and two had shoulder subluxation.

An important addition to this study was the use of the Western Ontario Shoulder Instability (WOSI) index, a validated quality-of-life index.[16,20,21] The authors found statistically significant differences at 33 months in disease-specific quality-of-life scores in patients treated surgically in comparison with those treated nonoperatively.[20] The authors also found that the nonoperatively treated patients had significantly more trouble with sports than the surgically managed group.[20] However, in the longer-term follow-up of these patients at 79 months with reexamination using the WOSI index, the previous statistically significant difference between the groups was lost.[21]

Another prospective, randomized trial of nonoperative treatment in comparison with arthroscopic stabilization used absorbable tacks to repair the labrum to the glenoid and shift the capsule to restore its tension. This study was presented in 2001 by the United States military.[25] These authors studied 21 active-duty military personnel with an average age of 22 (range 18–26). Twelve patients were treated with 4 weeks of immobilization followed by rehabilitation exercises. Nine of the 12 had sustained another dislocation at an average follow-up of 3 years. Six of these patients (75% of those with a recurrence, 50% of those treated nonoperatively) chose to have shoulder stabilization surgery. Of the nine patients randomized to the surgery group, only one (11%) had recurrent dislocation and underwent revision surgery. The authors also evaluated the patients using the validated L'Insalata shoulder evaluation,[61] the SANE evaluation, patient satisfaction score, and functional status rating. Scores using the L'Insalata scale and SANE evaluation were significantly better in the surgically treated group than in the nonoperative group (94 versus 73 and 88 versus 57, respectively). Of those treated nonoperatively, the nine with recurrent instability rated themselves as unsatisfactory (even though three did not opt for further surgery), and the three with no instability rated their shoulders as excellent. Of those treated surgically, six of the eight patients who were stable rated their shoulders as excellent, two as good, and the patient who redislocated as poor.

Wintzell *et al.* published a series of articles about a prospective, randomized study comparing nonoperative treatment without immobilization (except for comfort) with arthroscopic lavage (no fixation or repair of capsule or labrum).[22–24] The authors have published the results of 30 patients who were followed for two years and of 60 patients who were followed for one year (which includes the first 30 from the two year study).[22,24] The authors performed arthroscopic lavage of 200–400 mL within 10 days of injury until the shoulder was clear of hemarthrosis for the surgically treated group. Postoperatively, the patients used a sling for comfort. The other half of the patients in the study, the control group, were treated nonoperatively, using a sling for comfort only. All patients were under 30 years of age and had only one shoulder dislocation at the time they were randomized in the study.

Reviewing the results for the 60 patients followed for 1 year, the authors noted that this group averaged 23½ years of age.[22] The group treated with arthroscopic lavage had a recurrence rate of 13% (four of 30) at 1 year, in comparison with 43% (13/30) for the nonoperative group. Three of the 13 who had recurrences in the nonoperative group underwent shoulder stabilization surgery, while none of the three patients in the surgery group who had a recurrence opted for surgical intervention. The authors noted that the recurrence rate was high if the subjects were younger than 25. The redislocation rate was no different if the initial dislocation occurred during a sports activity in comparison with those whose dislocation did not occur during sports. However, the authors noted that individuals who gave up sports in both groups (seven of the 26 in the lavage group and eight of the 23 in the nonoperative group) were all involved in contact and overhead sports. The crank test was noted to be positive at follow-up in 57% of patients treated nonoperatively, and significantly less positive (23%) in patients treated with arthroscopic lavage. Using the Rowe scale, 24 of 30 patients (80%) were good to excellent in the lavage group, with only four (13%) rated as poor. This is to be compared with only 12 of 30 (40%) good to excellent results in the nonoperative group at the last follow-up and 17 (57%) rated as poor.

The results of the 2-year study by Wintzell *et al.* of 30 patients (26 men, four women, average age 24) are similar to those of the study just cited above, although the recurrence rate is greater.[23] In the lavage group, 20% of the patients experienced recurrent instability (three patients with an average 3.7 dislocations in a group of 15) in the lavage group. In the nonoperative group, 60% of the patients sustained recurrent instability (nine patients with an average 4.1 dislocations in a group of 15 patients). Three patients from the nonoperative group had already undergone shoulder stabilization surgery while another three were awaiting surgical stabilization (40% of the nonoperative group, 66% of those with recurrence). Two patients in the lavage group (13% of the lavage group, 66% of those with recurrent instability) elected to have shoulder stabilization surgery.

The crank test was positive in 53% (eight of 15 patients) of the lavage group and 75% (12 of 15) of patients in the nonoperative group. The difference in the Constant score between the two groups at 2 years was not statistically significant (91 for lavage versus 87 for nonoperative). The Rowe scale revealed 60% good to excellent results for the lavage group (with two poor, 13%) in comparison with 27% good to excellent results in the nonoperative patients (with eight poor, 53%).

Both groups did worse with time measured by instability episodes, apprehension measured by the crank test and Rowe scores. However, the results in the lavage group were better with respect to the Rowe scores, crank test, and rate of recurrence. The reason for this is not entirely clear. The joint effusion and hematoma after dislocation usually resolves within three to seven weeks after dislocation.[62] Though arthroscopic lavage does remove the hematoma, an effusion does reaccumulate.[62] This resolution of the joint effusion is 66% more rapid in the lavage group than in the control group. Removing the hematoma and fluid from the glenohumeral joint cavity by arthroscopic lavage may be the reason lavage appears to reduce the rate of redislocation.[22,23,63] One may deduce that a hematoma and joint effusion may compromise the healing of the Bankart lesion by pushing the anterior capsulolabral structures off the glenoid.

The results of the randomized studies (two from the same groups) are presented in Table 19.7 and Fig. 19.1. Although the estimated odds ratios appear to differ substantially (4.97, 3.85, 24) because of the small sample size in two of the studies, good evidence is lacking for heterogeneity. These numbers represent the odds of recurrent dislocation among the nonoperatively treated patients compared to the operatively treated patients. The combined Mantel–Haenszel estimated odds ratio is 5.63, with 95% confidence intervals of 2.42 to 13.19. Thus, the relative risk of recurrent dislocation is five times greater in the traditionally treated, nonoperative group in comparison with those who underwent early surgery ($P < 0.001$).

If the three nonrandomized papers from Table 19.6 are included, the combined estimated odds ratio is 12.22 (95% CI, 6.30 to 23.69). Given that the estimated odds ratios are so much larger in the nonrandomized studies (as would be expected), we feel that the results of the randomized studies (odds ratio 5.63; 95% CI, 2.42 to 13.19) represent a better estimate of the efficacy of surgical intervention over conservative treatment. Comparative studies indicate that surgical intervention results in a substantial reduction in the incidence of subsequent instability following index dislocation.

Appropriate criteria to determine the need for subsequent surgery are much less clear. The differences in the subsequent surgery rates between the control and surgery groups are 10% at 1 year, and 27%, 21%, and 39% at 2–3 years. For the nonrandomized comparative studies, the differences in subsequent surgery are 42% and 57%. Once again, the differences are expected to be greater in nonrandomized studies. In addition, the higher estimate for subsequent surgery among patients treated conservatively shown in Table 19.4 only serves to complicate any attempt to quantify this statistic. From our odds ratio calculations, treating all patients with surgery would result in operating on 75% of the patients who would not otherwise have needed surgery.

Separating the decision to operate from the technique

More than 250 operative techniques have been described for the treatment of anterior instability, all differing in their success rates and in the types and rates of complications. The surgical techniques can be classified into four basic groups: firstly, procedures that limit external rotation by tightening the anterior structures, such as the Magnuson–Stack[64] and Putti–Platt[65] procedures; secondly, bony blocks to prevent anterior humeral head translation, such as the Bristow procedure[66] and its variations; thirdly, osteotomies of the glenoid or rotational osteotomies of the humerus; and fourthly, anatomic reconstructions of the disrupted anteroinferior capsulolabral complex, such as the Bankart procedure[67] and capsular shift.[68] Because of its success in preventing recurrences (generally with success rates, with less than 5% recurrences)[69] the open Bankart repair and its modifications are generally considered the gold standard. Most of these open procedures are not without significant risk intraoperatively or postoperatively and have variable results with regard to returning the athlete to sports activity, depending on the procedure and on the sport played. Due to the risks involved and inconsistent results for athletes attempting to return to sports after shoulder stabilization, individuals advocating early surgical intervention for those with first-time shoulder dislocations did have many supporters until the advent of arthroscopy.

Table 19.7 Studies of prospective randomized comparisons of surgical and nonsurgical active or athletic populations

First author, ref.	Population	Mean follow-up	Mean age	n	Unstable		Surgery (n)	% Surgery after redislocation	% Surgery, total
					n	%			
Wintzell (1996)[24]	Lavage	6 mo	24	15	1	7	0	0	0
	Control	6 mo	24	15	7	47	1	14	7
Wintzell (1996)[24]	Lavage	1 y	24	15	2	13	0	0	0
	Control	1 y	24	15	8	53	3	38	20
Wintzell (1999)[23]	Lavage	2 y	24	15	3	20	2	67	13
	Control	2 y	24	15	9	60	6	67	40
Wintzell (1999)[22]	Lavage	1 y	24	30	4	13	0	0	0
	Control	1 y	24	30	13	43	3	23	10
Kirkley (1999)[20]	Arthroscopic stabilization	32 mo	22	19	5	26	3	60	16
	Traditional, control	36 mo	23	19	11	58	7	64	37
Kirkley (2005)[21]	Arthroscopic stabilization	83 mo	23	16	6	38	3	50	19
	Traditional, control	75 mo	23	15	11	73	7*	64	47
Bottoni (2002)[25]	Bankart repair	35 mo	22	9	1	11	1	100	11
	Control	37 mo	23	12	9	75	6	64	50

* One patient had surgery twice.

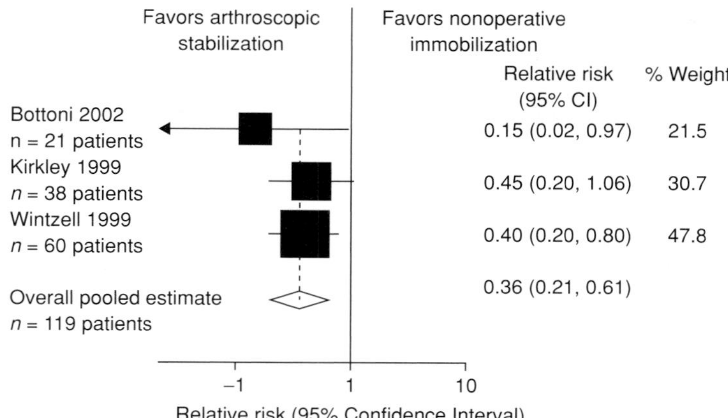

Figure 19.1 The effect of arthroscopic stabilization in comparison with nonoperative immobilization on recurrent instability.

Arthroscopic surgery has many potential advantages over comparable open procedures. Arthroscopy is relatively atraumatic, does not involve splitting or taking down the subscapularis muscle (resulting in less risk of injury or detachment of the subscapularis muscle-tendon unit), can be performed more easily and reliably as an outpatient procedure as compared with open procedures, and the patient notes quicker recovery from surgery (earlier return to work and fewer pain medications). However, the failure rate of arthroscopic stabilization is higher than the failure rate for open stabilization, ranging from 14–49% in some series.[70–76] Further, current arthroscopic stabilization procedures are technically demanding, possibly more so than open surgical stabilization.

The first generation of arthroscopic treatment of shoulder instability involved direct repair of the labrum to the glenoid without addressing capsular plastic deformation and residual laxity. The results of these early arthroscopic stabilization procedures were associated with high failure rates, particularly in contact athletes and in those with poor-quality capsular tissue. Due to the high recurrent dislocation rates and with the limited ability to re-tension the capsule, most advocates of arthroscopic shoulder stabilization suggested that this procedure should be performed in those with first-time shoulder dislocations, particularly early after the first dislocation, to prevent further capsular injury. This thought process has evolved to performing the surgery within 10 days from the first dislocation. It has been assumed that early surgery is better than surgery performed later, but this assumption has never been studied prospectively.

An explosion of technology has impacted arthroscopic shoulder stabilization surgery. This new technology has allowed many innovations and advancements in technique and in the ability to address all the pathology associated with shoulder dislocations. Newer techniques allow for tensioning of the capsule in addition to reattachment of the labrum to the glenoid rim. Arthroscopic stabilization techniques performed today are thus vastly different from the procedures that have been reported with medium-term follow-up periods, in which the results are not nearly as good as with open techniques. This constant evolution and innovation have perpetuated enthusiasm for this form of stabilization, though the data confirming its success are lacking. This era of innovation and advancement in surgical technique also brings light to the fact that possibly these procedures may not need to be done within 10 days from the injury, since capsular laxity may be addressed with current techniques and technology.

A recently published prospective, randomized controlled trial by Fabbriciani *et al.* compared open and arthroscopic shoulder stabilization for 60 individuals (30 in each group) with recurrent shoulder instability.[59] The authors found no recurrence with either technique, no intraoperative or postoperative complications and equal Constant scores. The only difference between the two groups was improved range of motion as assessed with the Constant score.[59]

Still yet to be studied, especially in a prospective, randomized fashion, is open versus arthroscopic stabilization for first-time shoulder dislocations. Any study forthcoming, however, may suffer from the fact that the arthroscopic technique performed in the study may be obsolete or may have been replaced by newer techniques by the time the subjects are followed for a minimum of 2 years and the data are eventually published. It must also be noted that these procedures, which are technically demanding, are being performed by surgeons who carry out the operations regularly; the resulting data may not always be applicable to orthopedic surgeons who do not conduct these technically demanding procedures as frequently as the clinician researchers.

Thus, there are no data to confirm if arthroscopic techniques are better or worse than open procedures for the treatment of first-time anterior dislocations of the shoulder and whether the timing of surgery has an important role. At present therefore, with no research to guide the physician, the technique utilized for shoulder stabilization should not play a role in the decision-making process on whether a young athlete with a first-time shoulder dislocation should undergo early surgery.

Complications of surgery

Any discussion of surgical intervention and the potential recommendation of surgery to alter the natural history of any disorder must address the risks of surgery, because surgical risk also plays a role in the cost–benefit ratio/comparison. Complication rates of shoulder stabilization surgery are highly dependent on the surgical technique utilized. Reported complications of open shoulder stabilization include infection, bleeding, injury to nerves (particularly the axillary and musculocutaneous nerves), loss of shoulder motion (the goal of many older open procedures, such as the Putti–Platt and Magnuson–Stack), recurrent instability (subluxation and/or dislocation; reports range from 3% to 50%),[77] hardware complications, arthritis (often due to loss of shoulder motion), subscapularis detachment/ disruption, pain, and weakness.

The reported complications of arthroscopic stabilization include infection, bleeding, injury to nerves (including the axillary, musculocutaneous, and suprascapular nerve), recurrent instability (subluxation and/or dislocation), hardware complications, loss of motion, pain, and weakness. Arthroscopic stabilization using lasers and radiofrequency probes includes the additional risks of thermal necrosis of articular cartilage, avascular necrosis, and necrosis and ablation of the glenohumeral ligaments and capsule. Essentially, arthroscopic stabilization has a higher recurrent dislocation rate and the added risks of injury to the suprascapular nerve from the posterior arthroscopy portal or from the transglenoid suture technique and thermal injury to the shoulder bony and soft-tissue structures. However, arthroscopic stabilization has a lower rate of stiffness/loss of motion and nearly no risk of subscapularis disruption/detachment. Complication rates vary with each individual surgical approach and technique, as well as with the experience of the surgeon.

Reviewing the prospective studies for the management of first-time shoulder dislocations, only one paper was found that did not list postoperative complications.[15] Considering adverse problems other than recurrent shoulder instability, three studies reported no complications for the combined population of 108 shoulders.[22,25,35] Kirkley *et al.*[20] noted one complication, joint sepsis, in their series of 19 patients treated surgically (5%). Arciero *et al.*[10] reported three complications for their 21 patients (14%): one suture abscess and two transient median nerve injuries due to traction.

Outcomes assessment

Most studies of patients with shoulder dislocation evaluate recurrent instability and/or the need for surgery. However, an important measurement tool is frequently absent from these studies—assessments of quality-of-life and quality-of-function outcomes. These tools may be very important in determining the treatment of the athlete with recurrent instability. An athlete may not have any recurrences but may give up athletics due to apprehension or concern about instability. Kirkley *et al.* evaluated their subjects in a prospective randomized study of first-time shoulder dislocations using the validated quality-of-life index, the WOSI index.[20] The importance of this information is highlighted by the fact that the authors found that quality-of-life scores were not normal, even for those individuals treated nonoperatively who did not have any further instability. The authors noted that the nonoperatively treated subjects who had no recurrences had a WOSI score of 14.5% less than normal, which is a similar score to those treated surgically (16% less than normal).[20]

Kirkley *et al.* also found in the initial report (with a 32-month follow-up) that those subjects treated nonoperatively measured 70% of normal on the WOSI index, while the surgically treated group measured 86% of normal on the WOSI index (statistically significant).[20] In other words, the surgery group's total WOSI scores were 16.5% better than the scores of the traditional group, demonstrating the difference between the two treatment groups. Further, Kirkley *et al.* specifically evaluated sports-specific capabilities and found that the nonoperatively treated group had significantly more trouble with sports than the surgically treated group (sports scores for the nonoperative group 20% below those of the surgical group). However, at a longer-term follow-up of 79 months, Kirkley *et al.* found that the surgically treated group's WOSI score remained at 86% of normal, while the conservatively treated group improved to 75% of normal.[21] The WOSI scores (and each subdomain) at over 6 years of follow-up were not statistically significantly different. However, in Kirkley's athletic patients treated nonoperatively at an average of over 6 years follow-up, the WOSI scores averaged 67% of normal.[21] Interestingly, when queried, all but one in each group (traditional and surgical) returned to all or most of their pre-injury level of activity. In their analysis of efficacy, Kirkley *et al.* noted that those in the traditional group who had not had surgery (n = 8, mean age 20.7) were not significantly different from the surgery group as a whole (WOSI scores: traditional 86.8, surgery 86.3; $P = 0.95$); however, those in the traditional group who had surgery (n = 7, mean age 21.5 y) had a significantly worse disease-specific quality of life than the surgery group as a whole (WOSI scores: traditional 38.8, surgery 86.3; $P = 0.025$).[21]

Sachs *et al.*, in a natural history study, had patients complete three outcome scores at their final follow-up: Constant scale, American Shoulder and Elbow Surgeons (ASES), and WOSI.[31] These three outcome scores were compared among three groups: 1, patients who became stable after their first dislocation; 2, patients who had recurrence of dislocation but chose to cope; and 3, patients who had recurrence and underwent successful Bankart repair. Patients who became stable after their first dislocation had outcome scores equivalent to patients who were unstable and had successful Bankart repair. Of interest is that patients who were unstable but who chose to cope had statistically significantly lower ASES, Constant, and WOSI scores than patients who were stable. All outcome scores were significant, but the WOSI most clearly differentiated between patients who were stable and those who were unstable.[31] Kirkley also noted the WOSI score to be more sensitive of difference between groups.[21]

Bottoni *et al.* also found that SANE scores (a nonvalidated questionnaire that correlates well with the Rowe and American Shoulder and Elbow Society Scales) and L'Insalata scores (a validated questionnaire) were significantly lower for nonoperatively treated shoulders with a first-time dislocation in comparison with those treated surgically.[25]

DeBerardino *et al.* found near-normal SANE scores and SF-36 scores for those who had surgery to stabilize their first-time shoulder dislocation and were stable at follow-up.[35]

Recommendation for treatment of the young athlete

The issue of how to best manage the shoulder of a young athlete with a first-time dislocation cannot be answered in a straightforward way. The answer is even more difficult to determine due to the lack of adequate data available. Determining the best management of the young athlete with a first-time shoulder dislocation depends on the physician and in large part on the goals of patient. The treatment recommendation may be at either end of the spectrum from surgery to "watchful waiting," depending on the outcome sought as well as the true natural history of first-time shoulder dislocation for this type of patient. The fundamental questions are: 1, is the natural history bad enough to warrant intervention; 2, will the proposed intervention alter the natural history; and 3, whether the cost–benefit ratio favors the intended intervention. The answer will likely vary with each physician and each individual athlete, on the basis of the individual's goals and motivation to return to the present sport or alternative sports. Possible outcome goals for intervention to alter the natural history are: 1, the ability to prevent re-dislocation; 2, the ability to avoid the need for subsequent surgery; 3, the effect on athletic participation; and 4, the effect on quality of life.

Table 19.4 summarizes the available data for the natural history of the young athlete with a first-time shoulder dislocation, with outcomes for recurrent instability and for eventual surgery when available. The current literature does not provide information on the long-term consequences of shoulder instability with regard to rotator cuff pathology and degenerative arthritis. Data regarding the quality of life impacted by shoulder instability as well as subsequent sporting activities are scarce. The best available published data refer to prevention of re-dislocation and subsequent surgery.

Surgical intervention has been shown to be effective in reducing the risk of re-dislocation. Young subjects with first-time shoulder dislocations are the highest-risk individuals, and the pooled data certainly suggest that young athletes may have the highest risk. However, it is important to note that 36–48% of young athletes with a first-time shoulder dislocation will likely not have a re-dislocation or instability episode. Thus, any recommendation to operate on all first-time dislocation patients will result in many young athletes being subjected to unnecessary surgery. It is highly unlikely that any such strategy would survive a rigorous cost–benefit analysis, even in cases in which the risks involved with the surgery itself were minimal. Any strategy involving surgery should be limited to a patient population in which the risks of recurrent instability are almost certain. Unfortunately, this population cannot be identified with the present data available.

As to the ability to prevent the need for subsequent surgery, there is a surprising paucity of data. The primary outcome evaluated in most of the studies is the occurrence of further instability episodes. Studies utilizing outcomes assessment tools are absent in the scientific literature. Further, there are no good-quality clinical studies (large, prospective, randomized, double-blinded clinical trials) studying the effect of immobilization for varying lengths of time and/or exercises on re-dislocation or subsequent surgery. This is especially true for the young athlete with a first-time shoulder dislocation.

The third and fourth considerations relate to the effects of the first-time shoulder dislocation with respect to the young athlete's quality-of-life measures and the quality of sports activity. Unfortunately, there is few data that include quality-of-life measures. More must be done. The little data that exist suggest that patients treated nonoperatively experience lower quality of life and sports.[20,25] Quality-of-life indices are an important indicator of the success of treatment or nontreatment. The possibility exists that the number of athletes treated nonoperatively who do not have a recurrent dislocation or surgery may be artificially low. The data may not reflect the experiences of subjects who may have avoided repeat injuries by giving up their sport or opting to compete at less capacity because they may have felt unstable, unsure of their shoulder, or unable to return to sports. This is suggested by the results presented by Salmon and Bell, who found that 29% of their patients complained of a lack of confidence in the shoulder even though they had no indication of subluxation or dislocation, and that 18% of their subjects did not return to sports because of this feeling of no confidence in their shoulder.[57]

Future studies are necessary and need to include quality-of-life measures such as the SF-36 and/or the WOSI index to allow for more critical evaluation of the effect of the first-time shoulder dislocation and its relationship to alternative treatment options. Even though patients may not have a recurrent dislocation, their quality of life and quality of sporting life may be diminished following a shoulder dislocation. Outcomes with regard to quality of life and sports activity must also be considered in the cost–benefit analysis for the individual athlete with a first-time shoulder dislocation, since not all athletes are equally committed to their sport (type, level, or amount of time participating).

Conclusion

The best way to manage a young athletic patient with a first-time shoulder dislocation is not an easy question to answer. Currently, the relatively small number of prospective, double-blind, randomized trials with a sufficient sample size means that recommendations for specific treatment following a first-time shoulder dislocation cannot be made with much confidence from an evidence-based medicine point of view. There are a few good studies published that help shed some light. In the randomized trials reported thus far, surgery does substantially reduce the incidence of recurrent shoulder instability in this subgroup of high-risk patients, and some studies do suggest that quality of life improves with surgical stabilization, allowing patients to return to sports. However, surgery does have risks and potential complications. Unless performed selectively, a large number of individuals may undergo an operation unnecessarily. A cost–benefit ratio must be determined, though ratios may vary among different patients and surgeons. As a result, management should be individualized on the basis of the athlete's personal goals, motivation, sports played, and willingness to undergo surgery with the known risks.

It is the opinion of the authors, on the basis of the best evidence available, that some younger athletes might benefit from surgical intervention following initial anterior dislocation of the shoulder. In many cases, surgical intervention results in a substantial reduction of subsequent re-dislocations, improved functional ability following surgery, and the possibility that up to one-fourth or more of the patients treated conservatively might still go on to subsequent surgery. However, what is entirely missing from all of these studies is any attempt to distinguish those patients who would require subsequent surgery from those who would not. To help determine which subgroup would benefit from surgical intervention at the time of the first encounter after initial shoulder dislocation, the authors of the existing publications must conduct and report more complete investigations of the athletes, especially in terms of why subsequent surgery was considered necessary and why those who had recurrent instability did not wish to undergo surgical stabilization. Without this information, the treating physicians will have to rely on their own judgment regarding the preferred treatment, rather than relying on conclusive and scientific evidence-based data. Perhaps a more extensive investigation of the patients' expectations and future intentions may be very helpful here. After reduction, immobilization for 3 weeks and possibly refraining from sports for another 3 weeks may reduce the rate of recurrence of shoulder dislocations in the young athlete.

In summary, at this point no conclusive evidence exists to recommend early surgical intervention for the young athlete with a first-time shoulder dislocation. There does appear to be a subgroup of young athletes (approximately 25% of young athletes with first-time anterior shoulder dislocation) who do need surgery. Currently, there is no evidence to predict who they are. As Sachs *et al.*[31] noted, the need for immediate surgery was not predictable with any accuracy in their population. Even in their high-risk subgroup of young, collision athletes, they could not, in retrospect, have predicted who would eventually ask for surgery. Taking that information together with a review of the literature, in which only 50% of patients with recurrences requested surgery, even though surgery can be shown to raise outcome scores, it remains hard at present to justify surgery in the acute setting.

Future large, double-blinded, prospective, randomized clinical trials evaluating the risk of recurrence with and without surgery are needed. Such studies should evaluate the results separately for different types of sports activity (collision sports, contact sports, etc.), for males and females, and for different age groups. These studies must include more details on the level of activity, validated scales to assess quality of life, and function scores such as the SF-36 and WOSI index, as well as details of surgical complications and cost considerations. Only then can the small subgroup of young athletic patients with a first-time anterior dislocation of the shoulder be identified who eventually need surgery. Once this group has been identified, we can then begin to answer the question of which patients (if any) would most benefit from surgery after their first shoulder dislocation.

Key messages

- Young patients have a higher rate of recurrent dislocations.
- Immobilization and exercises may not affect the rate of recurrent dislocations.

• Surgery reduces the rate of recurrent dislocations.
• Approximately half of those with recurrent shoulder dislocations request surgery.
• Those treated surgically and those treated nonoperatively without recurrent dislocations do not have normal scores for quality of life and sports scales.

Summary

Natural history of shoulder dislocations

• Young patients have a higher rate of recurrent dislocations.
• Young athletes may have a higher rate of recurrent dislocations in comparison with young nonathletes.
• Immobilization and exercises may not affect the rate of recurrent dislocations.
• Surgery reduces the rate of recurrent dislocations.
• Approximately half of those with recurrent shoulder dislocations request surgery.

Outcomes analysis

• Very little data.
• Those treated surgically and those treated nonoperatively without recurrent dislocations do not have normal scores for quality of life and sports scales.
• Need for use of validated rating scales for quality of life and sports for future prospective randomized studies.

Factors to consider

• Recurrence of dislocation.
• Need for surgery.
• Quality of life and sports.
• Individual's goals with regard to return to play, sports played, at what level to participate.
• Risks of surgery.

Sample examination questions

Multiple-choice questions (answers on page 602)

1 The most important predictor of recurrent shoulder dislocation is:
  A Age at the time of shoulder dislocation
  B Gender
  C Concomitant greater tuberosity fracture
  D Sport
  E Arm dominance
2 Validated shoulder quality-of-life scales include:
  A Constant score
  B American Shoulder and Elbow Society scale
  C Western Ontario Shoulder Instability index
  D Lysholm
  E All of the above

3 Factors proven to reduce the rate of dislocation include:
  A Immobilization
  B Exercises
  C Surgery
  D All of the above
  E None of the above

Essay questions

1 Describe what factors help determine the cost–benefit ratio when attempting to come to a conclusion about the best approach to manage a young athlete with a first-time shoulder dislocation.
2 Write the methodology for putting together a study to answer the questions of how to best manage a first-time dislocation of the shoulder in a young athlete.
3 Why is a discussion only of the effect of surgery versus the natural history not adequate in determining the optimal management of the young athlete who has dislocated his or her shoulder for the first time?

Case study 19.1

An 18-year-old female volleyball player dives for a ball, sustaining an anterior dislocation of the dominant shoulder. This is the first time she has dislocated her shoulder. After her shoulder has been reduced, she is placed in a sling by the trainer and referred to the team physician. What are your recommendations? Does your recommendation change if the athlete also swims competitively? Does it change if the dislocation is in the nondominant shoulder? Does it change if she is 28 years old?

Summarizing levels of evidence

Treatment strategies	Results	Level of evidence*
Natural history	48–90% recur	A1
1st-time dislocator < 22 years old	3 PRCTs, 3 controlled series (not randomized) 1 large prospective natural history study, none moderate size Pooled data shows high recurrence rate	
Surgery Less Recurrence 1st-time dislocators vs. Non-op	3 PRCTs, 3 controlled series (not randomized) None moderate size Pooled data show reduced dislocation rate	A1
Quality of life	1 small PRCT Not normal for any 1st-time dislocators, better if they have surgery or are treated nonoperatively and never have recurrences	A4
Nearly half of recurrent dislocators eventually undergo surgical stabilization	3 PRCTs, 3 prospective controlled Series (not randomized) 1 large prospective natural have surgery history study Pooled data show surgery in half of recurrent dislocators come to surgery	A1

Summarizing levels of evidence *(Continued)*

Treatment strategies	Results	Level of evidence*
Immobilization may reduce dislocation	No PRCT, 1 prospective study with small numbers favors physiotherapy/immobilization Other data conflicting Pooled data do not show benefit	C

PRCT, prospective, randomized, and controlled study.
* A1: evidence from large randomized controlled trials (RCTs) or systematic reviews (including meta- analysis).†
A2: evidence from at least one high-quality cohort.
A3: evidence from at least one moderate-sized RCT or systematic review.†
A4: evidence from at least one RCT.
B: evidence from at least one high-quality study of nonrandomized cohorts.
C: expert opinions.
† Arbitrarily, the following cut-off points have been used; large study size: ≥ 100 patients per intervention group; moderate study size: ≥ 50 patients per intervention group.

References

1 Kazar B, Relovsky E. Prognosis of primary dislocation of the shoulder. *Acta Orthop Scand* 1969; **40**:216–224.
2 Rowe CR, Sakellarides HT. Factors related to recurrences of anterior dislocations of the shoulder. *Clin Orthop Rel Res* 1961; **20**:40–47.
3 Hovelius L. Incidence of shoulder dislocation in Sweden. *Clin Orthop Rel Res* 1982; **166**:127–131.
4 Hovelius L. Shoulder dislocation in Swedish ice hockey players. *Am J Sports Med* 1978; **6**:373–377.
5 Hovelius L, Augustini BG, Fredin H, *et al.* Primary anterior shoulder dislocation of the shoulder in young patients: a ten-year prospective study. *J Bone Joint Surg Am* 1996; **78**:1677–1684.
6 Hovelius L, Erikkson K, Fredin H, *et al.* Recurrences after initial dislocation of the shoulder results of a prospective study of treatment. *J Bone Joint Surg Am* 1983; **65**:343–349.
7 McLaughlin HL, Cavallaro WU. Primary anterior dislocation of the shoulder. *Am J Surg* 1950; **80**:615–621.
8 Rowe CR. Prognosis of dislocations of the shoulder. *J Bone Joint Surg Am* 1956; **38**: 957.
9 Simonet WT, Cofield RH. Prognosis in anterior shoulder dislocation. *Am J Sports Med* 1984; **12**:19–24.
10 Arciero RA, Wheeler JH, Ryan JB, McBride JT. Arthroscopic Bankart repair versus non-operative treatment for acute, initial anterior shoulder dislocations. *Am J Sports Med* 1994; **22**:589–594.
11 Henry JH, Genung JA. Natural History of Glenohumeral Dislocation–Revisited. *Am J Sports Med* 1982; **10**:135–137.
12 Hoelen MA, Burger AM, Rozing DM. Prognosis of primary anterior shoulder dislocation in young adults. *Arch Orthop Trauma Surg* 1990; **110**:51–54.
13 Marans HL, Angel KR, Schemitsch EH, Wedge JH. The fate of traumatic anterior dislocation of the shoulder in children. *J Bone Joint Surg Am* 1992; **74**:1242–1244.
14 Vermeiren J, Handelberg F, Casteleyn PP, Opdecam P. The rate of recurrence of traumatic anterior dislocation of the shoulder: a study of 154 and a review of the literature. *Int Orthop* 1993; **17**:337–341.
15 Wheeler JH, Ryan JB, Arciero RA, Molinari RN. Arthroscopic versus non-operative treatment of acute shoulder dislocations in young athletes. *Arthroscopy* 1989; **5**:213–217.
16 Kirkley A, Griffin S, McClintock JH, Ng L. Development and evaluation of a disease specific quality-of-life measurement tool for shoulder instability. *Am J Sports Med* 1998; **26**:764–772.
17 Huston P. Cochrane Collaboration helping unravel tangled web woven by international research. *CMAJ* 1996; **154**:1389–1392.
18 Handoll HH, Almaiyah MA, Rangan A. Surgical versus non-surgical treatment for acute anterior shoulder dislocation. *Cochrane Database Syst Rev* 2004;(1):CD004325.

19 Handoll H, Hanchard N, Goodchild L, Feary J. Conservative management following closed reduction of traumatic anterior dislocation of the shoulder. *Cochrane Database Syst Rev* 2006;(1):CD004962.

20 Kirkley A, Griffin S, Richards C, Miniaci A, Mohtadi N. Prospective randomized clinical trial comparing the effectiveness of immediate stabilization versus immobilization and rehabilitation in first traumatic anterior dislocations of the shoulder. *Arthroscopy* 1999; **15**:507–514.

21 Kirkley A, Werstine R, Ratjek A, Griffin S. Prospective randomized clinical trial comparing the effectiveness of immediate arthroscopic stabilization versus immobilization and rehabilitation in first traumatic anterior dislocations of the shoulder: long-term evaluation. *Arthroscopy* 2005; **21**:55–63.

22 Wintzell G, Haglund-Akerlind Y, Ekelund A, *et al.* Arthroscopic lavage reduced the recurrence rate following primary anterior shoulder dislocation: a randomised multicentre study with 1-year follow up. *Knee Surg Sports Traumatol* 1999; **7**:192–196.

23 Wintzell G, Haglund-Akerlind Y, Nowak J, Larsson S. Arthroscopic lavage compared with non-operative treatment for traumatic primary anterior shoulder dislocation: a 2-year follow up of a prospective randomized study. *J Shoulder Elbow Surg* 1999; **8**:399–402.

24 Wintzell G, Haglund-Akerlind Y, Tidermark J, Wredmark T, Ericksson E. A prospective controlled randomized study of arthroscopic lavage in acute primary anterior shoulder dislocation: one year follow up. *Knee Surg Sports Traumatol* 1996; **4**:43–47.

25 Bottoni CR, Wilckens JH, DeBerardino TM, *et al.* A prospective, randomized evaluation of arthroscopic stabilization versus nonoperative treatment in patients with acute, traumatic, first-time shoulder dislocations. *Am J Sports Med* 2002; **30**:576–580.

26 Jakobsen BSJ. Primary repair after traumatic anterior dislocation of the shoulder joint. *Acta Orthop Scand Suppl* 1996; **272**:67.

27 Sandow M. [Personal communication.]

28 Sandow M. Arthroscopic repair for primary shoulder dislocation: a randomized clinical trial [abstract]. *J Bone Joint Surg Br* 1995; **77** (Suppl 1):67.

29 Sandow M, Liu SH. Acute arthroscopic Bankart repair for initial anterior shoulder dislocation: a prospective clinical trial [abstract]. *J Shoulder Elbow Surg* 1996; **5**:581.

30 Hovelius L. Anterior dislocation of the shoulder in teen-agers and young adults. *J Bone Joint Surg Am* 1987; **69A**:393–399.

31 Sachs RA, Lem D, Stone ML, Paxton L, Kuney M. Can the need for future surgery be predicted? A prospective study of patients following acute traumatic anterior shoulder dislocation. [Paper presented at the 72nd Annual Meeting of the American Academy of Orthopedic Surgeons, Washington, D.C., February, 2005.]

32 McLaughlin HL. Recurrent anterior dislocation of the shoulder, 1: morbid anatomy. *Am J Surg* 1960; **99**:626–631.

33 McLaughlin HL MacLellan DI. Recurrent anterior dislocation of the shoulder. *J Trauma* 1967; **7**:191–201.

34 Milgrom C, Mann G, Finestone A. A prevalence study of recurrent shoulder dislocations in young adults. *J Shoulder Elbow Surg* 1998; **7**:621–624.

35 DeBerardino TM, Arciero RA, Taylor DC, Uhorchak JM. Prospective evaluation of arthroscopic stabilization of acute, initial anterior shoulder dislocations in young athletes. *Am J Sports Med* 2001; **29**:586–592.

36 Verhagen AP, de Vet HC, de Bie RA, *et al.* The Delphi list: a criteria list for quality assessment of randomized clinical trials for conducting systematic reviews developed by Delphi consensus. *J Clin Epidemiol* 1998; **51**:1235–1241.

37 Berlin JA. Does blinding of readers affect the results of meta-analyses? University of Pennsylvania Meta-analysis Blinding Study Group. *Lancet* 1997; **350**:185–186.

38 Lill H, Verheyden P, Korner J, Hepp P, Josten C. [Conservative treatment after 1st traumatic shoulder dislocation; in German]. *Chirurg* 1998; **69**:1230–1237.

39 Hovelius L. The natural history of primary anterior dislocation of the shoulder in the young. *J Orthop Sci* 1999; **4**:307–317.

40 Tijmes J, Loyd HM, Tullos HS. Arthrography in acute shoulder dislocations. *South Med J* 1979; **72**:564–567.

41 Neviaser RJ, Neviaser TJ, Neviaser JS. Anterior dislocation of the shoulder and rotator cuff rupture. *Clin Orthop* 1993; **291**:103–106.

42 Te Slaa RL, Brand R, Marti RK. A prospective arthroscopic study of acute first-time anterior shoulder dislocation in the young: a five-year follow-up study. *J Shoulder Elbow Surg* 2003; **12**:529–534.
43 Cleeman E, Flatow EL. Shoulder dislocations in the young patient. *Orthop Clin North Am* 2000; **31**:217–229.
44 Hovelius L, Augustini BG, Fredin H, *et al.* Correspondence: reply. *J Bone Joint Surg Am* 1998; **80**:299–300.
45 Kiviluoto O, Pasila M, Jaroma H, Sundholm A. Immobilization after primary dislocation of the shoulder. *Acta Orthop Scand* 1980; **51**:915–919.
46 Aronen JG, Regan K. Decreasing the incidence of recurrence of first time anterior shoulder dislocations with rehabilitation. *Am J Sports Med* 1984; **12**:283–291.
47 Yoneda B, Welsh RP, MacIntosh DL. Conservative treatment of shoulder dislocation in young males. *J Bone Joint Surg Br* 1982; **64**:254–255.
48 Itoi E, Hatakeyama Y, Urayama M, *et al.* Position of immobilization after dislocation of the shoulder: a cadaveric study. *J Bone Joint Surg Am* 1999; **81**:385–390.
49 Itoi E, Sashi R, Minagawa H, *et al.* Position of immobilization after dislocation of the glenohumeral joint: a study with use of magnetic resonance imaging. *J Bone Joint Surg Am* 2001; **83**:661–667.
50 Baker CL Jr. Arthroscopic evaluation of acute initial shoulder dislocations. *Instr Course Lect* 1996; **45**:83–89.
51 Baker CL Jr, Uribe JW, Whitman C. Arthroscopic evaluation of acute initial shoulder dislocations. *Am J Sports Med* 1990; **18**:25–28.
52 Norlin R. Intra-articular pathology in acute, first-time anterior shoulder dislocation: an arthroscopic study. *Arthroscopy* 1993; **9**:546–549.
53 Miller BS, Sonnabend DH, Hatrick C, *et al.* Should acute anterior dislocations of the shoulder be immobilized in external rotation? A cadaveric study. *J Shoulder Elbow Surg* 2004; **13**:589–592.
54 Itoi E, Hatakeyama Y, Kido T, Sato T, Minagawa H, Wakabayashi I, Kobayashi MA new method of immobilization after traumatic anterior dislocation of the shoulder: a preliminary study. *J Shoulder Elbow Surg* 2003; **12**:413–415.
55 Burkhead WZ, Rockwood CA. Treatment of instability of the shoulder with an exercise program. *J Bone Joint Surg Am* 1992; **74**:890–896.
56 Boszotta H, Helperstorfer W. Arthroscopic Transglenoid suture repair for initial anterior shoulder dislocation. *Arthroscopy* 2000; **16**:462–470.
57 Salmon JM, Bell SN. Arthroscopic stabilization of the shoulder for acute primary dislocations using a transglenoid suture technique. *Arthroscopy* 1998; **14**:143–147.
58 Uribe JW, Hechtman KS. Arthroscopically assisted repair of acute Bankart lesions. *Orthopaedics* 1993; **16**:1019–1023.
59 Fabbriciani C, Milano G, Demontis A, *et al.* Arthroscopic versus open treatment of Bankart lesion of the shoulder: a prospective randomized study. *Arthroscopy* 2004; **20**:456–462.
60 Williams GN, Gangel TJ, Arciero RA, Uhorchak JM, Taylor DC. Comparison of the single assessment numeric evaluation method and two shoulder rating scales: outcomes measures after shoulder surgery. *Am J Sports Med* 1999; **27**:214–221.
61 L'Insalata JC, Warren RF, Cohen SB, Altchek DW, Peterson MGE. A self-administered questionnaire for assessment of symptoms and function of the shoulder. *J Bone Joint Surg Am* 1997; **79**:738–748.
62 Wintzell G, Hovelius L, Wikblad L, Saebo M, Larsson S. Arthroscopic lavage speeds reduction in effusion in the glenohumeral joint after primary anterior shoulder dislocation: a controlled randomized ultrasound study. *Knee Surg Sports Traumatol Arthrosc* 2000; **8**:56–60.
63 Mole D, Coudane H, Quievreux P, Rio B, Roche O. Acute primary anterior glenohumeral dislocation: arthroscopic evaluation of the lesions and prognostic factors [abstract]. *J Shoulder Elbow Surg* 1999; **5**:S81.
64 Magnuson PB, Stack JK. Recurrent dislocation of the shoulder. *JAMA* 1943; **23**:889–892.
65 Osmond-Clarke H. Habitual dislocation of the shoulder: the Putti–Platt operation. *J Bone Joint Surg Br* 1948; **30**:19–25.
66 Helfet AJ. Coracoid transplantation for recurring dislocation of the shoulder. *J Bone Joint Surg Br* 1958; **40**:198–202.
67 Bankart ASB. Recurrent or habitual dislocation of the shoulder joint. *Br Med J* 1923; **2**:1132–1133.
68 Payne LZ, Altchek DW. The surgical treatment of anterior shoulder instability. *Clin Sports Med* 1995; **14**:863–883.

69 Rowe CR. Acute and recurrent anterior dislocations of the shoulder. *Orthop Clin North Am* 1980; **11**:252–270.
70 Coughlin L, Rubinovich M, Johansson J, White B, Greenspoon J. Arthroscopic staple capsulorrhaphy for anterior shoulder instability. *Am J Sports Med* 1992; **20**:253–256.
71 Grana WA, Buckley PD, Yates CK. Arthroscopic Bankart suture repair. *Am J Sports Med* 1993; **21**:348–353.
72 Manta JP, Organ S, Nirschl RP, Pettrone FA. Arthroscopic transglenoid suture capsulolabral repair: five year follow-up. *Am J Sports Med* 1997; **25**:614–618.
73 Mologne TS, Lapoint JM, Morin WD, Zilberfarb J, O'Brien TJ. Arthroscopic anterior labral reconstruction using a transglenoid suture technique: results in active duty military patients. *Am J Sports Med* 1996; **24**:268–274.
74 Pagnani MJ, Warren RF, Altchek DW, Wickiewicz TL, Anderson AF. Arthroscopic shoulder stabilization using transglenoid sutures: a four year minimum follow up. *Am J Sports Med* 1996; **24**:459–467.
75 Walch G, Boileau P, Levigne C, *et al.* Arthroscopic stabilization for recurrent anterior shoulder dislocation: results of 59 cases. *Arthroscopy* 1995; **11**:173–179.
76 Youssef JA, Carr CF, Walther CE, Murphy JM. Arthroscopic Bankart suture repair for recurrent traumatic unidirectional anterior shoulder dislocations. *Arthroscopy* 1995; **11**:561–563.
77 Matsen FA III, Thomas SC, Rockwood CA Jr. Anterior glenohumeral stability. In: Rockwood CA Jr, Matsen FA III, eds. *The Shoulder,* vol. 1. Philadelphia: Saunders, 1990: 547–551.

CHAPTER 20

Are corticosteroid injections as effective as physiotherapy for the treatment of a painful shoulder?

Daniëlle van der Windt and Bart Koes

Introduction

Shoulder pain is a common problem. The prevalence of shoulder pain in the general population may be as high as 6–11% in those under the age of 50 years, increasing to 16–25% in the elderly.[1,2] Estimates of the annual incidence of shoulder disorders in general practice vary from seven to 12 per 1000 registered patients per year.[3–5] Inability to work, loss of productivity, and inability to carry out household activities can be a considerable burden to the patient as well as to society.[6]

Shoulder pain can be the result of a variety of disorders, including referred pain from the cervical spine or internal organs, neurovascular disorders, and systemic conditions of the musculoskeletal system. In the majority of cases, however, the symptoms are caused by benign soft-tissue lesions of the shoulder joint.[7–9] Fifty percent of all presented episodes resolve within 6 months, but in many patients pain and disability may last longer, for many months or even years.[10–15]

Because of the complex functional anatomy of the shoulder girdle, the diagnosis of shoulder pain constitutes a major challenge. Determination of the exact location of the involved structures is often problematic. Consequently, there is much confusion and lack of consensus regarding the classification of shoulder disorders. Diagnostic criteria may even vary for disorders straightforwardly labeled as rotator cuff tendinitis or adhesive capsulitis. Difficulties have been encountered when trying to classify patients with shoulder pain according to diagnostic guidelines.[16] Although interobserver agreement on the diagnostic classification of shoulder pain has been reported to be high in one study ($\kappa = 0.88$),[17] results from other studies indicate that interobserver agreement can be rather poor among (trained) physiotherapists, general practitioners, and rheumatologists.[18–20] Furthermore, in many patients symptoms and signs vary over time, further complicating the identification of the source of shoulder pain. These difficulties should be taken into account when assessing a patient with shoulder pain. This chapter, therefore, does not concern a specific medical diagnosis, such as rotator cuff tendinitis or adhesive capsulitis, but is generally aimed at patients with a painful shoulder due to soft-tissue disorders of the shoulder, for whom treatment with corticosteroid injections or physiotherapy is considered.

Most patients with a painful shoulder are treated in primary care. Several interventions have been suggested for their treatment. If analgesics or nonsteroidal anti-inflammatory drugs (NSAIDs) do not result in relief of symptoms, patients are often referred for physiotherapy or treated with local infiltration of a corticosteroid.[4] In this chapter, the available evidence for the effectiveness of physiotherapy and corticosteroid injections will be summarized in a systematic review of the medical literature. This review has been substantially updated since the first edition of *Evidence-Based Sports Medicine*. It is the aim of this chapter to pay specific attention to the comparison between the effectiveness of corticosteroid injections and physiotherapy (exercises and/or mobilizations) in the treatment of shoulder pain.

Summary

- A painful or stiff shoulder is a common problem, which is mainly encountered and dealt with in primary care.
- Shoulder pain remains a diagnostic challenge. The reliability of diagnostic classifications based on identification of the source of the lesion has been shown to be poor.
- Previous systematic reviews have shown that there is insufficient evidence to support or refute the effectiveness of injections and physiotherapy for the painful shoulder.

Methods

Search strategy

Relevant trial reports were identified in MEDLINE, EMBASE, and the Cochrane Databases. Searches were conducted in 1995 to harvest randomized controlled trials (RCTs) for two systematic reviews.[21,22] Updates for *Evidence-Based Sports Medicine* have been carried out in 2001, 2003, and 2005 using similar search strategies. For the identification of RCTs, the search strategy described by Alderson *et al.* in the Cochrane Handbook[23] was used. This strategy was combined with relevant keywords (Medical Subject Headings and free-text words) related to shoulder pain, injections, corticosteroids, physiotherapy, manipulative therapy, mobilizations, and exercise therapy. The references of all retrieved trials and other relevant publications, including reviews and meta-analyses, were screened for additional potentially relevant publications.

Selection criteria

We identified trial reports that met the following conditions:

- Patients had shoulder pain and/or restricted mobility of the shoulder joint at inclusion. Symptoms and signs were assumed to originate from disorders of the shoulder joint. Trials aimed at extrinsic causes of shoulder pain (for example, systemic neurological or rheumatological disorders, neoplastic disorders, or cervicobrachialgia) were not selected.
- Treatments were allocated by a random procedure.
- At least one of the study groups was treated with corticosteroid injections and/or physiotherapy (including mobilizations or exercises). Trials investigating the effectiveness of physical applications only (for example, ultrasound therapy, electrotherapy, or laser therapy) were not selected. Comparisons with placebo interventions were allowed as well as comparisons with no treatment or other types of active interventions.
- Relevant outcome measures were used, such as success rate, pain, mobility or functional status.
- Results were published as a full report in English, German, Dutch, or French before March 2005.

Box 20.1 Checklist for assessing the internal validity of randomized trials[25]

Each item is scored as either "yes," "no," or "unclear."

- V1: Was a method of randomization performed? (Random—unpredictable—generation of sequence. Stating only "randomization" is scored "unclear")
- V2: Was the treatment allocation concealed? (sealed envelopes, randomization by telephone, etc.) (Allocation of the intervention cannot be influenced by those responsible for determining eligibility.)
- V3: Were the intervention groups similar at baseline with regard to prognostic indicators (age, gender, duration of symptoms, previous episodes of shoulder pain) and baseline scores of outcome measures?
- V4: Was the care provider blinded to the allocated intervention?
- V5: Were co-interventions avoided or standardized?
- V6: Was the level of adherence to the intervention (compliance) acceptable in all groups?
- V7: Was the patient blinded to the allocated intervention?
- V8: Was the withdrawal/drop-out rate described and acceptable? (The number of drop-outs and reasons for withdrawal are specified. The reviewer determines whether withdrawal has led to substantial bias.)
- V9: Was the outcome assessor blinded to the allocated intervention?
- V10: Was the timing of outcome assessment comparable in both groups?

Assessment of quality

Differences in the quality of methods across studies may indicate that the results of some trials are more biased than those of others. It is therefore important to take the quality of a study into account when evaluating the effectiveness of an intervention.[24] The internal validity of each trial was scored by two reviewers independently, using the standardized set of validity criteria from the Amsterdam–Maastricht Consensus List for Quality Assessment (Box 20.1).[25] Although the Amsterdam–Maastricht consensus list is not exhaustive, it represents a high standard for internal validity of trial methods. Much emphasis (together representing five out of 10 criteria) is put on an adequate randomization procedure and sufficient blinding. Other criteria in this checklist refer to prognostic similarity of intervention groups at baseline, drop-out rate, and control for co-interventions and compliance. The number of positively scored validity items was denoted as the validity score. A trial receiving a score of at least 6 points was (arbitrarily) considered to be of adequate validity.

Data extraction and analysis

Details on selection criteria, interventions, outcome measures, length of follow-up, adverse reactions, study size, analysis, and data presentation were extracted for each trial. The results of data extraction were used mainly to consider the generalizability of study findings (external validity) and to evaluate clinical heterogeneity across trials. The Cochrane Q test and I^2 were used to detect the statistical heterogeneity of trial results. In case of statistical heterogeneity (Q test $P < 0.10$, and high values of I^2), potential sources of heterogeneity were explored. For these exploratory subgroup analyses, the following variables were considered: type of control group, type of corticosteroid, duration of symptoms at baseline, medical diagnosis, total validity score, and separate aspects of validity (blinding, randomization procedure, and drop-out rate). Pooled estimates of outcome were computed for trials that showed sufficient homogeneity with respect to interventions and outcome measures, using a random-effects model.[26–28]

Data concerning general improvement of symptoms were used to compute success rates for each study group. The operational definition of a treatment success may vary across trials depending on the instrument used, and will be presented for each trial. The differences in success rates between study groups were computed, together with the 95% confidence intervals (CI). Subsequently, the number needed to treat (NNT) was computed as $1/(Pi - Pc)$, with Pi = the proportion of successes in the intervention group, and Pc = the proportion of successes in the reference group.[29]

For outcomes evaluated on a continuous or interval scale (for example, visual analogue scales for pain), standardized mean differences (SMDs) were computed as the difference between the mean change in outcome since baseline in the compared groups, divided by their pooled standard deviation.[30]

Differences between study groups may be considered to be clinically important if differences in success rates between study groups exceed 20% (NNT < 5),[31] or standardized mean differences are larger than 0.5.[30,32] A negative NNT or a negative SMD indicated superior effects of the reference treatment.

Results

The search in 2001 resulted in the identification of 85 papers, of which 62 papers were excluded. A total of 23 RCTs were included in the first edition of this chapter: 15 comparing the effectiveness of corticosteroid injections with placebo, analgesics or no treatment for shoulder pain;[33–47] four trials on the effectiveness of physiotherapy (mobilization and/or exercises);[48–52] and four comparing the effectiveness of corticosteroid injections with physiotherapy.[53–57]

The updated searches in March 2005 resulted in another 163 hits in MEDLINE, 62 in EMBASE, and 54 in the Cochrane databases. Out of these 279 hits, 256 were excluded for the following reasons: no randomized allocation of interventions (n = 120), no shoulder pain according to the selection criteria (n = 69), no relevant contrast regarding physiotherapy or injection therapy (n = 62), no relevant outcome measure, or no results presented (n = 5). The 18 remaining hits referred to 10 relevant RCTs.[58–67] Two additional trials were identified through reference tracking.[68,69] This means that a total of 35 RCTs were included in this updated review: 19 RCTs comparing the effectiveness of corticosteroid injections with placebo, analgesics or no treatment for shoulder pain;[33–47,58–61] nine trials on the effectiveness of physiotherapy (mobilization and/or exercises);[48–52,59,62–65,68] and seven comparing the effectiveness of corticosteroid injections with physiotherapy.[53–57,66,67,69] The trial by Carette *et al.*[59] included four intervention groups (corticosteroid injections, physiotherapy, both injections and physiotherapy, and a placebo intervention) and is included in all relevant comparisons.

Methodological quality

Table 20.1 presents the results of the assessment of internal validity of the selected trials. The papers are ranked according to their validity score. Papers with equal scores are ranked in alphabetical order based on the first author's name. The median validity score was 5 points. Methodological shortcomings mainly concerned blinding of the care provider (V4), patient (V7), or outcome assessment (V9).

Table 20.1 Results of quality assessment of randomized trials on corticosteroid injections and/or physiotherapy for shoulder pain

First author, ref.	Diagnosis or complaint	Symptom duration	Validity score (max. 10)*
Corticosteroid injections versus placebo/no treatment/analgesics			
Alvarez[58]	Chronic rotator cuff tendinosis	> 6 weeks	9
Carette[59]	Adhesive capsulitis	< 1 year	9
De Jong[33]	Capsulitis	no restriction	8
Adebajo[34]	Rotator cuff tendinitis	≤ 3 months	7
Akgün[60]	Subacromial impingement syndrome	No restriction	7
Blair[35]	Subacromial impingement syndrome	≥ 3 months	7
McInerney[61]	Post-traumatic impingement	No restriction	7
Petri[36]	Painful shoulder	No restriction	7
Vecchio[37]	Rotator cuff tendinitis	≤ 3 months	7
Withrington[38]	Supraspinatus tendinitis	No restriction	7
Richardson[39]	Painful shoulder	> 6 months	6
Jacobs[40]	Capsulitis	No restriction	5
Rizk[41]	Adhesive capsulitis	≤ 3 months	5
Berry[42]	Shoulder cuff lesion	No restriction	4
Hollingworth[43]	Painful shoulder	No restriction	4
Plafki[44]	Subacromial impingement syndrome	≥ 3 months	4
White[45]	Rotator cuff tendinitis	≤ 3 months	4
Lee[46]	Periarthritis	No restriction	2
Ströbel[47]	Painful shoulder	No restriction	2
Physiotherapy (exercise/mobilizations) versus placebo/no additional treatment			
Carette[59]	Adhesive capsulitis	< 1 year	9
Bergman[62]	Shoulder pain and dysfunction	No restriction	8
Bang[48]	Shoulder impingement syndrome	No restriction	7
Pajareya[63]	Adhesive capsulitis	No restriction	7
Brox[49,50]	Rotator cuff disease	≥ 3 months	6
Conroy[51]	Shoulder impingement syndrome	No restriction	5
Ginn[52]	Shoulder pain	No restriction	5
Walther[64]	Shoulder impingement syndrome	No restriction	5
Ludewig[65]	Shoulder impingement syndrome	No restriction	4
Werner[68]	Subacromial impingement syndrome	No restriction	3
Corticosteroid injections versus physiotherapy (exercises/mobilizations)			
Carette[59]	Adhesive capsulitis	< 1 year	9
Hay[66]	Shoulder pain	No restriction	7
Van der Windt[53]	Painful stiff shoulder	No restriction	6
Ginn[67]	Unilateral shoulder pain	> 1 month	4
Arslan[69]	Adhesive capsulitis	No restriction	3
Bulgen[54]	Frozen shoulder	≥ 1 month	3
Dacre[55]	Painful stiff shoulder	≥ 1 month	3
Winters[56,57]	Synovial shoulder disorders†	≥ 1 week	3

* Number of positively scored validity criteria. The validity criteria are enumerated as in Box 20.1.
† This study also includes a randomized evaluation of exercises versus manipulative treatment for shoulder girdle problems, which is not included in this review.

Many publications provided insufficient information to allow a good evaluation of the study design. This frequently concerned the description of procedures used for the generation of a random sequence (V1), for concealment of the allocation of interventions (V2), and for evaluation of compliance (V6).

Study characteristics

Table 20.1 also presents details about the duration of symptoms and medical diagnosis in patients included in the selected trials. Most trials concerned patients with a diagnosis of rotator cuff tendinitis, impingement syndrome or cuff lesion (16 trials), or a more general diagnosis of painful shoulder or painful stiff shoulder (10 trials). In 21 trials, no limitations were defined regarding the duration of symptoms at inclusion. Other trials did use selection criteria concerning the length of symptoms, restricting participation to either patients with chronic shoulder pain[35,39,44,49] or more acute shoulder pain.[34,37,41,45]

Table 20.2 presents information about the interventions, short-term results (after 2–8 weeks) for success rate and pain, and the authors' conclusions. Long-term follow-up measurements (at least 6 months) were described for 13 trials.[41,44,47,50,53–55,57–59,62,63,66] The study sizes were generally small; only five trials compared study groups of at least 50 patients and were designed with sufficient power to detect a difference in success rate of approximately 25%.[49,53,62,63,66] The median group size was only 20 patients.

Effectiveness of corticosteroid injections

Corticosteroids compared to "placebo"

In 18 trials, the effectiveness of corticosteroid injections was compared with a treatment considered to be of little or no effectiveness, being either a local anesthetic,[34–37,41,44,47,58,60] saline injection,[38,39,59] low-dose corticosteroid,[33] trigger-point injection,[43] distension,[40] placebo ultrasound,[42] analgesics,[46] or no other treatment[61] (Table 20.2). Eleven trials received validity scores of at least 6 points. Seven of these 11 trials reported significantly better short-term outcomes for corticosteroids. We used differences in proportions of treatment success to study the magnitude of the treatment effect. Such data were not available for five trials.[40,44,46,59,60] Figure 20.1 presents the differences in success rates (and 95% confidence intervals) for 13 trials. The trials are ranked according to their validity score. There was wide statistical heterogeneity across trials (test for heterogeneity $P < 0.0001$, $I^2 = 81.3\%$), with differences in the success rate between corticosteroids and control ranging between –25% and 70%. Therefore, we refrained from statistical pooling of the results.

We considered it likely that some of this heterogeneity was explained by differences across trials regarding the definition of a treatment success. Quality of methods did not appear to strongly influence the outcome. The results of trials with relatively high validity scores were not consistently different from those of relatively poor quality (Figure 20.1). A significant influence of specific aspects of validity (drop-out rate, blinding, or randomization procedure) could not be found (data not shown). Subsequently, exploratory subgroup analyses were conducted to investigate the potential influence of clinically relevant variables, including the use of different corticosteroid suspensions (triamcinolone or other), duration of symptoms at baseline, and medical diagnosis. The subgroup analyses showed only a few homogeneous subgroups. Favorable results were found for the use of triamcinolone compared to other suspensions, for patients with a relatively short duration of symptoms at baseline (less than 3 months), and for a diagnosis of capsulitis: pooled differences in success rates were 42% (95% CI, 25% to 60%), 42% (95% CI, 5% to 80%), and 43% (95% CI, 28% to 59%), respectively. However, these subgroup effects were based on small subgroups of trials, and showed considerable unexplained heterogeneity.

Only four trials, all of good quality, presented sufficient data for standardized mean differences for pain to be computed.[33,34,36,59] The pooled SMD for the improvement of

Table 20.2 Interventions and short-term results of randomized trials comparing corticosteroid injections with placebo treatment, no treatment, or analgesics for shoulder pain

First author, ref.	Validity score	Study groups (number of patients)	Follow-up (last assessment)	Success rate per group ΔSR (95% CI), NNT	Pain	Authors' conclusions
Alvarez[58]	9	i 1 x subacromial betamethasone & xylocaine (31) ii 1 × 6 mg subacromial xylocaine (31)	3 months (6 months)	Improvement on the WORC excellent or good: i: 2/30 (6.7%); ii: 2/28 (7.0%) ΔSR = 0.3% (–0.14 to 0.13%), NNT = 333		No significant differences for quality of life, ROM or impingement sign
Carette[59]	9	i 1 × 40 mg intra-articular triamcinolone hexacetonide (23) ii 12 × physiotherapy: TENS, mobilization techniques, active exercises, and ice (26) iii 1 × 40 mg triamcinolone + physiotherapy (21) iv 1 × saline (23)	6 weeks (12 months)		SPADI-pain mean change (SD) i: 39.1 (26.9); iii: 48.7 (27.0); iv: 17.3 (26.9) SMD i vs iv = 0.80 (0.19 to 1.40) SMD iii vs iv = 1.14 (0.50 to 1.79)	Significant short-term differences for pain, ROM, and function in favor of injection and injection + physiotherapy
De Jong[33]	8	i 3 × 40 mg intra-articular triamcinolone (25) ii 3 × 10 mg triamcinolone (32)	6 weeks	No residual functional impairment: i: 10/24 (42%); ii: 1/28 (4%) ΔSR = 36% (17 to 59%), NNT = 3	VAS (0–100), mean change (SD) i: 49.3 (21.3); ii: 31.2 (49.3) SMD = 0.46 (–0.10 to 1.01)	Significant differences for ROM, pain, function, and sleep disturbance in favor of high-dose triamcinolone
Adebajo[34]	7	i 1 × 80 mg subacromial triamcinolone & lignocaine plus placebo diclofenac (20) ii 1 × subacromial lignocaine plus diclofenac 150 mg daily (20) iii 1 × subacromial lignocaine plus placebo diclofenac (20)	4 weeks	Improvement pain, ROM & function: i: 14/20 (70%); ii: 6/20 (30%); iii: 0%. ΔSR i vs iii: 70% (49 to 91%), NNT = 2 ΔSR i vs ii: 40% (12 to 68%), NNT = 3	VAS (0–10), mean change (SD) i: 4.95 (3.31); ii: 3.60 (3.00); iii: 1.35 (3.31) SMD i vs iii: 1.07 (0.40 to 1.73) SMD i vs ii: 0.42 (–0.21 to 1.05)	Significant difference for pain, ROM, functional status in favor of i and ii. Triamcinolone Injections showed largest improvement

Continued

Table 20.2 *(Continued)*

First author, ref.	Validity score	Study groups (number of patients)	Follow-up (last assessment)	Success rate per group ΔSR (95% CI), NNT	Pain	Authors' conclusions
Akgün[60]	7	i 2 × subacromial 40 mg methylprednisolone & lignocaine (16) ii 1 × subacromial methylprednisolone & lignocaine, 1 x subacromial lignocaine (16) iii 2 × subacromial lignocaine (16)	1 month (3 months)		VAS pain on activity (0–10), mean (SD): i: 1.1 (0.9); ii: 1.4 (1.1); iii: 1.7 (1.0)	Significant differences in favor of corticosteroids for pain disturbing sleep, and function
Blair[35]	7	i 1 × 40 mg subacromial triamcinolone & lidocaine (19) ii 1 × subacromial lidocaine (21)	? (12 to 52 weeks)	Pain decreased: i: 16/19 (84%); ii: 8/21 (38%) ΔSR = 46% (20 to 73%), NNT = 2	4-point ordinal scale, mean score: i: 1.2; ii: 2.0 ($P < 0.005$)	Significant differences in favor of triamcinolone for pain, and ROM, but not for function
McInerney[61]	7	i 1 × 40 mg subacromial methylprednisolone and bupivacaine plus home exercises (54) ii Home exercises only (44)	12 weeks	VAS score > 1: i: 16/49 (32.6%); ii: 13/40 32.5%) ΔSR = 0.1% (–0.19 to 0.20%), NNT = 1000	VAS (0–10), mean score: i: 1.38; ii: 1.38 Only graphical data presentation for measures of dispersion	No significant differences for pain or ROM
Petri[36]	7	i 1 × 40 mg intrabursal triamcinolone & lidocaine plus placebo naproxen (25) ii 1 × 40 mg intrabursal triamcinolone & lidocaine plus naproxen 1000 mg daily (25) iii 1 × intrabursal lidocaine plus placebo naproxen (25) iv 1 × intrabursal lidocaine plus naproxen 1000 mg daily (25)	4 weeks	Remission: i: 7/25 (28%); ii: 7/25 (28%); iii: 2/25 (8%); iv: 5/25 (20%) ΔSR i vs iii = 20% (0 to 41%), NNT = 5 ΔSR i vs iv = 8% (–16 to 32%), NNT = 13	5-point ordinal scale, mean change (SD): i: 2.04 (1.55); ii: 1.95 (1.75); iii: 1.00 (1.60); iv: 1.76 (1.55) SMD i vs iii: 0.65 (0.08 to 1.22) SMD i vs iv: 0.18 (–0.38 to 0.73)	Significant differences for pain, ROM, function, and a clinical index in favor of triamcinolone compared to placebo. No significant differences compared to NSAIDs

Vecchio[37]	7	i 1 × 40 mg subacromial methylprednisolone & lignocaine (28) ii 1 × subacromial lignocaine (27)	4 weeks (12 weeks)	Complete remission: i: 9/28 (32%); ii: 7/27 (26%). ΔSR i vs ii = 6% (–18 to 30%), NNT = 17	VAS (1–100), median change (IQR): i: 10 (5 to 15); ii: 8 (4 to 14) Median Δ = 2 (P = 0.36)	No significant differences for success rate, pain, and ROM
Withrington[38]	7	i 1 × supraspinatus tendon 80 mg methylprednisolone & lignocaine (12) ii 1 × supraspinatus tendon saline (13)	8 weeks	Responders according to observer: i: 5/12 (42%); ii: 3/13 (23%) ΔSR i vs ii = 19% (–18 to 55%), NNT = 5	VAS (0–10), mean change: i: 2.7; ii: 1.2 ($p > 0.05$) SMD: insufficient data	No significant differences for success rate, pain, and use of analgesics
Richardson[39]	6	i 2 × intra-articular & intrabursal 25 mg prednisolone acetate plus Distalgic (54) ii 2 × intra-articular & intrabursal saline plus Distalgic (47)	6 weeks	Definite improvement / complete recovery (pain): i: 29/54 (53%); ii: 22/47 (46%) ΔSR i vs ii = 7% (–13 to 26%), NNT = 14		Significant improvement in favor of corticosteroids for ROM, but only a trend for pain
Jacobs[40]	5	i 3 × 40 mg intra-articular triamcinolone (15) ii 3 × 40 mg intra-articular triamcinolone plus distension (18) iii distension only (14)	6 weeks (16 weeks)		Data only available for ROM	Significant differences for ROM in favor of triamcinolone; no significant differences between i and ii
Rizk[41]	5	i 3 × 40 mg intra-articular methylprednisolone & lidocaine (16) ii 3 × 40 mg intrabursal methylprednisolone & lidocaine (16) iii 3 × intra-articular lidocaine (8) iv 3 × intrabursal lidocaine (8)	4 weeks (24 weeks)	Some relief: i: 10/16 (63%); ii: 10/16 (63%); 1/8 (13%); iv: 1/8 (13%) ΔSR (i + ii vs iii + iv) = 50% (27 to 73%), NNT = 2	6-point ordinal scale, mean score: i: 3.9; ii: 3.7; iii + iv: 3.9	No significant differences for pain and ROM

Continued

Table 20.2 *(Continued)*

First author, ref.	Validity score	Study groups (number of patients)	Follow-up (last assessment)	Success rate per group ΔSR (95% CI), NNT	Pain	Authors' conclusions
Berry[42]	4	i 1 × 40 mg intra-articular methyl-prednisolone & lignocaine plus placebo tolmetin sodium (12) ii 1 × 40 mg methyl-prednisolone & lignocaine plus tolmetin sodium 1200 mg daily (12) iii acupuncture (12) iv ultrasound therapy (12) v placebo ultrasound plus placebo tolmetin (12)	4 weeks	Success (no need for injection): i: 6/12 (50%); ii: 5/12 (42%); iii: 5/12 (42%); iv: 6/12 (50%); v: 9/12 (75%). ΔSR i vs v: –25% (–62 to 12%), NNT = –4	VAS (0–100), mean score (SD): i: 26.6 (22.5); ii: 29.2 (24.3); iii: 34.1 (27.2); iv: 41.2 (36.6); v: 22.0 (28.6)	No significant differences for success rates, pain, and ROM
Hollingworth[43]	4	i 40 mg methylprednisolone functional (39) ii 40 mg methylprednisolone + lignocaine tender or trigger point injection (38) Cross-over study	2 weeks (8 weeks)	Mild/no symptoms (after cross-over): i: 41/69 (59%); ii: 12/63 (19%) ΔSR = 40% (25 to 56%), NNT = 3		Significant difference for success rates in favor of functional injection
Plafki[44]	4	i 1 × 10 mg subacromial triamcinolone & bupivacaine (20) ii 1 × subacromial bupivacaine (10) iii 1 × 4 mg subacromial dexamethasone (20)	6 weeks (26 weeks)	Trial stopped for group ii (poor results) Excellent results: i: 8/20 (40%); iii: 11/20 (55%) ΔSR = –15% (–46 to 16%), NNT = –7		Trial had to be stopped in placebo group. No significant differences between suspensions

White[45]	4	i 1 × 40 mg intrabursal triamcinolone acetonide plus placebo indomethacin (20) ii 1 × intrabursal saline plus indomethacin 100 mg daily (20)	? 3 to 6 weeks	Responders (low global score): i: 9/20 (45%); ii: 10/20 (50%) ΔSR = –5% (–36 to 26%), NNT = –20	VAS (0–100), mean change (SD): i: 4.3 (5.2); ii: 5.5 (8.3) SMD = –0.17 (–0.79 to 0.45)	No significant differences for global assessment, pain, and ROM
Lee[46]	2	i 1 × 25 mg intra-articular hydrocortisone acetate plus exercise therapy (20) ii 1 × 25 mg biceps tendon sheath hydrocortisone plus exercise therapy (20) iii infra-red irradiation plus exercise therapy (20) iv analgesics only (20)	6 weeks		Graphical data presentation for ROM only	No significant differences, but less improvement for ROM in group receiving analgesics only
Ströbel[47]	2	i 1 × 20 mg subacromial triamcinolone & mepivacaine plus exercises (14) ii 1 × subacromial mepivacaine plus exercises (17)	2 weeks (12 months)	Able to work since treatment: i: 6/14 (43%); ii: 1/17 (6%) ΔSR = 37% (9 to 65%), NNT = 3	4-point ordinal scale, mean reduction of pain: i: 70%; ii: 60%	Significant differences in favor of triamcinolone for pain (after 90 days) and function

CI, confidence interval; IQR, interquartile range; NNT, number needed to treat; ROM, range of movement; SD, standard deviation; SMD, standardized mean difference; SPADI, Shoulder Pain and Disability Index; SR, success rate; TENS, transcutaneous electrical nerve stimulation; VAS, visual analogue scale; WORC, Western Ontario Rotator Cuff Index.

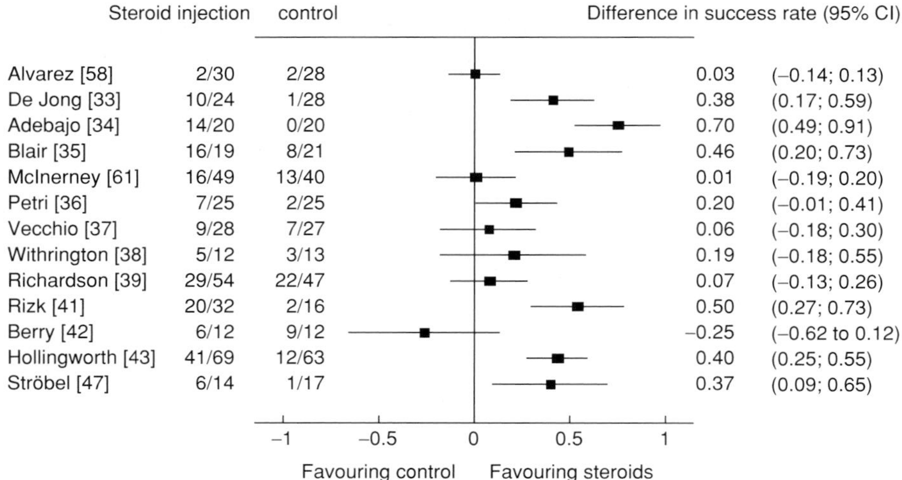

Figure 20.1 Estimates of differences in the success rate (short-term follow-up) for randomized trials comparing corticosteroid injection to placebo for shoulder pain.

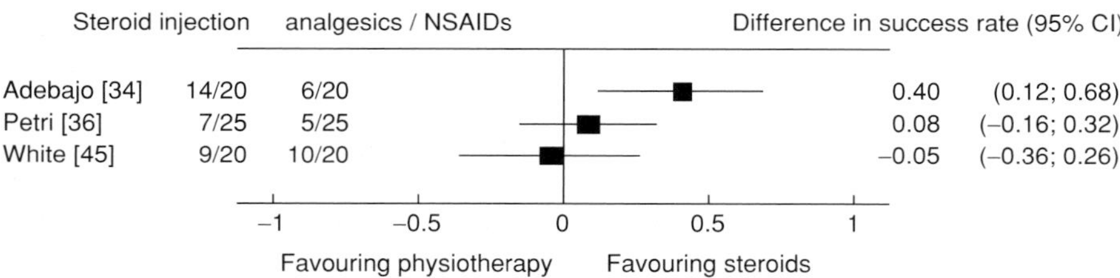

Figure 20.2 Estimates of differences in the success rate (short-term follow-up) for randomized trials comparing corticosteroid injection to nonsteroidal anti-inflammatory drugs (NSAIDs) for shoulder pain.

pain in patients treated with corticosteroid injections was 0.71 compared to placebo (95% CI, 0.42 to 1.01; test for heterogeneity, $P = 0.57$, $I^2 = 0\%$).

Corticosteroids compared to NSAIDs or analgesics

Four trials compared the effectiveness of corticosteroid injections with NSAIDs or analgesics.[34,36,45,46] One of the trials with a relatively high validity score[34] reported significant findings in favor of corticosteroids, whereas the other trials could not demonstrate significant differences. Three trials provided sufficient data to enable a quantitative analysis (Figure 20.2). Results for differences in success rate showed considerable heterogeneity, with estimates ranging between –5% and 40% (test for heterogeneity: $P = 0.09$, $I^2 = 59.4\%$). Differences in improvement of pain were small and not statistically significant (pooled SMD 0.14, 95% CI, –0.20 to 0.49; test for heterogeneity: $P = 0.42$, $I^2 = 0\%$).

Effectiveness of physiotherapy (exercises and mobilizations)

In Table 20.3, details regarding the interventions and results of 10 trials on the effectiveness of physiotherapy are presented. The results of six trials comparing physiotherapy with no treatment or a placebo intervention[49,50,52,59,63–65] are presented separately from those investigating the added value of manipulations or mobilizations.[48,51,62,68]

Four out of six trials (two with adequate validity scores) showed significant differences in favor of physiotherapy in comparison with no treatment or some form of placebo. Success rates were reported by two trials, showing differences of 16% (95% CI, 1% to 32%)[63] and 48% (95% CI, 30% to 67%)[52] in favor of physiotherapy. Three trials reported information regarding improvement of pain.[59,63,65] The pooled SMD for pain was statistically significantly in favor of physiotherapy: 0.54 (95% CI, 0.22 to 0.86, test for heterogeneity: $P = 0.25$, $I^2 = 28.9\%$). Exercise training was also reported to be of equal effectiveness in comparison with decompression surgery in patients with rotator cuff disease.[49]

Four trials evaluated the additional value of mobilizations or manipulative therapy to exercises or standardized GP care.[48,51,62,68] Three trials, two with high validity scores, reported larger improvements of pain for those treated with additional mobilizations. Pooling of these results was not possible due to insufficient data presentation by two of the trials.

Effectiveness of corticosteroid injections versus physiotherapy

It was the main objective of this chapter to investigate the more pragmatic comparison between injections and physiotherapy for shoulder pain. The number of trials investigating this comparison has increased over the past five years, from only four to eight randomized trials (Table 20.4). Only three of these trials appear to be of adequate validity.[53,59,66] The results of the trials are inconsistent. Three out of eight trials (two of adequate validity) reported significant and relevant differences in favor of corticosteroid injection for pain, function, and range of motion. One recently published large trial of adequate validity could not demonstrate any significant differences between injections and physiotherapy.[66]

Figure 20.3 shows the differences in short term success rates for four trials that provided information on this outcome measure. Statistical heterogeneity precluded statistical pooling of these results. The wide differences in outcome may be explained by variation in

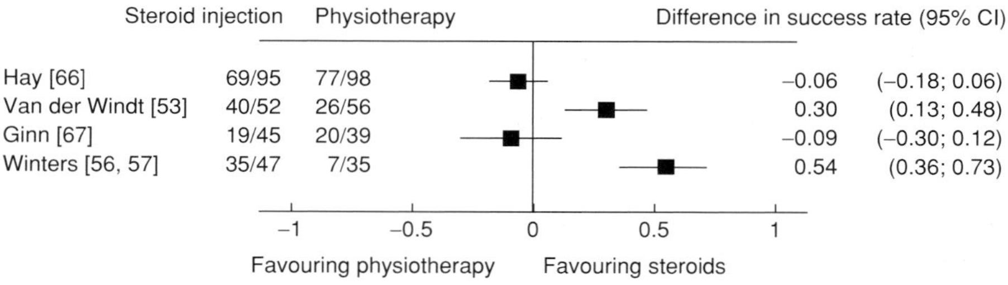

Figure 20.3 Estimates of differences in the success rate (short-term follow-up) for randomized trials comparing corticosteroid injection to physiotherapy for shoulder pain.

Table 20.3 Interventions and short-term results of randomized trials comparing physiotherapy (exercises/mobilizations) with placebo or no treatment for shoulder pain

First author, ref.	Validity score	Study groups (number of patients)	Follow-up (final assessment)	Success rate per group ΔSR (95% CI), NNT	Pain	Authors' conclusions
Physiotherapy versus control						
Carette[59]	9	i 1 × 40 mg intra-articular triamcinolone hexacetonide (23) ii 12 × physiotherapy: TENS, mobilization techniques, active exercises, and ice (26) iii 1 × 40 mg triamcinolone + physiotherapy (21) iv 1 × saline (23)	6 weeks (12 months)		SPADI-pain mean change (SD) ii: 21.8 (27.0); iv: 17.3 (26.9) SMD ii vs iv = 0.16 (−0.40 to 0.73)	No significant short-term differences for pain, ROM, and function
Pajareya[63]	7	i 9 × short-wave diathermy, mobilization and exercises plus ibuprofen & advice (61) ii ibuprofen (3 × 400 mg) & advice only (61)	3 weeks (24 weeks)	Full recovery or no interference with function: i: 21/60 (35%); ii: 11/59 (18.6%) ΔSR = 16% (1 to 32%), NNT = 6	SPADI mean change (SD) i: 20.5 (15.4); ii: 11.9 (14.2) SMD i vs ii = 0.58 (0.21 to 0.94)	Significant differences in favor of physiotherapy for pain, function and ROM
Brox[49,50]	6	i 3–6 months exercise training (58) ii Arthroscopic subacromial decompression (58) iii 12 × placebo laser therapy (34)	3 months (2.5 years)		Interim analysis, mean change Neer score: i: 10.8; ii: 20.2; iii:−0.3 median difference i vs iii: 13.0 (7 to 20) ($P < 0.001$) Randomization to placebo stopped.	Significant differences in favor of exercises and surgery compared to placebo. No differences between i and ii
Ginn[52]	5	i 4–10 × stretching/strengthening exercises, motor retraining (38?) ii No treatment (waiting list control) (28?)	1 month	Improved a lot: i: 21/38 (55%); ii: 2/28 (7%) ΔSR = 48% (30 to 67%), NNT = 2	VAS, median score: i: 1; ii: 21 ($P = 0.10$)	Significant differences in favor of exercises for function, ROM, and self-rated improvement, but not for pain

Walther[64]	5	i Standardized self-training, max 4 × supervision (20) ii 10 x conventional physiotherapy (20) iii Functional brace (20)	6 weeks (12 weeks)		Graphical data presentation, no measures of dispersion	No significant differences for pain, strength, or ROM
Ludewig[65]	4	i 8-week home exercise programme (34) ii No treatment (33)	10 weeks		Work-related pain (0–10), mean change (SD): i: 1.95 (1.63); ii: 0.48 (1.98) SMD = 0.80 (0.30 to 1.30)	Significant differences in favor of home exercises for pain and function
Additional mobilizations/manipulation						
Bergman[62]	8	i 6 × manipulative therapy (manipulations and mobilizations), 12 weeks plus GP treatment (79) ii GP treatment: NSAIDs, corticosteroid injection if needed, physiotherapy if needed (71)	3 months (12 months)	Very large improvement / full recovery: i: 34/79 (43%); ii: 15/71 (21%) ΔSR = 22% (7 to 36%), NNT = 5	Main complaint, VAS (0–10) mean change (SD): i: 4.4 (3.0); ii: 2.9 (3.4) SMD = 0.47 (0.14 to 0.79)	Significant differences in favor of manipulative therapy for pain and symptoms
Bang[48]	7	i 6 × manual therapy (Maitland mobilization) plus flexibility/strengthening exercises (28) ii 6 × exercises only (24)	Appr. 4 weeks (2 months)		Functional pain (9 × VAS), mean score (SD) i: 98 (107.4); ii: 226.7 (194.7)	Significant differences in favor of manual therapy for strength, pain, and function
Conroy[51]	5	i 9 × Maitland mobilization plus hot packs, exercises, friction, massage (7) ii 9 x hot packs, exercises, friction, massage (7)	Appr. 4 weeks		VAS (0–100), mean score (SD) i: 12.0 (14.4); ii: 44.1 (32.0)	Significant differences in favor of mobilization for pain, but not for function or ROM
Werner[68]	3	i 10 × exercises and mobilization (20) ii 5 × per week home exercises + max. 4 × supervision (20)	6 weeks (12 weeks)		Mean change Constant score: i: 5.5; ii: 9 (no measure of dispersion presented)	No significant differences for Constant score

CI, confidence interval; NNT, number needed to treat; ROM, range of movement; SD, standard deviation; SMD, standardized mean difference; SPADI, Shoulder Pain and Disability Index; SR, success rate; TENS, transcutaneous electrical nerve stimulation; VAS, visual analogue scale.

Table 20.4 Interventions and short-term results of randomized trials comparing corticosteroid injections with physiotherapy for shoulder pain

First author, ref.	Validity score	Study groups (number of patients)	Follow-up (final assessment)	Success rate per group ΔSR (95% CI), NNT	Pain	Authors' conclusions
Carette[59]	9	i 1 × 40 mg intra-articular triamcinolone hexacetonide (23) ii 12 × physiotherapy: TENS, mobilization techniques, active exercises, and ice (26) iii 1 × 40 mg triamcinolone + physiotherapy (21) iv 1 × saline (23)	6 weeks (12 months)		SPADI-pain mean change (SD): i: 39.1 (26.9); ii: 21.8 (27.0); SMD i vs ii = 0.63 (0.15 to 0.92)	Significant short-term differences for pain, ROM, and function in favor of injection and injection + physiotherapy
Hay[66]	7	i 1 × 40 mg subacromial methylprednisolone and lidocaine (104) ii 8 × physiotherapy: advice + exercises, plus ultrasound / mobilization if necessary (103)	6 weeks (6 months)	Recovery or improvement: i: 69/95 (79%); ii: 77/98 (79%) ΔSR = −6% (−18 to 6%), NNT = 17	VAS (0–10), median score (IQR): i: 3 (1–5); ii: 3 (1–4)	No significant differences for pain, function, ROM, or quality of life
Van der Windt[53]	6	i Max. 3 × 40 mg intra-articular triamcinolone (53) ii Max. 12 × exercises and mobilizations (56)	7 weeks (12 months)	Much improvement/complete recovery: i: 40/52 (77%); ii: 26/56 (46%) ΔSR = 31% (13 to 48%), NNT = 3	VAS (0–100), mean change (SD): i: 35 (20); ii: 23 (24) SMD = 0.54 (0.15 to 0.94)	Significant differences in favor of injections for pain, function, and ROM
Ginn[67]	4	i 1 × 40 mg subacromial methylprednisolone plus lignocaine (48) ii Home-based daily exercise programme, supervision by physiotherapist 1/week, 5 weeks (48) iii 10 × passive joint mobilization, electrophysical modalities plus daily ROM exercises (42)	5 weeks	Perceived change in symptoms: i: 19/45 (43%); ii: 19/43 (44%); iii: 20/39 (52%) ΔSR i vs ii = −2% (−23 to 19%), NNT = −50 ΔSR i vs iii = −9% (−30 to 12%), NNT = −11	Pain (0–10), median (95% CI): i: 0.2 (0 to 1.7; ii: 0.3 (0 to 2.3); iii: 1.0 (0 to 2.5)	No significant differences for pain, function or ROM

Arslan[69]	3	i 1 × 40 mg intra-articular methylprednisolone and lidocaine (10) ii Physiotherapy: hot packs, ultrasound, exercises (10)	12 weeks		VAS (0–10), mean score (SD): i: 2.3 (2.5); ii: 2.7 (2.6)	No significant differences for pain or ROM
Bulgen[54]	3	i 3 × 20 mg intra-articular plus intrabursal methylprednisolone and lignocaine (11) ii Maitland mobilizations (11) iii Ice packs plus proprioceptive neuromuscular facilitation (12) iv Pendular exercises, analgesics, diazepam (8)	6 weeks (6 months)		Insufficient data (graphical data for ROM only)	No significant differences for ROM
Dacre[55]	3	i 1 × 20 mg triamcinolone (22) ii 4 to 6 weeks physiotherapy (mainly mobilizations) (20) iii 1 × 20 mg triamcinolone plus physiotherapy (20)	6 weeks (6 months)		Insufficient data (graphical presentation of pain and ROM only	No significant differences for pain or ROM
Winters[56,57]	3	i Max. 3 × 40 mg triamcinolone multiple locations (47) ii Appr. 12 × exercises, physical applications and massage (35) iii Max. 6 × manipulative treatment (32)	6 weeks (2 to 3 years)	Feeling cured: i: 35/47 (75%); ii: 7/35 (20%); iii: 13/32) 40% ΔSR i vs ii: 55% (36 to 73%), NNT = 2 ΔSR i vs iii: 34% (13 to 55%), NNT = 3	Composite pain score, mean score (SD): i: 9.2 (3.7); ii: 12.6 (5.1); iii: 11.5 (4.4)	Significant differences for time to recovery in favor of injections

CI, confidence interval; IQR, interquartile range; NNT, number needed to treat; ROM, range of movement; SD, standard deviation; SMD, standardized mean difference; SPADI, Shoulder Pain and Disability Index; SR, success rate; TENS, transcutaneous electrical nerve stimulation; VAS, visual analogue scale.

characteristics of the study population (duration of symptoms, clinical diagnosis), content of treatment (number of injections and suspension used for injections, content of physiotherapy), or definition of outcome measures (various definitions of success, different measures for pain and function).[66,70]

Long-term outcomes

Most trials included only a short-term outcome assessment. Long-term follow-up measurements conducted at least six months after randomization were presented for 13 trials.[41,44,47,50,53–55,57–59,62,63,66] Beneficial long-term effects of corticosteroids were only reported by Ströbel,[47] who described long-term superior effects of corticosteroids on pain and work disability after 12 months' follow-up. It must be noted, however, that the study size was small, and that the trial was considered to be of rather poor quality (validity score 2). The positive short-term effects of corticosteroids reported by three other trials did not persist after 6–18 months of follow-up.[53,57,59]

The trial by Brox *et al.* showed that results of exercise treatment were not as good as those of surgery after 2.5 years' follow-up, but the differences were not statistically significant and only minor changes were observed after 6 months.[50] Interestingly, Bergman *et al.*[62] reported long-term beneficial effects of manipulative therapy as an addition to usual primary care. After 12 months of follow-up, the success rates and improvement of pain were significantly larger in patients treated with manipulative therapy in comparison with those receiving only usual care.

Summary

• The majority of trials of adequate validity report statistically significant and clinically relevant beneficial short-term effects of corticosteroid injections, but the available evidence is not consistent.
• Corticosteroid injections may be more effective than nonsteroidal anti-inflammatory drugs in the short term, but the differences are not very large and not statistically significant.
• Existing evidence on long-term outcomes indicates that beneficial effects of corticosteroid injection do not persist after 6 months, with similar outcomes regardless of treatment.
• Exercise therapy may be more effective for shoulder pain than placebo or no treatment. Effects are statistically significant, yet modest in most available trials.
• Physiotherapy, including passive mobilizations or manipulation, appears to be more effective than exercises only or usual primary care.
• The existing evidence is inconsistent regarding the short-term effects of corticosteroid injections in comparison with physiotherapy.

Adverse reactions

Eleven of the 26 trials investigating injection therapy included information about adverse reactions to corticosteroids. Adverse reactions were generally mild, and mainly consisted of some pain and discomfort following the injection.[33,34,53,61] Adverse reactions seemed to be particularly frequent in women, who may report facial flushes or abnormal menstrual bleeding.[33,36,40,53] Other reactions attributed to corticosteroids were headache, rashes, and skin depigmentation. Adverse reactions were rarely reported for physiotherapy. Only one study reported extra pain persisting for more than 2 hours following treatment in some patients.[63]

Discussion

The objective of this systematic review was to investigate the effectiveness of corticosteroid injections and physiotherapy for shoulder pain. We identified 35 relevant trials that met our selection criteria. Eight of these RCTs were pragmatic trials, directly comparing injection therapy with physiotherapy for shoulder pain.

Search strategy

It is not very likely that we have missed large or influential randomized trials that would have substantially modified our conclusions, but some additional relevant trials may not have been detected. Titles or abstracts do not always clearly describe the design and/or objective of a study. Furthermore, we may have failed to identify trials which were published in journals that are difficult to retrieve, or were excluded due to our language restrictions. Moher *et al.*[71] showed that there are no significant differences between trials published in English or other languages with regard to methods scores or completeness of reporting. Their results encourage the inclusion of all trial reports in systematic reviews, irrespective of the language in which they are published. Furthermore, we cannot rule out the risk of publication bias, although our review did include several small trials with negative results. Retrieval of unpublished data requires a huge effort that was not within the scope of this review.

Methodological quality

The Amsterdam–Maastricht Consensus list is one of the many scales and checklists that have been designed to assess quality of randomized trials.[24] Most of these scales and checklists, including the one we used, are based on generally accepted principles of intervention research. Nevertheless, we consider quality assessment to be important and believe that relatively more weight should be attached to the outcomes of trials that reported and used adequate methods. Several studies have provided empirical evidence that trials with inadequate methods, particularly concerning concealment of treatment allocation and blinding, report different estimates of treatment effect.[72–74] In our review, however, the quality of methods did not seem to have a strong influence on the outcome. The heterogeneity of the results of the included trials could not be explained by differences in total validity score, nor by differences in scores on important specific aspects of validity (concealed randomization, blinding and drop-out rate).

Insufficient reporting of trial methods sometimes hampered the quality assessment in this review, especially for the trials with publications dates before 1995. Journal style or editorial decisions may partly be the reason for the lack of information on important items. A more complete and informative trial report may result in higher validity scores, but could also reveal additional flaws in design or conduct.

Effectiveness of corticosteroid injections and physiotherapy

Previous systematic reviews on the effectiveness of corticosteroid injections or physiotherapy for shoulder disorders[21,22,28] have emphasized the necessity for research on the effectiveness of exercises and mobilization. Despite their common use in clinical care, evidence for these interventions was scant. For this second edition of *Evidence-Based Sports Medicine*, we identified 10 additional randomized trials investigating the effectiveness of physiotherapy for shoulder pain. This has added substantial information in comparison with the previous edition of this chapter.

The estimates for short-term differences in success rate of high quality trials ranged between 0% and 70% for corticosteroid injections in comparison with control, and between −10% and 55% for injections in comparison with physiotherapy. It did not seem sensible to compute a pooled estimate for such widely varying results. Pooled estimates were presented in the previous edition of this chapter, but recently published high-quality RCTs[58,59,66] have provided conflicting evidence for the effects of corticosteroid injection, with widely varying estimates. We used quantitative analyses to explore potential sources of heterogeneity. Subgroup analyses, which were only feasible for placebo-controlled trials on the effectiveness of corticosteroid injections, could not explain most of the heterogeneity across trials. There was evidence for subgroup effects favoring triamcinolone over other suspensions, for larger effects of corticosteroids in patients with a relatively short duration of symptoms at presentation, and in patients with a diagnosis of capsulitis. However, given persisting statistical heterogeneity we must urge caution in the interpretation of these pooled subgroup effects. It is likely that part of the remaining heterogeneity is explained by differences among trials regarding the definition of a treatment success. The influence of these differences was difficult to analyze because of the wide variety of definitions, but readers may consult Tables 20.2–20.4 for the definitions used in the analyses.

It is important to consider not only the statistical significance of individual trial results and pooled estimates, but also the magnitude of the treatment effect. Pooling of many small studies will eventually produce statistically significant results, but if the size of the treatment effect is small, the costs of treatment may easily outweigh its benefits. Deciding on the magnitude of a clinically important difference is difficult and certainly arbitrary, as it depends on several factors, including the natural history of the condition, the reference treatment, potential adverse reactions and inconvenience of therapy, treatment preferences, and costs (including costs of personnel, equipment, and time spent on therapy).[75] In addition, it should be noted that the absolute difference in success rates between intervention groups may depend on the baseline success rate in a population, which limits the possibilities of extrapolating an NNT outside the context of a trial.[76,77]

Conclusions

Despite the considerable number of trials available, there still seems to be no definitive answer as to the effectiveness of corticosteroid injections. This systematic review clearly shows that there is conflicting evidence regarding the short-term effects of corticosteroid injections for the painful shoulder in comparison with placebo injection or physiotherapy. Research into the long-term effectiveness of corticosteroid injections is relatively scarce, but the existing evidence indicates that any beneficial effects do not persist after 3 months, with similar outcomes regardless of the treatment.

Evidence seems to be mounting that exercise treatment appears to be more effective than a placebo intervention or a waiting list control. Furthermore, physiotherapy that includes passive mobilizations seems to be more effective than a treatment consisting of exercises only.

The number of pragmatic trials of adequate validity that directly compare treatments as they are offered to patients in everyday care is increasing. Such trials may show some methodological limitations, as blinding of patients and care providers is usually not possible, but the external validity of pragmatic trials is high, facilitating implementation of the findings in clinical practice. Additional research is necessary to confidently answer the main question of our review: are corticosteroid injections as effective as physiotherapy for the painful shoulder? One explanation for the conflicting evidence regarding treatment effects may be the inability to define subgroups most likely to respond to a particular intervention. Future trials should be of adequate internal validity, include a long-term outcome assessment, and have sufficient statistical power to detect clinically relevant differences. The results in relevant subgroups of patients, for example patients with either acute or chronic shoulder pain, should be analyzed and presented separately, in order to provide more evidence on the important question of "what works for whom."

Summary

- Adverse reactions to corticosteroid injections are usually mild, and mainly consist of temporary pain and discomfort, facial flushes, and abnormal menstrual bleeding in women.
- Additional research is needed to establish the effectiveness of corticosteroid injections compared to physiotherapy, particularly in relevant subgroups of patients.
- Future trials should be of relatively high internal validity, enrol a sufficient number of patients, include a long-term follow-up, and present results for relevant subgroups of patients separately.

Key messages

- In patients with a painful shoulder, significantly better short-term effects have been reported for corticosteroid injections in comparison with placebo injection. The differences result mainly from a comparatively fast relief of symptoms occurring after corticosteroid injection. However, recently published trials of adequate validity produce conflicting evidence.
- Doctors and patients should be aware of mild but sometimes troublesome adverse reactions to corticosteroid injection.
- There is, as yet, no evidence for long-term beneficial effects of corticosteroid injections. This should be taken into account when deciding on treatment in patients with shoulder pain.
- There is increasing evidence to support the use of physiotherapy for the painful shoulder. Physiotherapy that includes both exercises and passive mobilization techniques may be preferred to exercises alone.

Sample examination questions

Multiple choice questions (answers on page 602)

1 What are the most important shortcomings of research on the effectiveness of corticosteroid injections and physiotherapy for shoulder pain?
   A Insufficient blinding, high drop-out rate, poor description of interventions
   B High drop-out rate, small study size, selection criteria not clear
   C Insufficient blinding, small study size, no long-term follow-up
   D Poor compliance, no long-term follow-up, poor description of interventions
   E Study groups not similar at baseline, poor compliance, no long-term follow-up

2 Which statement correctly reflects currently available evidence for the effectiveness of corticosteroid injections for shoulder pain?
   A Available evidence is conflicting; several studies of adequate validity show beneficial short-term effects of corticosteroid injections, whereas other studies demonstrate no differences with placebo or other control treatment
   B The effectiveness of injections is superior to other conservative treatments at any moment of follow-up
   C Injections are no better than physiotherapy for the painful shoulder, but superior to placebo treatment or analgesics
   D Injections consistently show better short-term effects compared to other conservative treatments, but there is little evidence for long-term benefits
   E The available evidence shows little or no beneficial effects of corticosteroid injections for shoulder pain
3 Trials comparing the effects of corticosteroid injections with physiotherapy show widely varying results. Which factors might explain these differences?
   A Differences in the quality of research methods
   B Differences in the selection or definition of outcome measures
   C Differences in characteristics of the study population
   D Variation in the content of treatment (e.g., number of injections, content of physiotherapy)
   E All of the factors mentioned above

Essay questions

1 When reading a paper on the effectiveness of corticosteroid injections or physiotherapy for shoulder pain, we should try to take the methodological quality of the study into account. What are important aspects of the design of a randomized clinical trial?
2 Over the past 10 years, several studies have evaluated the effectiveness of exercise treatment and passive mobilizations for the painful shoulder. What are the most important results of these studies?
3 Many questions regarding the effectiveness of corticosteroid injections and physiotherapy for the painful shoulder remain unanswered, and further research is needed. In your opinion, what are the most important research questions, and which studies should be given a high priority on the research agenda?

Case study 20.1

A female laboratory worker (35 years old) consults her general practitioner with shoulder pain. The pain is aggravated by repeated movements and by moving the arm above shoulder level. She is unable to continue her laboratory work. The pain has been present for 3 months, has gradually increased, and is now quite severe. The pain started after she painted a ceiling in her new house. Physical examination shows pain during abduction (with painful arc) and during external rotation, and seems to indicate a lesion of the subacromial structures. The woman is treated with corticosteroid injections (40 mg triamcinolone acetonide), one given immediately, one 3 weeks later. She reports facial flushes and some abnormal menstrual bleeding following the injections. The complaints resolve within 6 weeks. However, 6 months after presentation, she reports again with recurrent symptoms of a similar nature and severity.

Summarizing the evidence: injections or physiotherapy for painful shoulder

Comparison	Trials	Results	Level of evidence*
Corticosteroid injection versus placebo/no treatment	18 RCTs, none of moderate size 11 of adequate validity (≥ 6 points)	—Available evidence is inconsistent —Significant results in favor of injection: 10 RCTs —Pooling of results is not possible due to heterogeneity of populations, and outcomes	A1
Corticosteroid injections versus NSAIDs or analgesics	4 RCTs, none of moderate size 2 of adequate validity (≥ 6 points)	—Significant results in favor of injection: 1 RCT —Pooled estimate for pain is small and not statistically significant	A1
Physiotherapy versus placebo/no treatment	6 RCTs, 1 of moderate size 3 of adequate validity (≥ 6 points)	—Significant results in favor of physiotherapy: 4 RCTs —Pooled estimate for pain is clinically relevant and statistically significant	A1
Physiotherapy including manipulation or mobilization compared to exercises only/usual primary care	4 RCTs, 1 of moderate size 2 of adequate validity (≥ 6 points)	—Significant results of additional manipulation or mobilizations: 3 RCTs —Pooling of results is not possible due to insufficient data presentation	A3
Corticosteroid injection versus physiotherapy	8 RCTs, one moderate, -sized one large 3 of adequate validity (≥ 6 points)	—Available evidence is inconsistent —Significant results in favor of injection: 3 RCTs —Pooling of results is not possible due to heterogeneity of populations, interventions and outcomes	A3

* A1: evidence from large randomized controlled trials (RCTs) or systematic review (including meta-analysis).†
A2: evidence from at least one high-quality cohort.
A3: evidence from at least one moderate-size RCT or systematic review.†
A4: evidence from at least one RCT.
B: evidence from at least one high-quality study of nonrandomized cohorts.
C: expert opinions.
† Arbitrarily, the following cut-off points have been used; large study size: ≥ 100 patients per intervention group; moderate study size ≥ 50 patients per intervention group.

Case study 20.2

A 62-year-old man reports to his general practitioner with shoulder pain. Over the past 5 years, he has had several episodes of shoulder pain, which were treated with physiotherapy or injections. There is no clear precipitating cause of the symptoms. The pain is moderate, and movements above shoulder level are limited. Physical examination shows a restriction of external rotation of 40° in comparison with the healthy shoulder. Abduction is slightly painful, but only mildly restricted. The patient is referred for physiotherapy and receives 11 treatments, consisting mainly of exercise therapy and passive mobilization. The severity of symptoms gradually decreases. After 6 months, the shoulder complaints no longer limit daily activities.

References

1 Badley EM, Tennant A. Changing profile of joint disorders with age: findings from a postal survey of the population of Calderdale, West Yorkshire, United Kingdom. *Ann Rheum Dis* 1992; **51**:366–371.
2 Bjelle A. Epidemiology of shoulder problems. *Baillière's Clin Rheumatol* 1989; **3**:437–451.
3 Croft P. Soft tissue rheumatism. In: Silman AJ, Hochberg MC, eds. *Epidemiology of the Rheumatic Diseases.* Oxford: Oxford Medical Publications, 1993: 375–421.
4 Van der Windt DAWM, Koes BW, De Jong BA, Bouter LM. Shoulder disorders in general practice: incidence, patient characteristics, and management. *Ann Rheum Dis* 1995; **54**:959–964.
5 Bot SDM Terwee CB, Van der Windt DAWM, Bouter LM, Dekker J. Incidence of complaints of the neck and upper extremity in general practice. *Ann Rheum Dis* 2005; **64**:118–123.
6 Nygren A, Berglund A, Von Koch M. Neck-and-shoulder pain, an increasing problem: strategies for using insurance material to follow trends. *Scand J Rehabil Med Suppl* 1995; **32**:107–112.
7 Uhthoff HK, Sarkar K. An algorithm for shoulder pain caused by soft-tissue disorders. *Clin Orthop* 1990; **254**:121–127.
8 Zuckerman JD, Mirabello SC, Newman D, Gallagher M, Cuomo F. The painful shoulder, part 1: extrinsic disorders. *Am Fam Physician* 1991; **43**:119–128.
9 Zuckerman, JD, Mirabello SC, Newman D, Gallagher M, Cuomo F. The painful shoulder, 2: intrinsic disorders and impingement syndrome. *Am Fam Physician* 1991; **43**:497–512.
10 Van der Windt DAWM, Koes BW, Boeke AJP, *et al.* Shoulder disorders in general practice: prognostic indicators of outcome. *Br J Gen Pract* 1996; **46**:519–523.
11 Winters JC, Sobel JS, Groenier KH, Arendzen JH, Meyboom-de Jong B. The long-term course of shoulder complaints: a prospective study in general practice. *Rheumatology* 1999; **38**:160–163.
12 Croft P, Pope D, Silman A. The clinical course of shoulder pain: prospective cohort study in primary care. *BMJ* 1996; **313**:601–602.
13 Shaffer B, Tibone JE, Kerlan RK. Frozen shoulder: a long term follow-up. *J Bone Joint Surg Am* 1992; **74**:738–746.
14 Chard MD, Satelle LM, Hazleman BL. The long-term outcome of rotator cuff tendinitis: a review study. *Br J Rheumatol* 1988; **27**:385–389.
15 Vecchio PC, Kavanagh RT, Hazleman BL, King RH. Community survey of shoulder disorders in the elderly to assess the natural history and effects of treatment. *Ann Rheum Dis* 1995; **54**:152–154.
16 Winters JC, Groenier KH, Sobel JS, Arendzen HH, Meyboom-de Jongh B. Classification of shoulder complaints in general practice by means of cluster analysis. *Arch Phys Med Rehabil* 1997; **78**:1369–1374.
17 Pellecchia GL, Paolino J, Connell J. Inter-tester reliability of the Cyriax evaluation in assessing patients with shoulder pain. *J Orthop Sports Phys Ther* 1996; **23**:34–38.
18 De Winter AF, Jans MP, Scholten RJPM, *et al.* Diagnostic classification of shoulder disorders: inter-observer agreement and determinants of disagreement. *Ann Rheum Dis* 1999; **58**:272–277.
19 Liesdek C, Van der Windt DAWM, Koes BW, Bouter LM. Soft-tissue disorders of the shoulder: a study of inter-observer agreement between general practitioners and physiotherapists and an overview of physiotherapeutic treatment. *Physiotherapy* 1997; **83**:12–17.
20 Bamji AN, Erhardt CC, Price TR, Williams PL. The painful shoulder: can consultants agree? *Br J Rheumatol* 1996; **35**:1172–1174.

21 Van der Heijden GJMG, Van der Windt DAWM, Kleijnen J, Koes BW, Bouter LM. The efficacy of steroid injections for shoulder disorders: a systematic review of randomized clinical trials. *Br J Gen Pract* 1996; **46**:309–316.

22 Van der Heijden GJMG, Van der Windt DAWM, De Winter AF. Physiotherapy for patients with soft tissue shoulder disorders: a systematic review of randomised clinical trials. *BMJ* 1997; **315**:25–30.

23 Alderson P, Green S, Higgins JPT, eds. MEDLINE highly sensitive search strategies for identifying reports of randomized controlled trials in MEDLINE. *Cochrane Reviewers' Handbook* 4.2.2 [updated March 2004], Appendix 5b. Chichester: Wiley/Cochrane Organization, 2004.

24 Moher D, Jadad AR, Tugwell. Assessing the quality of randomized controlled trials. *Int J Technology Assessment Health Care* 1996; **12**:195–208.

25 Van Tulder MW, Assendelft WJJ, Koes BW, Bouter LM. Methodologic guidelines for systematic reviews in the Cochrane Collaboration Back Review Group for Spinal Disorders. *Spine* 1997; **22**:2323–2330.

26 DerSimonian R, Laird N. Meta-analysis in clinical trials. *Contr Clin Trials* 1986; **7**:177–188.

27 Fleiss JL. The statistical basis of meta-analysis. *Stat Methods Med Res* 1993; **2**:121–145.

28 Green S, Buchbinder R, Glazier R, Forbes A. Systematic review of randomized controlled trials of interventions for painful shoulder: selection criteria, outcome assessment, and efficacy. *BMJ* 1998; **316**:354–356.

29 Laupacis A, Sackett DL, Roberts RS. An assessment of clinically useful measures of the consequences of treatment. *N Engl J Med* 1988; **318**:1728–1733.

30 Cohen J. *Statistical Power Analysis for the Behavioral Sciences*, 2nd ed. Hillsdale, New Jersey: Erlbaum, 1988.

31 Goldsmith CH, Boers M, Bombardier C, Tugwell P. Criteria for clinically important changes in outcomes: development, scoring and evaluation of rheumatoid arthritis patients and trial profiles. *J Rheumatol* 1993; **20**:561–565.

32 Brønfort G. Efficacy of spinal manipulation and mobilisation for low back pain and neck pain: a systematic review and best evidence synthesis. In: Brønfort G. *Efficacy of Manual Therapies of the Spine* [thesis]. Amsterdam: Thesis Publishers, 1997: 117–146.

33 De Jong BA, Dahmen R, Hogeweg JA, Marti RK. Intra-articular triamcinolone acetonide injection in patients with capsulitis of the shoulder: a comparative study of two dose regimens. *Clin Rehabil* 1998; **12**:211–215.

34 Adebajo OA, Nash P, Hazleman BL. A prospective double blind dummy placebo controlled study comparing triamcinolone hexacetonide injection with oral diclofenac 50 mg TDS in patients with rotator cuff tendinitis. *J Rheumatol* 1990; **17**:1207–1210.

35 Blair B, Rokito AS, Cuomo F, Jarolem K, Zuckerman JD. Efficacy of injections of corticosteroids for subacromial impingement syndrome. *J Bone Joint Surg Am* 1996; **78**:1685–1689.

36 Petri M, Dobrow R, Neiman R, Whiting-O'Keefe Q, Seaman WE. Randomised, double-blind, placebo-controlled study of the treatment of the painful shoulder. *Arthr Rheum* 1987; **30**:1040–1045.

37 Vecchio PC, Hazleman BL, King RH. A double-blind trial comparing subacromial methylprednisolone and lignocaine in acute rotator cuff tendinitis. *Br J Rheumatol* 1993; **32**:743–745.

38 Withrington RH, Girgis FL, Seifert MH. A placebo-controlled trial of steroid injections in the treatment of supraspinatus tendonitis. Scand *J Rheumatol* 1985; **14**: 76–78.

39 Richardson AT. The painful shoulder. *Proc R Soc Med* 1975; **68**:731–736.

40 Jacobs LG, Barton MA, Wallace WA, *et al.* Intra-articular distension and corticosteroids in the management of capsulitis of the shoulder. *BMJ* 1991; **302**:1498–1501.

41 Rizk TE, Pinals RS, Talaiver AS. Corticosteroid injections in adhesive capsulitis: investigation of their value and site. *Arch Phys Med Rehabil* 1991; **72**:20–22.

42 Berry H, Fernandes L, Bloom B, Clark RJ, Hamilton EB. Clinical study comparing acupuncture, physiotherapy, injection and oral anti-inflammatory therapy in shoulder-cuff lesions. *Curr Med Res Opin* 1980; 7:121–126.

43 Hollingworth GR, Ellis RM, Hattersley TS. Comparison of injection techniques for shoulder pain: results of a double blind, randomised study. *BMJ* 1983; **287**: 1339–1341.

44 Plafki C, Steffen R, Willburger RE, Wittenberg RH. Local anaesthetic injection with and without corticosteroids for subacromial impingement syndrome. *Int Orthop* 2000; **24**:40–42.

45 White RH, Paull DM, Fleming KW. Rotator cuff tendinitis: comparison of subacromial injection of a long acting corticosteroid versus oral indomethacin therapy. *J Rheumatol* 1986; **13**:608–613.

46 Lee PN, Haq AMMM, Wright V, Longton EB. Periarthritis of the shoulder: a controlled trial of physiotherapy. *Physiotherapy* 1973; **59**:312–315.

47 Ströbel G. [Long-term therapeutic effect of different intra-articular injection treatments of the painful shoulder: effect on pain, mobility and work capacity; in German.] *Rehabilitation* 1996; **35**:176–178.

48 Bang MD, Deyle GD. Comparison of supervised exercise with and without manual physical therapy for patients with shoulder impingement syndrome. *J Orthop Sports Phys Ther* 2000; **30**:126–137.

49 Brox JI, Staff PH, Ljunggren AE, Brevik JI. Arthroscopic surgery compared with supervised exercises in patients with rotator cuff disease (stage II impingement syndrome). *BMJ* 1993; **307**:899–903.

50 Brox JI, Gjengedal E, Uppheim G, *et al.* Arthroscopic surgery versus supervised exercises in patients with rotator cuff disease (stage II impingement syndrome): a prospective, randomized, controlled study in 125 patients with a 2 1/2-year follow-up. *J Shoulder Elbow Surg* 1999; **8**:102–111.

51 Conroy DE, Hayes KW. The effect of joint mobilization as a component of comprehensive treatment for primary shoulder impingement syndrome. *J Orthop Sports Phys Ther* 1998; **28**:3–14.

52 Ginn KA, Herbert RD, Khouw W, Lee R. A randomized, controlled clinical trial of a treatment for shoulder pain. *Phys Ther* 1997; **77**:802–809.

53 Van der Windt DA, Koes BW, Deville W, *et al.* Effectiveness of corticosteroid injections versus physiotherapy for treatment of painful stiff shoulder in primary care: randomised trial. *BMJ* 1998; **317**:1292–1296.

54 Bulgen DY, Binder AI, Hazleman BL, Dutton J, Roberts S. Frozen shoulder: prospective clinical study with an evaluation of three treatment regimens. *Ann Rheum Dis* 1984; **43**:353–360.

55 Dacre JE, Beeney N, Scott DL. Injections and physiotherapy for the painful stiff shoulder. *Ann Rheum Dis* 1989; **48**:322–325.

56 Winters JC, Sobel JS, Groenier KH, Arendzen HJ, Meyboom-de Jong B. Comparison of physiotherapy, manipulation, and corticosteroid injection for treating shoulder complaints in general practice: randomised, single blind study. *BMJ* 1997; **314**:1320–1325.

57 Winters JC, Jorritsma W, Groenier KH, *et al.* Treatment of shoulder complaints in general practice: long term results of a randomised, single blind study comparing physiotherapy, manipulation, and corticosteroid injection. *BMJ* 1999; **318**:1395–1396.

58 Alvarez CM, Litchfield R, Jackowski D, Griffin S, Kirkley A. A prospective, double-blind, randomized clinical trial comparing subacromial injection of betamethasone and xylocaine to xylocaine alone in chronic rotator cuff tendinosis. *Am J Sports Med* 2005; **33**:255–262.

59 Carette S, Moffet H, Tardif J, *et al.* Intraarticular corticosteroids, supervised physiotherapy, or a combination of the two in the treatment of adhesive capsulitis of the shoulder: a placebo-controlled trial. *Arthritis Rheum* 2003; **48**:829–838.

60 Akgün K, Birtane M, Akarirmak U. Is local subacromial corticosteroid injection beneficial in subacromial impingement syndrome? *Clin Rheumatol* 2004; **23**:496–500.

61 McInerney JJ, Dias J, Durham S, Evans A. Randomised controlled trial of single, subacromial injection of methylprednisolone in patients with persistent, post-traumatic impingement of the shoulder. *Emerg Med J* 2003; **20**:218–221.

62 Bergman GJ, Winters JC, Groenier KH, *et al.* Manipulative therapy in addition to usual medical care for patients with shoulder dysfunction and pain: a randomized, controlled trial. *Ann Intern Med* 2004; **141**:432–439.

63 Pajareya K, Chadchavalpanichaya N, Painmanakit S, *et al.* Effectiveness of physical therapy for patients with adhesive capsulitis: a randomized controlled trial. *J Med Assoc Thai* 2004; **87**:473–480.

64 Walther M, Werner A, Stahlschmidt T, Woelfel R, Gohlke F. The subacromial impingement syndrome of the shoulder treated by conventional physiotherapy, self-training, and a shoulder brace: results of a prospective, randomized study. *J Shoulder Elbow Surg* 2004; **13**:417–423.

65 Ludewig PM, Borstad JD. Effects of a home exercise programme on shoulder pain and functional status in construction workers. *Occup Environ Med* 2003; **60**:841–849.

66 Hay EM, Thomas E, Paterson SM, Dziedzic K, Croft PR. A pragmatic randomised controlled trial of local corticosteroid injection and physiotherapy for the treatment of new episodes of unilateral shoulder pain in primary care. *Ann Rheum Dis* 2003; **62**:394–399.

67 Ginn K, Cohen M. Exercise therapy for shoulder pain aimed at restoring neuromuscular control: a randomized comparative clinical trial. *J Rehabil Med* 2005; **37**:115–122.

68 Werner A, Walther M, Ilg A, Stahlschmidt T, Gohlke F. [Self-training versus conventional physiotherapy in subacromial impingement syndrome; in German.] *Z Orthop Ihre Grenzgeb* 2002; **140**:375–380.

69 Arslan S, Celiker R. Comparison of the efficacy of local corticosteroid injection and physical therapy for the treatment of adhesive capsulitis. *Rheumatol Int* 2001; **21**:20–23.

70 Van der Windt DAWM, Bouter LM. Physiotherapy or corticosteroid injection for shoulder pain [editorial]. *Ann Rheum Dis* 2003; **62**:385–387.

71 Moher D, Fortin P, Jadad AR, *et al.* Completeness of reporting of trials published in languages other than English: implication for conduct and reporting of systematic reviews. *Lancet* 1996; **347**:363–366.

72 Chalmers TC, Celano P, Sacks HS, Smith H. Bias in treatment assignment in controlled clinical trials. *N Engl J Med* 1983; **309**:1358–1361.

73 Colditz GA, Miller JN, Mosteller F. How study design affects outcomes in comparison of therapy. *Stat Med* 1989; **8**:441–454.

74 Schulz KF, Chalmers I, Hayes RJ, Altman DG. Empirical evidence of bias: dimensions of methodological quality associated with estimates of treatment effects in controlled trials. *JAMA* 1995; **273**:408–412.

75 Cook DJ, Guyatt GH, Laupacis A, Sackett DL. Rules of evidence and clinical recommendations on the use of antithrombotic agents. *Chest* 1992; **102**:305S–311S.

76 Cook RJ, Sackett DL. The number needed to treat: a clinically useful measure of treatment effect. *BMJ* 1995; **310**:452–454.

77 Chatellier G, Zapletal E, Lemaitre D, Menard J, Degoulet P. The number needed to treat: a clinically useful monogram in its proper context. *BMJ* 1996; **312**:426–429.

CHAPTER 21

How should you treat tennis elbow? An updated scientific evidence-based approach

Alasdair J.A. Santini, Michael J. Hayton, Simon P. Frostick

Introduction

Since we originally wrote this chapter, there have been a number of new high-quality publications on the treatment options available. Some of these have been prospective and randomized, giving us quality information with regard to the scientific evidence available to judge our therapeutic regimens. In particular, two interesting treatment modalities have been discussed in greater detail in the literature, namely extracorporeal shock-wave therapy (ESWT) and botulinum toxin treatment, and we have incorporated these into this updated chapter.

Lateral epicondylitis or tennis elbow is one of the commoner pathologies of the arm encountered by surgeons. Despite its name, it occurs more commonly in nonathletes than athletes. Its peak incidence is in the fifth decade, with an equal male to female ratio.[1,2]

It was first described by Runge in 1873, and since then over 30 different conditions have been described as possible etiologies.[1,3,4] The term "epicondylitis" suggests an inflammatory etiology, but Boyer and Hastings commented that there was no evidence of acute or chronic inflammation in all but one of the publications examining pathological specimens of patients operated on for this condition.[5] The pathology is more likely to be angiofibroblastic degeneration in the origin of the extensor carpi radialis brevis rather than an inflammatory process, and the term "epicondylosis" is therefore a more correct one. It may be a normal part of aging or a response to the stress of overload and overuse.[6–8]

There are many treatment options available to the clinician, which are often based on anecdotal evidence. The treatments include various anti-inflammatory medications, ultrasound, physical therapy, steroid injections, ESWT, and botulinum toxin. A large number of operations have also been described, with varying results of success. Although the literature is wide-ranging, there is still a general paucity of high-quality scientific evidence to support any one treatment protocol over any other. In this chapter, we will discuss the anatomy, pathology, and treatment options and review the literature. We will propose that the term "tennis elbow" is antiquated and that the term "epicondylitis" should be replaced with "epicondylosis." We will also critically review the available literature and offer an evidence-based treatment plan for lateral epicondylosis.

Methodology

A comprehensive search of scientific papers was undertaken in medical, sporting, and rehabilitation journals, using MEDLINE database utilities. The search was initiated using the words "lateral epicondylitis," "lateral epicondylosis," and "tennis elbow." The searches were limited to peer-review journals of high standing, published in English in the past 30 years, with the exception of those of historical interest. A total of 939 papers were assessed by abstract. Case reports, epidemiological studies, imaging and diagnostics, and generalized upper limb pathologies were rejected. Where studies of similar scientific merit and content had been published, we rejected the older papers. The references of key papers were also accessed and edited in the same manner. Ideally, only prospective, randomized trials would be included, but these are unfortunately in small numbers and hence papers were individually assessed as to their scientific merit at the discretion of the authors. Where review articles have summarized large numbers of papers, we have not individually referenced these papers.

As clinicians usually reach for a textbook to gain information, we have also used standard textbooks as a basis for the treatment protocols. Quoted papers in various chapters were cross-referenced and added to the pool described above. By doing this, we hope to discuss the evidence available based on the protocols that a clinician may already work with.

Anatomy

The standard teaching places the pathology at the origin of the extensor carpi radialis brevis.[1,6,9] The origin of the extensor carpi radialis brevis is covered by both the extensor carpi radialis longus and the extensor communis origin, and is found just distal to the midpoint of the lateral epicondyle. Figure 21.1 shows the anatomy of the elbow with the muscle attachments.

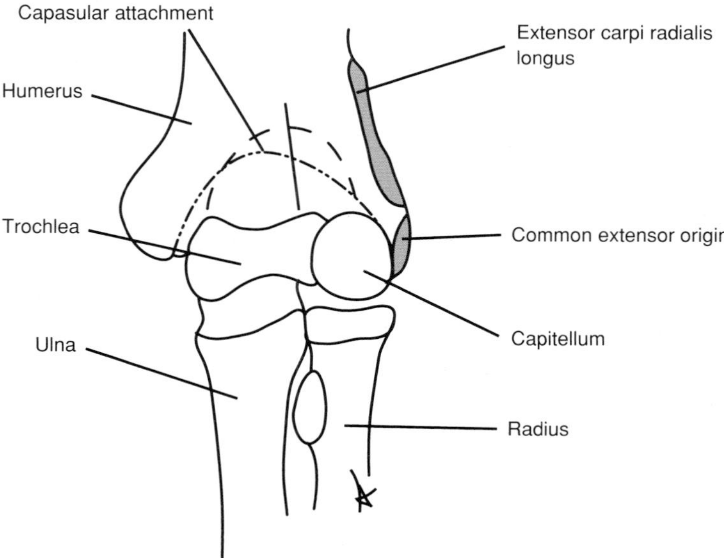

Figure 21.1 The anterior anatomy of the elbow with muscle attachments.

Common extensor origin

The origin of the common extensor is from the smooth area in front of the lateral epicondyle and consists of the fused tendons of the extensor carpi radialis brevis, extensor digitorum, extensor digiti minimi, and extensor carpi ulnaris. All four muscles pass to the posterior surface of the forearm. When the forearm is extended and supinated, they spiral around the upper end of the radius. In the flexed and semipronated, working position of the forearm, the muscles pass straight from the front of the lateral epicondyle to the forearm.[10]

Extensor carpi radialis longus

This muscle takes its origin from the lower third of the lateral supracondylar ridge of the humerus, and passes down the forearm, behind the brachioradialis and deep to the thumb muscles, to the base of the second metacarpal. It is supplied by the radial nerve (C6/7). It is an extensor and abductor of the wrist and assists in flexion of the elbow. It is indispensable to the action of making a fist, acting as a synergist during finger flexion. It is tested with the forearm pronated and the wrist extended and abducted against resistance; the muscle is palpated below and behind the lateral side of the elbow.[10]

Extensor carpi radialis brevis

This muscle runs from the common extensor origin behind and deep to the extensor carpi radialis longus and inserts into the third metacarpal, which is the same metacarpal as for the flexor carpi radialis muscle. It is supplied by the posterior interosseous nerve (C7/8). Its action, like that of the longus, is in making a fist.[10]

An anatomical study by Greenbaum *et al.* highlighted the difficulty in isolating the origin of extensor carpi radialis brevis.[11] In 40 cadaveric specimens, 10 showed the brevis tendon to be running under the muscle bellies of the extensor carpi radialis longus and extensor communis, such that its origin on the condyle was not identifiable. The remaining 30 specimens showed that the smaller tendon of the brevis interdigitated with that of communis at its origin, forming a large aponeurosis. The center of this coalescence was found consistently over the most prominent and lateral portion of the condyle. In all dissections, there was a lack of a definitive separation of the brevis and communis at the osseotendinous junction. The histological analysis confirmed the macroscopic lack of separation between the two tendons. This paper questioned the "tennis elbow" symptoms being ascribed to the extensor carpi radialis brevis and suggested it be ascribed to the common extensor origin.

Histopathology

The exact pathophysiology of lateral epicondylitis is controversial. The pathology is likely to be a hypoxic degeneration in the origin of the extensor carpi radialis brevis and not an inflammatory process, as suggested by the term "epicondylitis."[6] Histopathological studies have shown that specimens of tendon obtained from areas of chronic overuse do not contain large numbers of macrophages, lymphocytes, or neutrophils.[7] The condition may be a normal part of aging or can be a response to overload stress. Overloading and overuse leads to an incomplete healing response characterized by a vascular and fibrous proliferation in areas of poor vascularity.[6]

Kannus and Jozsa compared 891 ruptured tendons with a controlled group of cadaveric specimens. They were all repaired operatively and histologically analyzed. None of these were of a healthy structure, but 66% of the controls were ($P < 0.001$). Ninety-seven percent of the pathological changes were of a degenerative type, including hypoxic degenerative tendinopathy, mucoid degeneration, tendolipomatosis and calcifying tendinopathies, either alone or in combination. These changes occurred in 34% of controls ($P < 0.001$). Kannus concluded that degenerative changes are common in people over 35 years and are associated with spontaneous rupture of tendons.[12]

Chronic tendon injuries result from multiple microtraumatic events causing disruption of the internal structure and degeneration of the cells and matrix, which then fail to mature into a normal tendon. This injury pattern may result in tendinosis.[7,8,13]

The theory is that when a tendon is injured by a cyclically applied, cumulative type of force, the injury is perceived by the body's immune system as subclinical, because of the lack of involvement of the hemopoietic system. The normal sequence of inflammatory response is bypassed and instead, tendon intrasubstance proliferates, leading to degeneration in a poorly vascularized area. This is characterized, histologically, by cellular atrophy, diminished protein synthesis, and cyst proliferation. As the degenerative areas enlarge, the tendon weakens and eventually microruptures. Only at this stage is the classic inflammatory response and healing cascade initiated.[8] The whole histological pattern is of dense populations of fibroblasts, vascular hyperplasia, and disorganized collagen. This has been termed "angiofibroblastic hyperplasia."[7,8] Kraushaar and Nirschl[7] and Nirschl and Pettrone[13] have described tendinosis as the disruption of normally ordered tendon fibers by a characteristic pattern of invasion by fibroblasts and vascular granulation tissue. They termed this "angiofibroblastic tendinosis," as the angiofibroblastic tissue was found to be insinuating itself through abnormal hypercellular regions and extending focally into adjacent normal-appearing tendon fibers.

Nirschl has classified the stages of repetitive microtrauma into four groups.[14] The first stage is a minor injury, resulting in an inflammatory response. This is not associated with any pathological alteration and therefore resolves. The second stage is one of pathological alterations such as angiofibroblastic degeneration and tendinosis. The third stage is associated with more severe pathological changes, leading to structural failure of the tendon and hence rupture. The fourth stage shows the features of stage two and stage three with the addition of further pathologies such as fibrosis, soft-tissue calcification and hard osseous calcification. Nirschl suggested that this stage may be related to the use of cortisone. Thus, the overuse injuries and sport-induced injuries that are called "tennis elbow" would seem to represent stage two in Nirschl's classification.

It would be fair to comment that the sequence of events and the resulting histological findings are incompletely understood. It is not clear why tendinosis is painful, given the absence of inflammatory cells. Is it due to some chemical characteristic within the healing matrix such as the pH level or the level of prostaglandins?[7] Nor is it clear why the collagen fails to mature. Is it due to a vascular abnormality and a relative hypoxic state?[7] Kraushaar and Nirschl suggest that shear forces within the tendon may either signal the mechanoreceptors (integrins) on the surface of the resting tenocyte, or actually harm the cells when a cleavage plane is formed between the tendon fascicles. The activated fibroblast begins to multiply and starts to produce collagen locally. However, it is the lack of an effective vascular system that leads to the failure of the healing cycle in tendinosis. Instead of the classic immune-based inflammatory response, the mesenchymal cell-based process in tendinosis lacks the chemical guidance that normally would lead to maintenance of the matrix and the expected remodeling phase of tendon healing.[7,8]

The terms "epicondylitis" and "tendonitis" are commonly used to describe tennis elbow. However, the histopathological studies, as mentioned above, have shown that the condition is not an inflammatory condition; rather, it is a fibroblastic and vascular response called angiofibroblastic degeneration. It should more correctly be labeled *tendinosis*.[7,8,13,14] Using the correct nomenclature may allow us a better understanding of the pathology. With this knowledge, we may be able to implement better treatment plans.

Summary of histopathology

- Tennis elbow is *not* an inflammatory condition.
- Overload and overuse cause an incomplete healing response.
- There is a fibroblastic and abnormal vascular response to injury.
- This is termed "angiofibroblastic degeneration."
- It is a tendinosis rather than a tendonitis.

Treatment options

The principle of any successful management plan should be to identify the causative pathological process and aim to correct this. As we have discussed, the pathology is one of angiofibroblastic degeneration. Therefore, the aim should be to promote normal vascularization and collagen production to promote healing.[7]

The treatment options and ensuing results are varied and often based on the personal experience of the treating clinician, rather than sound scientific evidence. An attempted meta-analysis in 1992 reviewed the 185 articles published on this subject since 1966.[15] Only 18 of the reviewed papers were randomized, controlled trials, assessing treatment protocols. The papers were assessed using the "Chalmers" quality index method, which evaluates design, conduct, and the analysis of scientific research. The index is expressed as a percentage. An arbitrary score of 70% is considered to be the minimum required for a good-quality design for controlled therapeutic trials. The average score for the 18 controlled trials was 33%, with a range of 6% to 73%. Only one paper reached the required 70% level. The authors concluded that there was insufficient scientific evidence to support any single current method of treatment. This paper highlights that although many authors publish good results for treatment protocols, the pure scientific evidence is poor. A better understanding and classification of the pathology may help future treatment protocols.

Over 90% of patients are said to respond to conservative treatments, such as avoiding overuse, wearing braces, strengthening exercises, and steroid injections.[1,3,7,9,13,14,16–18] In carefully selected groups, over 90% of those who require surgery do well.[1,13] With these levels of response, it is not surprising that many clinicians insist on a prolonged period of active conservative treatment.[3,7,17] It is important that the symptoms of pain are relieved and maintenance of function is achieved, but equally that the clinician identifies the pathology and administers an appropriate treatment protocol. We will describe some of the various treatment options that are available and discuss the scientific evidence published to support their use. We will then discuss an evidence-based method of treatment.

Physical therapy

Although lateral epicondylosis is more common in nonathletes, it remains the commonest problem in the United Kingdom in athletes and is due to overuse or overtraining. In elite athletes, 90% of instances of lateral epicondylosis occur in athletes using backhand strokes. This is due to an overloading of the extensor muscles that extend the wrist on backhand. The cause is multifactorial, due to improper stroke mechanics; weakness of the wrist extensors; inflexibility of the wrist musculature; and posterior shoulder weakness.[19] Physiotherapy focusing on strength and flexibility exercises for wrist extensors and flexors has been shown to be effective in the prevention of tennis elbow-type symptoms.[18] If an athlete can increase the strength of the wrist extensors, this allows the muscles to absorb a greater force, hence lessening the force transferred to the elbow. Similarly, flexibility of these muscles also causes less force to be transmitted to the elbow; and strong posterior shoulder muscles allow more rapid movement in the arm and wrist through the hitting zone, decreasing the tensile load on the elbow. Regardless of the actual cause of initial trauma, achievement of normal strength and flexibility is a major component of both the preventive and rehabilitative program for lateral epicondylosis in athletes.[19] This method of therapy can be used for nonathletes who have the same pathology, although often brought on by a different cause.

Manipulation therapy has been offered as a similar method to physiotherapy. It is, however, not the same. Wadsworth describes the use of "manipulation therapy" in patients resistant to more conservative treatments. The results appear anecdotal, with no scientific evidence to provide support them.[3]

Ultrasound

There have been a number of trials comparing ultrasound therapy with placebo for the treatment of soft-tissue lesions including lateral epicondylosis. Unfortunately, many of the trials are of insufficient scientific standard to support the evidence for ultrasound over placebo in the treatment of lateral epicondylosis.[15]

Laser therapy

Laser therapy is a widespread but controversial treatment, based on the theory that laser radiation, at intensities too low to produce significant heating, produces clinically meaningful improvements in a variety of soft-tissue conditions. The mechanism is only partially understood and is believed to be due to cellular changes secondary to heat production.[20] Basford *et al.* ran a double-masked, placebo-controlled, randomized trial to assess this. Fifty-two patients with symptomatic lateral epicondylosis were randomized into two groups. They underwent radiation for 60 seconds at seven points along the symptomatic forearm, three times a week for 4 weeks, with a treatment probe of continuous-wave laser emitting 204 mW/cm^2. This was active for treated subjects and inactive for the control subjects. The patients were assessed for pain, tenderness to palpation, various grip strengths, medication usage, and a subjective perception of benefit. There was no significant difference between the groups in any of the parameters. These results support other studies suggesting that this form of treatment has no proven beneficial effect.[15]

Oral anti-inflammatory tablets

There are inadequate trials to show the benefit of oral anti-inflammatory tablets over any other modality of treatment.[15] Given that the pathology is not one of inflammation, but rather one of angiofibroblastic degeneration, this is perhaps not surprising. However, in many patients there is a beneficial effect after taking such medication. Kraushaar and

Nirschl propose two methods to explain this. The first is that the anti-inflammatory effect will reduce inflammation in any surrounding tissues, which are indirectly involved. This may make it easier to rehabilitate the injured muscle–tendon groups and hence aid therapy. Secondarily, nonsteroidal anti-inflammatory drugs increase protein synthesis by fibroblasts, which may benefit the remodeling phase of repair.[7]

Extracorporeal shock-wave therapy (ESWT)

Numerous investigators have recommended extracorporeal shock-wave therapy as an alternative treatment for chronic lateral epicondylosis of the elbow. Ko *et al.* reported 31% of patients rated as "excellent" at 6 weeks after ESWT treatment, with further improvement up to 6 months and with no side effects.[21] This suggests that shock-wave therapy may offer a safe nonoperative treatment for lateral epicondylosis; however, recommendations have been based largely on observational or nonrandomized trials.

The mode of action of ESWT is uncertain. It has been used by urologists in the treatment of urinary calculi for over 20 years and more recently in orthopedics for calcific tendonitis, plantar fasciitis, and nonunion of fractures, amongst other conditions. It may work by relieving pain by hyperstimulation analgesia, ascribed to mechanisms in the brain stem exerting a descending inhibitory control of transmission, but the details of the electrophysiological pathways and molecular mechanisms of the antinociceptive effect are still unknown.

The Extracorporeal Shock-Wave Therapy Clinical Trial Group randomized 272 patients with chronic symptoms to receive local anesthetic and then either extracorporeal shock-wave therapy or placebo therapy. The success rate was 25.8% in the group treated with ESWT and 25.4% in the placebo group. None of the measured criteria showed any significant difference between the groups, but two-thirds of the patients in both groups showed improvement at 12 months. The authors concluded that "extracorporeal shock wave therapy" was ineffective in the treatment of lateral epicondylitis."[22] In the group's various trials, totalling 399 ESWT and 402 placebo treatments, there were more side effects documented with ESWT. Twenty-one percent of patients had transitory reddening of the skin, and other side effects included pain, hematomas, migraine, and syncope.[22,23]

Speed *et al.* randomized 75 patients with chronic tennis elbow to receive either ESWT or sham therapy.[24] The symptoms lasted for a mean of 16 months in the ESWT group and 12 months in the sham group. Both groups showed improvements in mean pain scores from 3 months, but these were not significantly different. The authors concluded that there appeared to be "a significant placebo effect of moderate-dose ESWT" and that there was "no evidence of added benefit of treatment when compared to sham therapy."

Crowther *et al.* prospectively randomized 93 patients, with chronic tennis elbow, to either a single injection of triamcinolone and lignocaine or ESWT.[25] Only 73 completed the study, with 48 receiving ESWT and 25 receiving injections. At 6 weeks, using pain scores, the improvement with the injection group was significantly greater than in the ESWT group. After 3 months, 84% of patients with the injection treatment were considered to have had successful treatment, compared with 60% of patients with ESWT. The authors concluded that "in the medium term, local injection of steroid is more successful and 100 times less expensive than ESWT in the treatment of tennis elbow."

One can critically analyze all of the above papers with regard to their design, and in some with regard to the addition of local anesthetic to the area of pain—are we testing

ESWT or just the response to local anesthetic? However, the designs are largely of high quality, and local anesthetic is widely used in addition to ESWT in clinical practice. Hence, we conclude that although there are many recommendations for the efficacy of ESWT in the treatment of lateral epicondylosis, there is little scientific evidence to support its use as a treatment modality.

Steroid injections

In the previous edition of this book, we concluded that there was no evidence to support the long-term efficacy of steroid injections in the treatment of tennis elbow, despite its common use in clinical practice.[7,15,26] Hay *et al.* showed, in a randomized controlled trial of 164 patients comparing corticosteroid injections versus naproxen versus placebo tablets, that at 4 weeks, there was a significant improvement in the injection group in comparison with the naproxen and placebo groups. However, at 1 year, all three groups had responded well and there was no significant difference between them.[26] Since then there have been three publications that have reexamined this treatment form.

Newcomer *et al.* undertook a randomized, controlled, double-blinded study comparing a corticosteroid injection and early rehabilitation, with a control injection and rehabilitation.[27] They recruited 39 patients, all of whom had had symptoms for less than 4 weeks. Nineteen received a sham injection, with 20 receiving a corticosteroid injection; all 39 had rehabilitation. The authors found no significant differences between the two groups, with the exception of an improvement in the visual analogue pain scale in the corticosteroid group. In both groups, outcome measurements improved significantly over time, and over 80% of the subjects reported improvements from baseline to 6 months for all scales. The authors concluded that a corticosteroid injection did "not provide a clinically significant improvement . . . and rehabilitation should be the first line of treatment in patients with a short duration of symptoms."

Nirschl *et al.* undertook a randomized, double-blinded, placebo-controlled study comparing a dexamethasone injection with a placebo injection, in both medial and lateral epicondylosis.[28] A total of 169 patients were recruited to receive six injections of either active or placebo treatment. Using a 100-mm visual analogue scale, patients who had had the dexamethasone injection produced a significant 23-mm improvement, compared with a 14-mm improvement for the placebo injections at 2 days, and 24 mm compared with 19 mm at 1 month. At 2 days, 52% of those treated with dexamethasone scored "moderate" or better, compared with 33% of those treated with placebo. At 1 month, the difference was not significant, with 54% of the steroid group scoring "moderate" or better, compared to 49% of the placebo group. It was noted that patients completing six treatments in 10 days or less had better results than those treated over a longer period. The authors concluded that "iontophoresis treatment was well tolerated by most patients and was effective in reducing symptoms of epicondylitis at short-term follow-up."

The Dutch College of General Practitioners recommend a "wait-and-see" policy rather than steroid injections or physiotherapy for the treatment of tennis elbow. Smidt *et al.* assessed this policy by randomizing 185 patients to 6 weeks of treatment with either corticosteroid injections; physiotherapy and ultrasound, or a wait-and-see policy.[29] At 6 weeks, corticosteroid injections were significantly better than the other therapy options for all outcome measures, with success rates of 92% compared with 47% for physiotherapy and 32% for the wait-and-see policy. However, the recurrence rate in the injection group was high, and success rates at 52 weeks were 69% for injections, 91% for physiotherapy, and 83% for the wait-and-see policy. The latter two groups showed no significant difference. The authors concluded that "patients should be properly informed about the advantages and disadvantages of the treatment options for lateral epicondylitis" and that "the decision to treat with physiotherapy or to adopt a wait-and-see policy might depend on available resources, since the relative gain of physiotherapy is small."

These three new papers support the previously documented evidence that steroid injections may offer improvement of symptoms in the short term, but have little long-term benefit, with a high recurrence rate and no additional benefit over less invasive treatment forms.[2,15,17,26] Steroids have well documented side effects and should not be used without due care and attention. It has been proposed that the benefit that some patients gain from steroid injections is due to direct damage from the needle itself, which causes an inflammatory response to be mounted that aids muscle and tendon healing.[7]

Botulinum toxin therapy

Botulinum toxin is used in the treatment of various spastic and muscle tone disorders, such as torticollis, strabismus, and fissura ani. The toxin irreversibly binds to specific receptors at the presynaptic cholinergic end-plate membrane and inhibits the release of acetylcholine at the neuromuscular junction, leading to paresis. New axons sprout and form new junctions and lead to a full recovery in 2–6 months. The theory behind the therapy regime is that complete rest of extensor carpi radialis brevis, through botulinum toxin–induced paralysis, may lead to a normal repair mechanism of the muscle by preventing continued tensile forces acting through the abnormal tissue.

Keizer *et al.* published a prospective and randomized pilot study comparing treatment with botulinum toxin infiltration and surgery.[30] The authors recruited 40 patients who had had symptoms for over 6 months and had failed to respond to conservative measures. Twenty patients underwent surgery, and 20 patients were treated with botulinum toxin. At 1 year, 13 patients in the botulinum toxin group and 15 patients in the surgical group had "good" or "excellent" results. At 2 years, 15 patients in the botulinum toxin group and 17 patients in the surgical group had "good" or "excellent" results. Four patients required surgical intervention after initial treatment with botulinum toxin. The authors found no differences between the two forms of treatment and concluded that "botulinum toxin infiltration, a less invasive technique, may be an alternative for surgical treatment of tennis elbow."

Hayton *et al.* ran a prospective, randomized, double-blinded trial to compare botulinum toxin injections with placebo injections.[31] Forty patients with chronic, unremitting symptoms were randomized into two groups. Eighteen received 50 units of botulinum toxin, and 19 received normal saline. Three patients withdrew before completion of the study. At 3 months after the injection, there was no significant difference between the two groups, although the botulinum toxin group had a greater improvement in grip strength. The authors concluded that there was no evidence to "propose the use of botulinum toxin treatment over placebo."

These two papers are well designed, but have small numbers, as both are pilot studies. However, both show no benefit of botulinum toxin over surgery or placebo. This may represent the small numbers involved (type 2 or beta error) and suggests that conclusions cannot be drawn until a larger trial is undertaken—a minimum of 300 patients would be required to show a difference in Hayton's trial. However, from the data available, botulinum toxin does not offer any advantage in treatment over placebo or surgery.

Acupuncture

Acupuncture has long been used in China and more recently in Western countries as a first-line treatment for various musculoskeletal disorders. The evidence to support acupuncture has been assessed by Green *et al.* for the Cochrane database.[32] They included four small randomized controlled trials by Molsberger, Haker (two trials) and Wang, but due to flaws in the study designs and clinical differences between the trials, data could not be combined in a meta-analysis. Molsberger found that needle acupuncture resulted in relief of pain for significantly longer than placebo and was more likely to result in a 50% or greater reduction in pain after one treatment. Haker demonstrated needle acupuncture to be more likely to result in an overall improvement as reported by the participant than placebo in the short term, but no significant differences were found after 3 or 12 months. In a separate trial by Haker, there was no difference between laser acupuncture and placebo with respect to overall benefit. Wang demonstrated no difference between vitamin B_{12} injection plus acupuncture with vitamin B_{12} injection alone.

The conclusions from this review were that there was "insufficient evidence to either support or refute the use of acupuncture (either needle or laser) in the treatment of lateral elbow pain." The review demonstrated needle acupuncture to be of short-term benefit with respect to pain, but this was based on the results of two small trials, "the results of which were not able to be combined in meta-analysis." Hence, no substantial "conclusions can be drawn regarding the effect of acupuncture on tennis elbow."

Surgical options

There have been numerous publications on the surgical treatment of lateral epicondylosis. Many of these are historical, many retrospective, many poorly designed, many with inadequate patient numbers, and many with combinations and permutations of all of these. No prospective, randomized trials have been published. Although many report good results, this may be due to factors other than the operation itself. The surgical options fall into two broad groups. The first is a tenotomy of varying degree; the second is an attempt to excise the pathological tissue causing the symptoms.

Tenotomy

Bosworth's classic paper of 1965 described varying surgical techniques in 62 patients based on the division of the common extensor origin (with or without repair) and resection of the orbicular (annular) ligament. The results, obtained retrospectively, suggested that patients improved more quickly if the orbicular ligament was resected and the common extensor origin not repaired.[33]

Grundberg and Dobson[16] described a percutaneous release of the common extensor origin through a 1-cm incision just distal to the lateral epicondyle in 323 patients in whom nonoperative treatment had failed. The procedure resulted in a 1-cm displacement of the common extensor origin from the lateral epicondyle, and this could be palpated through the skin. An immediate postoperative therapy regime was undertaken. The patients were reviewed after an average of 26 months. Twenty-six elbows were rated as excellent and three rated as good; the pain was relieved in an average of 9 weeks. Three elbows were rated as poor.

Verhaar *et al.* described exposing the extensor origin and dividing it transversely close to its attachment on the epicondyle allowing it to retract distally. This was done under local anesthetic so that the surgeon could monitor the completeness of the release by asking the patients to dorsiflex the wrist. The release was continued to the synovial membrane of the radiohumeral joint, which was breached to allow removal of any intra-articular lesions. Only the subcutaneous tissues and the skin were sutured.[34] Early, nonstressful movements were encouraged for 6 weeks, at which time physical therapy was introduced. Initially, 62 patients were assessed at 1 year, with 47 of these having no pain or slight pain. Fifty-seven were reexamined at 5 years, and 52 of them had no pain or slight pain. Thirty-two of the elbows were described as excellent and 19 as good.

Tissue excision

Goldberg *et al.* described identifying the common extensor origin and releasing the extensor carpi radialis brevis, extensor digitorum communis, and extensor digiti minimi, but preserving the extensor carpi radialis longus. The muscle mass was allowed to slide for around 1 cm. Any pathological tissue found at the site of the release was excised, and a 2-mm thick fragment of lateral epicondyle was removed. Active elbow motion was encouraged from the first day. Retrospective analysis showed that 25 of 34 patients had complete pain relief at an average of 4 years. A further eight had minimal symptoms. All but one patient returned to regular work at an average of 5 weeks postoperatively.[4]

Coonrad and Hooper retrospectively reviewed 1000 patients, 39 of whom required surgery. The procedure, done under local anesthetic, involved dissecting down to the tendinomuscular area, and when there was a gross tear of scar tissue replacement, a "V" excision of the degenerative or torn area was carried out. The remaining parts of the tendons were sutured. The results are reported as satisfactory in all 39 patients; they all returned to their preoperative occupations and activities in a recovery period of 3 months to a year.[9]

Nirschl and Pettrone[13] described a surgical technique aimed to specifically treat the angiofibroblastic hyperplasia. The origin of the extensor carpi radialis brevis tendon was incised from the anterior edge of the lateral epicondyle to reveal the pathological tissue, and all fibrous and granulation tissue was excised and removed. In contrast to the paper by Greenbaum *et al.*,[11] the authors stated that it is the brevis that is involved, rather than any aspect of the extensor digitorum communis aponeurosis. A small area of the exposed lateral condyle was decorticated to improve blood supply. The extensor carpi radialis brevis origin was not repaired, as it did not retract, hence the only repair was to the interface between the extensor carpi radialis longus and the anterior edge of the extensor aponeurosis. Eighty-two patients, including five who had previously had a failed Bosworth procedure, underwent this technique. Sixty-six were rated as excellent (full return to all activity with no pain), nine as good (full return to all activity with occasional mild pain), 11 as fair (normal activity with no pain or significant pain with heavy activity) and two as having failures. Overall, 97.7% improved, with 85.2% returning to full activity, including rigorous sports.

Summary of treatment options

- Oral anti-inflammatory medications
- Physical therapy
- Soft-tissue manipulation therapy (ultrasound and laser therapy)
- Steroid injections
- Botulinum toxin
- Extracorporeal shock-wave therapy (ESWT)

• Acupuncture
• Surgery

An evidence-based treatment protocol

We have described a number of treatment options from a mixture of anecdotal, retrospective, and prospective papers. However, the clinician requires a protocol to follow in this group of patients to aid their treatment. Hence, we propose a treatment regimen based on the available scientific evidence, but note that the evidence is generally poor.

Initial pain symptoms

The initial presenting complaint is usually pain, with loss of function as the secondary effect. The standard treatment would be one of rest, ice, splinting, and analgesia. This allows the tissues to settle down after the initial insult. As the pathology is one of angiofibroblastic degeneration, nonsteroidal anti-inflammatory medication should have little effect. However, some patients do receive some benefit. This is perhaps due to the reduction of inflammation in surrounding tissues and perhaps due to nonsteroidal anti-inflammatory drugs having an effect on increasing protein synthesis by fibroblasts, which may benefit the remodeling phase of repair. Cortisone injections have no proven effect on healing and should be avoided unless absolutely necessary.[7,27–29]

Muscle exercises

After the initial pain has been controlled, the patient requires an active rehabilitation program to align collagen fibers and improve tensile strength. The initial pathology was caused by a repetitive, cyclically applied, cumulative type of force.[8] Hence, the patient should avoid this and concentrate on controlled exercises of low velocity with gradual application of increasing resistance, under the supervision of a physiotherapist with an understanding of the pathology.[7,18,19]

Surgery

The vast majority of compliant patients respond to the nonoperative forms of treatment. This, however, leaves a small group of patients who require surgical intervention. There are numerous surgical reports, few of which are prospective and none of which are randomized. However, the results support procedures that identify and remove the pathological tissue that represents the angiofibroblastic degeneration. This allows the healing process to be reinitiated and gives better results. Hence Verhaar, Goldberg, Coonrad and Nirschl all describe techniques that are based on the histopathology and have good results. Less interventional techniques do not address the histopathology and may work purely by exciting an inflammatory response.[4,7,8,13,34] It must be noted that there is little hard scientific evidence to support this philosophy.

Summary of evidence-based treatment protocol

• Initial control of pain and surrounding inflammatory tissues (rest, ice, splinting, and analgesia).
• A specifically targeted physical therapy program.
• Surgery for the small group not responding to conservative measures, specifically aimed at excising the pathological tissue of angiofibroblastic degeneration.

Conclusions

Tennis elbow or lateral epicondylosis is not necessarily a pathology of tennis players, or indeed an inflammatory pathology. The pathology is one of angiofibroblastic degeneration, and the term "lateral epicondylosis" is therefore a more correct one. The term "tennis elbow" is also inaccurate, probably antiquated, and really should not be used—although it will probably remain in medical parlance for some time.

The vast majority of patients improve with nonoperative therapy, as long as this is tailored to the underlying pathology. Initially, simple measures to relieve pain and reduce inflammation in surrounding tissues are required. A specifically aimed physical therapy rehabilitation program may be useful for those who do not settle. Over 90% of patients will respond to these measures. Some patients do require surgery, and the procedures that give the best results are the ones that identify and excise the area of angiofibroblastic degeneration.

It must be remembered that the majority of studies are weak on pure scientific evidence, and hence one cannot fully recommend any one technique over any other.[15] Ideally, a true randomized, prospective controlled trial with large numbers of patients is required to fully answer the difficult question of the treatment of lateral epicondylosis.

Summary

- Tennis elbow is a non-inflammatory process of degenerative change in the extensor tissues at the elbow.
- The clinical course seems to be unchanged by a variety of standard non-surgical interventions perhaps due to its non-inflammatory aetiology and relapsing nature. Hence many clinicians to adopt a wait-and-see policy.
- There are new trials studying extracorporeal shock-wave therapy and botulinum toxin administration but none of these have shown significant evidence to favor any of the above regimens over any other.
- The mechanism of ESWT is still unknown and the procedure has a number of mild side effects.
- Botulinum toxin can also have significant short-term side effects.
- As both injections and operations can lead to potential side-effects it seems that the wait-and-see policy may still be appropriate.

Sample examination questions

Multiple-choice questions (answers on page 602)

1 With regard to the anatomy of the elbow:
   A The posterior interosseous nerve has roots C7 and C8
   B The extensor carpi radialis brevis is supplied by the median nerve
   C The working position of the forearm is a position of extension and supination
   D The extensor carpi radialis brevis lies deep to the extensor carpi radialis longus
   E The extensor carpi radialis brevis inserts into the second metacarpal

2 With regard to surgery in tennis elbow:
   A The majority of published surgical trials are retrospective and of poor scientific design
   B The technique described by Nirschl to specifically treat the angiofibroblastic hyperplasia has a success rate of over 97%

C Surgery is not possible under a local anesthetic
D Over 50% of patients will eventually require some type of surgical procedure
E The surgical procedures can be broadly divided into two main groups—a tenotomy or an excision of the pathological tissue

3 With regard to the nonsurgical treatment of tennis elbow:
A ESWT works in relieving pain by hyperstimulation analgesia
B The side effects of ESWT include pain, hematoma, and migraines
C Steroid injections have little short-term benefit over physiotherapy, but provide better long-term benefit
D Botulinum toxin injections give significantly better results at 3 months than placebo injections
E There is insufficient evidence either to support of refute the use of acupuncture in lateral epicondylosis

Essay questions

1 Is there a role for extracorporeal shock-wave therapy (ESWT) in the treatment of lateral epicondylosis?
2 What treatment does one offer to a 30-year-old secretary with lateral elbow pain in her dominant arm, whose hobbies include playing squash?
3 What is the evidence for botulinum toxin being a treatment option in lateral epicondylosis and how does it work in theory?

Case study 21.1

A 40-year old right-handed man presents to the clinic with a 12-month history of pain in his right elbow. He is a construction worker, describing his work as “strenuous manual labor.” His job had changed about 18 months previously to one involving more upper limb work. More recently he had become unable to do the gardening at the weekend due to elbow pain, prompting his referral.

He had localized pain on the lateral side of the elbow and was maximum over the extensor origin. He had slightly reduced elbow extension. Resisted extension of the wrist was painful in the lateral elbow region. He described this as severe. Radiographs of the elbow were normal when taken in the clinic.

He was treated with simple measures of rest, splinting, and analgesics. Once his acute symptoms had settled, he underwent a specific physiotherapy program aimed at improving the tensile strength of the muscle. He made a full improvement after a couple of months. He returned to this job.

Summarizing the evidence

Comparison/treatment strategies	Results	Level of evidence*
Physiotherapy	2 observational studies	C
Ultrasound	Several poorly constructed studies	B
Laser	1 prospective randomized trial	A3
Surgery	2 retrospective studies, moderate numbers	
	4 expert opinions	C
ESWT	3 prospective randomized controlled trials	A1
Botulinum toxin	2 prospective randomized controlled trials	A3
Steroids	3 prospective randomized controlled trials	A1
Acupuncture	4 small randomized controlled trials	A3

* A1: evidence from large randomized controlled trials (RCTs) or systematic review (including meta-analysis).†
A2: evidence from at least one high-quality cohort.
A3: evidence from at least one moderate-size RCT or systematic review.†
A4: evidence from at least one RCT.
B: evidence from at least one high-quality study of nonrandomized cohorts.
C: expert opinions.
† Arbitrarily, the following cut-off points have been used; large study size: ≥ 100 patients per intervention group; moderate study size ≥ 50 patients per intervention group.

References

1 Canale ST, ed. *Campbell's Operative Orthopaedics*, 9th ed. St. Louis: Mosby, 1998.
2 Frostick SP, Mohammad M, Ritchie DA Sports injuries of the elbow. *Br J Sports Med* 1999; **33**:301–311.
3 Wadsworth TG. Tennis elbow: conservative, surgical, and manipulative treatment. *BMJ* 1987; **294**:621–624.
4 Goldberg EJ, Abraham E, Siegel I. The surgical treatment of chronic lateral humeral epicondylitis by common extensor release. *Clin Orthop Relat Res* 1988; **233**:208–212.
5 Boyer MI, Hastings H 2nd. Lateral tennis elbow: "is there any science out there?" *J Shoulder Elbow Surg* 1999; **8**:481–491.
6 Regan W, Wold LE, Coonrad R, Morrey BF. Microscopic histopathology of chronic refractory lateral epicondylitis. *Am J Sports Med* 1992; **20**:746–749.
7 Kraushaar BS, Nirschl RP. Tendinosis of the elbow (tennis elbow): clinical features and findings of histological, immunohistochemical, and electron microscopy studies. *J Bone Joint Surg Am* 1999; **81**:259–278.
8 Nirschl RP. Elbow tendinosis/tennis elbow. *Clin Sports Med* 1992; **11**:851–870.
9 Coonrad RW, Hooper WR. Tennis elbow: its course, natural history, conservative and surgical treatment. *J Bone Joint Surg Am* 1973; **55**:1177–1182.
10 McMinn RMH, ed. *Last's Anatomy: Regional and Applied*, 8th ed. Edinburgh: Churchill Livingstone, 1993: 61–64, 70–71.
11 Greenbaum B, Itamura J, Vangsness CT, Tibone J, Atkinson R. Extensor carpi radialis brevis. *J Bone Joint Surg Br* 1999: **81**:926–929.
12 Kannus P, Jozsa L. Histopathological changes preceding spontaneous rupture of a tendon: a controlled study of 891 patients. *J Bone Joint Surg Am* 1991; **73**:1507–1525.
13 Nirschl RP, Pettrone FA. Tennis elbow: the surgical treatment of lateral epicondylitis. *J Bone Joint Surg Am* 1979; **61**:832–839.
14 Nirschl RP. Prevention and treatment of elbow and shoulder injuries in the tennis player. *Clin Sports Med* 1988; 7:289–308.
15 Labelle H, Guibert R, Joncas J, *et al.* Lack of scientific evidence for the treatment of lateral epicondylitis of the elbow. *J Bone Joint Surg Br* 1992; **74**:646–651.

16 Grundberg AB, Dobson JF. Percutaneous release of the common extensor origin for tennis elbow. *Clin Orthop Relat Res* 2000; **376**:137–140.
17 Sevier TL, Wilson JK. Treating lateral epicondylitis. *Sports Med* 1999; **28**:375–380.
18 Kuland DN, McCue FC 3rd, Rockwell DA, Gieck JH. Tennis injuries: prevention and treatment. A review. *Am J Sports Med* 1979; **7**:249–253.
19 Kreider RB, Fry AC, O'Toole ML. *Overtraining in Sport.* Champaign IL: Human Kinetics 1998, 177–179.
20 Basford JR, Sheffield CG, Cieslak KR. Laser therapy: a randomised, controlled trial of the effects of low intensity Nd:YAG irradiation on lateral epicondylitis. *Arch Phys Med Rehabil* 2000; **81**:1504–1510.
21 Ko JY, Chen HS, Chen LM. Treatment of lateral epicondylitis of the elbow with shock waves. *Clin Orthop* 2001; **387**:60–67.
22 Haake M, Konig IR, Decker T, *et al.* Extracorporeal shock wave therapy in the treatment of lateral epicondylitis: a randomized multicenter trial. *J Bone Joint Surg Am* 2002; **84**:1982–1991.
23 Haake M, Boddeker IR, Decker T, *et al.* Side-effects of extracorporeal shock wave therapy (ESWT) in the treatment of tennis elbow. *Arch Orthop Trauma Surg* 2002; **122**:222–228.
24 Speed CA, Nichols D, Richards C, *et al.* Extracorporeal shock wave therapy for lateral epicondylitis: a double blind randomised controlled trial. *J Orthop Res* 2002; **20**:895–898.
25 Crowther MA, Bannister GC, Huma H, Rooker GD. A prospective, randomised study to compare extracorporeal shock-wave therapy and injection of steroid for the treatment of tennis elbow. *J Bone Joint Surg Br* 2002; **84**:678–679.
26 Hay EM, Paterson SM, Lewis M, Hosie P. Pragmatic randomised controlled trial of local corticosteroid injection and naproxen for treatment of lateral epicondylitis of elbow in primary care. *BMJ* 1999; **319**:964–968.
27 Newcomer KL, Laskowski ER, Idank DM, McLean TJ, Egan KS. Corticosteroid injection in early treatment of lateral epicondylitis. *Clin J Sport Med* 2001; **11**:214–222.
28 Nirschl RP, Rodin DM, Ochiai DH, Maartmann-Moe C. Iontophoretic administration of dexamethasone sodium phosphate for acute epicondylitis: a randomized, double-blinded, placebo-controlled study. *Am J Sports Med* 2003; **31**:189–195.
29 Smidt N, van der Windt DA, Assendelft WJ, *et al.* Corticosteroid injections, physiotherapy, or a wait-and-see policy for lateral epicondylitis: a randomised controlled trial. *Lancet* 2002; **359**:657–662.
30 Keizer SB, Rutten HP, Pilot P, *et al.* Botulinum toxin injection versus surgical treatment for tennis elbow: a randomized pilot study. *Clin Orthop* 2002; **401**:125–131.
31 Hayton MJ, Santini AJA, Hughes PJ, *et al.* Botulinum toxin injection in the treatment of tennis elbow. *J Bone Joint Surg Am* 2005; **87**:503–507.
32 Green S, Buchbinder R, Barnsley L, *et al.* Acupuncture for lateral elbow pain. *Cochrane Database Syst Rev* 2002; (1):CD003527.
33 Bosworth DM. Surgical treatment of tennis elbow: a follow-up study. *J Bone Joint Surg Am* 1965; **47**:1533–1536.
34 Verhaar J, Walkenkamp G, Kester A, van Mameren H, van der Linden T. Lateral extensor release for tennis elbow. *J Bone Joint Surg Am* 1993; **75**:1034–1043.

SECTION 5
Injuries to the groin and knee

CHAPTER 22

How reliable is the physical examination in the diagnosis of sports-related knee injuries?

Anthony Festa, William R. Donaldson, and John C. Richmond

Introduction

The clinical diagnosis of knee injuries continues to be a topic for active study and debate. As a large, complex joint without inherent bony stability, the knee must rely on soft-tissue structures to provide structural stability. Soft-tissue structures, such as the capsule, ligaments, and menisci, are subject to large forces delivered by the long lever arms of the lower extremity. The high frequency of sports-related injuries is, therefore, not surprising. The exact incidence of knee injuries varies with gender from one sport to another. However, the frequency is considered to be in the range of 15–30% of all athletic injuries. In this setting, the sports-medicine physician is frequently called upon to diagnose and treat knee injuries. Accurate diagnosis is the cornerstone of an appropriate treatment plan. Newer diagnostic modalities, including magnetic resonance imaging (MRI), can be helpful, but involve delay in diagnosis and can increase cost. With increasing pressures for cost containment and "throughput," physicians are being asked to closely examine the direct patient benefit, relative to cost, of all diagnostic and therapeutic measures. In this light, it is appropriate to critically analyze the various components of the physical examination for evidence of their effectiveness. In this manner, we may better appreciate the statistical likelihood of a given diagnosis, and when it is appropriate to proceed with further modalities, such as MRI, examination under anesthesia, or arthroscopic evaluation. Part of surgical education and practice is based on tradition grounded in emulation—physical examination included. Evaluating which components of the physical examination are based on scientific evidence can lead to more accurate diagnosis and better care of the patient.

Methods

This review is based on systematic searches of the various journal and texts familiar to the physician interested in sports medicine. Internet searches were performed using PubMed and OVID search engines, as well as localized queries on individual journal web sites. The journals included *Arthroscopy; Journal of Arthroscopic and Related Surgery; American Journal of Sports Medicine; Journal of Bone and Joint Surgery* (American and British editions); *Journal of the American Academy of Orthopaedic Surgeons; Journal of Orthopaedic and Sports Physical Therapy; Journal of Orthopaedic Trauma; Knee Surgery, Sports Traumatology, Arthroscopy;* and *Annals of the Royal College of Surgeons.* The Medical

Table 22.1 Summary of Medical Subject Headings (MeSH) terms

- Knee joint
- Knee injuries/diagnostic
- Physical examination
- Ligaments, articular
- Menisci, tibial/injuries
- Arthroscopy
- Magnetic resonance imaging
- Sports medicine
- Diagnosis, differential
- Sensitivity and specificity
- Joint instability
- Patella
- ACL, PCL
- MCL, LCL

ACL, anterior cruciate ligament; LCL, lateral collateral ligament; MCL, medial collateral ligament; PCL, posterior cruciate ligament.

Subject Headings (MeSH) are noted in the summary box below. A variety of widely available texts were used for background information and additional references.

In general, the accuracy of clinical examination and MRI has been established by comparison with arthroscopy. By not including patients who were treated nonoperatively or who were not diagnosed as having the index condition, finding both true-negatives and false-negatives will be underrepresented in the calculation of accuracy, sensitivity, and specificity. The results of studies using arthroscopic findings to assess the accuracy of the preoperative examination should therefore be viewed with caution. Unfortunately, this will likely remain a constant feature of most clinical studies, in which only selected patients are brought to surgery and no control population is available for comparison (Table 22.1).

Physical examination

The physical examination should start with general observations, then proceed to an examination of the contralateral, uninjured knee, and lastly, to the injured extremity. General observations of age, sex, height, weight, and overall physical fitness should be made. In stance, one should observe for pelvic obliquity, leg length discrepancy, and lower extremity alignment in both coronal and sagittal planes. The patient should then be observed in gait, noting any irregularities, or the need for walking aids (i.e., crutches). The examination should then proceed with inspection for effusion, ecchymosis, or localized tenderness. One should systematically palpate all bony and soft-tissue prominences. Hughston *et al.* found that point tenderness will localize the site of injury 76% of the time.[1] Active and passive range of motion should be gently assessed and compared with the contralateral side. The knee can then be tested for ligamentous stability. The neurologic examination should include muscle strength, sensation, and reflex testing. Finally, the examiner should perform specialized tests for any individual areas of interest.

Meniscal examination

The myriad of tests for meniscal injury suggests that no single test can be relied on to define meniscal pathology. Most examinations include some combination of palpation of the joint line at rest, and with motion, rotation, or a combination of the two. McMurray's test is performed by moving the knee from flexion to extension with applied rotation of the tibia. With external rotation, medial-sided pain and a palpable "click" or "clunk" are said to be positive for a medial meniscal tear. Applied internal rotation is said to be provocative for a lateral meniscal tear. If findings occur near flexion, the tear is considered to be more posterior. Pain with passive hyperflexion loads the posterior horns of the menisci and may cause pain. The Apley grind test is performed with the patient prone and the knee in 90° of flexion. If rotation with axial loading is more painful than with joint distraction, the test is said to be suggestive of a meniscal tear.

Discussion

The accuracy of the physical examination of the meniscus has been the topic of numerous studies. While some studies compare the accuracy of examination findings with MRI, the standard by which the examination is assessed continues to be the arthroscopic examination.

The clinical signs commonly considered to be indicative of a meniscal tear include joint line tenderness, a positive McMurray's test, a positive Apley test, and posterior medial or posterior lateral joint line pain with hyperflexion.

Fowler *et al.* conducted a prospective study of 161 consecutive patients to evaluate the predictive value of five common clinical tests for meniscal tear.[2] All patients underwent a preoperative examination, including tests for joint line tenderness, pain on forced flexion, McMurray, Apley, and distraction tests, and block to extension. The patients then underwent an arthroscopic evaluation, and the findings were compared with the results of the clinical examination. With an intact anterior cruciate ligament (ACL), Fowler *et al.* found that joint line tenderness had an 86% sensitivity for detecting a meniscal repair, but a specificity of only 29%. Pain on forced flexion showed a sensitivity of 50% but a specificity of 68%. The McMurray test and extension block had a high correlation with meniscal tears, with specificities of 95% and 85% respectively. The Apley compression and distraction tests correlated poorly with meniscal lesions.

In a prospective study of 104 patients with suspected meniscal lesion, Eren correlated medial and lateral joint line tenderness with arthroscopic results for respective meniscal tears.[3] Medial joint line tenderness showed 74% accuracy, 86% sensitivity, and 67% specificity, while lateral joint line tenderness showed 96% accuracy, 92% sensitivity, and 97% specificity.

Shelbourne *et al.* analyzed the efficacy of joint line tenderness in patients with acute ACL tears.[4] They examined 173 patients with acute ACL injuries for joint line tenderness, and then observed for meniscal tears during arthroscopic ACL reconstruction. They found that in the knee with and acute ACL injury, joint line tenderness was neither sensitive nor specific for a meniscal tear.

The McMurray test is commonly believed to have low sensitivity and high specificity for meniscal tears. Evans *et al.* evaluated the McMurray test for the diagnosis of meniscal tears by comparing examination results with arthroscopic findings in a prospective study of 104 consecutive patients.[5] They also analyzed the interexaminer reliability of the McMurray test. With fair interexaminer reliability, the only significant McMurray sign found to correlate with meniscal lesion was a "thud" elicited on the medial joint line. This sign showed 16% sensitivity and 98% specificity. In a similar study, Corea *et al.* evaluated the McMurray test in a group of 93 patients undergoing surgery.[6] They found a sensitivity of 59%, a specificity of 93%, and a positive predictive value of 83%.

In a prospective study of 150 consecutive patients, Akseki *et al.* evaluated the diagnostic value of a newly described weight-bearing test, McMurray's test, and joint line tenderness.[7] All patients were evaluated with arthroscopic examinations. With regard to joint line tenderness, the accuracy, sensitivity, and specificity for medial/lateral meniscal tears were 71%/77%, 88%/67%, and 44%/80%, respectively. The accuracy, sensitivity, and sensitivity of the McMurray test for medial/lateral tears were 60%/82%, 67%/53%, and 69%/88%, respectively.

A variety of studies have compared the accuracy of clinical examination and MRI in the diagnosis of meniscal pathology. While some studies show MRI to be more accurate than the examination, others reveal no clear advantage. Rose and Gold conducted a prospective and retrospective study of 100 patients to evaluate the accuracy of clinical examination and MRI scan for the diagnosis of meniscal injury.[8] All patients underwent physical examination and MRI prior to arthroscopy. The study found that clinical examination had an accuracy of 79% for detecting meniscal lesions, in comparison with 72% for MRI. The authors concluded that MRI was not a cost-effective tool. Miller also evaluated the accuracy of the clinical examination and MRI in detecting meniscal lesions in 57 consecutive knees.[9] The study revealed the accuracy of the examination and MRI to be 81% and 74%, respectively. He concluded that MRI did not prevent unnecessary surgery.

In a prospective study of 61 knees, Munk *et al.* compared MRI and clinical findings to arthroscopic findings.[10] In contrast to the above studies, they found the accuracy and positive predictive value of MRI to be twice that of clinical examination. In similar studies by Fischer *et al.* and Muellner *et al.*, comparing MRI with arthroscopic results, MRI was found to have accuracy rates of 89% and 95%, respectively[11,12] (Tables 22.2–22.4).

Table 22.2 Summary of meniscal tests

- Joint line tenderness
- McMurray test
- Apley grind test
- Passive hyperflexion

Table 22.3 McMurray's test (Evans *et al.*[5])

Sensitivity	16%
Specificity	98%
Positive predictive value (PPV)	83%
Negative predictive value (NPV)	65%

Table 22.4 Joint line tenderness (Eren[3])

	Medial	Lateral
Sensitivity	86%	92%
Specificity	67%	97%
Positive predictive value (PPV)	59%	92%
Negative predictive value (NPV)	90%	97%
Accuracy	74%	96%

Patellofemoral examination

Examination of the patellofemoral joint should begin with overall observation of leg alignment and length. One should evaluate femoral version, tibial torsion, and foot position, as well as the femorotibial angle (anatomic axis) and the Q angle. The Q angle is defined by the intersection of a line from the tibial tubercle to the center of the patella, and a line from the center of the patella to the anterior superior iliac spine. Quadriceps status is evaluated by noting visual atrophy, palpating the muscle during contraction, and measurements of thigh circumference. The patella and corresponding soft-tissue insertions, such as the quadriceps and patellar tendons and medial and lateral retinaculum, should be palpated for evidence of localized tenderness. Next, patellar mobility can be tested. Lateral retinacular tightness can be assessed by medial and lateral (Sage) glide tests. This Sage test is often described by the number of quadrants the patella can be displaced medially from its resting position with the knee in 20° of flexion. One quadrant is said to indicate tightness, and three quadrants to indicate laxity. The tilt test also measures lateral retinacular tightness, and is defined as the ability to elevate the lateral border of the patella to neutral or slightly beyond with the knee in extension. The apprehension test is performed by laterally translating the patella. The "apprehension sign" is positive when the patient recognizes instability symptoms. Further assessment includes observation of patellar tracking with knee extension and flexion. Finally, the examiner should assess for pain and/or crepitus with direct patellar compression at various degrees of flexion. This is a useful time to evaluate for an effusion.

Discussion

Evaluation of the patellofemoral joint requires examination not only of the extensor mechanism but also of the entire lower extremity. Patellofemoral disorders are multifactorial. Mathematic modeling and instrumented specimens have increased understanding of pathology in the patellofemoral joint and allowed the development of more rational treatment programs. The function of the patellofemoral joint is affected by bone morphology and soft-tissue influences from the hip to the foot.

With regard to the technique for Q angle measurement discussed above, studies have shown that measurements of the Q angle can be affected by patient and lower extremity positioning. In a study of 526 college-aged men and women, Woodland *et al.* found significant differences in Q angle measurement done in the supine and standing position. He attributed the greater values found while standing were to increased valgus angulation forces on the knee during weight-bearing.[13] While it is generally accepted that the degree of valgus alignment of the knee affects patellar alignment, Olerud *et al.* showed that foot positioning can as well.[14] In a study of 34 healthy patients, they found that the Q angle increased as the foot shifted from outward to inward rotation, and conversely decreased as the foot shifted from pronation to supination. Although Q angle measurement is an integral part of most clinicians' patellofemoral examination, there is no direct correlation with the incidence of patellofemoral symptoms or disorders. In a review of the clinical evaluation of patellofemoral disorders, Post analyzed previous studies by Insall and Aglietti that compared Q angle measurements in patients with patellofemoral pain.[15] He noted that 60% of Aglietti's and 52% of Insall's patients with patellofemoral pain had Q angles within their original definition of normal. These findings are supported in a study by Fairbank *et al.*[16] In a study of 446 adolescents, they found no significant difference in Q angle measurements when comparing patients with and without knee pain.

While there is no direct correlation between the Q angle and patients' symptoms, there does seem to be agreement that the factors which serve to increase patellofemoral joint reaction force or to decrease surface contact area will result in cartilage degeneration and arthrosis. The Q angle is a measurement of the lateral vector acting on the patella. Huberti and Hayes tested 12 cadaveric knee joints using a loading fixture to test flexion angle and Q angle for contact pressure.[17] This was measured on pressure sensitive film and demonstrated a balanced distribution of pressure on the medial and lateral facets at all angles of flexion. They studied the effect on the distribution and amount of contact pressure with changes in the Q angle. A 10° increase or decrease in the Q angle was associated with a nonuniform pressure distribution and increases in peak stress observed.

Increased femoral anteversion may affect alignment by displacing the trochlear groove medially. Lee *et al.* studied human cadaveric knees for patellofemoral contact pressure due to fixed rotational deformity of the femur.[18] They demonstrated increased patellofemoral pressures in the presence of increased femoral anteversion. Using computed tomography (CT) evaluation to measure femoral anteversion, Eckoff *et al.* compared 20 adult patients with anterior knee pain to 10 controls. They found that patients with anterior knee pain demonstrated significantly more anteversion than controls (23° vs. 18°).[19]

A number of studies have suggested an association between lateral placement of the tibia tubercle and anterior knee pain. Using CT scans to determine the tibial tubercle position relative to the intercondylar notch (tubercle sulcus angle), Muneta *et al.* demonstrated the association of lateral placement with patellofemoral pain and CT documented tilt.[20] In a similar study, Jones *et al.* measured anatomic relationships of tibial tubercle lateralization in 50 patients.[21] The study confirmed that patients with anterior knee pain secondary to malalignment demonstrated significantly greater lateralization of the tubercle than asymptomatic controls.

The glide (Sage) and tilt tests are methods of assessing the patellar mobility and the tightness of the medial and lateral retinaculum. The findings with these examinations are often difficult to quantify and often exhibit poor interobserver reliability. In a study of 66 patients, Fitzgerald and McClure evaluated the reliability of four tests for patellofemoral alignment, including medial/lateral displacement and medial/lateral tilt, when performed by 12 different examiners.[22] The study revealed fair to poor interobserver reliability with these tests. In a study of 99 knees, Watson *et al.* examined the reliability of the patellar tilt test. As in Fitzgerald and McClure's study, it exhibited poor interobserver reliability.[23] Some researchers have used instrumented measuring devices to improve the accuracy, precision, and reliability of patellar mobility testing. Using a hand-held patella pusher, Fithian *et al.* examined 94 uninjured athletes and 22 athletes with unilateral patellar dislocations for patellar laxity.[24] In comparison with controls, the study showed increased laxity not only in the dislocated knees, but also in the contralateral uninjured knee, suggesting possible predisposition to injury. Using an instrumented device, they also showed good intraobserver and interobserver reliability. Reider *et al.* used an instrumented measuring device to measure medial/lateral displacement during active flexion and extension.[25] The study compared 50 athletes who complained of patellar pain or instability (subluxation or dislocation) with 50 controls. In comparison with the control group, the group with pain exhibited similar laxity. The instability groups, however, exhibited increased laxity in comparison with the controls.

With regard to patellar instability, studies have been performed to evaluate the soft-tissue restraints on lateral patellar translation. Desio *et al.* biomechanically tested nine cadaveric

Table 22.5 Patellofemoral examination

- Observe:
  - —Muscle atrophy
  - —Knee alignment (Q angle)
  - —Femoral version
  - —Tibial tubercle position
  - —Foot position
- Palpate bony and soft-tissue structures
- Patellar mobility
- Patellar tracking
- Compression (pain)
- Crepitus

knees to identify and quantify the soft-tissue restraints on lateral patellar translation.[26] The knees were tested at 20° of flexion. The contribution of each structure was identified by sectioning restraints in a predetermined order. The medial patellofemoral ligament was found to be the primary restraint on lateral patellar translation, contributing 60% of the total restraining force. In a similar study, Conlan *et al.* performed biomechanical testing on 25 knees to evaluate medial soft-tissue restraints to lateral patellar translation.[27] Again, the medial patellofemoral ligament was found to be the major medial soft-tissue restraint, contributing an average of 53% of the total force.

Compression of the patella into the trochlea at various degrees of flexion is thought to produce pain and crepitus when the area of abnormal cartilage contacts the femur. In a study of 100 knees, Niskanen *et al.* assessed four such compressive tests, including the inhibition and the tracking tests.[28] The results of these tests were then compared with arthroscopic findings. In general, the tests showed low sensitivity, specificity, accuracy, and predictive values. In a study by Johnson *et al.*, the authors carried out a comprehensive clinical assessment of 100 women and 110 men with asymptomatic knees.[29] The patients underwent a thorough medical history, physical examination, and plain-film radiographs. Interestingly, the authors found crepitus in 94% of women and 45% of men who had never had knee complaints (Table 22.5).

Ligament and capsule: study technique

The functional stability of the knee depends on both static and dynamic factors. The musculature that crosses the knee provides dynamic support. The joint reactive forces and ligaments provide static stabilization. In order to be useful, the clinical examination should define abnormal limits of motion in the knee in such a way that injury to specific structures is defined. Only then can a rational approach be developed.

It must first be established that manual testing does correlate both with anatomic integrity and functional instability. In performing the physical examination, the passive restraint provided by the ligaments is being tested at much lower values than *in vivo* forces. This, coupled with the qualitative manner of testing, may create a significant disparity between the joint examination and *in vivo* joint function.[30]

The study of knee biomechanics can be classified into three broad categories: mathematical modeling, ligament-cutting studies, and ligament force measurements.[31]

Ligament-cutting studies can be performed in one of two ways. First, the displacement resulting from applied load is measured before and after sectioning the ligament under study. This is analogous to the clinical laxity examination, in which the amount of displacement to an applied load is estimated. Measurement of laxity changes after sectioning of a ligament gives an indication of changes in joint stability after injury and therefore is useful in evaluating the sensitivity of knee laxity tests. Beynnon categorized the above as flexibility tests.[31]

The second type of ligament-cutting study is described by Beynnon as the stiffness approach.[31] The method involves measuring changes in the amount of load required to produce a given amount of displacement of the joint before and after ligament sectioning. According to Noyes *et al.*, this technique allows ligaments to be classified as primary and secondary stabilizers of the knee and is independent of the order in which ligaments are sectioned.[30] The primary stabilizers provide most of the restraint on motion and protect the secondary stabilizers, which will experience greater loads following injury to the primary stabilizers. This approach gives a better indication of ligament function than the laxity studies described above.

The third approach to the study of ligament function includes anatomic description, as well as *in situ* measurements of both ligament force and strain. Knee ligaments are most effective at controlling motion parallel to the orientation of their fibers. Therefore, knowledge of its anatomic attachments will provide an understanding of which forces it can best resist. Strain gauges applied directly to ligaments have allowed *in vitro* assessment of displacement under load, as have placement of markers at ligament ends.

The diagnosis of ligament and capsular defects requires the use of selective laxity tests for which the primary and secondary ligamentous restraints have been experimentally determined.

Ligament examination

The clinical diagnosis of ligament injury is based on the demonstration of pathologic knee motion.[32] The increased limits of motion resulting from applied forces should be described in relation to the three rotational and three translational axes (six degrees of freedom) of motion. Frequently, the abnormal motions take place on more than one axis (coupled) and may result in both pathologic motion and abnormal joint positioning (subluxation).[33] The demonstration of abnormal motion first requires an assessment of constitutional laxity, defined most commonly by recurvatum at the elbow, ability to touch the abducted thumb to the forearm, and hyperextension at the metacarpal–phalangeal joints of the fingers. The demonstration of abnormal motion should therefore always be based on an assessment of the contralateral uninjured knee. Clinical laxity tests must be performed in a consistent manner in order to minimize intraobserver and interobserver error. Measurement of tibial displacement should be made in relation to the femur. The starting position is the neutral resting position, with the joint surfaces in contact.[32]

There are a variety of clinical tests to assess the integrity of the anterior cruciate ligament (ACL) and secondary stabilizers. The Lachman test is performed with the femur stabilized, by placing an anterior force on the proximal tibia without constraining rotation. Both the amount of displacement and the end-point stiffness are graded. The end point should be described as firm, soft, or absent. The displacement can be further quantified with the use of an instrumented laxity testing device (e.g., KT 2000). A side-to-side difference of more than 3 mm is considered pathologic. The anterior drawer test is performed with the knee flexed 90°, by applying an anterior force to the proximal tibia. Care must be taken to ensure a neutral starting point with these tests. Otherwise, one might interpret posterior sag from a posterior cruciate ligament (PCL) injury as anterior subluxation due to ACL injury. Various pivot shift tests have been described. These demonstrate an increased internal rotation and anterior subluxation of the lateral tibial plateau as a result of ACL injury.

Examination of the PCL starts with an observation of the resting position of the knee in 90° of flexion compared to the contralateral knee. With an intact PCL, the tibia will not sag and cannot be displaced posteriorly more than the opposite knee. Damage to the PCL will produce a posterior subluxation, which can be quantified by comparing the relationship of the anterior tibia to the femoral condyle or by the posterior displacement from the neutral joint position and graded one plus for each 5 mm of displacement. Contraction of the quadriceps with the foot fixed will tend to reduce the posterior subluxation (quadriceps active test).[32] The posterior drawer is performed with the knee flexed 90° by applying a posterior force to the proximal tibia.

The abduction stress test evaluates the medial collateral ligament (MCL) and medial capsular structures. This is performed with restraint of tibial rotation and starting with the joint surfaces in contact. A valgus force, applied to the tibia in 30° of flexion, tests the MCL alone, and an extension tests the MCL and posteromedial capsule. Both the amount of displacement and the end point are graded.

The adduction or varus stress test evaluates the lateral collateral ligament (LCL) and lateral capsular structures. A varus force applied to the tibia at 30° of flexion tests the LCL alone, and in extension tests the LCL and posterolateral capsule. Again, the amount of displacement and end point are graded.

The Slocum test involves carrying out the anterior drawer in both neutral and external rotation.[34] Injury to the posteromedial capsule in association with ACL injury is thought to result in increased anterior excursion of the tibia in external rotation. Signs of injury to the posterolateral complex include increased external rotation of the tibia at 30° and 90° of flexion (dial test), external rotation recurvatum, posterolateral drawer, and the reverse pivot shift. The external rotation recurvatum test is performed by elevation of the leg in extension by lifting at the great toe. This will allow external tibial rotation, creating apparent varus and hyperextension. The posterolateral drawer demonstrates external rotation of the lateral tibial plateau in 30° of flexion. Placing the patient prone with the knees together allows accurate assessment of differences in available external rotation of the tibia at 30° and 90°. The reverse pivot shift as described by Jacob begins with the knee flexed and externally rotated.[35] As the knee is extended, the tibia accelerates from a subluxed to a reduced position, often with a clunk.

ACL and PCL discussion

The anterior cruciate ligament (ACL) is the primary restraint on anterior translation of the tibia in relation to the femur. Cadaveric studies have shown that the ACL provides approximately 85% of the restraint to an anterior shear load at 90° and 87% at 30° of flexion. After ACL transaction, the remaining ligamentous structures provide little restraint on anterior subluxation of the tibia.[36]

In 1976, Torg *et al.* first described the Lachman test.[37] In this study, 250 knee examinations were retrospectively reviewed and compared with intraoperative findings. Of these knees, 136 had ACL ruptures documented with Lachman tests. The Lachman test was positive in 96%. The authors concluded that the Lachman test is a simple, reliable, and reproducible method for demonstrating ACL instability. Of note, the original test was described with the knee in 15° of flexion.

Donaldson *et al.* performed a retrospective study on 100 patients documented during surgery to have ACL ruptures.[38] Of these 100 patients, 37 had isolated ACL injuries, whereas the remainder had ACL injuries coupled with meniscal and/or collateral ligament injuries. Both the preoperative examination and the examination under anesthesia were compared with findings at surgery. When the preoperative examination (no anesthesia) was analyzed for patients with isolated ACL injuries, the authors found that 98% of the Lachman tests, 54% of the anterior drawer tests, and 27% of the pivot shift tests were positive. When the examination under anesthesia was analyzed for these isolated injuries, authors found that 100% of the Lachman tests, 81% of the anterior drawer tests, and 100% of the pivot shift tests were positive. Notably, they performed the Lachman test at 30° of flexion. In a retrospective study of ACL tears confirmed by arthroscopy, Katz and Fingeroth analyzed the Lachman, anterior drawer, and pivot shift tests when performed with the patients under anesthesia.[39] For all ACL injuries, the Lachman test was 81.8% sensitive and 96.8% specific, the anterior drawer sign was 40.9% sensitive and 95.2% specific, and the pivot shift test was 81.8% sensitive and 98.4% specific.

In a study of 147 patients with arthroscopically documented chronic ACL injuries, Kim *et al.* evaluated the clinical examination under anesthesia.[40] Interestingly, in 19 of these cases, the proximal end of the torn ACL had reattached to the PCL. Overall, the sensitivities of the Lachman test, the anterior drawer sign, and the pivot shift test were 98.6%, 79.6%, and 89.8%, respectively. When the 19 ACL reattached knees were evaluated, the sensitivities differed. The sensitivities were 89.5% for the Lachman test, 68.4% for the anterior drawer sign, and 63.2% for the pivot shift test.

With regard to the clinical examination of the ACL, a study by Oberlander *et al.* warrants discussion.[41] In this study, the physical examination of the knee was compared to arthroscopic finding in 296 knees. Arthroscopy revealed 48 ACL ruptures. After physical examination, 32 knees were suspected for ACL injury, of which 30 were confirmed arthroscopically. The diagnostic accuracy was 94%. However, an additional 18 ACL injuries were discovered at surgery that had not been suspected on examination. These knees were operated on for other reasons and were found incidentally to have ACL ruptures. This then resulted in a sensitivity and specificity of 63% and 93%, respectively, for the physical examination. Although the authors did not comment on which examination techniques were used, this study acknowledges inherent biases found in the literature, particularly selection bias. Many studies calculate values on the basis of a retrospective analysis of patients documented by arthroscopy to have a certain injury. They often do not include patients who were incorrectly diagnosed.

Studies have also compared the accuracy of clinical examination and MRI in diagnosing ACL injuries. Rose and Gold performed a retrospective study of 100 patients to evaluate the accuracy of clinical examination and MRI scan for the diagnosis of ACL tears.[8] All patients underwent physical examination and MRI prior to arthroscopy. The accuracy of MRI was 98%, while the accuracy of the physical examination was 99%. The authors concluded that MRI was an unnecessary diagnostic test for patients with a suspected ACL tear.

The posterior cruciate ligament (PCL) is the primary restraint to posterior translation of the tibia in all degrees of flexion, where it provides 94% of the restraining force on posterior displacement.[36] The secondary restraints include the posterolateral capsule, the popliteus complex, and the medial collateral ligament. Sectioning of the PCL alone produced an increase in straight posterior translation, with no change in the rotation or varus and valgus rotation.[42] The maximum displacement was at 90° of flexion. Therefore, the

Table 22.6 Anterior cruciate ligament (ACL) and posterior cruciate ligament (PCL) tests

- ACL Lachman, anterior drawer, pivot shift
- PCL Posterior drawer, quadriceps active, posterior sag

Table 22.7 Examination of the anterior cruciate ligament (Katz and Fingeroth[39])

	Sensitivity	Specificity	Positive predictive value (PPV)	Negative predictive value (NPV)
Lachman test	81.8%	96.8%	90.0%	93.8%
Anterior drawer test	40.9%	95.2%	75.0%	82.2%

Table 22.8 Examination of the posterior cruciate ligament (Rubinstein *et al.*[43])

	Sensitivity	Specificity
Posterior drawer test	90%	99%
Quadriceps active test	54%	97%

posterior drawer test would be most sensitive at 90°, with no change in varus or external rotation. In a study of 75 knees, Rubinstein *et al.* assessed the effectiveness of the clinical examination of the knee in the setting of a posterior cruciate ligament injury. Of the 75 patients, 19 had chronic PCL-deficient knees.[43] These were confirmed by MRI, since the majority of patients at the institution were treated nonoperatively. The accuracy of the overall examination for an isolated PCL injury was 96%, whereas the sensitivity and specificity of the posterior drawer examination were 90% and 99%, respectively. Notably, the sensitivity and specificity of the quadriceps-active test were 54% and 97%, respectively. In a study of patients with isolated PCL injuries confirmed by arthroscopy or arthrotomy, Dale *et al.* evaluated the quadriceps active test to diagnose PCL disruption and measure posterior laxity of the knee.[44] The test was positive in 41 of 42 patients with documented and isolated disruption of the PCL. The test was not positive for the contralateral, normal knee in the same subjects, patients with isolated ACL injuries, or normal subjects (Tables 22.6–22.8).

Medial collateral ligament and medial capsule

The diagnosis of superficial medial collateral injury is made by performing the abduction stress test in 30° of flexion. Evidence for this comes from ligament-cutting studies in cadaver models. By performing ligament-cutting studies, Grood *et al.* identified the superficial medial collateral ligament as the primary restraint to abduction force, and the posterior oblique and cruciate ligaments as secondary stabilizers.[45] They only observed a 5-mm medial opening after the MCL was sectioned. This small amount of displacement was considered a result of the restraint provided by the secondary stabilizers, as well as the small forces involved during clinical testing. The MCL provided 57% of the medial restraint at 5° of flexion and 78% at 25°. The greater restraint at 25° was due to relaxation

Table 22.9 Stress tests

Medial collateral ligament (MCL)	Abduction stress, 30° flexion
Lateral collateral ligament (LCL)	Adduction stress, 30° flexion
Posteromedial capsule	Abduction stress, 0°, Slocum
Posterolateral complex	Adduction stress, 30°, external rotation 30° (dial), external rotation recurvatum, reverse pivot shift

of the posterior medial capsule, which is a secondary stabilizer in extension. At 5°, the deep capsular ligament provided 8% of restraint, while the posterior oblique ligament accounted for 18%. At 25°, these two ligaments each accounted for 4% of the restraint. Grood supported the idea that the cruciates were important restraints on abduction only with pathologic amounts of laxity.[45] Other investigators, however, have concluded that the ACL is a more important stabilizer to abduction.[46] They speculated that this could explain the good functional stability after MCL injury with an intact ACL.

Lateral collateral ligament and posterolateral capsule

The diagnosis of LCL injury is made by performing the adduction stress test in 25–30° of knee flexion, with restraint to eliminate rotation. According to Grood *et al.*, axial rotation with valgus and varus testing can lead to overestimation of joint opening.[45] In studies analogous to those performed on the medial side, they evaluated the contribution of the lateral ligaments using the stiffness approach. The LCL was found to provide 55% of the restraint to varus rotation at 5° of flexion, and 69% at 25°. The increase in restraint at 25° was attributed to decreased involvement of the posterolateral capsule.

Gollehou *et al.* studied the contribution of the LCL, posterolateral complex, and PCL in cadaver ligament-cutting studies.[47] The LCL was identified as the primary restraint on varus rotation in all degrees of knee flexion, with maximum displacement at 30°. However, increases in varus rotation were small. Additional sectioning of the deep ligament complex (arcuate ligament, popliteus tendon, fabellofibular ligament, and posterolateral capsule) produced an increase in varus rotation, as well as external rotation. Maximum values were obtained at 30° of flexion for both. If the LCL, posterolateral complex, and PCL are sectioned, further increases in both varus and external rotation are noted at 60–90°. Therefore, isolated injuries to the posterolateral complex will be most evident at 30°. When combined with PCL injuries, maximum displacement is observed at 60–90° (Table 22.9).

Summary

- The knee is a commonly injured body part in sports-related activity, representing 15 to 30% of all athletic injuries.
- The sports medicine doctor is frequently called upon to diagnose and treat these injuries.
- The physical exam is one basic tool these physicians use to obtain a diagnosis.
- Studies examining the accuracy of clinical examination after injury have found the correct diagnosis is made preoperatively from 56% to 83% of the time.
- By analyzing the components of the physical exam, and utilizing those proven effective by evidence-based studies, physicians will be able to improve their diagnostic capabilities.

Sample examination questions

Multiple-choice questions (answers on page 602)

1 Isolated medial joint-line opening with valgus stress at only 30° of flexion is indicative of injury to what structure?
   A LCL
   B MCL
   C ACL
   D PCL
   E Medial meniscus

2 Which condition is most likely associated with lateral placement of the tibial tubercle?
   A ACL laxity
   B Torn medial meniscus
   C Patellofemoral pain
   D Quadriceps weakness
   E Collateral ligament laxity

3 Which ligament is the primary restraint on posterior translation of the tibia?
   A ACL
   B MCL
   C LCL
   D POL
   E PCL

4 Which is the most sensitive test for meniscal injury?
   A McMurray test
   B Apley grind test
   C Lachman test
   D Posterior drawer
   E Joint line tenderness

Essay questions

1 Describe how to perform the physical examination tests for assessing ligamentous stability of the knee.

2 Compare the effectiveness of the physical examination versus MRI in diagnosing meniscal tears.

3 Describe how the position/alignment of the lower extremity can affect the patellofemoral examination.

Case study 22.1

A 20-year-old male collegiate basketball player presents with a 2-week history of knee instability, pain, and swelling. While cutting during a game, he felt a "pop" in his knee. This was followed by diffuse pain and progressive swelling. Since the injury, he has experienced several episodes of his knee "giving way," causing him to fall on one occasion. Physical examination reveals a moderate effusion with a positive Lachman and anterior drawer sign. Pivot shift and posterior drawer sign are negative. There is no joint line tenderness, and McMurray's test is negative. The knee is stable to varus and valgus stress at 0°, 30°, and 90°. This patient likely has an isolated ACL rupture. Routine radiographs should be obtained to rule out fracture. An MRI is not necessary for diagnosis. Given the patient's age and level of sports involvement, he is a good candidate for ACL reconstruction.

Case study 22.2

A 45-year-old recreational tennis player developed painful swelling of his knee following a weekend of gardening 6 weeks previously. He recalls no prior injury or recent traumatic episode to this knee. He is aware of frequent pain and clicking on the medial side of the knee. Physical examination reveals a moderate effusion, tenderness along the medial joint line, a negative Apley grind test, and pain and a clunk with McMurray's test. No instability was appreciated. Routine radiographs, including weight-bearing views, should be obtained to assess for degenerative joint disease. MRI evaluation is not necessary given the high likelihood of meniscal tear. If resolution does not occur with observation and physiotherapy, arthroscopic evaluation with partial meniscal resection is warranted.

References

1 Hughston JC, Andrews JR, Cross MJ, Mochi A. Classification of knee ligament instabilities, part I. *J Bone Joint Surg Am* 1976; **85**:159–172.
2 Fowler PJ, Lublimer JA. The predictive value of five clinical signs in the evaluation of meniscal pathology. *Arthroscopy* 1989; **5**:184–186.
3 Eren OT. The accuracy of joint line tenderness by physical examination in the diagnosis of meniscal tears. *Arthroscopy* 2003; **19**:850–854.
4 Shelbourne KD, Martini DJ, McCarroll JR, Van Meler CD. Correlation of joint line tenderness and meniscal lesions in patients with acute anterior cruciate ligament tears. *Am J Sports Med* 1995; **23**:166–169.
5 Evans PJ, Bell GD, Frank C. Prospective evaluation of the McMurray test. *Am J Sports Med* 1993; **21**:604–608.
6 Corea JR, Mousa M, Othman A. McMurray's test tested. *Knee Surg Sports Traumatol Arthrosc* 1994; **2**:70–72.
7 Akseki D, Ozcan O, Boya H, Pinar H. A New weight-bearing meniscal test and a comparison with McMurray's test and joint line tenderness. *Arthroscopy* 2004; **20**:951–958.
8 Rose NE, Gold SM. A comparison of accuracy between clinical examination and magnetic resonance imaging in the diagnosis of meniscal and anterior cruciate tears. *Arthroscopy* 1996; **12**:398–405.
9 Miller GK. A prospective study comparing the accuracy of clinical diagnosis of meniscus tears with magnetic resonance imaging and its effect on clinical outcome. *Arthroscopy* 1996; **12**:406–413.
10 Munk B, Madsen F, Lundorf E, *et al.* Clinical magnetic resonance imaging and arthroscopic findings in knees: a comparative prospective study of meniscus anterior cruciate ligament and cartilage lesions. *Arthroscopy* 1998; **14**:171–175.
11 Fischer SP, Fox JM, DelPizzo W, Friedman SJ, *et al.* Accuracy of diagnosis from magnetic resonance imaging of the knee: a multi-center analysis of one thousand and fourteen patients. *J Bone Joint Surg* 1991; **73**:2–10.
12 Muellner T, Weinstabl R, Schabus R, Vecsei V, Kainberger F. The diagnosis of meniscal tears in athletes: a comparison of clinical and magnetic resonance imaging investigations. *Am J Sports Med* 1997; **25**:7–12.
13 Woodland LH, Francis RS. Parameters and comparisons of the quadriceps angle of college-aged men and women in supine and standing positions. *Am J Sports Med* 1992; **20**:208–211.
14 Olerud C, Berg P. The variation of the Q angle with different positions of the foot. *Clin Orthop* 1984; **191**:162–165.
15 Post WR. Current concepts: clinical evaluation of patients with patellofemoral disorders. *Arthroscopy* 1999; **15**:841–851.
16 Fairbank JC, Pynsent PB, Van Poortvliet JA, Phillips H. Mechanical factors in the incidence of knee pain in adolescents and young adults. *J Bone Joint Surg Br* 1984; **66**:685–693.
17 Huberti HH, Hayes WC. Patellofemoral contact pressures. *J Bone Joint Surg Am* 1984; **66**:715–724.
18 Lee TW, Anzel SH, Bennett KA, Pang D, Kin WC. The influence of fixed rotational deformities of the femur on the patellofemoral contact pressures in human cadaver knees. *Clin Orthop* 1994; **302**:69–74.

19 Eckhoff DG, Montgomery WK, Kilcoyne RF, Stamm ER. Femoral morphometry and anterior knee pain. *Clin Orthop* 1994; **302**:64–68.
20 Muneta T, Yammamoto H, Ishibashi T, Asahina S, Furuya K. Computerized tomographic analysis of tibial tubercle position with painful female patellofemoral joint. *Am J Sports Med* 1994; **22**:67–71.
21 Jones RB, Barlett EC, Vainright JR, Carroll RG. CT determination of tibial tubercle lateralization in patients presenting with anterior knee pain. *Skeletal Radiol* 1995; **24**:505–509.
22 Fitzgerald GK, McClure PW. Reliability of measurements obtained with four tests for patellofemoral alignment. *Phys Ther* 1995; **75**:84–92.
23 Watson C, Leddy H, Dynjan T, Parham J. Reliability of the lateral pull test and tilt test to assess patellar alignment in subjects with symptomatic knees: student raters. *J Orthop Sports Phys Ther* 2001; **31**:368–374.
24 Fithian DC, Mishra DK, Balen PF, Stone ML, Daniel DM. Instrumented measurement of patellar mobility. *Am J Sports Med* 1995; **23**:607–615.
25 Reider B, Marshall JL, Warren RF. Clinical characteristics of patellar disorders in young athletes. *Am J Sports Med* 1981; **9**:270–274.
26 Desio SM, Burks RT, Bachus KN. Soft tissue restraints to lateral patellar translation in the human knee. *Am J Sports Med* 1998; **26**:59–65.
27 Conlan T, Garth WP, Lemons JE. Evaluation of the medial soft-tissue restraints of the extensor mechanism of the knee. *J Bone Joint Surg* 1993; **75**:682–693.
28 Niskanen R, Paavilainen P, Jaakkola M, Korkala O. Poor correlation of clinical signs with patellar cartilaginous changes. *Arthroscopy* 2001; **17**:307–310.
29 Johnson LL, Van Dyk GE, Green JR, *et al.* Clinical assessment of asymptomatic knees: comparison of men and women. *Arthroscopy* 1998; **14**:347–359.
30 Noyes RF, Grood ES, Butler DL, Maler M. Clinical laxity tests and functional stability: biomechanical concepts. *Clin Orthop* 1990; **146**:84–89.
31 Beynnon BD. Anatomy and biomechanics of the knee. In: Garret WE, Speer KP, Kirendall DT, eds. *Principles and Practice of Sports Medicine.* Philidelphia: Lippincott, Williams and Wilkins, 2000: 623–644.
32 Daniel, D. Diagnosis of a ligament injury. In: Daniel D, Akeson W, O'Connor J, eds. *Knee Ligaments.* New York: Raven Press, 1990: 3–10.
33 Grood ES, Noyes FR. Diagnosis of knee ligament injuries: biochemical precepts. In: Feagin J (ed): *The Crucial Ligaments*, Churchill Livingstone: New York, NY, 1988: 114–134.
34 Slocum DB, Larson RL. Rotary instability of the knee. *J Bone Joint Surg Am* 1978; **50**:211.
35 Jakob RP, Hassler H, Straeobli HU. Observations of rotary instability of the lateral compartment of the knee. *Acta Orthop Scand* 1981; **191**:1–32.
36 Butler DL, Noyes FR, Grood ES. Ligamentous restraints to anterior–posterior drawer in the human knee: a biomechanical study. *J Bone Joint Surg Am* 1980; **62**:259–270.
37 Torg JS, Conrad W, Kalen V. Clinical diagnosis of anterior cruciate ligament instability in the athlete. *Am J Sports Med* 1976; **4**:84–93.
38 Donaldson WF, Warren RF, Wickiewicz T. A comparison of acute anterior cruciate ligament examinations: initial versus examination under anesthesia. *Am J Sports Med* 1985; **13**:5–10.
39 Katz JW, Fingeroth RJ. The diagnostic accuracy of ruptures of the anterior cruciate ligament comparing the Lachman test, the anterior drawer sign, and pivot shift test in acute and chronic knee injuries. *Am J Sports Med* 1986; **14**:88–91.
40 Kim SJ, Kim HK. Reliability of the anterior drawer, the pivot shift test, and the Lachman test. *Clin Orthop* 1995; **317**:237–242.
41 Oberlander MA, Shalvoy RM, Hughston JC. The accuracy of the clinical knee examination documented by arthroscopy: a prospective study. *Am J Sports Med* 1993; **21**:773–778.
42 Grood ES, Stowers SF, Noyes FR. Limits of movement in the human knee. *J Bone Joint Surg Am* 1988; **70**:88–97.
43 Rubinstein RA, Shelbourne DK, McCarroll JR, VanMeter CD, Rettig AC. The accuracy of the clinical examination in the setting of posterior cruciate ligament injuries. *Am J Sports Med* 1994; **22**:550–557.
44 Dale DM, Stone ML, Barnett P, Sachs R. Use of the quadriceps active test to diagnose posterior cruciate-ligament disruption and measure posterior laxity of the knee. *J Bone Joint Surg Am* 1988; **70**:386–391.
45 Grood ES, Noyes FR, Butler NL, Suntay WJ. Ligamentous and capsular restraints preventing straight medial and lateral laxity in intact human cadaver knees. *J Bone Joint Surg Am* 1981; **63**:1257–1269.

46 Inoue M, McGruk-Burleson E, Hollis IM, Woo S. Treatment of medial collateral ligament injury. *Am J Sports Med* 1987; **15**:15–21.
47 Gollehou DL, Torzilli PA, Warren RF. The role of the posterolateral and cruciate ligaments in the stability of the human knee. *J Bone Joint Surg Am* 1987; **69**:233–242.
48 O'Shea KJ, Murphy KP, Heekin RD, Herzwurm PJ. The diagnostic accuracy of the history, physical examination and radiographs in evaluation of traumatic knee disorders. *Am J Sports Med* 1996; **24**:164–167.

CHAPTER 23

What is the optimal treatment of acute anterior cruciate ligament injury?

Graham Bailie and Ian Corry

Background

"I was running with no one near me. My studs caught and my knee twisted. I heard a crack and I fell to the ground with a sudden pain. My knee became very swollen, and the next day I could not fully straighten it. I went to hospital, where I was told that my X-ray was normal. They gave me crutches and a bandage."

If the patient is fortunate, this is the story of a recent injury told to a doctor or physiotherapist who can recognize the probability of an acute anterior cruciate ligament (ACL) tear. If the patient is unfortunate, this is the story of an injury several years ago. Subsequently, there may have been frequent episodes of giving way followed by locking and arthroscopic surgery. After meniscectomy with or without a diagnosis of ACL injury, the history may have been presented at a tertiary referral to a surgeon with an interest in sports medicine and knee surgery.

The latter presentation is frequent at a sports-medicine knee practice, and delay in diagnosis continues to be a problem in the UK. A recent study showed that delay in diagnosis led to an increased incidence of meniscal tears. The mean time from injury to ACL reconstruction was 23 months.[1] A previous study reported 119 consecutive "clinically obvious" ACL ruptures presenting to a specialist knee clinic with a mean delay from injury to diagnosis of 22 months. Most of the patients had been injured playing sport, and the majority had been discharged from a hospital casualty department at the time of their injury. Thirty percent of the patients had been seen by an orthopedic surgeon and 28% had undergone an arthrotomy or arthroscopy without diagnosis.[2]

In a related study from the same center in 2004 (V. Veysi and S. Bollen, unpublished observations), the correct diagnosis of ACL injury was made in only 13% of cases assessed at accident and emergency departments, 30% of family practitioner cases, and 57% of orthopedic consultant cases.

The patient presenting acutely can only be described as "fortunate" if earlier recognition of ACL injury leads to an improved outcome by earlier commencement of treatment. The optimal treatment of the isolated acute ACL injury with evidence to support current principles of treatment is the focus of this chapter. Management of the late presentation or chronic ACL injury is not considered.

The anterior cruciate ligament has a very poor capacity for intrinsic repair, and current approaches to treatment are either conservative (nonoperative) with functional adaptation or surgical reconstruction. *Conservative* management includes activity modification, rehabilitation, and functional bracing. The issues in *surgical* management include the timing of surgery, the operative technique for reconstruction, and the postoperative rehabilitation program. Specific treatment depends on many factors, including associated injuries, degree of disability, and the age and functional expectations of the patient. For the purposes of this chapter, it is assumed that the correct diagnosis has been made. There is some reference to the positive or negative role of early arthroscopy without reconstruction.

Methods

The literature on ACL injury is extensive, with many retrospective and some prospective studies published on almost all aspects of management. A literature search was performed using the MEDLINE database via the PubMed interface with the search term "anterior cruciate ligament" from 1960 to the end of March 2006, identifying 6768 publications, of which 665 were considered to be reviews. This search was narrowed by trying to answer the question: "In the isolated ACL-deficient knee, does surgical intervention lead to a better outcome than conservative management?" The term "acute" was included, and the search was limited to "human subjects," to reveal 568 papers. To further modify the literature review towards papers on clinical trials, the 568 papers were searched using the terms "randomized" or "randomised," and a similar search was carried out on the 6768 papers for the terms "randomised/randomized" and "controlled." Duplicate papers and reviews were excluded, leaving 62 randomized controlled trials (Table 23.1). These were subsequently examined to provide evidence for treatment within conservative or surgical subgroups and to extract relevant papers referring to clinical/functional outcome or management following acute injury in order to be used for this review.

Only two randomized trials that dealt directly with the issue of surgical versus nonsurgical treatment were identified.[3,4] The trials were published in 1991 and 1987, and differed considerably in trial design. No other randomized studies comparing conservative treatment with surgical treatment were identified.

An additional search of recent review articles from the last 5 years highlighted 247 articles, which were analyzed for relevant and important reviews, particularly those referring to treatment of injury. Reviews referring mainly to specific technical detail such as operative technique or graft selection were not directly included. Hence, the most comprehensive were selected as having come from large eminent institutions in order to obtain further references about the topic.[5–11]

Table 23.1 Principal area of intervention in anterior cruciate ligament injury, assessed by published randomized controlled trials (RCTs)

Subject area of RCT	n
Operative technique/graft selection	17
Rehabilitation and physiotherapy	14
Functional bracing	5
Anesthesia and analgesia	22
Timing to surgery	1
Surgical vs. nonsurgical treatment	3
Total	62

A further search of PubMed identified a number of recent important meta-analyses on the subject, principally relating to graft selection, which are summarized in Table 23.2.[12–20]

The Wiley Interscience web site was used to search the Cochrane Library Database, using the term "anterior cruciate ligament" without restrictions. The numbers of references obtained in the subsections were as listed in Table 23.3.

These papers were scanned to identify those directly relevant to this review. In particular, one important Cochrane Review on surgical versus conservative interventions for ACL injury has been published recently and was used for this review.[21] Also included was a review and recent update of rehabilitation programs after ACL injury[22,23] and one paper on the cost-effectiveness of ACL reconstruction in comparison with nonoperative care in young adults.[24]

Finally, there are several papers widely familiar to those commonly treating this injury that would be a part of any review on the subject.[25–34] The recent Best Practice Guidelines advice on ACL Reconstruction from the British Orthopaedic Association have been included.[35]

Main results

It is obvious from the literature review that, whilst there is a large amount written about the anterior cruciate ligament, there are few controlled trials of conservative management versus reconstruction, and it remains the case that there are no well-designed prospective randomized controlled trials. Such a trial would be difficult to achieve, as there is a lack of consensus on what exactly constitutes an optimal result after ACL injury, and the trial design would be complicated. A long-term trial with degenerative change as an outcome would require the conservative and surgical groups to be matched for activity level after treatment. Since the main feature of conservative management is activity modification to avoid instability, and the main feature of surgical management is an attempt to regain peak activity, the post-treatment activity regimes differ significantly and are difficult to match. Furthermore, a high dropout rate would be expected in the conservative group as more and more patients became dissatisfied with their instability. Equal matching would require those with successfully stabilized knees to behave as if they were still unstable, largely avoiding vigorous activity. Patient compliance would become an obvious problem. Whilst it is not entirely satisfactory to prejudge a potential clinical trial in this way, at present we must rely on slightly more circumstantial evidence of long-term difference in outcome.

Using activity level rather than degenerative change as the outcome measure, the study by Andersson *et al.*[3] randomized 167 subjects to one of three groups—conservative management, repair only, or repair with augmentation—and showed convincing evidence of a higher functional knee score (Lysholm) after repair with augmentation compared to the other two groups after an average 55-month follow-up. Sixty three percent returned to competitive sport against 32% in the repair-only group and 27% in the conservatively managed group. There was also a 17% subsequent transfer of patients from conservative management to operative management, confirming the problem of defaulting patients in a controlled study.[3,36] Sandberg *et al.*[4] included 157 subjects with ACL injury randomized to conservative treatment or primary repair without augmentation. They found that conservative treatment led to more rapid recovery but a similar functional outcome for both treatment groups, and less objective knee instability in the surgical group. Neither study reported radiological assessment or post-traumatic arthritis.

Table 23.2 Summary of published meta-analyses relevant to treatment of anterior cruciate ligament (ACL) injury

First author, ref.	Date	Subject	Principal findings
Prodromos[12]	Oct 2005	Hamstring versus patellar tendon graft and fixation type in ACL reconstruction	64 studies, multiple study types included. Four-strand hamstring ACL reconstruction produces higher stability rates than bone–patellar tendon–bone, and stability is fixation-dependent
Thompson[13]	Aug 2005	Patellofemoral pain and functional outcome after ACL reconstruction	No significant functional difference between use of patellar tendon and hamstring
Goldblatt[14]	Jul 2005	Patellar tendon versus 3- or 4-strand hamstring for ACL reconstruction	11 randomized or prospective studies included. No difference in instability. Trend towards less kneeling pain and less patellofemoral crepitus in hamstring group
Forster[15]	Jun 2005	Patellar tendon or 4-strand hamstring in ACL reconstruction	6 randomized controlled trials, 475 patients. No difference in knee scores, return to sport, or graft rupture. Greater chance of extension loss and trend to patellofemoral joint pain with patellar tendon graft. Hamstring weakness and trend to increased pivot with 4-strand hamstring graft
Herrington[16]	Jan 2005	Hamstring vs. bone patellar tendon bone in ACL reconstruction	13 studies included. No significant evidence to indicate one graft is superior, with both improving performance both suitable for ACL recon.
Freedman[17]	Jan 2003	Hamstring vs. patellar tendon graft in ACL reconstruction	34 studies, multiple study types included, 1976 patients, significantly lower graft failure + better static knee stability with patellar tendon, but increased rate of anterior knee pain compared to hamstring graft
Raynor[18]	Apr 2005	Cryotherapy after ACL reconstruction	7 randomized clinical trials. Significantly lower postoperative pain with cryotherapy, but no difference in range of motion or postoperative drainage
Hinterwimmer[19]	May 2003	Operative or conservative treatment of ACL rupture	11 studies (only two randomized). Results in the operative groups were generally better than conservative in all but one study
Martinek[20]	Jun 1999	The effectiveness of knee braces after ACL reconstruction	Braces have a limited function in lowering shear stress below physiological load, but no effect on postoperative outcome after ACL reconstruction

Table 23.3 Search results for "anterior cruciate ligament" in all fields of the Cochrane Database

Systematic reviews	19
Abstracts of reviews of effectiveness	12
Central Register of Controlled Trials	502
Methodology reviews	Nil
Methodology register	Nil
Health Technology Assessment Database	2
NHS Economic Evaluation Database	15

NHS, National Health Service (United Kingdom).

It is important to note that these studies were carried out during the 1980s and that both conservative and surgical approaches to ACL injury have changed significantly since then. There are no well-designed prospective studies comparing modern methods of conservative and surgical treatment.

Trial design would be further complicated by selection bias, as patients often do not present after ACL injury until they have instability. Therefore, studies reporting on those presenting with instability or, at the very least, a proven ACL injury, tend to be studies on the more severely affected individuals and not on the total population of ACL-deficient knees. Patients with less severely affected or asymptomatic ACL-deficient knees may not be included, since they have not requested treatment. Conclusions on the optimal management of a patient presenting prior to the onset of instability should recognize the limitations of the evidence. It is generally based on treatment of those who already have instability and the outcomes are in nonmatched, poorly controlled clinical trials. They usually include more than one type of surgery, different patterns of injury, and patients with a heterogeneous mixture of age and activity levels. Since the evidence will always be limited by conclusions drawn after some unproven assumptions, the best estimate of ideal treatment will always have an empirical element. The remainder of this chapter outlines the circumstantial evidence that gives us some objective grounds for advising and treating our patients.

Early management

After recognition of the likely diagnosis, early management should be similar both for surgical and conservative groups. The question of conservative or surgical management may be left to the subacute period (> 4–6 weeks from injury) after initial urgent management.

Primary *repair* is not considered a good option, since without augmentation or reconstruction, there is a high incidence of failure.[37–39] Immediate *reconstruction* is associated with a higher incidence of stiffness.[34,40,41] The exceptions are displaced bony avulsions, which may heal if replaced, and which may prevent full extension if left displaced,[42–44] and the multiple ligament injury or at worst the dislocated knee, which may do better with early repair and reconstruction.[45–49] If the ACL injury is combined with one other collateral ligament injury, an argument for early repair at least of the collateral could be made. However, the evidence is inconclusive when associated medial collateral ligament (MCL) injury is considered. Reconstruction of the ACL alone in this combination has had good results,[50,51] although additional MCL repair may be more appropriate if the MCL tear is complete and extending into the posterior capsule.[52]

Many knees with acute ACL injuries have incomplete extension—i.e., they are "locked." This may be due to the injury and a hemarthrosis, or due to a true mechanical block, which is either a displaced meniscal tear or the ACL remnant. There is evidence that resolution of incomplete extension is likely in the ACL-deficient knee.[53] Jomha found that two-thirds of acute ACL injuries had an extension loss of more than 3°, but only 5% of these had a true mechanical block found at subsequent arthroscopic ACL reconstruction (2% displaced meniscus and 3% ACL stump). In this small subgroup with persistent loss of extension after a period of 4–6 weeks, arthroscopy to remove the potential mechanical block should be offered. For the displaced meniscal tear, there is evidence that an unstable and repairable meniscal lesion combined with ACL deficiency is an indication for early combined ACL reconstruction and meniscal repair rather than meniscectomy alone.[35]

Following this initial 4–6-week period after injury, the question of conservative versus operative management may be posed.

Outcome of conservative management

The natural history of the ACL-deficient knee has been examined in isolation and in comparison with surgical treatment, although not in well-designed randomized controlled trials. Absolute data on the natural history have not been obtained, because asymptomatic "carriers" of ACL deficiency are not identified. The natural outcome is based only on those known to have ACL deficiency, who are by implication more severely affected. In practical terms, this information is still useful, since the patients we are asked to treat are those who have presented. However, as public awareness of the injury becomes more widespread, diagnosis of those affected in a more minimal way will be inevitable. We must be aware that advice about their treatment may be based on outcome studies of more severely affected patients.

Patients with ACL deficiency managed conservatively have an increased risk of subsequent meniscal tear.[25,28,31,35,53] This can only be estimated, but may be 15–20% over 8 years.[30] Daniel *et al.* found a 20% meniscal injury incidence over 5 years.[26]

It is well documented that ACL instability itself has a higher risk of degenerative change.[30,32,54–57] Cartilage thinning due to rotational changes in the knee caused by ACL deficiency has been demonstrated by Andriacchi *et al.*, suggesting that progression of osteoarthritis after ACL injury is due to abnormal load bearing of the articular surface.[58] Meniscal tear with meniscectomy causes this degenerative process to occur more quickly.[35,57] The studies by McDaniel and Dameron suggested that 20% would have significant degenerative change at a mean 9.9-year follow-up, rising to 35% at a mean 14-year follow-up.[31,59] The conclusions from these studies further emphasized that the degenerative changes seemed to be related to the meniscal injuries.

Lesions of the articular surface are also more common in the ACL-deficient knee. Murrell *et al.* reported a six-fold greater area of articular surface cartilage loss in those presenting beyond 2 years compared with those presenting within 2 months, and a further threefold increase if there had been meniscal loss.[60] There is evidence that delay in diagnosis increases the prevalence of meniscal tears.[1,35] There is also evidence that the development of articular cartilage lesions is time-dependent in the symptomatic ACL-deficient knee.[8] It must be remembered that some of these studies are biased towards symptomatic knees, and it could be argued that asymptomatic knees with a deficiency of similar duration had not presented.

The biomechanics of ACL-deficient knee movement has been evaluated by studies on dynamic magnetic resonance imaging, which has confirmed greater anterior subluxation of the lateral tibial plateau in comparison to the medial plateau. This could contribute to these degenerative changes.[9]

Conservative management with bracing

There is no evidence to show that bracing alters the risk of degenerative change in the ACL-deficient knee. However, Fleming *et al.* showed, in a small biomechanical study, that functional bracing reduces the anterior–posterior shear loading in the weight-bearing knee, which may be protective,[61] but subsequently showed that this reduction does not occur during the transition from non–weight-bearing to weight-bearing, suggesting only limited benefit.[62] Bracing does help the functional ability of the ACL-deficient patient by giving confidence, preventing hyperextension, and protecting the tibia from forward translation on the femur at low levels of load. Bracing does not appear to prevent such translation nor to protect the ACL at the loads of vigorous activity.[29,63,64] The conclusion is that bracing may be helpful in lower-demand patients, but does not appear beneficial for high levels of activity. The evidence for the role of bracing in both conservative and surgical treatment after acute ACL injury is summarized in Table 23.4.[65–69]

Table 23.4 Randomized controlled trials on the role of bracing in the knee with an injured anterior cruciate ligament

First author, ref.	Date	Subject of trial	Principal findings	Level of evidence
Harilainen[65]	Feb 2006	RCT, rehabilitation knee brace for 12 weeks vs. no brace after ACL reconstruction	60 patients with 5-y follow-up. No difference in knee scores, activity, or laxity	A4
Pforringer[66]	Sep 2005	RCT, brace in full extension vs. brace in 20° flexion after ACL reconstruction	46 patients, 12-month follow-up. Full extension group had less postoperative pain and swelling, with better clinical outcome and activity level	A4
Swirtun[67]	Sep 2005	RCT, functional bracing for 12 weeks in acute ACL-deficient knee vs. no brace	42 patients, 6-month follow-up. Positive subjective effect and less sense of instability in brace group. No difference in objective assessment using knee scores	A4
McDevitt[68]	Dec 2004	RCT, brace for sport for 1 y vs. no brace after ACL reconstruction	100 patients, 2-y follow-up. No significant difference for stability, function, knee scores, or re-injury	A3
Sitler[69]	May 1990	RCT, use of brace to reduce knee injury during 1 y of sport versus no brace	1396 patients, 1-y duration. Use of brace did not reduce frequency or severity of ACL injury, but did reduce overall incidence of knee injury	A1

ACL, anterior cruciate ligament ; RCT, randomized controlled trial.

Functional considerations

Functional ability is an important aspect in decision-making when considering the ACL-deficient knee, and this has been estimated in terms of quality-adjusted life-years to establish a cost-effective approach to management.[24] The difference in quality-adjusted life-years (QALY) between surgical reconstruction and nonoperative management has been estimated and recognized in the Cochrane database.[24] This study was based on functional outcomes and did not take into account degenerative change in the longer term. The authors concluded that the operative strategy (using patellar tendon graft) provided 5.1 quality-adjusted life-years versus 3.49 years for nonoperative treatment in adults under 30 years old. From its low expense per QALY, it could be inferred that ACL reconstruction is a cost-effective method of treatment for acute tears in young adults. The strength of this evidence is improved considering that the article excluded studies that had patients who awaited the onset of symptoms before recruitment. Also, the treatment of the ACL was exclusively acute rather than chronic. Interpretation of the evidence is helped by using a 5-point grading system, in which comparisons can be made with other interventions and technologies. Grade A technologies are the most favorable, most effective, and least expensive, and grade E is the least favorable. ACL reconstruction in this age group would rank as a grade B—i.e., "strong evidence for adoption and appropriate utilization."[70]

Gottlob *et al.*[24] also analyzed expected functional outcome in ACL tears for nonoperative management compared to reconstruction. Activity level was graded from 0 to 5. The outcome probabilities in each of these grades for mean activity levels from five separate trials of nonoperative treatment[55,71–74] and six trials of operative treatment[75–80] are summarized in Table 23.5.[24] The table demonstrates how the expected functional outcome for individual patients can assist in decision-making when determining the most appropriate management of acute ACL tears in young adults. Only 18% of ACL injuries treated conservatively could expect a functional outcome that would allow participation in very stressful sports, compared to 66.5% for those treated operatively. Other more general studies have also noted the decrease in activity level with ACL deficiency,[25,27,32] although inevitably slightly overestimated by failure to count asymptomatic cases.

Occupational disability was the subject of a large population-based study by Dunn *et al.*[81] Of the 2192 ACL injuries included in the study, 9.5% resulted in a permanent disability discharge from the military. The principal factors relating to disability discharge were psychosocial. The type of treatment was not a factor associated with occupational

Table 23.5 Expected functional outcome after anterior cruciate ligament tear for nonoperative treatment in comparison with reconstruction[24]

Class	Expected functional outcome	Nonoperative treatment (% of patients)	ACL reconstruction (% of patients)
0	Death	0	0
1	Symptomatic with ADLs	15.0	3.3
2	Tolerates ADLs only	21.8	1.4
3	Play mildly stressful sports	21.3	11.8
4	Play moderately stressful sports	23.8	17.0
5	Play very stressful sports	18.1	66.5

ACL, anterior cruciate ligament; ADL, activity of daily living.

disability, 43% of patients having had conservative management, and 57% having ACL reconstruction. This study provides evidence of the importance of taking psychosocial factors into consideration in the management of the ACL-deficient knee.

The benefits of conservative management are avoiding surgery and its potential complications or poor results. It will always be an individual matter of judgment if the associated risks of conservative management are preferred to those of surgical management. Minimizing the risks of further injury by lifestyle modification and functional adaptation is thought to be a reasonable option for some patients but without published evidence.

Outcome of surgical management

Given the natural history of the ACL-deficient knee outlined above, for surgery to be worthwhile, the results of operative intervention should offer a better alternative, either in terms of long-term degenerative change or in terms of lifestyle. If only the benefit to lifestyle is proven, then there should be little or no significant adverse long-term effect of reconstruction in comparison with nonoperative management.

Does ACL reconstruction cause osteoarthritis?

There is ongoing debate in the literature about the influence of ACL reconstruction on the development of osteoarthritis (OA) in the knee. One major study has shown an increase in late degenerative change after ACL reconstruction.[26] However, this probably indicates that conservative management is protective to the knee, by inhibiting activity in patients who "cope" with an ACL-deficient knee. This reduced level of activity, as a means of reducing late degenerative change, is not always acceptable to the young and active individual. Subsequent reports of prospective studies examining the incidence of OA have shown either no difference or only marginal differences between reconstructed and conservatively treated knees.[82–84] Interpretation of this published literature is difficult as most studies include some degree of bias.

The exact incidence of degenerative change is also uncertain. A randomized controlled trial comparing three different surgical techniques of ACL reconstruction with a minimum 6-year follow-up of 225 patients showed only 11.6% with radiological evidence of degenerative change, not influenced by the surgical technique.[85] A 50% incidence of radiological evidence of early degenerative change at 5–9 years has been reported following ACL reconstruction.[86] This is confirmed by a small case series with 13 years' follow-up, in which the radiological incidence of degenerative change was 79% (associated with meniscectomy), but with minimal clinical consequences, as 96% of the patients reported normal or near normal function.[87]

Is ACL reconstruction protective to menisci?

There is still no direct evidence that ACL reconstruction can reduce the incidence or progression of degenerative change, but several studies have shown that stabilization seems to reduce the incidence of meniscal pathology.[1,3,26,35] It is reasonable to conclude that this will have a protective effect on the knee for the future.

About 30% of acute ACL injuries coming to reconstruction are isolated.[88] Few studies have separated those with isolated ACL injury from those with associated injury, especially meniscal. Those that have done so seem to have shown a protective effect of reconstruction on the menisci if the menisci were intact at the time of ACL surgery.[89,90] The medium-term outcome, in terms of reduced degenerative change at 7 years in these patients, is very supportive of this treatment.[91] An intact meniscus at surgery could therefore be seen as a good prognostic indicator, given that 17 of 20 subjects in the Jomha *et al.* series with intact menisci had normal radiographs at the 7-year follow-up, whilst none of the 16 subjects who had meniscectomy had normal radiographs after 7 years.[89] There was also an interesting trend that showed early reconstruction after acute injury was more protective of menisci compared to reconstruction in a chronic ACL-deficient knee. This concept of protecting the meniscus needs further evaluation by clinical trial. In a five to fifteen year outcome study by Shelbourne and Gray (mean 8.6 years), the International Knee Documentation Committee (IKDC) rating was normal or nearly normal in 87% of those with intact menisci, 70% with lateral meniscectomy, 63% with medial meniscectomy, and 60% with both menisci removed.[90] In a further study with a 13-year follow-up after reconstruction using patellar tendon, radiological evidence of degenerative change was strongly associated with meniscectomy.[87] This indirect evidence gives additional support for early ACL reconstruction, especially if the menisci are intact.

Should meniscal tears be repaired in the ACL-deficient knee?

In the ACL-deficient knee, associated meniscal tears may be suitable for repair at the time of an initial arthroscopy or ACL reconstruction, but the long-term survival of meniscal repair with ACL reconstruction is unknown. Where repair is undertaken, it is generally accepted that any meniscal repair in the ACL-deficient knee should be protected by subsequent ACL reconstruction to reduce the rate of re-tear.[92] Success of isolated meniscal repair is approximately 76% at 10 years in knees with intact ligaments,[93] although the overall success rate of meniscal repair with ACL reconstruction may be slightly less in the longer term.[94] This has been reported as high as 89% at three-year follow-up;[95] however, Shelbourne and Carr[96] and Shelbourne and Dersam[97] have reported that meniscal repair with ACL reconstruction does no better than partial meniscectomy for subjective knee and IKDC scores at 6–8 years' follow-up. Definitive conclusions and recommendations on the role of meniscal repair cannot be made on the basis of current evidence, as longer-term follow-up is required, but meniscal preservation should be considered where possible.[98]

If there is nonrepairable meniscal or articular damage, it would seem that degenerative change is almost inevitable, and evidence showing a reduction in this following ACL reconstruction is unlikely to emerge. Surgery for these patients must be justified only by evidence of an improvement in lifestyle or function. There are plenty of outcome studies showing such improvement, but none with an adequate control group. The patients entering these outcome studies are usually heavily preselected by their need or demand for surgery. This means that they tend to be towards the more severely affected end of the spectrum. However, to use the example of the study by Shelbourne and Gray,[90] even in the severely affected group with both menisci removed or partly removed, there was still an IKDC rating of 60% normal or nearly normal after a medium-term to long-term follow-up of reconstructed knees.

When should ACL reconstruction be recommended?

From the current evidence available, ACL reconstruction is indicated for symptomatic instability to restore more physiological knee function, help preserve the menisci, and reduce the potential for cartilage thinning. Meniscal repair should be considered if a tear is present. As the incidence of meniscal injury increases with time from ACL injury with symptomatic instability, surgical reconstruction should be undertaken early rather than late. Furthermore, even with menisci that remain intact, instability is associated with articular cartilage lesions, thinning of articular cartilage, and subsequent degenerative change. Earlier reconstruction may also reduce this.

Combined injuries

Where the ACL tear is part of a combined meniscal or ligamentous injury, reconstruction is indicated for those who cannot function at an adequate level, due to episodes of instability. These patients may require early arthroscopy to assess and treat the accompanying pathology (e.g., displaced meniscal tear), and may have reconstruction at the same time to avoid a second operation. However, this decision is based on the surgeon's judgment and patient's preference, rather than objective evidence. There is good evidence that the majority of these patients will maintain an improvement at least in the medium term.

Technique of reconstruction

Many techniques for ACL reconstruction have been proposed and tested, including prosthetic ligament, allograft, autograft, graft with prosthetic augmentation, and extra-articular reconstruction. Outcome studies following ACL reconstruction have included simple assessment of a particular technique and comparison of one surgical technique with another or others. Autografts of patellar tendon (PT) or hamstring tendon (HT) are now preferred by most surgeons, and extra-articular reconstruction is rarely used.[29] Furthermore, studies have shown no difference in the results when an extra-articular augmentation was added to an intra-articular PT reconstruction.[99,100] Prosthetic ligaments have been associated with an unacceptably high failure rate (40–78% over 15 years).[101]

Open versus arthroscopic techniques of graft substitution have been compared without significant differences in outcome, although the arthroscopic hamstring technique was not assessed.[102–104]

The optimal method of graft fixation has been investigated extensively. Suspensory methods (i.e., fixation outside the tunnel) and aperture methods (i.e., with an interference screw close to the origin and insertion) have been described. Biomechanically, there is increased stiffness in the construct for grafts held anatomically by direct graft tissue aperture fixation rather than using a suspensory method,[105–108] and the importance of a high-stiffness construct for postoperative stability has been emphasized.[109] Aperture fixation is now considered important in ACL reconstruction, in view of the biological and cellular integration of the graft to the bone tunnel required for long-term stability using this technique.[110] Pinczewski *et al.* examined the histology at the bone–tendon junction of two specimens retrieved from patients undergoing revision surgery at 12 and 15 weeks following reconstruction for traumatic mid-substance hamstring graft rupture at 6 and 10 weeks.[111] Integration of the hamstring tendon ACL autograft was demonstrated by observation of collagen fiber continuity between bone and tendon. The histology plus the low overall incidence of early graft failure together imply that the strength of the bone–tendon junction, supported by the interference screw, is adequate for rehabilitation forces below the threshold for provocation of mid-substance rupture. For biomechanical testing in the dog, Rodeo *et al.*[112] used a snug-fit tendon in a tibial tunnel secured with stainless-steel sutures, allowing postoperative exercise *ad libitum*. They noted failure by tendon "pull-out" from the tunnel at up to 8 weeks after surgery. By 12 weeks, all "pull-out" tests resulted in graft slippage from the clamp or graft rupture, implying that the tunnel–graft interface was no longer the weakest link. Song *et al.* reported that failure of osteointegration of tendon graft to bone caused early clinical failure.[113] More recently, there is a trend towards investigating the role of growth factors and their potential for a positive influence on healing and structural properties of grafts.[9,110]

Hamstring or patellar tendon for ACL reconstruction?

There are many reports in the literature of comparisons between groups having patellar tendon or hamstring tendon grafts,[76,79,114–117] and the optimum choice remains controversial.[9] Earlier reports[76,116,117] showed some differences in outcome between the two groups, but the studies contained confounding variables other than graft choice. Marder *et al.*[79] compared patellar tendon versus hamstring in well-matched groups and with little difference in outcome. Corry *et al.*[118] had groups matched for all features except graft type (PT or HT) and also showed little outcome difference, although the subjects were sequential rather than randomized. Several randomized controlled trials have been published recently comparing bone–patellar tendon–bone with two- or four-strand hamstring grafts, with equivalent results for functional outcome with each technique.[119–124] However, increased kneeling pain is often seen in the patellar tendon groups, and slightly increased laxity on objective measurement has been seen in the hamstring groups. A number of meta-analyses have now been published on graft choice (see Table 23.2),[12–17] and the overall conclusion from this literature is that both hamstring and patellar tendon provide excellent clinical results in ACL reconstruction. The choice of graft is therefore down to the preferences of the individual patient and surgeon.

Graft placement is as important as graft selection. The ideal bony tunnel position has been worked out by collective clinical experience rather than by trial, with anterior placement of tibial or femoral tunnels the commonest error. This can lead to impingement of the graft in the femoral notch in extension or overconstraint of knee motion. The review by Fu *et al.* gives a good summary.[6] Techniques of ACL reconstruction are being further enhanced and refined using computer-assisted surgery and computer navigation to optimize tunnel and graft positioning. Navigated ACL reconstruction may reduce the rate of revision surgery, and early results in the literature are encouraging.[125–127]

What is the best rehabilitation after ACL reconstruction?

Accelerated rehabilitation is now well established after ACL reconstruction. This approach has been shown to have results as good as older methods of more cautious postoperative care[33] and has been confirmed in a randomized controlled trial.[128] Regaining muscle control is an essential part of recovery from ACL injury, and there are various strategies for assisting with return to pre-injury levels of activity. However, there is insufficient evidence to support one exercise intervention over another.[22,23] Relevant published trials and the evidence for rehabilitation in ACL injury are summarized in Table 23.6.[18,23,128–135]

Conclusions

The evidence for treatment of acute ACL injury supports an immediate first-aid period of 4–6 weeks to allow the hemarthrosis to settle and allow restoration of the range of movement. After this, successful reconstruction in the patient with an isolated ACL injury and symptomatic instability reduces the rate of subsequent meniscectomy and may reduce medium-term degenerative change.

Table 23.6 Summary of recently published evidence relevant to rehabilitation after anterior cruciate ligament injury

First author, ref.	Date	Subject of study	Principal findings	Level of Evidence
Grant[129]	Sep 2005	Home vs. physical therapy-supervised rehabilitation programs after ACL reconstruction	RCT, 145 patients. Minimally supervised rehabilitation was more effective in achieving acceptable knee ROM in 3 months than standard program	A3
Cooper[130]	Jul 2005	Comparison of 6-week proprioceptive and balance exercise program with 6-week strengthening program after ACL reconstruction	RCT, 29 patients. No significant difference on hop testing. The strengthening group had better function scores in the early phase	A4
Cooper[131]	Apr 2005	Systematic review of proprioceptive and balance exercise on ACL-deficient knees or reconstructed. Short-term outcomes assessed	5 studies included. Some evidence that proprioceptive + balance exercises improve outcome in ACL-deficient knees. No real benefit compared to standard rehabilitation for reconstructed knees	A1
Perry[132]	Jul 2005	Closed vs. open chain knee extensor resistance training at 8–12 weeks after ACL reconstruction	RCT, 49 patients. No significant difference in knee laxity or leg function between the groups. Open chain is safe	A4
Perry[133]	Nov 2005	Closed vs. open chain knee extensor resistance training over 6 weeks in ACL-deficient knees	RCT, 64 patients. No significant differences between groups for knee laxity or leg function	A4
Shaw[134]	2005	Effects of early quads exercises (first 2 weeks postoperatively) on outcomes after ACL reconstruction	RCT, 91 patients, 6-month follow-up. Better knee scores + faster recovery of ROM and stability with quads exercises, but did not reach statistical significance	A4
Beynnon[128]	Mar 2005	Rehabilitation with accelerated or nonaccelerated program after ACL reconstruction	RCT, 25 patients, 24-month follow-up. No difference for knee laxity, patient satisfaction or functional performance	A4
Zatterstrom[135]	Jun 2000	Efficacy of 2 programs of rehabilitation in ACL-deficient knees. Self-monitored training compared to supervised training program	RCT, 100 patients, 12-month follow-up. 50% of patients in self-monitored group required supervision by 6 weeks. Supervised group did better at 3 + 12 months	A3

Continued

Table 23.6 (*Continued*)

First author, ref.	Date	Subject of study	Principal findings	Level of Evidence
Raynor[18]	Apr 2005	Effectiveness of cryotherapy after ACL reconstruction	Meta-analysis of 7 RCTs. Cryotherapy has significant benefit in postoperative pain control; no difference in ROM or drainage	A1
Trees[23]	Oct 2005	Cochrane review of effectiveness of exercise used in rehabilitation after isolated ACL injury in adults	9 RCTs included 391 patients. Insufficient evidence to support one exercise intervention over another	A1

ACL, anterior cruciate ligament; ROM, range of movement.

If there is meniscal or articular surface damage, stability and therefore function can be improved. Degenerative change in the medium term is no greater, but long-term degenerative change may be more than with conservative management, which involves reduction in activity levels.

If conservative management is selected, patients must be counseled against high-risk activities to prevent recurrent injury. Whilst there is no evidence that functional bracing changes the long-term outcome, it may allow an increased exercise level in lower-demand patients.

Based on the available evidence, the current practice is to advise activity modification to avoid giving way episodes, or to have an ACL reconstruction. The reconstruction should be performed using a biologically compatible graft, anatomically placed, with near-aperture fixation and accelerated postoperative rehabilitation. If conservative management is selected, a brace may be used for low-demand exercise but is not suitable for high-demand activity.

Summary

- There is good biochemical, clinical and histological evidence to support ACL reconstruction.
- A biologically compatible graft should be used, either 4 strand hamstring or patellar tendon.
- The graft should be anatomically placed and held by near anatomical fixation.
- Accelerated rehabilitation is likely to achieve best results from current techniques available.
- After isolated ACL reconstruction approximately 90% of patients can return to their previous level of activity.

Key messages

- Modify activity to suit the knee, or modify the knee to suit activity.
- In the isolated ACL injury, reconstruction helps protect the menisci.

• In the presence of associated meniscal or articular damage, the functional outcome should be improved following reconstruction but the chance of long term degenerative change may be greater.
• Reconstruct using a biological graft, anatomically placed, with near-aperture fixation and accelerated rehabilitation.
• In the multiple-ligament injury, repair and reconstruct early.

Clinical implications

• The isolated ACL injury in an active person who wishes to continue with potentially unstable exercise should be reconstructed early.
• The ACL injury combined with other knee ligamentous injury, meniscal injury, or chondral damage should be treated empirically, taking multiple factors into consideration. These include the age and the exercise demands of the patient, the pattern of injury, and the surgical skills available.
• A decision to manage conservatively should be reviewed when the patient has reached the peak level of activity. The decision can be changed to perform reconstruction if instability becomes evident at that time.

Sample examination questions

Multiple-choice questions (answers on page 602)

1 In the isolated acute ACL injury:
  A The history may be a simple weight-bearing twist
  B Subsequent meniscal tear is common
  C A mid-substance ACL tear is likely to heal if repaired
  D Incomplete extension should be treated by urgent arthroscopy
  E Stiffness is less if the reconstruction is performed as soon as possible
2 In ACL reconstruction:
  A The knee must be immobilized postoperatively
  B Arthroscopic reconstruction has better long-term results than open
  C An additional extra-articular procedure significantly improves the result
  D Patellar tendon and hamstring tendon grafts give similar outcomes
  E Subsequent meniscal tear is unusual
3 In conservative management of ACL injuries:
  A Return to vigorous side-stepping sport is not possible
  B Future degenerative change is likely only if there is a meniscal tear
  C Incomplete extension will usually resolve
  D Bracing prevents tibial translation in vigorous activity
  E 50% of patients will have instability in activities of daily living

Essay questions

1 What are the risks in the natural history of the ACL-deficient knee?
2 Outline the potential benefits of ACL reconstruction.
3 Discuss the different types of ACL reconstruction and comment on their relative merits.

Case study 23.1

A 23-year-old competitive downhill female skier returned from skiing after a significant knee injury. Whilst skiing, one of her skis had caught on a turn, forcibly twisting her knee and causing her to fall. She felt immediate pain in her knee and could not continue skiing. On her return home, she sought advice from her doctor, who referred her for physiotherapy, and advised her to return if the knee failed to improve. After 4 weeks of physiotherapy, her pain and swelling settled, and a reasonable range of movement was regained. However, she felt her knee was weak and would not support her, and it had given way on one occasion when she was walking over uneven ground.

The physiotherapist recommended returning to the doctor, who referred the patient for an orthopedic opinion. The orthopedic surgeon made a clinical diagnosis of anterior cruciate ligament rupture, confirmed with a magnetic resonance imaging (MRI) scan, and the surgeon recommended early anterior cruciate ligament reconstruction using hamstring graft. After surgery and a supervised rehabilitation program, the patient made a successful recovery and returned to skiing within 10 months.

Case study 23.2

A 35-year-old office worker injured his left knee when he jumped off a wall and landed awkwardly, twisting the knee on landing. Initial pain and swelling failed to settle, so he attended his doctor. The doctor was suspicious of a torn meniscus, and the patient was referred for orthopedic opinion and MRI scan. The scan identified intact menisci, but a rupture of the anterior cruciate ligament. The surgeon recommended a period of physiotherapy and rehabilitation before making a decision on reconstruction.

Within 4 months, the patient had successfully returned to his pre-injury level of activity, which included occasional golf; he did not have any symptoms of instability or giving way, and he wished to continue with a conservative approach to his knee.

Case study 23.3

A 42-year-old police officer injured his left knee during a recreational football game. He was tackled from the side, another player fell onto him, and he felt something give way in his knee as he fell. He couldn't take weight on the leg, he was unable to continue playing, and his leg "felt wobbly."

He was initially told he had a medial collateral ligament tear, given advice about range of movement exercises, and treated in a Zimmer splint. Six weeks later, he complained to his doctor that he had been unable to return to work, as his leg did not feel right and felt unstable, particularly when he tried to turn quickly. The doctor suspected an anterior cruciate ligament injury, and after assessment by an orthopedic surgeon, the diagnosis of ACL-deficient right knee was confirmed and surgery was recommended. He underwent ACL reconstruction using patellar tendon graft, with an accelerated rehabilitation program, and was fit to return to full duties as a police officer within 9 months.

Summarizing the evidence

Comparison/treatment strategies	Results	Level of evidence*
Conservative versus operative management	2 moderate sized RCTs 1 Cochrane Database systematic review Insufficient evidence from randomized trials to determine whether surgery or conservative management was best for ACL injury in the 1980s	A3

Summarizing the evidence *(Continued)*

Comparison/treatment strategies	Results	Level of evidence*
Conservative versus operative management (outcome: activity level)	One moderate-sized unequally randomized study and one systematic review showing increased activity level following repair plus augmentation	A3
Conservative versus operative management (outcome: meniscal tear)	Two cohort studies showing low meniscectomy rate following reconstruction. Several natural history studies showing high meniscectomy rate following conservative management	B
Bracing versus no bracing (ACL-deficient)	2 small RCTs. Results in favor of bracing for positive subjective effect, no difference in objective assessment	A4
Acute versus delayed reconstruction	1 small RCT in favor of reconstruction at 8–12 weeks rather than within first 2 weeks (outcome measure: scores, ROM) Other nonrandomized cohorts in favor of early surgery rather than acute reconstruction (outcome measure: stiffness)	A3 B
Repair versus reconstruction	One moderate-sized RCT and other nonrandomized cohorts, pooled results in favor of reconstruction (outcome measure: measured laxity and return to sports)	A3
Four-strand hamstring or patellar tendon for ACL reconstruction	6 RCTs, one large and several moderate-sized 6 meta-analyses. In favor of either patellar tendon or 4-strand hamstring, as excellent clinical outcomes with both. Trend towards kneeling pain with patellar tendon, and hamstring weakness with hamstring grafts	A1 A1
Bracing versus no bracing (ACL reconstruction)	3 RCTs, one of moderate size 1 meta-analysis. Pooled results in favor of no brace after ACL reconstruction	A3 A1

* A1: evidence from large randomized controlled trials (RCTs) or systematic review (including meta-analysis).†
A2: evidence from at least one high-quality cohort.
A3: evidence from at least one moderate-size RCT or systematic review.†
A4: evidence from at least one RCT.
B: evidence from at least one high-quality study of nonrandomized cohorts.
C: expert opinions.
† Arbitrarily, the following cut-off points have been used; large study size: ≥ 100 patients per intervention group; moderate study size ≥ 50 patients per intervention group.

References

1 De Roeck NJ, Lang-Stevenson A. Meniscal tears sustained awaiting anterior cruciate ligament reconstruction. *Injury* 2003; **34**:343–345.

2 Bollen SR, Scott BW. Anterior cruciate ligament rupture: a quiet epidemic? *Injury* 1996; **27**:407–409.

3 Andersson C, Odensten M, Gillquist J. Knee function after surgical or nonsurgical treatment of acute rupture of the anterior cruciate ligament: a randomized study with a long-term follow-up period. *Clin Orthop* 1991; **264**:255–263.

4 Sandberg R, Balkfors B, Nilsson B, Westlin N. Operative versus non-operative treatment of recent injuries to the ligaments of the knee: a prospective randomized study. *J Bone Joint Surg Am* 1987; **69**:1120–1126.

5 Gotlin RS, Huie G. Anterior cruciate ligament injuries: operative and rehabilitative options. *Phys Med Rehab Clin* 2000; **11**:895–928.

6 Fu FH, Bennett CH, Lattermann C, Ma CB. Current trends in anterior cruciate ligament reconstruction, part 1: biology and biomechanics of reconstruction. *Am J Sports Med* 1999; **27**:821–830.

7 Fu FH, Bennett CH, Ma CB, Menetrey J, Lattermann C. Current trends in anterior cruciate ligament reconstruction, part 2: operative procedures and clinical correlations. *Am J Sports Med* 2000; **28**:124–130.

8 Maffulli N, Binfield PM, King JB. Articular cartilage lesions in the symptomatic anterior cruciate ligament-deficient knee. *Arthroscopy* 2003; **19**: 685–690.

9 Montgomery SC, Miller MD. What's new in sports medicine. *J Bone Joint Surg Am* 2005; **87**:686–694.

10 Beynnon BD, Johnson RJ, Abate JA, Fleming BC, Nichols CE. Treatment of anterior cruciate ligament injuries, part I. *Am J Sports Med.* 2005; **33**:1579–1602.

11 Beynnon BD, Johnson RJ, Abate JA, Fleming BC, Nichols CE. Treatment of anterior cruciate ligament injuries, part 2. *Am J Sports Med.* 2005; **33**:1751–1767.

12 Prodromos CC, Joyce BT, Shi K, Keller BL. A meta-analysis of stability after cruciate ligament reconstruction as a function of hamstring versus patellar tendon graft and fixation type. *Arthroscopy* 2005; **21**:1202.

13 Thompson J, Harris M, Grana WA. Patellofemoral pain and functional outcome after anterior cruciate ligament reconstruction: an analysis of the literature. *Am J Orthop* 2005; **34**:396–399.

14 Goldblatt JP, Fitzsimmons SE, Balk E, Richmond JC. Reconstruction of the anterior cruciate ligament: meta-analysis of patellar tendon versus hamstring tendon autograft. *Arthroscopy* 2005; **21**:791–803.

15 Forster MC, Forster IW. Patellar tendon or four-strand hamstring? A systematic review of autografts for anterior cruciate ligament reconstruction. *Knee* 2005; **12**:225–230.

16 Herrington L, Wrapson C, Matthews M, Matthews H. Anterior cruciate ligament reconstruction, hamstring versus bone–patella tendon–bone grafts: a systematic literature review of outcome from surgery. *Knee* 2005; **12**:41–50.

17 Freedman KB, D'Amato MJ, Nedeff DD, Kaz A, Bach BR Jr. Arthroscopic anterior cruciate ligament reconstruction: a metaanalysis comparing patellar tendon and hamstring tendon autografts. *Am J Sports Med* 2003; **31**:2–11.

18 Raynor MC, Pietrobon R, Guller U, Higgins LD. Cryotherapy after ACL reconstruction: a meta-analysis. *J Knee Surg* 2005; **18**:123–129.

19 Hinterwimmer S, Engelschalk M, Sauerland S, Eitel F, Mutschler W. [Operative or conservative treatment of anterior cruciate ligament rupture: a systematic review of the literature; in German.] *Unfallchirurg* 2003; **106**:374–379.

20 Martinek V, Friederich NF. [To brace or not to brace? How effective are knee braces in rehabilitation? In German.] *Orthopäde* 1999; **28**:565–570.

21 Linko E, Harilainen A, Malmivaara A, Seitsalo S. Surgical versus conservative interventions for anterior cruciate ligament ruptures in adults. *Cochrane Database Syst Rev* 2005; (**2**):CD001356.

22 Thomson LC, Handoll HH, Cunningham A, Shaw PC. Physiotherapist-led programmes and interventions for rehabilitation of anterior cruciate ligament, medial collateral ligament and meniscal injuries of the knee in adults. *Cochrane Database Syst Rev* 2002; (**2**):CD001354.

23 Trees AH, Howe TE, Dixon J, White L. Exercise for treating isolated anterior cruciate ligament injuries in adults. *Cochrane Database Syst Rev* 2005; (**4**):CD005316.

24 Gottlob CA, Baker CL Jr, Pellissier JM, Colvin L. Cost effectiveness of anterior cruciate ligament reconstruction in young adults. *Clin Orthop* 1999; **367**:272–282.

25 Arnold JA, Coker TP, Heaton LM, *et al.* Natural history of anterior cruciate tears. *Am J Sports Med* 1979; 7:305–313.

26 Daniel DM, Stone ML, Dobson BE, *et al.* Fate of the ACL-injured patient: a prospective outcome study. *Am J Sports Med* 1994; **22**:632–644.

27 Feagin JA, Curl WW. Isolated tear of the anterior cruciate ligament: 5 year follow up study. *Am J Sports Med* 1976; **4**:95–100.

28 Finsterbush A, Frankl U, Matan Y, *et al.* Secondary damage to the knee after isolated injury of the anterior cruciate ligament. *Am J Sports Med* 1990; **18**:475–479.

29 Johnson RJ, Beynnon BD, Nichols CE, *et al.* Current concepts review. The treatment of injuries of the anterior cruciate ligament. *J Bone Joint Surg Am* 1992; **74**:140–151.

30 Kannus P, Jarvinen M. Conservatively treated tears of the anterior cruciate ligament. Long term results. *J Bone Joint Surg Am* 1987; **69**:1007–1012.

31 McDaniel WJ, Dameron TB. Untreated ruptures of the anterior cruciate ligament: a follow-up study. *J Bone Joint Surg Am* 1980; **62**:696–705.

32 Noyes FR, Mooar PA, Matthews DS, *et al.* The symptomatic anterior cruciate-deficient knee. Part I: the long term disability in athletically active individuals. *J Bone Joint Surg Am* 1983; **65**:154–162.

33 Shelbourne KD, Nitz P. Accelerated rehabilitation after anterior cruciate ligament reconstruction. *Am J Sports Med* 1990; **18**:292–299.

34 Shelbourne KD, Wilckens JH, Mollabashy A, DeCarlo M. Arthrofibrosis in acute anterior cruciate ligament reconstruction: the effect of timing of reconstruction and rehabilitation *Am J Sports Med* 1991; **19**:332–336.

35 British Orthopaedic Association. *Best Practice for Primary Isolated Anterior Cruciate Ligament Reconstruction.* London: British Orthopaedic Association, July 2001. Available online at: http://www.boa.ac.uk/PDF%20files/BASK/ACL%20best%20practice.pdf (accessed June 2005).

36 Odensten M, Hamberg P, Nordin M, Lysholm J, Gillquist J. Surgical or conservative treatment of the acutely torn anterior cruciate ligament: a randomized study with short-term follow-up observations. *Clin Orthop* 1985; **198**:87–93.

37 Engebretsen L, Renum P, Sundalsvoll S. Primary suture of the anterior cruciate ligament: a 6-year follow-up of 74 cases. *Acta Orthop Scand* 1989; **60**:561–564.

38 Grontvedt T, Engebretsen L, Benum P, *et al.* A prospective, randomized study of three operations for acute rupture of the anterior cruciate ligament. *J Bone Joint Surg Am* 1996; **78**:159–168.

39 Sgaglione NA, Warren RF, Wickiewicz TL, *et al.* Primary repair with semitendinosus tendon augmentation of acute anterior cruciate ligament injuries. *Am J Sports Med* 1990; **18**:64–73.

40 Waselewski SA, Covall DJ, Cohen S. Effect of surgical timing on recovery and associated injuries after anterior cruciate ligament reconstruction. *Am J Sports Med* 1993; **21**:338–347.

41 Harner CD, Irrgang JJ, Paul J, *et al.* Loss of motion after ACL reconstruction. *Am J Sports Med* 1992; **20**:499–505.

42 Edwards PH Jr, Grana WA. Physeal fractures about the knee. *J Am Acad Orthop Surg* 1995; **3**:63–69.

43 Lo IK, Bell DM, Fowler PJ. Anterior cruciate ligament injuries in the skeletally immature patient. *Instr Course Lect* 1998; **47**:351–359.

44 Micheli LJ, Foster TE, Acute knee injuries in the immature athlete. *Instr Course Lect* 1993; **42**:473–481.

45 Ibrahim SA. Primary repair of the cruciate and collateral ligaments after traumatic dislocation of the knee. *J Bone Joint Surg Br* 1999; **81**:987–990.

46 Frassica FJ, Sim FH, Staeheli JW, Pairolero PC. Dislocation of the knee. *Clin Orthop* 1991; **263**:200–205.

47 Sisto DJ, Warren RF. Complete knee dislocation: a follow-up study of operative treatment. *Clin Orthop* 1985; **198**:94–101.

48 Klimkiewicz JJ, Petrie RS, Harner CD. Surgical treatment of combined injury to anterior cruciate ligament, posterior cruciate ligament, and medial structures. *Clin Sports Med* 2000; **19**:479–492.

49 Fanelli GC. Treatment of combined anterior cruciate ligament–posterior cruciate ligament–lateral side injuries of the knee. *Clin Sports Med* 2000; **19**:493–502.

50 Ballmer PM, Ballmer PT, Jakob RP. Reconstruction of the ACL alone in the treatment of a combined instability with complete rupture of the MCL: a prospective study. *Arch Orthop Trauma Surg* 1991; **110**:139–141.

51 Indelicato PA. Injury to the medial capsuloligamentous complex. In: Feagin JA, ed. *The Crucial Ligaments: Diagnosis and Treatment of Ligamentous Injuries about the Knee.* New York: Churchill Livingstone, 1988: 197–206.
52 Shapiro MS, Markolf KL, Finerman GA, Mitchell PW. The effect of section of the medial collateral ligament on force generated in the anterior cruciate ligament. *J Bone Joint Surg Am* 1991; **73**:248–256.
53 Jomha NM, Clingeleffer A, Pinczewski L. Intra-articular mechanical blocks and full extension in patients undergoing anterior cruciate ligament reconstruction. *Arthroscopy* 2000; **16**:156–159.
54 Fetto JF, Marshall JL. The natural history and diagnosis of anterior cruciate ligament insufficiency. *Clin Orthop* 1980; **147**:29–38.
55 Hawkins RJ, Misamore GW, Merritt TR. Follow-up of the acute nonoperated isolated anterior cruciate ligament tear. *Am J Sports Med* 1986; **14**:205–210.
56 Jacobsen K. Osteoarthritis following insufficiency of the cruciate ligaments in man. *Acta Orthop Scand* 1977; **48**:520–526.
57 Sherman MF, Warren RF, Marshall JL. A clinical and radiographical analysis of 127 anterior cruciate deficient knees. *Clin Orthop* 1988; **227**:229–237.
58 Andriacchi TP, Briant PL, Bevill SL, Koo S. Rotational changes at the knee after ACL injury cause cartilage thinning. *Clin Orthop Relat Res* 2006; **442**:39–44.
59 McDaniel W Jr, Dameron TB Jr. The untreated anterior cruciate ligament rupture. *Clin Orthop* 1983; **172**:158–163.
60 Murrell GA, Maddali S, Horovitz L, Oakley SP, Warren RF. The effects of time course after anterior cruciate ligament injury in correlation with meniscal and cartilage loss. *Am J Sports Med* 2001; **29**:9–14.
61 Fleming BC, Renstrom PA, Beynnon BD, Engstrom B, Peura G. The influence of functional knee bracing on the anterior cruciate ligament strain biomechanics in weightbearing and nonweightbearing knees. *Am J Sports Med* 2000; **28**:815–824.
62 Beynnon BD, Fleming BC, Churchill DL, Brown D. The effect of anterior cruciate ligament deficiency and functional bracing on translation of the tibia relative to the femur during nonweightbearing and weightbearing. *Am J Sports Med* 2003; **31**:99–105.
63 Cawley PW, France E, Paulos LE. The current state of functional knee bracing research: a review of the literature. *Am J Sports Med* 1991; **19**:226–233.
64 Beynnon B, Wertheimer C, Fleming B, *et al.* An in-vivo study of the anterior cruciate ligament strain biomechanics during functional knee bracing. *Trans Orthop Res Soc* 1990; **15**:223.
65 Harilainen A, Sandelin J. Post-operative use of knee brace in bone–tendon–bone patellar tendon anterior cruciate ligament reconstruction: 5-year follow-up results of a randomized prospective study. *Scand J Med Sci Sports* 2006; **16**:14–18.
66 Pforringer W, Kremer C. [Subsequent treatment of surgically managed, fresh, anterior cruciate ligament ruptures: a randomized, prospective study; in German.] *Sportverletz Sportschaden* 2005; **19**:134–139.
67 Swirtun LR, Jansson A, Renstrom P. The effects of a functional knee brace during early treatment of patients with a nonoperated acute anterior cruciate ligament tear: a prospective randomized study. *Clin J Sport Med* 2005; **15**:299–304.
68 McDevitt ER, Taylor DC, Miller MD, *et al.* Functional bracing after anterior cruciate ligament reconstruction: a prospective, randomized, multicenter study. *Am J Sports Med* 2004; **32**:1887–1892.
69 Sitler M, Ryan J, Hopkinson W, Wheeler J, *et al.* The efficacy of a prophylactic knee brace to reduce knee injuries in football: a prospective, randomized study at West Point. *Am J Sports Med* 1990; **18**:310–315.
70 Laupacis A, Feeny D, Detsky AS, Tugwell PX. How attractive does a new technology have to be to warrant adoption and utilization? Tentative guidelines for using clinical and economic evaluations. *Can Med Assoc J* 1992; **146**:473–481.
71 Barrack RL, Bruckner JD, Kneisl J, Inman WS, Alexander AH. The outcome of nonoperatively treated complete tears of the anterior cruciate ligament in active young adults. *Clin Orthop* 1990; **259**:192–199.
72 Bonamo JJ, Fay C, Firestone T. The conservative treatment of the anterior cruciate deficient knee. *Am J Sports Med* 1990; **18**:618–623.
73 Engebretsen L, Tegnander A. Short-term results of the nonoperated isolated anterior cruciate ligament tear. *J Orthop Trauma* 1990; **4**:406–410.
74 Satku K, Kumar VP, Ngoi SS. Anterior cruciate ligament injuries. To counsel or to operate? *J Bone Joint Surg Br* 1986; **68**:458–461.

75 Aglietti P, Buzzi R, D'Andria S, Zaccherotti G. Long-term study of anterior cruciate ligament reconstruction for chronic instability using the central one-third patellar tendon and a lateral extraarticular tenodesis. *Am J Sports Med* 1992; **20**:38–45.

76 Aglietti P, Buzzi R, Zaccherotti G, *et al.* Patellar tendon versus doubled semitendinosus and gracilis tendons for anterior cruciate ligament reconstruction. *Am J Sports Med* 1994; **22**:211–218.

77 Bach BR Jr, Jones GT, Sweet FA, Hager CA. Arthroscopy-assisted anterior cruciate ligament reconstruction using patellar tendon substitution: two- to four-year follow-up results. *Am J Sports Med* 1994; **22**:758–767.

78 Harner CD, Marks PH, Fu FH, *et al.* Anterior cruciate ligament reconstruction: endoscopic versus two-incision technique. *Arthroscopy* 1994; **10**:502–512.

79 Marder RA, Raskind JR, Carroll M. Prospective evaluation of arthroscopically assisted anterior cruciate ligament reconstruction: patellar tendon versus semitendinosus and gracilis tendons. *Am J Sports Med* 1991; **19**:478–484.

80 Shelbourne KD, Whitaker HJ, McCarroll JR, Rettig AC, Hirschman LD. Anterior cruciate ligament injury: evaluation of intraarticular reconstruction of acute tears without repair. Two to seven year followup of 155 athletes. *Am J Sports Med* 1990; **18**:484–489.

81 Dunn WR, Lincoln AE, Hinton RY, Smith GS, Amoroso PJ. Occupational disability after hospitalization for the treatment of an injury of the anterior cruciate ligament. *J Bone Joint Surg Am* 2003; **85**:1656–1666.

82 Fink C, Hoser C, Hackl W, Navarro RA, Benedetto KP. Long-term outcome of operative or nonoperative treatment of anterior cruciate ligament rupture: is sports activity a determining variable? *Int J Sports Med* 2001; **22**:304–309.

83 Lohmander LS, Ostenberg A, Englund M, Roos H. High prevalence of knee osteoarthritis, pain, and functional limitations in female soccer players twelve years after anterior cruciate ligament injury. *Arthritis Rheum* 2004; **50**:3145–3152.

84 Von Porat A, Roos EM, Roos H. High prevalence of osteoarthritis 14 years after an anterior cruciate ligament tear in male soccer players: a study of radiographic and patient relevant outcomes. *Ann Rheum Dis* 2004; **63**:269–273.

85 O'Neill DB. Arthroscopically assisted reconstruction of the anterior cruciate ligament: a follow-up report. *J Bone Joint Surgery Am* 2001; **83**:1329–1332.

86 Ruiz AL, Kelly M, Nutton RW. Arthroscopic ACL reconstruction: a 5–9 year follow-up. *Knee* 2002; **9**:197–200.

87 Salmon LJ, Russell VJ, Refshauge K, *et al.* Long-term outcome of endoscopic anterior cruciate ligament reconstruction with patellar tendon autograft: minimum 13-year review. *Am J Sports Med* 2006; **34**:721–732.

88 Sgaglione NA, Warren RF, Wickiewicz TL, *et al.* Primary repair with semitendinosus tendon augmentation of acute anterior cruciate ligament injuries. *Am J Sports Med* 1990; **18**:64–73.

89 Jomha NM, Pinczewski LA, Clingeleffer A, Otto DD. Arthroscopic reconstruction of the anterior cruciate ligament with patellar-tendon autograft and interference screw fixation: the results at seven years. *J Bone Joint Surg Br* 1999; **81**:775–779.

90 Shelbourne KD, Gray T. Results of anterior cruciate ligament reconstruction based on meniscus and articular cartilage status at the time of surgery: five- to fifteen-year evaluations. *Am J Sports Med* 2000; **28**:446–452.

91 Jomha NM, Borton DC, Clingeleffer AJ, Pinczewski LA. Long-term osteoarthritic changes in anterior cruciate ligament reconstructed knees. *Clin Orthop* 1999; **358**:188–193.

92 Kim HJ, Rodeo SA. Approach to meniscal tears in anterior cruciate ligament reconstruction. *Orthop Clin North Am* 2003; **34**:139–147.

93 Johnson MJ, Lucas GL, Dusek JK, Henning CE. Isolated arthroscopic meniscal repair: a long-term outcome study (more than 10 years). *Am J Sports Med* 1999; **27**:44–49.

94 Horibe S, Shino K, Nakata K, *et al.* Second-look arthroscopy after meniscal repair: review of 132 menisci repaired by an arthroscopic inside-out technique. *J Bone Joint Surg Br* 1995; **77**:245–249.

95 Spindler KP, McCarty EC, Warren TA, Devin C, Connor JT. Prospective comparison of arthroscopic medial meniscal repair technique: inside-out suture versus entirely arthroscopic arrows. *Am J Sports Med* 2003; **31**:929–934.

96 Shelbourne KD, Carr DR. Meniscal repair compared with meniscectomy for bucket-handle medial meniscal tears in anterior cruciate ligament-reconstructed knees. *Am J Sports Med* 2003; **31**:718–723.

97 Shelbourne KD, Dersam MD. Comparison of partial meniscectomy versus meniscus repair for bucket-handle lateral meniscus tears in anterior cruciate ligament reconstructed knees. *Arthroscopy* 2004; **20**:581–585.
98 Wu WH, Hackett T, Richmond JC. Effects of meniscal and articular surface status on knee stability, function, and symptoms after anterior cruciate ligament reconstruction: a long-term prospective study. *Am J Sports Med* 2002; **30**:845–850.
99 O'Brien SJ, Warren RF, Pavlov H, *et al.* Reconstruction of the chronically insufficient anterior cruciate ligament with the central third of the patellar ligament. *J Bone Joint Surg Am* 1991; **73**:277–281.
100 Strum GM, Fox JM, Ferkel RD, *et al.* Intraarticular versus intraarticular and extraarticular reconstruction for chronic anterior cruciate ligament instability. *Clin Orthop* 1989; **245**:188–198.
101 Frank CB, Jackson DW. The science of reconstruction of the anterior cruciate ligament. *J Bone Joint Surg Am* 1997; **79**:1556–1576.
102 Gillquist J, Odensten M. Arthroscopic reconstruction of the anterior cruciate ligament. *Arthroscopy* 1988; **4**:5–9.
103 Raab DJ, Fischer DA, Smith JP, Markman AW, Steubs JA. Comparison of arthroscopic and open reconstruction of the anterior cruciate ligament: early results. *Am J Sports Med* 1993; **21**:680–684.
104 Fremerey R, Lobenhoffer P, Skutek M, Gerich T, Bosch U. Proprioception in anterior cruciate ligament reconstruction: endoscopic versus open two-tunnel technique. A prospective study. *Int J Sports Med* 2001; **22**:144–148.
105 Ishibashi Y, Kim HS, Rudy T, *et al.* Robotic evaluation of the effect of the tibial fixation level on ACL reconstructed knee stability. [Paper presented at the ORS Annual Meeting, Orlando, Florida, 1995.]
106 Kurosaka M, Yoshiya S, Andrish JT. A biomechanical comparison of different surgical techniques of graft fixation in anterior cruciate ligament reconstruction. *Am J Sports Med* 1987; **15**:225–229.
107 Northrup T, Linter D, Farmer J, *et al.* Biomechanical evaluation of interference screw fixation of hamstring and patellar tendon grafts used in ACL reconstruction. [Paper presented at the AAOS Annual Meeting, San Francisco, 1997.]
108 Steiner ME, Hecker AT, Brown CH, *et al.* Anterior cruciate ligament graft fixation comparison of hamstring and patellar tendon grafts. *Am J Sports Med* 1994; **22**:240–247.
109 Karchin A, Hull ML, Howell SM. Initial tension and anterior load-displacement behavior of high-stiffness anterior cruciate ligament graft constructs. *J Bone Joint Surg Am* 2004; **86**:1675–1683.
110 Deehan DJ, Cawston TE. The biology of integration of the anterior cruciate ligament. *J Bone Joint Surg Br* 2005; **87**:889–895.
111 Pinczewski LA, Clingeleffer AJ, Otto DD, *et al.* Integration of hamstring tendon graft with bone in reconstruction of the anterior cruciate ligament. *Arthroscopy* 1997; **13**:641–643.
112 Rodeo SA, Arnoczky SP, Torzilli PA, *et al.* Tendon-healing in a bone tunnel: a biomechanical and histological study in the dog. *J Bone Joint Surg Am* 1993; **75**:795–1803.
113 Song EK, Rowe SM, Chung JY, Moon ES, Lee KB. Failure of osteointegration of hamstring tendon autograft after anterior cruciate ligament reconstruction. *Arthroscopy* 2004; **20**:424–428.
114 Harter RA, Osternig LR, Singer K. Instrumented Lachman tests for the evaluation of anterior laxity after reconstruction of the anterior cruciate ligament. *J Bone Joint Surg Am* 1989; **71**:975–983.
115 Holmes PF, James SL, Larson RL, *et al.* Retrospective direct comparison of three intraarticular anterior cruciate ligament reconstructions. *Am J Sports Med* 1991; **19**:596–560.
116 O'Neill DB. Arthroscopically assisted reconstruction of the anterior cruciate ligament: a prospective randomized analysis of three techniques. *J Bone Joint Surg Am* 1996; **78**:803–813.
117 Otero AL, Hutcheson L. A comparison of the doubled semitendinosus/gracilis and central third of the patellar tendon autografts in arthroscopic anterior cruciate ligament reconstruction. *Arthroscopy* 1993; **9**:143–148.
118 Corry IS, Webb JM, Clingeleffer AJ, Pinczewski LA. Arthroscopic reconstruction of the anterior cruciate ligament: a comparison of patellar tendon autograft and four-strand hamstring tendon autograft. *Am J Sports Med* 1999; **27**:444–454.
119 Feller JA, Webster KE. A randomized comparison of patellar tendon and hamstring tendon anterior cruciate ligament reconstruction. *Am J Sports Med* 2003; **31**:564–473.
120 Laxdal G, Kartus J, Hansson L, *et al.* A prospective randomized comparison of bone–patellar tendonbone and hamstring grafts for anterior cruciate ligament reconstruction. *Arthroscopy* 2005; **21**:34–42.

121 Aglietti P, Giron F, Buzzi R, Biddau F, Sasso F. Anterior cruciate ligament reconstruction: bone–patellar tendon–bone compared with double semitendinosus and gracilis tendon grafts. A prospective, randomized clinical trial. *J Bone Joint Surg Am* 2004; **86**:2143–2155.
122 Beard D, Anderson JL, Davies S, Price AJ, Dodd CA. Hamstrings vs. patella tendon for anterior cruciate ligament reconstruction: a randomised controlled trial. *Knee* 2001; **8**:45–50.
123 Jansson KA, Linko E, Sandelin J, Harilainen A. A prospective randomized study of patellar versus hamstring tendon autografts for anterior cruciate ligament reconstruction. *Am J Sports Med* 2003; **31**:12–18.
124 Shaieb MD, Kan DM, Chang SK, Marumoto JM, Richardson AB. A prospective randomized comparison of patellar tendon versus semitendinosus and gracilis tendon autografts for anterior cruciate ligament reconstruction. *Am J Sports Med* 2002; **30**:214–220.
125 Valentin P, Hofbauer M, Aldrian S. Clinical results of computer-navigated anterior cruciate ligament reconstructions. *Orthopedics* 2005; **28** (10 Suppl):S1289–1291.
126 Ishibashi Y, Tsuda E, Tazawa K, Sato H, Toh S. Intraoperative evaluation of the anatomical double-bundle anterior cruciate ligament reconstruction with the OrthoPilot navigation system. *Orthopedics* 2005; **28** (10 Suppl):S1277–1282.
127 Koh J. Computer-assisted navigation and anterior cruciate ligament reconstruction: accuracy and outcomes. *Orthopedics* 2005; **28** (10 Suppl):S1283–1287.
128 Beynnon BD, Uh BS, Johnson RJ, *et al.* Rehabilitation after anterior cruciate ligament reconstruction: a prospective, randomized, double-blind comparison of programs administered over 2 different time intervals. *Am J Sports Med* 2005; **33**:347–359.
129 Grant JA, Mohtadi NG, Maitland ME, Zernicke RF. Comparison of home versus physical therapy-supervised rehabilitation programs after anterior cruciate ligament reconstruction: a randomized clinical trial. *Am J Sports Med* 2005; **33**:1288–1297.
130 Cooper RL, Taylor NF, Feller JA. A randomised controlled trial of proprioceptive and balance training after surgical reconstruction of the anterior cruciate ligament. *Res Sports Med* 2005; **13**:217–230.
131 Cooper RL, Taylor NF, Feller JA. A systematic review of the effect of proprioceptive and balance exercises on people with an injured or reconstructed anterior cruciate ligament. *Res Sports Med* 2005; **13**:163–178.
132 Perry MC, Morrissey MC, King JB, Morrissey D, Earnshaw P. Effects of closed versus open kinetic chain knee extensor resistance training on knee laxity and leg function in patients during the 8- to 14-week post-operative period after anterior cruciate ligament reconstruction. *Knee Surg Sports Traumatol Arthrosc* 2005; **13**:357–369.
133 Perry MC, Morrissey MC, Morrissey D, *et al.* Knee extensors kinetic chain training in anterior cruciate ligament deficiency. *Knee Surg Sports Traumatol Arthrosc* 2005; **13**:638–648.
134 Shaw T, Williams MT, Chipchase LS. Do early quadriceps exercises affect the outcome of ACL reconstruction? A randomized controlled trial. *Aust J Physiother* 2005; **51**:9–17.
135 Zatterstrom R, Friden T, Lindstrand A, Moritz U. Rehabilitation following acute anterior cruciate ligament injuries: a 12 month follow-up of a randomized clinical trial. *Scand J Med Sci Sports* 2000; **10**:156–163.

CHAPTER 24

What is the most appropriate treatment for patellar tendinopathy?

Jill L. Cook and Karim M. Khan

Introduction

In this millennium, we have abandoned the inflammatory paradigm as the primary pathology in tendinopathy.[1] Abandoning this paradigm has left sports medicine practitioners without a clear model of pathology and repair on which to base treatments. As little research has been conducted on treatments based on other models, clinicians have limited treatment options.

After abandoning inflammation, the primary model of pathology has been degeneration,[2] but an alternative concept of a failed healing response may be more fitting.[3] Other concepts such as compression[4] and stress-shielding[5] have been hypothesized, although they have little data to support them at this time.

In all these models, treatment that maintains or encourages the appropriate healing response in the tendon may be appropriate. Both surgical and conservative treatments may fulfill this role. There is now clear evidence that tendon is responsive to mechanical loading and that exercise stimulates tendon healing.[6] Surgical intervention appears to stimulate tendon repair by initiating the triphasic response of inflammation, proliferation, and repair.[7]

The limited literature on the pathology and repair of tendon tissue may not be of critical clinical significance, as the primary clinical issue is tendon pain. On the basis of the response in other soft tissues, it is widely surmised that resolving acute pathology will correspondingly improve pain. This is often not so in tendons, as pain is not related to pathology either in the acute or chronic stage. Most treatments reviewed in this chapter are hypothesized to affect pathology, but the goal of all clinical treatment programs is to reduce pain. As pain is the presenting feature of this condition, and outcome measures are mainly pain-based, most treatments do not measure changes in the underlying pathology of tendinopathy.

The conservative treatment recorded in the literature of patellar tendinopathy includes combinations of rest, exercise (especially eccentric exercise), modalities including ultrasound, heat and cryotherapy, frictions, biomechanical adjustment, nutritional supplements, sclerosing injections, and pharmaceutical treatment. Different conservative treatments may have a cumulative effect, and investigations often include more than one aspect to the intervention as well as other activity and treatments—making it difficult to delineate the most effective part of the treatment.

The surgical management of patellar tendinopathy traditionally follows when conservative treatment fails. Surgical treatment includes several different operative procedures and postoperative rehabilitation protocols and research that defines the best surgical option is absent. The quality of surgical intervention trials are constrained by low subject numbers, data that suggest that a suboptimal outcome is common,[8] multiple surgical techniques, and the absence of a reasonable model for appropriate intervention on which to base study hypotheses.

As the literature has shifted from an inflammatory model, studies of the treatment of patellar tendinopathy have focused on exercise, and most of the new studies included in this edition include an exercise-based treatment. This chapter will summarize the limited evidence on the effectiveness of treatments for patellar tendinopathy.

Methodology

Search methods

Databases searched were MEDLINE, EMBASE, CINAHL, Current Contents, AMED, and PubMed. The search was limited to the English language, and although there are several publications in other languages, our inability to review them satisfactorily led us to exclude them from the review. Primary terms used in the search included: jumper's knee, patellar tendon, tendinitis, tendonitis, tendinosis, and tendinopathy. Secondary terms included: treatment, surgery, and conservative. Citation tracking of available papers was also performed.

Inclusion criteria and quality assessment

Studies were reviewed if all included subjects had patellar tendinopathy, and the study design was a randomized trial or was prospective in nature. Due to the low number of studies meeting the inclusion criteria and the wide range of studies encompassing different participants, outcomes and treatments, no attempt was made to exclude studies by using a quality assessment evaluation.

Results

The eight randomized trials that met the inclusion criteria studied the effect of exercise on the patellar tendon (n = 5), the effects of medications (n = 2), and the effect of local massage (n = 1). Prospective studies were also sparse, with six studies having a prospective experimental design, on the surgical (n = 3), exercise-based (n = 2), or pharmacological treatment (n = 1) of this condition.

Conservative treatment

Exercise

There are six papers that document the effectiveness of exercise on patellar tendinopathy. These can be divided into two groups: those studies that investigated exercises on a decline board and those using other exercises.

Three papers suggest an effect from exercise-based interventions such as squatting, isokinetics, and weights on patellar tendinopathy (Table 24.1).[9–11] Similar in many ways, these studies focus on strengthening of the muscles around the knee in those subjects with jumper's knee, and measuring changes in strength, pain and function after a 4-week, 8-week, or 12-week intervention. Only the study by Stasinopoulos and Stasinopoulos[9]

Table 24.1 Conservative exercise-based studies

First author, ref.; study design	Intervention	Diagnostic criteria	No. starting/ completing study	Minimum symptoms before study	No of treatments/ study length	Outcome measures—when taken	Results	Authors stated limitations of the study	Conclusion
Jensen[10] Randomized controlled trial	Eccentric exercise on isokinetic equipment	Orthopod referral, palpation	31/31	6 weeks	3 × week/ 8 weeks	Pain intensity and occurrence (5-point scale) Eccentric work of quadriceps Baseline and at 4 and 8 weeks	Improved strength in exercise group both control and tendinitis	Gender make-up of groups may skew results. Tendinitis may limit strength increase due to pain	Eccentric exercise results in strength gains in both normal and tendinitis limbs. Tendinitis pain may limit strength gains
Cannell[11] Randomized single blind trial comparing 2 treatments	Strengthening with either squats or weights	Pain, palpation	19/19	4 weeks	5 × week/ 12 weeks	VAS, return to sport Baseline, 6 and 12 weeks	Both groups had reduced pain, improved hamstring strength Neither group improved in quads strength	Small sample size	Both squat and weight exercises reduces pain of jumper's knee
Stasinopoulos[9] Randomized controlled trial	Eccentric squat exercise and stretching, or ultrasound or transverse frictions	Palpation and decline squat pain	30/30	3 months	3 × week for 4 weeks	Change pain; worse, no change better no pain. 4, 8 and 12 weeks	Exercise program improved pain more than US or frictions	Small samples, outcome measures not validated, no control group, heterogeneous sample and no power analysis	Exercise program was better than US and frictions

Purdam[13] Prospective, nonrandomized pilot study	Eccentric squat on or off the decline board	Pain with load, palpation, imaging abnormality	17/17	3 months	Exercise twice daily, 12 weeks	VAS during loading, return to previous activity Baseline, 12 weeks, 15 months	Decline squat: 6 subjects return to activity and decreased pain Standard squat: one subject return to activity, no change in pain	Nonrandomized, small subject numbers, limited outcome measures	Decline squat indicated for chronic patellar tendinopathy
Young[14] Randomized controlled trial	Eccentric exercise on decline board or on step	Pain limiting sport, palpation and load pain, VISA less than 80, abnormal ultrasound	17/17	Not stated	Exercise twice daily 12 weeks	Compliance, VISA, VAS Recruitment, baseline, 12 weeks, 12 months	Both groups improved. Improvement of more than 20 VISA points 94% likely in decline group and 41% likely in step group at 12 months	Each intervention had several parts and which aspect was most effective is not known	Decline squat effective for patellar tendinopathy as a preseason program in athletes who train and play with pain
Visnes[15] Randomized controlled trial	Eccentric exercise on a decline or normal training	Pain on palpation, pain with sport. VISA less than 80	29/27	3 months	Exercise twice daily 12 weeks	Compliance, VIS, jump performance and change score Baseline, 12 weeks	No change in either group	Study may have been underpowered	Eccentric exercise on a decline is not beneficial during competition season

US, ultrasound; VAS, visual analogue scale; VISA, Victorian Institute of Sport Assessment (score).

extended outcome measures beyond the intervention period, but they limited their outcomes to pain change from baseline.

A reduction in pain in the study period was apparent in two studies.[9,11] However, quadriceps strength gains were not apparent[11] or not measured.[9] The lack of strength gains in the study by Cannell *et al.*[11] may be due to measurement strategies, as concentric strength measurements were used and the intervention was directed at improving eccentric strength. Eccentric strength training does not necessarily lead to gains in concentric strength, and gains in eccentric strength may not have been measured. Conversely, the study by Jenson and Di Fabio[10] showed improvement in quadriceps work in the study period, but it is unclear if there was a concurrent reduction in pain.

The recent literature has provided three studies that investigated the effectiveness of exercise on a decline board. This is based on the earlier research by Purdam *et al.*,[12] who documented a better discriminative ability of the decline to load the extensor mechanism of the knee. Squats on a 25° decline board improved the specificity of the squat, as the decline decreases the contribution of the calf muscle and passive ankle structures to the control of the squat. This study showed that the single-leg decline squat was a superior objective test for patellar tendinopathy to either normal squat, step-ups, or double-leg tests.

Further studies have investigated exercise on the decline board. These include one prospective study[13] and two randomized trials.[14,15] Two trials reported improvements in outcome measures—return to sport, visual analogue scale (VAS), Victorian Institute of Sport Assessment (VISA) score, change in pain, jump performance—with exercise, although time frames for improvement varied. Purdam *et al.*[12] reported improvement both at the end of the intervention and after a follow-up period. Young *et al.*[14] reported no difference between groups at the end of the intervention (both improved), but a greater clinically important difference in the decline-squat group at 12 months. Visnes *et al.*,[15] whose intervention occurred during competition, reported no improvement in pain or jump performance in comparison with those who undertook no exercise.

Massage/frictions (Table 24.2)

Two studies compared massage/frictions with other treatments.[9,16] The study by Wilson *et al.*[16] used a massage device and compared outcomes with those treated traditionally. The intervention differed between groups in several ways, as did the number of treatments. The main outcome measure used in this study was a patellofemoral joint evaluation scale,[17] not validated for studies in patellar tendinopathy. Results indicated that the main outcome measures did not differ between groups, and those outcomes that were significantly different are not fully documented in the paper. It is difficult to conclude from this study that massage offered a better outcome than the traditional treatment.

Stasinopoulos and Stasinopoulos[9] compared frictions with exercise or ultrasound, and found that frictions provided a reduction in pain for more participants (20%) than therapeutic ultrasound (0%), but that significantly fewer participants improved in comparison with the exercise group (100%).

Pharmacotherapy (Table 24.3)

There have been three studies of pharmacotherapy in the treatment of patellar tendinopathy. Two studies investigated corticosteroids using iontophoresis, phonophoresis, or injection,[18,19] and one study investigated the effect of sclerosing injections.[20]

Table 24.2 Other conservative interventions

First author, ref.; study design	Intervention	Diagnostic criteria	No. starting/completing study	No. of treatments/study length	Minimum symptoms before study	Outcome measures when taken	Results	Authors stated limitations of the study	Conclusion
Wilson[16] Randomized single-blind, cross-over trial	Massage/frictions	History and physical examination	38/20	Not stated	3 × week controls, 2 × week intervention group/4 weeks	Patellofemoral joint evaluation scale, Blazina scale, functional tests Baseline, 6 and 12 weeks	No difference in groups on reported outcome measures	Diagnosis (no imaging), nonstandardized traditional treatment, different no. of treatments, large drop-out, limited outcome measures, small sample size	Frictions improved clinical outcome
Panni[24] Prospective clinical trial	Cryotherapy, electrical currents, magnetic field, ultrasound, laser, strengthening exercise, stretches	Pain, palpation, muscle atrophy, ultrasound and radiograph	42	Not stated/ 6 months	4 weeks to 6 months	Excellent, good, fair, poor (EGFP) Baseline and 6 months	Excellent or good results in 33 (79%) patients	Not stated	Adequate nonoperative management should be attempted before surgery

Table 24.3 Pharmacological interventions

Study	Intervention	Diagnostic criteria	No. starting/ completing study	No. of treatments/ study length	Length of symptoms before study	Outcome measures when taken	Results	Authors stated limitations of the study	Conclusion
Pellechia[18] Randomized cross-over trial comparing 2 treatments	Iontophoresis (dexamethasone–lidocaine) vs. heat, cold frictions, phonophoresis (hydrocortisone)	Pain, palpation	48/42	6/2–3 weeks	3 days to 10 years	VAS, palpation, step-ups, functional index Baseline, after 6 and 12 treatments	Iontophoresis improved all outcome measures significantly Frictions and modalities only improved step ups	Small sample size, uncontrolled exercise	Iontophoresis recommended for treatment of infrapatellar pain
Capasso[19] Randomized double blind controlled trial comparing 2 treatments	Injected methylprednisolone and lidocaine vs. aprotinin and lidocaine vs. placebo (saline)	Clinical and ultrasound criteria	116/103	2–4 injections fortnightly/ 12 months	Not stated	Excellent, good, fair, poor Baseline, at completion, 1 month and 1 year after study	Aprotinin had better outcome than corticosteroid, which had a better outcome than placebo	Not stated	Aprotinin offers short-term benefits but needs further investigation
Alfredson[20] Prospective trial	Polidocanol injections	Pain and abnormal imaging	15/15	Up to 5 treatments	Mean 23 months	VAS, return to sport	12/15 improved and returned to sport	Not stated	Sclerosing injections cures pain

Iontophoresis with corticosteroids improved the outcome in comparison with phonophoresis, as it may introduce corticosteroids into target tissue more effectively than phonophoresis.[18] Capasso *et al.*[19] reported that aprotinin offered a better outcome than either corticosteroids or a placebo. The time from onset of patellar tendinopathy to recruitment into the study was not stated, hence some subjects may have the short-term symptoms that may respond to anti-inflammatory medication. Outcome measures in this study were based on the Kelly grading system,[21] and the study used an unblinded clinical investigator.

Neovascularization is a cornerstone of tendon pathology and was the target of treatment by Alfredson and Ohberg.[20] This prospective trial investigated sclerosing injections on pain and function in the patellar tendon. Eighty percent returned to their previous level of competition, and pain reductions were also significant (VAS reduced from 81 to 10). The authors suggest that the results of this treatment on those with long-term tendon pain (mean 23 months) challenges the need for surgery for patellar tendinopathy.

Surgical treatment (Table 24.4)

There are no randomized studies of surgical treatment in patellar tendinopathy. Three studies have a prospective design. Khan *et al.*[22] showed that 73% of the subjects who underwent surgery for patellar tendinopathy had good results. The VISA score[23] in this group improved significantly, which reflected improvement in pain, function, and sporting capacity. The primary outcome of this study was that there was no correlation between clinical outcome and imaging appearance in postsurgical subjects.

Panni *et al.*[24] included both conservative and surgical treatment in their study. Subjects who had failed the conservative treatment were operated on, and all of these subjects were reported to have a good or excellent outcome.

Testa *et al.*[7] investigated the efficacy of percutaneous tenotomy, and reported that the technique was more effective for treatment of mid-tendon pathology than it was for proximal tendon pathology. The diagnosis of a mid-tendon lesion was made on clinical grounds (palpation) and seven subjects had normal imaging. Nearly 40% of participants in this study reported poor results, and isokinetic testing revealed persistent strength deficits. Given that mid-tendon pathology is relatively rare, this study may have limited clinical utility.

Discussion

Patellar tendinopathy investigations have been limited by the relatively small number of patients (compared with, for example, a medical condition such as hypertension or osteoporosis), the wide range of clinical presentations, and the possibility of multiple conservative and surgical interventions available. There have been a larger number of quality studies in the last few years, and more are clearly needed before treatment of this condition has a clear evidence base.

Conservative treatment

Studies of patellar tendinopathy have been reported in the literature for 30 years. Many of these studies have suggested that it is resistant to treatment and recurrent in nature.[25] Similarly, many authors suggest the need to exhaust conservative treatment options before proceeding to surgery.[26,27]

Table 24.4 Surgical trials

Study	Intervention	Diagnostic criteria	No. starting/ completing study	Study length	Length of symptoms before study	Outcome measures when taken	Results	Authors stated limitations of the study	Conclusion
Testa[7] Prospective surgical trial	Percutaneous longitudinal tenotomy	Pain, palpation	38/34	6 months	11–57 months	EGFP, strength test Baseline, 6 weeks, 6 and 24 months	Excellent or good results in 25 (74%) of patients Work and average power significantly lower in the operated limb (as it was preoperatively)	Study not randomized	Procedure not recommended in insertional tendinopathy
Khan[22] Prospective surgical trial	Surgical debridement	Pain and tenderness	13/13	12 months	9–96 months	Ultrasound, MRI, EGFP, VISA score Baseline, 3, 6, 9, and 12 months	Excellent or good results in 73%. VISA score improved from a mean of 22 presurgery to 69 at 12 months. US and MRI did not predict clinical outcome	Subject inclusion restricted geographically	Management after surgery should be clinical and not based on imaging appearance
Panni[24] Prospective surgical trial	Surgical debridement, longitudinal tenotomy and drilling of the insertion	Pain, palpation, muscle atrophy, ultrasound and radiograph	9	6 months	> 6 months	EGFP Baseline and 6 months	Excellent or good results in all patients	Not stated	Surgery should include all the techniques described in this study

EGFP, excellent, good, fair, poor (scale); MRI, magnetic resonance imaging; US, ultrasound; VISA, Victorian Institute of Sport Assessment (score).

Studies on the conservative treatment of patellar tendinopathy are difficult to design and implement, as the subjects are often elite, young sports people and need to return to their activity as soon as possible.[18,28] On the basis of the literature reviewed for this paper, conservative treatment based on an eccentric exercise program conducted on a decline board is the best treatment for patellar tendinopathy.

Surgical treatment

No studies on the surgical treatment of patellar tendinopathy fully met the criteria outlined in the methods section. When prospective studies were included, only three surgical studies were appropriate to review, all with relatively small numbers. None of the studies offers great insight as to the effectiveness of surgery on this tendon. In these three studies, the excellent and good outcomes were 100%,[24] 73%,[22] and 62%.[7]

The paper by Khan *et al.*[22] had imaging as a primary outcome and does not clarify treatment options other than to describe rather mediocre results in that particular cohort. The study by Panni *et al.*[24] reported the success of surgery in all the patients treated and complete recovery in muscle strength, although the technique of measuring this was not documented fully. The study by Testa *et al.*[7] appears most effective in the mid-tendon tendinopathy, a clinical and imaging phenomenon seen much less often than pathology and pain at the insertions of the tendon. Hence, the clinical relevance of this procedure may be low. The literature does not offer any indication of the effectiveness or otherwise of surgical treatment for patellar tendinopathy.

Study design

Several issues consistently compromise the conclusions that can be drawn from all of the studies summarized in this chapter. Two of them include the inconsistency of the diagnostic criteria and the appropriateness of some of the outcome measures.

Diagnostic criteria

Diagnostic criteria for patellar tendinopathy varied among studies; most authors used clinical assessment for diagnosis, and only six studies used confirmatory tendon imaging. The presence of abnormal imaging does not indicate absolutely that the pain is coming from the tendon, and it can be argued that imaging is not necessary to diagnose patellar tendinopathy.[29] Nevertheless, as clinical tendon assessment is also not 100% accurate, imaging at least confirms that the tendon is a potential source of pain.

Pain and palpation tenderness were almost exclusively used to diagnose patellar tendinopathy; only three studies documented pain on resistance of muscle contraction or other functional testing.[9,13,18] Two studies used a reliable outcome measure (VISA score) to quantify inclusion pain and function levels,[14,15] to ensure that participants had a minimal level of pain and incapacity on entry into the study. Palpation as a diagnostic criterion is a reliable, but not necessarily valid, diagnostic test for this condition, as it does not correlate with either imaging changes or symptoms.[30]

As there is no criterion measure for the diagnosis of patellar tendinopathy, future studies should include multiple subjective and objective tests and report these fully in the paper. At a minimum, inclusion criteria should include the patient having symptoms with objective loading, the pain documented to be correctly located on a pain map, a quantifiable score with a validated outcome measure, as well as diagnostic imaging (either magnetic resonance imaging or diagnostic ultrasound). Confirmation of pathology within the tendon in conjunction with clinical tests and validated outcome measures would guarantee that the best diagnostic criteria are used, and future studies should include these as a minimum standard of tests needed to confirm the diagnosis and quantify the participant's entry level pain and capacity. This, along with the distribution of pain on a pain map, would help ensure the diagnostic homogeneity of the study participants.

Outcome measures

Outcome measures specifically for patellar tendinopathy have only recently been developed. Studies published prior to this used unvalidated[18] or adapted knee pain scales,[10] or scales not specifically designed for tendinopathy.[16] It is likely that these and other scales lacked specificity and sensitivity in quantifying the outcome after treatment for patellar tendinopathy.

Similarly, the use of palpation as an outcome measure lacks validity.[30] The use of a gauge to standardize and quantify palpation tenderness[31] may improve the validity of this outcome measure, but normative data in tendons are still required.

The most appropriate tests to use when conducting clinical trials of this condition are the VISA score, as a subjective measure of pain and function, and the decline squat, as an objective loading test for patellar tendinopathy. In studies investigating the decline squat as a treatment, other outcome measures must be used.

Duration of symptoms

Duration of tendon symptoms before an intervention also varied widely. Some studies included patients with short-term tendon symptoms (subjects in the study had symptoms of less than 5 days[18]) or did not state the duration of symptoms,[16,19,32] whereas seven studies excluded those with short-term symptoms (subjects in the study had symptoms > 3 months). It could be argued that these two opposing exclusion criteria are therefore investigating subjects with different conditions.

Those studies that include short-term symptoms risk including tendons without overuse tendinopathy, and any treatment efficacy demonstrated in these studies would need to be interpreted with caution as there may not have been a true tendinopathy in the first instance. Such a fear would be exacerbated if the study also has poorly documented and restricted diagnostic criteria.

Participants

Patellar tendinopathy is usually treated when the person presents with symptoms severe enough to require medical intervention. Participants in two studies[14,15] in this review were from a nonclinical population—that is, athletes who had pain but who were continuing to play and train. The results of these studies may not be comparable to a clinical population, in that the baseline pain and possibility to improve may be less. Both these studies quantified symptoms and function at recruitment, excluding those with VISA scores higher than 80 points and limiting participants to those with more severe symptoms.

These two studies used a similar type of participant, but the timing of the intervention was different, and this appears to affect the outcome. Exercise-based treatments in a clinical population are always completed when the person is resting from activities, and this was similar in the study by Young *et al.*,[14] who completed the intervention in the off-season. Visnes *et al.*,[15] however, completed the exercise program during a competitive season, and as the outcomes were poorer than other exercise-based treatments, future studies should investigate exercise interventions while the participant is not actively undertaking sport.

Study numbers

Studies in this review had relatively low subject numbers; one study had more than 100 subjects, the remaining studies had fewer than 50 subjects. It is possible these studies would have a type 2 statistical error. No studies report making a prior estimate of the patient numbers required to demonstrate statistical power[33] or calculating power from the effect size of the study.

Study length: treatment and follow-up

The treatment protocol was appropriate in most studies, and studies of exercise interventions lasted 6–12 weeks. Only four conservative studies, three of them exercise-based studies, extended the follow-up beyond the end of treatment,[9,13,14,19] with subjects being evaluated up to 15 months after the completion of treatment. As patellar tendinopathy is a recurrent condition,[25] these studies provide some evidence about the long-term efficacy of these treatments.

Recommendations

Carefully conducted randomized trials of both conservative and surgical treatments with large participant numbers are still needed. Multicenter trials may offer the best way to increase participant numbers in intervention trials. We recommend the wider use of quantifiable subjective measures designed for this condition, such as the VISA scale,[23] in future studies. For between-study comparison, the use of the 11-point or 100-mm VAS is also recommended. The development and testing of more objective tests is also recommended. Conservative treatments require clarification of the best strength protocols for this condition.

Surgically, there is a need to compare surgical techniques, to identify whether the outcome of any one technique is superior to another. Coleman *et al.*[8] reviewed 25 patellar tendon surgery papers and identified methodological flaws in many of them. Their criticism of the literature suggests that future studies must be at least prospective in nature, that bias in subject recruitment and data collection should be controlled, that outcome measures should be improved, and that postoperative regimens should be standardized.

Conclusions

Patellar tendinopathy affects athletes in many sports and at all levels of participation, but has a particular association with elite, jumping athletes. These athletes can endure months of frustratingly slow rehabilitation, with treatment based on limited investigations into the conservative or surgical treatment of patellar tendinopathy.

The studies examined in this review indicate that exercise-based treatment is recommended for this condition. There are no data to suggest that any one surgical treatment offers a better outcome than any other, and all surgical techniques require further investigation.

Recommendations for further studies

- Objective diagnostic criteria: imaging (ultrasound, magnetic resonance), pain maps, functional tests.
- Subjective outcome measures: VISA scale, 100-mm VAS.
- Objective outcome measures: decline squat.
- Length of symptoms > 3 months.
- Follow-up: extended beyond the end of the study.

Key messages

- Exercise-based conservative treatment appears to be the most appropriate treatment.
- Massage has a limited effect on pain.
- There is limited evidence to support surgical treatment of patellar tendinopathy.

Summary

- Patellar tendinopathy is common in sports involving jumping and change of direction.
- Conservative management should include exercise and pharmacological intervention.
- Eccentric exercise is best done on a decline board during the off-season.
- Sclerosing injections offer pain relief in the majority of cases.
- There is limited evidence on which to base surgical management.

Sample examination questions

Multiple-choice questions (answers on page 602)

1 Conservative treatment of patellar tendinopathy is likely to result in:
   A Resolution of pain only
   B Resolution of pathology
   C Resolution of both pain and pathology

2 Treatments that are based on the current model of tendon pathology are:
   A Nonsteroidal anti-inflammatory medication
   B Eccentric exercise
   C Corticosteroid medication

3 Exercise interventions have been shown to result in improved outcomes in comparison with:
   A Massage
   B Frictions
   C Both of the above

Essay questions

1 Plan an algorithm of conservative management of patellar tendinopathy that is scaled from the treatments with the most evidence to the treatment with the least evidence.

2 Discuss the pharmacotherapies investigated in the studies in this chapter in relation to the current understanding of tendon pathology and pain.

3 Write a research proposal that would result in a study worthy of inclusion in the next edition of this book to investigate surgical treatment of patellar tendinopathy.

Summarizing the evidence

Treatment	Results	Level of evidence*
Conservative treatment		
Exercise	4 RCTs, small size, favor exercise. 1 RCT found no improvement	A3
Massage	2 RCTs, results show little improvement	A4
Pharmacology	2 RCTs show benefit from treatment	A4
Surgical treatment	No RCTs; surgery may offer symptomatic improvement	B

* A1: evidence from large randomized controlled trials (RCTs) or systematic review (including meta-analysis).
A2: evidence from at least one high quality cohort.
A3: evidence from at least one moderate sized RCT or systematic review.†
A4: evidence from at least one RCT.
B: evidence from at least one high quality study of nonrandomized cohorts.
C: expert opinion
† Arbitrarily, the following cut-off points have been used; large study size: ≥ 100 patients per intervention group; moderate study size ≥ 50 patients per intervention group.

References

1 Khan K, Cook J, Kannus P, Maffulli N, Bonar SF. Time to abandon the "tendinitis" myth. *BMJ* 2002; **324**:626–627.
2 Józsa L, Reffy A, Kannus P, Demel S, Elek E. Pathological alterations in human tendons. *Arch Orthop Trauma Surg* 1990; **110**:15–21.
3 Clancy W. Failed healing responses. In: Leadbetter W, Buckwater J, Gordon S, eds. *Sports-Induced Inflammation: Clinical and Basic Science Concepts.* Park Ridge, IL: American Orthopedic Society for Sports Medicine, 1989:573–575.
4 Hamilton B, Purdam C. Patellar tendinosis as an adaptive response: a new hypothesis. *Br J Sports Med* 2003; **38**:758–761.
5 Almekinders LC, Weinhold PS, Maffulli N. Compression etiology in tendinopathy. *Clin Sports Med* 2003; **22**:703–710.
6 Kjaer M. Role of extracellular matrix in adaptation of tendon and skeletal muscle to mechanical loading. *Physiol Rev* 2004; **84**:649–698.
7 Testa V, Capasso G, Maffulli N, Bifulco G. Ultrasound guided percutaneous longitudinal tenotomy for the management of patellar tendinopathy. *Med Sci Sport Exerc* 1999; **31**:1509–1515.
8 Coleman BD, Khan KM, Maffulli N, Cook JL, Wark JD. Studies of surgical outcome after patellar tendinopathy: clinical significance of methodological deficiencies and guidelines for future studies. *Scand J Med Sci Sports* 2000; **10**:2–11.
9 Stasinopoulos D, Stasinopoulos I. Comparison of effects of exercise programme, pulsed ultrasound and transverse friction in the treatment of patellar tendinopathy. *Clin Rehabil* 2004; **18**:347–352.
10 Jensen K, Di Fabio RP. Evaluation of eccentric exercise in treatment of patellar tendinitis. *Phys Ther* 1989; **69**:211–216.
11 Cannell LJ, Taunton JE, Clement DB, Smith C, Khan KM. A randomised clinical trial of the efficacy of drop squats or leg extension/leg curl exercises to treat clinically diagnosed jumper's knee in athletes: pilot study. *Br J Sports Med* 2001; **35**:60–64.
12 Purdam C, Cook J, Hopper D, Khan K. Discriminative ability of functional loading tests for adolescent jumper's knee. *Phys Ther Sport* 2003; **4**:3–9.
13 Purdam CR, Johnsson P, Alfredson H, *et al.* A pilot study of the eccentric decline squat in the management of painful chronic patellar tendinopathy. *Br J Sports Med* 2004; **38**:395–397.

14 Young M, Cook J, Purdam C, Kiss ZS, Alfredson H. Conservative treatment of patellar tendinopathy: a 12-month prospective randomised trial comparing two treatment protocols. *Br J Sports Med* 2005; **39**:102–105.
15 Visnes H, Hoksrud A, Cook J, Bahr R. No effect of eccentric training on jumper's knee in volleyball players during the competitive season: a randomized clinical trial. *Clin J Sport Med* 2005; **15**:227–234.
16 Wilson JK, Sevier TL, Helfst R, Honong E, Thomann A. Comparison of rehabilitation methods in the treatment of patellar tendinitis. *J Sport Rehabil* 2000; **9**:304–314.
17 Karlsson J, Thomee R, Sward L. Eleven year follow-up of patello-femoral pain syndrome. *Clin J Sport Med* 1996; **6**:22–26.
18 Pellecchia G, Hamel H, Behnke P. Treatment of infrapatellar tendinitis: a combination of modalities and transverse friction massage versus iontophoresis. *J Sport Rehabil* 1994; **3**:315–345.
19 Capasso G, Testa V, Maffulli N, Bifulco G. Aprotinin, corticosteroids and normosaline in the management of patellar tendinopathy in athletes: a prospective randomized study. *Sports Exerc Inj* 1997; **3**:111–115.
20 Alfredson H, Ohberg L. Neovascularisation in chronic painful patellar tendinosis: promising results after sclerosing neovessels outside the tendon challenge the need for surgery. *Knee Surg Sports Traumatol Arthrosc* 2005; **13**:74–80.
21 Kelly DW, Carter VS, Jobe FW, *et al.* Patellar and quadriceps ruptures: jumper's knee. *Am J Sports Med* 1984; **12**:375–380.
22 Khan KM, Visentini PJ, Kiss ZS, *et al.* Correlation of US and MR imaging with clinical outcome after open patellar tenotomy: prospective and retrospective studies. *Clin J Sports Med* 1999; **9**:129–137.
23 Visentini PJ, Khan KM, Cook JL, et al. The VISA score: an index of the severity of jumper's knee (patellar tendinosis). *J Sci Med Sport* 1998; **1**:22–28.
24 Panni A, Tartarone M, Maffuli N. Patellar tendinopathy in athletes: outcome of nonoperative and operative management. *Am J Sports Med* 2000; **28**:392–397.
25 Cook JL, Khan K, Harcourt PR, *et al.* A cross-sectional study of 100 cases of jumper's knee managed conservatively and surgically. *Br J Sports Med* 1997; **31**:332–336.
26 Colosimo AJ, Bassett FH. Jumper's knee: diagnosis and treatment. *Orthop Rev* 1990; **29**:139–149.
27 Ferretti A, Puddu G, Mariani P, Neri M. The natural history of jumper's knee: patellar or quadriceps tendinitis. *Int Orthop* 1985; **8**:239–242.
28 Penderghest C, Kimura I, Gulick D. Double-blind clinical efficacy study of pulsed phonophoresis on perceives pain associated with symptomatic tendinitis. *J Sport Rehabil* 1998; **7**:9–19.
29 Cook JL, Khan KM, Harcourt PR, *et al.* Patellar tendon ultrasonography in asymptomatic active athletes reveals hypoechoic regions: a study of 320 tendons. *Clin J Sports Med* 1998; **8**:73–77.
30 Cook J, Khan K, Kiss S, Purdam C, Griffiths L. Reproducibility and clinical utility of tendon palpation to detect patellar tendinopathy in young basketball players. *Br J Sports Med* 2001; **35**:65–69.
31 McCarty D, Gatter R, Phelps P. A dolorimeter for quantification of articular tenderness. *Arthritis Rheumatol* 1965; **8**:551–559.
32 Young M, Cook J, Purdam C, Kiss ZS, Alfredson H. Conservative treatment of patellar tendinopathy: a 12-month prospective randomised trial comparing two treatment protocols. *Br J Sports Med* 2004; **39**:102–105.
33 Chalmers TC, Smith H Jr, Blackburn B, *et al.* A method for assessing the quality of a randomized control trial. *Control Clin Trials* 1981; **2**:31–49.

CHAPTER 25
How do you treat chronic groin pain?

Peter A. Fricker and Greg Lovell

Introduction

Groin pain presents a problem for both the patient and therapist. Experience shows that diagnoses abound (Table 25.1) and that symptomatology becomes ever more varied and confusing. With increased participation in sport (in terms of duration, frequency, and intensity of activity, and as much by females as males in number), groin pain is a common problem, and it is important for the practitioner to have a reasonable approach to clinical management of the presenting condition.

Necessarily, evidence-based practice is the cornerstone of good management, and this chapter attempts to underpin clinical recommendations with sound research.

We are fortunate that recent improvements in imaging and information processing (and communication) have helped to untangle the knot of musculoskeletal and neurological complaints that affect the groin in athletes. Much of the literature cited in this chapter relies on the association between symptoms and signs and findings in diagnostic imaging, with a diagnosis confirmed by surgery in many cases, or with resolution of the clinical problem after some therapeutic intervention. This is as good as it gets and, although patchy, clinical research is making our understanding of groin pain easier.

Table 25.1 Common causes of groin pain in athletes

- Osteitis pubis
- Incipient direct inguinal hernia (sportsman's hernia, conjoint tendon lesion)
- Adductor muscle strain
- Adductor tendinopathy
- Stress fracture in the inferior pubic ramus
- Osteomyelitis of the pubic ramus or symphysis
- Iliopsoas muscle strain and/or bursitis
- "Snapping hip" syndrome
- Ilioinguinal neuropathy
- Iliohypogastric neuropathy
- Obturator neuropathy
- Rectus femoris strain
- Perthes disease, avascular necrosis of the femoral head
- Slipped femoral capital epiphysis
- Stress fracture in the neck of the femur
- Synovitis, osteoarthritis of the hip joint
- Hip labral and chondral lesions
- Iliolumbar ligament lesion
- Sacroiliac ligament lesion
- Spine pathology (radicular neuropathy, L1–L2 disk pathology, L4–L5 zygapophysial joint pathology)
- Pelvic and lower urinary tract disorders

This chapter outlines the approach taken by the authors to the management of groin pain in athletes and considers the patterns of pain, biomechanical factors, anatomical structures, and diagnostic tests (clinical and technical) that are all relevant. Groin pain in the athlete refers to the discomfort noted around the area of the lower abdomen anteriorly, the inguinal regions, the area of the adductors and perineum and, by extension, the upper anterior thigh and hip. The broad scope of diagnoses is discussed and management plans are outlined. It should be recognized that while there is an emphasis on evidence-based management, much of our practice is still empirical, requiring all of us to pursue an understanding of groin pain through thoughtful scientific endeavor.

Methods

This chapter is an expanded and updated version of papers published in 1991 and 1997,[1,2] an initial literature search using medicine and SportDiscus databases for the period 1990–1997 (February), a literature search using the National Sports Information Center Easy Search (Australian Sports Commission) specifying the period 1982–2000 (December), and a recent literature search using the above databases over 1997–2005 (April). Literature in English was specified, and combinations of keywords used for both the initial review and this chapter included groin pain, athletes, osteitis pubis, conjoint tendon, hernia, adductor, stress fracture, footballers, injury, and imaging. The authors' own collections of papers and personal correspondence have also been used.

References have been selected on the basis of each paper's individual contribution to understanding the nature, pathomechanics, and management of chronic groin pain in athletes. Outcomes of management protocols were especially considered. There have been no meta-analyses (level I grade evidence) in this area and only a few randomized controlled trials (level II). Most recommendations are therefore made on level III and IV evidence. Anecdotal reports were taken into account, but the preference was for larger, well-designed studies.

Background

A thorough understanding of regional anatomy, its relevant functions, and associated patterns of pain is essential. The reader is referred to an excellent review of this subject by O'Brien and Delaney[3] and to reviews particularly on the anatomy of the inguinal area by Skandelakis *et al.*[4] and on adductor longus by Tuite *et al.*[5] Akita *et al.* have also provided a thorough understanding of the cutaneous nerves in the inguinal region.[6] Knowledge of the symphysis pubis, the inguinal canal, the hip joint, and the musculature about the anterior pelvis is fundamental.

An understanding of the normal mechanics and pathomechanics of the pelvis and sacrum is also desirable, because many of the injuries described in this chapter are associated with (if not resultant from) abnormal forces applied around the pelvis. Understanding the behavior of the pelvis in this context sets the template for appropriate treatment, especially where rehabilitation is concerned. Prather[7] has provided a thoughtful and thorough review of pelvis and sacral dysfunction in sports and exercise, and this is also commended to the reader.

Finally, understanding particular aspects of technique peculiar to individual sports lays the groundwork for appropriate diagnosis and management. Familiarity with the range of sports or activities seen in sports medicine clinics is a *sine qua non* for the well-prepared practitioner.

History and examination

Groin pain may originate from muscles, tendons, bursae, fascial structures, nerves, and joints. It may present acutely or otherwise, and may arise from more than one source.[8,9] It may herald a localized injury in the groin, a disease process, or be referred in nature. There have been no reports on the relationship of presenting symptoms and final diagnoses, although one of the authors has suggested a diagnostic framework for differential diagnosis based on specific criteria for the diagnosis of chronic groin pain.[9] Derman has presented several algorithms in his clinic's approach to clinical diagnosis and management of athletes with chronic groin pain.[10] Recently there have been several reports on the reliability and value of examination in athletes with groin pain. In a very good randomized and controlled study (level II) on clinical examination, Holmich *et al.*[11] have shown good intraobserver and interobserver reliability for reproducing groin pain with: 1, bilateral adduction against resistance; 2, palpation of adductor longus, the pubic symphysis, rectus abdominis, and iliopsoas; 3, passive stretching of the adductors and iliopsoas; and 4, functional testing of abdominal muscle strength. The authors noted that strength testing of iliopsoas was not reliable. Verrall *et al.*[12] have described three pain provocation tests (single-leg resisted femoral adduction, "squeeze" test of femoral adduction in hip and knee flexion, and the bilateral resisted femoral adduction test in knee extension and slight hip flexion) as having good predictive value in footballers with pubic groin pain. Croft *et al.* found that measurement of the range of movement of the hip is reliable between medical practitioners when using a plurimeter.[13] Byrd and Jones have indicated that while hip examination is useful for detecting intra-articular hip pathology, it is not able to discriminate between various intra-articular hip lesions.[14] In a study comparing ultrasound and magnetic resonance imaging (MRI) examination with clinical examination for the detection of groin (inguinal) hernia, Van den Berg *et al.* found a sensitivity and specificity of 75% and 96% for clinical examination.[15]

Diagnosis

The pattern of pain is important. Pain that emanates from the area of the pubic symphysis into the area of the lower rectus abdominis, the upper adductors of the thigh, and the scrotum is probably from the symphysis and suggests osteitis pubis.[2] The pathology of this condition is still uncertain, leading some authors to suggest using alternative labels such as "adductor-related groin pain,"[16] "pubic symphysis stress injury,"[17] or "pubic bone stress injury."[18] The pain may be unilateral or bilateral, may involve one or more sites from time to time, and may present acutely or, more often, subacutely or by gradual onset.[2] It typically presents during or after kicking and running, and is seen most often in footballers (soccer and Australian football players), in whom limitation of rotation of the hip is thought to be a contributing factor.[19,20]

A symptom described for osteitis pubis but not commonly seen is that of a painful clicking at the symphysis on certain movements (such as rolling over in bed).[21] It may reflect instability of the symphysis, which is often visible radiographically (in the "flamingo view," discussed below).

Local tenderness of the symphysis, painful resisted hip (femoral) adduction and loss of rotation (particularly internal) of the hips are the hallmark clinical signs of osteitis pubis, and a technetium-99m (^{99m}Tc) bone scan typically shows increased isotope uptake on the delayed views of one or both margins of the symphysis. Plain radiography of the symphysis reveals characteristic changes of widening of the cleft, and erosive changes of either or both symphyseal margins.[22] Changes affect the lower end of the joint initially. Harris and Murray[21] initially noted a relationship between changes at the pubic symphysis and sports activity, and Besjakov *et al.*[23] have confirmed this finding and presented a grading system for the bony radiological changes seen. The "flamingo view" is so called because the patient stands first on one leg and then on the other during plain radiography of the pelvis, to ascertain any shift across the symphysis. This was first described by Chamberlain as evidence for sacroiliac joint slip.[24] Movement across the joint of more than 2 mm is significant[24,25] and heralds pubic instability. This is not an inevitable sequel to osteitis pubis and may be asymptomatic.

MRI of the symphysis has attracted some attention recently. MRI with gadolinium enhancement in athletes with pubic pain revealed lesions of the pubis (characterized by low signal on T1-weighted images, high signal on fat-suppressed T2-weighted images, and enhancement of pubic symphysis cartilage) in those deemed to be affected by chronic microtraumatic osteitis pubis.[26] Another study has reported a good correlation between parasymphysial bone-marrow edema and chronic groin pain, and suggests that a stress injury to the bone may be the source of pain in osteitis pubis.[18] It should, however, be noted that in this study, some of the asymptomatic athletes had significant pubic bone marrow edema on MRI scanning. In a separate study by the same authors, biopsy of the pubic symphysis at the site of bone-marrow edema on MRI found woven bone and no sign of inflammation.[27] MRI of the symphysis in cases of peripartum rupture has also been described.[28] Changes include effusions and hemorrhage within the secondary clefts of symphyseal cartilage and ligaments, with preservation of the surrounding ligaments of the joint. As there may be a subgroup of athletes with osteitis pubis who have a pre-existing obstetric or gynecological history,[2] similar changes may be seen in the athletic context, particularly if the condition has presented acutely.

Osteitis pubis can be a difficult diagnosis in an athlete with chronic groin pain, and recently one author has recommended a protocol to include exclusion of other diagnoses, such as sports hernia (see below), gynecological, urological, and general surgical conditions, and recommends imaging with plain radiographs, flamingo views, and MRI and bone scan results combined with laboratory investigations such as rheumatologic and infection studies.[29] De Paulis *et al.* have stated that their imaging protocol for osteitis pubis is plain radiography with flamingo views and MRI, but with selected computed tomography (CT) in some cases.[30] While the pathophysiological process of osteitis pubis in athletes remains elusive, the diagnosis will inevitably continue to lack an evidence base.

A problem seen often in footballers, and in association with osteitis pubis, is incipient direct inguinal hernia (otherwise known as sportsman's hernia,[31] conjoint tendon lesion[2]) or inguinal groin pain (sometimes termed pubalgia[32] or primary abdominal musculofascial abnormality, PAMA[33]). Pain from a weakness of the posterior wall of the inguinal canal at its medial end is typically local, but it may radiate to the area of the lower rectus abdominis and perhaps to the ventral surface of the scrotum and proximal ventromedial surface of the thigh.[6]

There is local pain, often associated with activity, and tenderness, which is emphasized if the patient half sits up while local pressure is maintained over the area of the medial end of the inguinal canal. There may also be a palpable small direct inguinal hernia at the site.[34] It must be remembered that such hernias may be bilateral.

Investigation is difficult, but promising work has been carried out with ultrasonography, which can demonstrate a defect in the medial posterior inguinal wall in real-time (dynamic) imaging in young (male) athletes with no clinical sign of hernia.[35] Herniography by peritoneal imaging has also proven useful, but this technique is not without morbidity and it is technically demanding.[36,37] When performed, it can demonstrate filling defects in the posterior inguinal wall and can confirm that hernia repair in an athlete is warranted. More recently, MRI has been used in athletes with "unclear" groin pain.[33,38,39] Leander *et al.*[38] found that MRI is not as useful for detecting inguinal wall weakness as herniography but that it is useful for detecting other musculoskeletal abnormalities, while Albers *et al.*[33] found MRI "very important when the diagnosis was ambiguous." The latter group of authors proposed that the bulging of the abdominal wall musculature may represent a very early stage in the continuum of hernia development from incipient hernia to frank hernia. This would accord with the most commonly reported surgical findings, revealing a weakness of the posterior inguinal wall (see the section on management below).

Adductor strain is relatively easy to diagnose. The patient usually provides a clear history of pain at the site of the lesion (usually the adductor longus) associated with activities involving rapid adduction of the thigh—for example, kicking across the body—which may present acutely or with a gradual onset, and which tends not to radiate much beyond the area of injury.[40] Importantly, the clinician must decide whether the injury affects the tenoperiosteal attachment of the upper adductor or involves the musculotendinous junction or muscle belly proper. This distinction is necessary because the management varies. Local tenderness and pain on resisted adduction confirm the diagnosis. Ultrasound imaging can be useful in delineating the lesion, as can MRI,[41] but these are not usually necessary.

Other causes of groin pain include stress fracture of the (usually inferior) pubic ramus[42] and osteomyelitis of the anterior bony pelvis.[43]

Stress fractures typically present as gradually evolving pain and tenderness at the site of the fracture. Most often, the inferior ramus is involved, and the condition is seen in female marathon runners in particular.[42] As with all stress fractures, the cause is repetitive physical activity, and the onset is related to periods of heavy training or competition.

There is local tenderness on examination (which may be nauseating in intensity), and often the patient may complain of pain when standing on one leg (on the ipsilateral side of the lesion).[42] Running and jumping may, of course, be difficult. ^{99m}Tc bone scanning confirms the diagnosis readily in most cases, whereas plain radiography may be unhelpful.

Osteomyelitis is reportedly a rare condition in healthy athletes,[43] but it demands prompt recognition and management. Osteomyelitis of the symphysis is manifest by severe bony pain, local tenderness, and the development of systemic symptoms such as fever, malaise, and lassitude. Pain may radiate across the symphysis and mimic the bilateral pain of osteitis pubis. Weight-bearing becomes difficult. The diagnosis is confirmed by finding positive blood cultures of *Staphylococcus aureus* in particular, or a culture of pathogenic organisms obtained by needle aspiration or open biopsy. In the early stages, the patient may be active, and the erythrocyte sedimentation rate, bone scan, and radiography may be unhelpful.[43]

Bacterial osteitis pubis has also been described.[44] The clinical presentation is similar to that of osteomyelitis, with systemic symptoms, and signs of tenderness and irritability of the symphysis. Radiography may be normal, but blood tests positive for staphylococcus aureus are reported.

Of recent interest has been neurogenic groin pain, and McCrory and Bell have provided an overview of nerve entrapment syndromes of the hip, groin, and buttock.[45] In particular, Lovell[9] discussed the clinical presentation of ilioinguinal neuralgia in a series of athletes with groin pain and noted that the diagnosis is made on finding pain in the area over the iliac fossa, tenderness at the point in the anterior abdominal wall where the ilioinguinal nerve passes through the musculature (near the anterior superior iliac spine), and that injection of 2–5 mL of local anesthetic at this site relieves the pain.

Similarly, entrapment of the iliohypogastric nerve by the external oblique aponeurosis may cause groin pain.[46] In this context, tenderness may be noted just superior to the deep inguinal ring and groin pain may be exacerbated by kicking, rolling over in bed, coughing, and sneezing.

Obturator nerve entrapment has also been described as a cause of groin pain in athletes.[47] This diagnosis relies on noting exercise induced medial thigh pain over the area of the adductors, particularly after kicking and twisting. There may also be adductor muscle weakness and/or paresthesia of the medial thigh after exercise. Electromyography demonstrates chronic denervation changes in the adductor muscles and the lesion is thought to result from nerve compression by fascial entrapment of the obturator nerve where it enters the thigh (at the adductor brevis).

Referred pain, as in radicular neuropathy at the level of L1 or L2 in particular, may manifest as groin pain. Macnab[48] suggests that posterior joint damage produced by degenerative changes of the L4–L5 disk may also produce pain referred to the groin, and more recently Bogduk and Twomey[49] have cited research showing that noxious stimulation of lumbar zygapophysial joints can cause referred pain in various regions of the lower limbs, including the groin.

Bursitis, particularly associated with the iliopsoas muscle of the hip, may also produce groin pain in athletes.[50,51] This structure is irritated by repeated activity involving hip flexors and may therefore be a problem for runners, jumpers, hurdlers, and footballers. The diagnosis of iliopsoas bursitis may be extended to include inflammation of the iliopsoas muscle or tendon,[52] or, if symptoms are acute, a strain of these structures. Inflammation of these structures produces deep groin or anterior hip pain, which the patient finds difficult to localize and the clinician finds frustrating because of the lack of a point of deep tenderness in many cases. Resisted hip flexion may reproduce the symptoms, and a lunge in which the affected groin and hip are forced into extension may be painful. Ultrasound examination of deep hip structures can identify fluid collection at the site of a bursa, and on MRI this is seen as a well-defined area with high signal on T2-weighted images.[53]

"Snapping hip" syndrome is a common condition, characterized by an audible snapping sensation during certain hip movements, but less than one-third of patients have associated pain.[54] Hip intra-articular and extra-articular causes have been described,[51,54] and the final diagnosis will necessarily require a thorough clinical examination and possibly extensive imaging investigation with plain radiography, ultrasound, arthrography, and MRI. Management will be dictated by the determined cause of the hip discomfort.

Rectus femoris strain is easily diagnosed because of this muscle's relatively superficial location and because the history of pain and its whereabouts are usually quite definite.

Local tenderness, irritability of the muscle (with or without evident weakness), and confirmation of the lesion by ultrasonography if needed,[53] all make the diagnosis. Intramuscular tears can be associated with significant bleeding (and the risk of calcification or myositis ossificans), and thorough evaluation of the extent of any injury of this muscle is warranted. Myositis ossificans can be detected early in its course by MRI and later by plain radiography and CT scan.[53]

Hip joint pathology may present as exercise-related groin pain. The differential diagnosis includes Perthes disease and slipped capital femoral epiphysis in the young, synovitis of the hip at all ages, and stress fracture of the neck of femur, osteoarthritis (or osteoarthrosis), and avascular necrosis of the head of the femur in the older patient. The reader is referred to an excellent review of common hip injuries in sport by Boyd *et al.*[55] Recently, hip arthroscopy has been developed and has been found useful for diagnosis and treatment in a number of case series reports on athletes.[56–59] The advent of this technique has opened up a new area of management, to such an extent that a complete review of current hip intra-articular injuries is beyond this chapter; however, the reader is referred to papers by Narvani *et al.* on the features of acetabular labral tears,[60] current indications for hip arthroscopy by Kelly *et al.*,[61] hip arthroscopy technique by Dienst,[62] and hip arthroscopy in athletes by Byrd.[63] The diagnosis depends on a careful history and examination,[64] although several authors have noted that the diagnosis of intra-articular hip lesions is difficult and may require a diagnostic injection of intra-articular anesthetic.[14,58] Overuse contributes to the development of stress fracture and synovitis in particular, while osteoarthritic change is seen in those who have participated in vigorous sports, such as squash, or contact sports such as football or rugby. Perthes disease, slipped capital femoral epiphysis, and avascular necrosis of the head of the femur are notoriously insidious in onset and may only be discovered late, after the development of permanent changes. The universal caution to be aware of the child or adolescent who walks with a limp and complains of leg or knee pain applies.

Appropriate clinical examination includes assessment of hip rotation (both hips), leg length discrepancy, and gait, supported by imaging of the joint by plain radiography, CT scanning, ^{99m}Tc bone scanning, or MRI. Ultrasonography can demonstrate fluid in the hip joint and is therefore useful in diagnosing arthritis or synovitis.[52] Other lesions show morphological changes in the head of the femur and hip joint that are characteristic and well described. Stress fracture of the neck of the femur and avascular necrosis may be discovered by changes on bone scan or MRI early in their development, with radiographic changes evident at later stages.[53]

Kiuru *et al.* have recommended MRI of the pelvis and proximal femur in all patients presenting with stress-related groin pain.[65] In their review of 340 military conscripts, MRI revealed bone stress injuries in 40%, with 60% of those located in the proximal femur. This is perhaps important in the light of several reports of negative bone scans with femoral neck stress fractures,[66–69] and it strongly suggests that MRI should be considered if the clinical suspicion is high.

Posterior pelvic structures such as the iliolumbar ligament and posterior sacroiliac ligaments can also produce groin pain. Lesions of these structures produce local pain, which radiates into the groin and upper adductor areas, as well as down the lateral thigh and posteriorly down the leg in the case of sacroiliac ligament lesions.[70] Diagnosis is made on an appropriate history of low back and/or sacroiliac pain, together with local tenderness of involved ligamentous structures. Local injection of Xylocaine should relieve symptoms and confirm the diagnosis.

Other causes of groin pain include pelvic, gynecological, and urinary tract conditions. Some conditions occur commonly, and athletes are prone to the same range of ills as the rest of the population.

Management

Once the diagnosis has been made, there are useful steps in management for each clinical situation.

Osteitis pubis is perhaps the most difficult of the groin problems. The following regimen suggests a number of positive measures which may assist the affected athlete's outlook as much as their recovery. Firstly, osteitis pubis is a self-limited disease, and every patient should expect to get better.[2,22] Secondly, it is as yet unclear whether continued activity delays recovery, and so, at least for now, patients can be encouraged to maintain activity for fitness, such as swimming, cycling, and rowing, while avoiding those activities that are painful or that may worsen the condition (or delay recovery), such as vigorous kicking or lots of running. Running in deep water ("pool running") may be a useful substitute for athletes wanting to maintain running fitness. Rodriguez *et al.* recently described a clinical grading system (I, mild to IV, severe) used in their series of 44 cases and found a marked difference in return- to sport-times with the different grades of injury.[71] They found average times of return to sport of 3.8 weeks in 25 grade I cases, 6.7 weeks in nine grade II cases, and 10 weeks in their one grade III case, while the nine grade IV cases required surgical intervention. This would suggest that early intervention may be worthwhile and that this condition would fit with a bone stress injury model. In the only randomized controlled trial on rehabilitation, Holmich *et al.* have provided strong evidence for an active treatment protocol aimed at improving strength and coordination of the pelvic musculature.[72] Although the authors preferred the term adductor-related groin pain, all the patients in this study had evidence suggestive of osteitis pubis either clinically or on investigation. A more thorough description of the exercise program was presented in 2000, with avoidance of pain recommended as an important indicator of exercise progression.[73] This program consisted of two phases over 8–12 weeks. The initial phase involved two static and two dynamic adductor exercises three times a week. The second phase consisted of an additional seven exercises involving the hip adductors, abductors, flexors and extensors, the lower back and side-skating movements three times per week. No stretching of the adductors was allowed, and if exercises were painful the intensity was reduced. Jogging was allowed after 6 weeks, provided it did not provoke pain. A similar program has also been described by Hogan, along with clinical criteria for assessment of exercise progression.[74,75] Further, an EMG study by Cowan *et al.* has shown that transversus abdominis activation onset is delayed in athletes with chronic groin pain;[76] lower abdominal exercise retraining may therefore be important in osteitis pubis rehabilitation. These programs have now laid the foundation for a consistent conservative program of exercise progression, with return to sport over 3–5 months.

Most authors feel that improving flexibility of the hips (especially in rotation) is vital, as is correcting any limitation of movement in the sacroiliac or lumbosacral joints (which promotes excess movement at the symphysis),[7] however in the only randomized controlled trial, Holmich *et al.*[72] noted in the active treatment group that hip range of motion returned to normal without specific stretching exercises.

Wearing supportive compressive shorts has been shown by McKim and Taunton to significantly reduce groin pain and would therefore be a useful adjunct in the recovery phase of osteitis pubis.[77]

Medication for osteitis pubis is contentious, but most authors recommend at least a short trial of nonsteroidal anti-inflammatory drugs.[2]

Corticosteroid treatment (either by injection or orally) could be counterproductive. Corticosteroids are catabolic, and there is at least the theoretical risk of loosening the symphysis by using these agents. Corticosteroid injection to the symphysis of athletes in the acute phase (less than 2 weeks) of osteitis pubis may hasten recovery;[78] O'Connell *et al.*[79] felt that injection was useful for both diagnosis and treatment in 16 athletes with osteitis pubis, but larger studies need to be carried out to confirm these findings.

A recent pilot study has reported a very positive effect on return to sport when dextrose was injected into the thigh adductor origins, suprapubic abdominal insertions, and pubic symphysis in athletes with chronic groin pain.[80] This study was not controlled or randomized, and imaging data were not presented; the authors note that while these results are promising, larger controlled trials are needed. Similarly, Maksymowych *et al.* reported on the successful use of intravenous pamidronate in three (nonathletic) patients with refractory symphysitis pubis.[81] A recent case report on the treatment of tibial stress fractures with this treatment[82] would suggest that a formal trial of bisphosphonate therapy in osteitis pubis may be worthwhile.

The role of surgery in the management of osteitis pubis is also debated. In a thoughtful paper by Williams *et al.*,[83] seven rugby players who had undergone at least 13 months of nonoperative therapy were provided with arthrodesis of the pubic symphysis by bone grafting, supplemented by a compression plate. At a mean follow-up of 52.4 months (range 10 months to 12 years), all of the patients were free of symptoms and flamingo views were normal, implying no pubic instability. The mean time to return of full match fitness was 6.6 months (range 5–9 months). The authors pointed out that arthrodesis was to be a last resort after failed nonoperative measures had been undertaken.

Wedge resection of the symphysis has also been described for the management of osteitis pubis,[84] but this report refers to an older, nonsporting, female cohort of subjects. In addition, three of the patients were not satisfied with their result and one other required a further procedure to stabilize the sacroiliac joints for painful posterior instability. This latter complication has also been cited by Moore *et al.*[85] in reference to resection of the symphysis for the treatment of osteitis pubis. In a report on two cases of recalcitrant groin pain, Mulhall *et al.*[86] have described successful curettage of the symphysis as a promising procedure requiring limited surgical exposure and with the potential for early return to sport, while Paajanen *et al.* have described a novel approach using a preperitoneal retropubic mesh insertioplasty successfully in five athletes with osteitis pubis.[87]

Most cases of osteitis pubis resolve with a structured rehabilitation program, although delineation of the prognostic implications for athletes with pubic instability apart from those with osteitis pubis would be very useful but has not yet been reported. All authors have noted that surgical intervention should only be considered for cases that are disabling and recalcitrant to conservative measures and after a thorough work-up, such as described by Mandelbaum and Mora.[29] Although the evidence is limited and it is clear that the role of surgery needs cautious definition, symphyseal curettage or the placement of retropubic mesh would appear to be the most promising procedures in recalcitrant cases of osteitis

pubis while arthrodesis and bone grafting is more suitable for patients with disabling pubic instability.

Lesions of the inguinal canal do not appear to recover in athletes who continue their athletic activity. In a study assessing abdominal muscle strength in 16 patients (males less than 40 years of age) with "posterior abdominal wall deficiency," Hemingway *et al.* found a significant abdominal oblique strength deficit that improved after surgical open mesh repair and a 6-week abdominal and hip exercise program.[88] Despite considerable controversy,[89] there is no doubt that surgery is effective for such patients, with return to activity in about 6 weeks.[31,90] These early reports of surgical success have been followed by over 20 successful (but uncontrolled) case series reports. More importantly, Ekstrand and Ringborg[91] have now provided clear evidence of benefit in a randomized, controlled (level II) study comparing surgical intervention (Bassini-type repair with ilioinguinal and iliohypogastric neurectomy), two rehabilitation groups, and a control group. In this study, the surgical intervention group showed a marked benefit in reduction of symptoms at 3 and 6 months' follow-up, while none of the conservatively managed groups improved over the trial period. In a study comparing open and laparoscopic inguinal repair procedures, Ingolby showed that both were effective, although the return to sport was faster in the laparoscopic group.[92] More recently, endoscopic preperitoneal procedures have also been described in athletes.[93,94] From the numerous case series reports, the most common surgical finding has been a weakness of the posterior inguinal wall, which can be strengthened using different surgical procedures. There is also the question of whether repair of an asymptomatic posterior wall defect should be performed for those who have been investigated for groin pain and for whom such an incidental finding has been reported. This may occur particularly in athletes with one symptomatic lesion but with bilateral defects evident on imaging studies. If repair is advised for the symptomatic lesion, then bilateral repair is probably appropriate, given the natural history of the condition. Some authors have also described performing adductor tenotomy at the same time as repair to the inguinal/rectus abdominis region, with good results.[95–97]

Adductor strain is treated differently depending on the site of the lesion, either at the tenoperiosteal attachment or within the muscle (the musculotendinous junction or muscle belly). Despite the common occurrence of adductor strains, there are no evidence-based reports on the management of acute or chronic adductor injuries. Acute strain at the tenoperiosteal attachment should be rested until pain and local tenderness have settled, with gentle stretching and strengthening to follow over a period of weeks. Running or sprinting should be encouraged as symptoms permit, with rapid changes of direction and kicking introduced towards the end of recovery.

Muscle strain within the belly or at the musculotendinous junction can be managed more aggressively, provided bleeding has been stopped and the risks of muscle hematoma, calcification, or myositis ossificans have been addressed appropriately. Stretching, strengthening, and the return to activity follow standard practice guidelines for the management of muscle injury.[98,99] Nicholas and Tyler have suggested a specific three-phase program which, although anecdotal, appears to be effective.[100] This consisted of an acute phase of tissue injury management with early submaximal isometric adduction exercises, followed by more specific concentric and eccentric adductor exercises before a final sport-specific rehabilitation phase. A recent paper[72] on the effectiveness of active physical training as treatment for long-standing (median 9 months) adductor-related groin pain in athletes, which did not differentiate between chronic adductor tendon injuries and osteitis pubis, found that active exercises that involved strengthening (but not stretching) and muscular coordination to improve postural stability of the pelvis was better than physiotherapy that included stretching, massage, heat or cold application, and ultrasound therapy. Interestingly, as noted earlier, the range of motion at the hip improved in the "nonstretching" group as much as in those who stretched.

Nonsteroidal anti-inflammatory drugs and corticosteroid injections may be used judiciously when inflammation is apparent, but it should be recognized that there is no clinical evidence to recommend their use *per se*.[101]

Successful surgical intervention with adductor tenotomy in the management of chronic groin pain has been described in only a small number of published case series reports in the English-language literature.[95–97,102] Furthermore, as noted above, several of these studies have included inguinal surgery as part of the same procedure, thus making evidence-based recommendations difficult.[95–97]

Stress fractures of the inferior pubic ramus settle over 2–5 months with rest from running.[103] Stress fracture of the neck of femur demands prompt attention, vigilance, and caution. Stress fracture of the upper cortex of the neck of femur requires immediate non-weight-bearing (bed rest) and orthopedic attention to guard against the risk of complete fracture, displacement, and avascular necrosis of the femoral head.[104] Stress fracture of the inferior cortex requires non-weight-bearing on crutches for 3–4 weeks, followed by gradual resumption of full weight-bearing over the ensuing weeks.[55]

Osteomyelitis is managed according to standard principles and involves the appropriate use of specific antibiotics, both intravenously and orally, supported by bed rest as necessary and analgesics. Surgery may be required where conservative measures fail. Return to sport is usually delayed and averages about 5 months.[43]

Nerve entrapments are relieved by appropriate surgical decompression (for a definitive cure). This applies particularly to the obturator neuropathy described above, whereby the thick fascia overlying the adductor brevis anteriorly is divided.[47] Ilioinguinal nerve entrapment can respond to decompression, and neurolysis if necessary,[105,106] and repair of the external oblique aponeurosis has been advocated for relief of symptoms attributed to associated entrapment of the terminal branches of the iliohypogastric nerve.[46]

The management of spinal conditions that contribute to groin pain is beyond the scope of this chapter, but there are many excellent texts available on this subject.

Iliopsoas muscle strain and associated bursitis are managed by anti-inflammatory medication and modalities, together with appropriate stretching and strengthening of the iliopsoas muscles as outlined by Dahan.[99] Surgery to the iliopsoas tendon and bursa has been shown to be effective in recalcitrant cases.[107,108] Corticosteroid injection can be tried, but difficulty in placement of the injection would require this procedure to be done under direct imaging. Return to activities such as kicking and lunging should be cautious and promoted carefully within the limits of pain. Again, there is little evidence to support treatment guidelines, but Johnston *et al.* have provided a good review of the current diagnosis and management of iliopsoas bursitis and tendonitis.[51]

Strain of the rectus femoris is managed along the principles outlined above, with similar precautions applied to the return to kicking or jumping movements. Hematomas in the quadriceps complex must be managed carefully to minimize rebleeding and/or calcification (myositis ossificans). This implies appropriate anti-inflammatory medication (typically 6 weeks of indomethacin) and modalities, and the avoidance of premature stretching (particularly passive stretching) and of vigorous massage in particular.[55]

Hip joint pathology should involve early referral to an orthopedic surgeon for the management of Perthes disease, avascular necrosis of the head of the femur, slipped femoral capital epiphysis, and stress fracture of the neck of femur. All of these conditions are prone to debilitating sequelae and should never be underestimated. Conservative management can be tried in many of these conditions but the decision to intervene surgically is critical and not for the inexperienced or untrained practitioner.

Synovitis of the hip can be managed with rest and anti-inflammatory modalities, but the clinician must always have a diagnosis in mind. Synovitis of the hip is often secondary to a disease process and not necessarily an overuse or benign self-limiting condition. The management of osteoarthritis of the hip depends on the clinical state of the joint and can vary from simple measures of appropriate symptom relief and rehabilitative exercise (for strength and flexibility), to surgical intervention and joint replacement.[55] Successful management of intra-articular hip lesions such as labral tears and chondral injuries has been described in recent case reports,[56,57] but Byrd has noted that little is understood about their natural history, that it is unknown whether early diagnosis requires early intervention, and that it is uncertain whether lesions identified on MRI may settle and become asymptomatic.[63] Despite this, this is an exciting new field that will hopefully develop some good evidence-based management.

Management of posterior pelvic problems such as iliolumbar ligament sprain and posterior sacroiliac ligament sprain depends upon attention to causative factors such as trauma and/or faulty mechanics, together with the traditional forms of therapy including mobilization, soft-tissue massage, and anti-inflammatory modalities. Sacroiliac hypermobility is a difficult problem, and prolotherapy (to induce fibrosis of ligaments and thus restrict joint motion) has been proposed, but no prospective controlled studies exist to substantiate this recommendation. Management of sacroiliac dysfunction is discussed more fully by Prather.[7]

Risk factors

Identifying risk factors for specific injuries is always difficult and sometimes controversial, and this has not been any different for injuries to the groin region. Most of the studies have looked at the risk factors for adductor strain injuries. The main risk factors that have been identified in a number of prospective cohort studies are reduced hip adduction strength[109,110] (although contradictory findings were reported in one study[111]), reduced hip abduction,[112,113] pre-existing groin injury,[110–112] low levels of preseason sports specific training,[111] reduced strength ratio of hip muscles,[110,114] increased body mass[114] and decreased femur diameter.[114]

Conclusions

Groin pain in the athlete is a difficult clinical problem because of the range of possible diagnoses. Much of the "theory" of groin pain is based on supposition and assumption, with little clinical evidence to validate the therapeutic interventions currently employed in management. Nevertheless, the clinician should be prepared to apply the principles outlined in this chapter to provide relief if not a cure to the majority of patients.

The recommended diagnostic approach is anatomical, supported by judicious selection of diagnostic imaging techniques. Understanding the biomechanics of sport, and therefore possible pathomechanics, as presented by each patient then provides a direction for management in terms of prescribed rest (or modified activity), technique correction and a measure of recovery (in terms of return of normal function).

Treatment modalities such as anti-inflammatory medication, corticosteroid injection, electrotherapy devices, local applications of cold and heat, and the manual techniques of physiotherapy must all be considered in context. Anti-inflammatory modalities have their place relatively early in the period of recovery, whilst stretching and strengthening of injured tissue or muscle that has been affected by disuse must be prescribed carefully to allow for healing and promote normal function as early as possible.

Return to sport must only take place once normal function has been demonstrated.

If return to full activity is impossible despite optimal therapy—then surgery may be considered. A complete post-operative rehabilitation program is implicit.

Patients should be reminded that there are no short cuts and precipitate return to sport is not worth the risk in most cases.

Summary: groin pain in athletes

- Groin pain is common and affects male and female athletes.
- Groin pain may result from a number of simultaneous conditions.
- Radiography, ultrasound, ^{99m}Tc bone scanning, CT, and MRI may be helpful in confirming a diagnosis.
- Understanding sport techniques is an important part of diagnosis and planning rehabilitation.
- Beware of hip disease manifesting as groin pain.

Summary: radiological investigation for groin pain

- Plain radiography and flamingo views are useful investigations for bony pathology and pubic instability.
- ^{99m}Tc triple-phase bone scan is useful for stress fractures, osteomyelitis and osteitis pubis.
- Ultrasound examination is useful for sportsman's hernia, musculotendinous injuries and bursitis/synovitis.
- MRI may help in difficult cases in which bone edema is involved (osteitis pubis, stress fracture), in muscle/tendon injuries and in hip injuries.

Key messages

- Groin pain can be difficult to manage and can involve multiple pathologies.
- Appropriate clinical examination and investigation will determine the best approach to a sound management plan.
- Current evidence supports a conservative rehabilitation program for osteitis pubis or adductor-related groin pain and a surgical approach for the management of inguinal pathology.
- Both nonsteroidal anti-inflammatory drugs and corticosteroids (particularly via local injection) have an adjunctive role at best in the management of specific conditions.
- Hip arthroscopy is providing an additional tool for the diagnosis and management of athletes with hip-related groin pain.
- A wide range of risk factors have been identified, but more evaluation is required in order to provide clinicians with preventative strategies for groin injuries.

Sample examination questions

Multiple-choice questions (answers on page 602)

1 Sportsman's hernia:
  A Refers to a tear of the rectus abdominis muscle
  B May be seen on ultrasound examination
  C Usually affects the medial end of the inguinal canal
  D Is an indirect incipient inguinal hernia
  E Responds well to surgical repair in athletes

2 Osteitis pubis:
  A Presents in males and females in equal numbers
  B Is a result of overuse rather than acute injury
  C Is characterized by pain radiating into the medial thigh and scrotum
  D Is always bilateral
  E None of the above

3 Imaging in groin pain:
  A May involve peritoneal imaging in the diagnosis of sportsman's hernia
  B Is best done with MRI rather than CT scan
  C May use ultrasound imaging for the diagnosis of bursitis
  D None of the above
  E All of the above

Essay questions

1 Briefly outline the symptoms and signs that differentiate osteitis pubis from sportsman's hernia (incipient inguinal hernia) in a 25-year-old male soccer player.
2 Briefly outline the diagnostic features of adductor muscle injury and indicate which imaging techniques might be useful.
3 What is a "flamingo view" and why is it done?

Case study 25.1

A 19-year-old 10-km runner has recently increased his mileage from 50 km per week to 100 km per week and has developed an ache from the perineum into the left adductor area. He has noted this ache is gradually worsening over recent weeks. There is some discomfort and tenderness around the symphysis pubis and medial inferior ramus on the left at rest. There is no history of fever, weight loss, acute episodes of pain, or recent trauma.

(Differential diagnosis: osteitis pubis, stress fracture of the pubic ramus, osteomyelitis, tumor).

Summarizing the evidence

Recommendation (see text)	Grade of evidence
• An active training program is effective in comparison with a conventional physiotherapy program (without active training) in the treatment of adductor related groin pain in athletes	A
• Surgical repair of the inguinal wall is of significant benefit in comparison with rest or active rehabilitation programs in athletes with groin pain from sports hernia/incipient inguinal hernia	A
• Compression shorts are a useful adjunct in the rehabilitation and management of athletes recovering from osteitis pubis	A
• Examination techniques of the groin are reliable	A
• A grading scale of radiographic findings for changes at the pubic symphysis may be a useful descriptive tool for physicians and radiologists	B
• Radiological studies (plain radiography, flamingo views, bone scan, ultrasound, herniography and MRI) are useful investigations in athletes with hip and groin pain	B
• Athletes with chronic groin pain may have multiple pathologies contributing to their groin pain	B
• Risk factors for groin injuries include: reduced hip adduction strength, reduced hip abduction range, preexisting groin injury, low levels of preseason sport-specific training, change in the strength ratio of the hip muscles, increased body mass, and decreased femur diameter	B
• Drug therapy that may be useful in osteitis pubis includes NSAIDs, corticosteroids, bisphosphonates, dextrose prolotherapy	C/D
• Surgery may be useful for recalcitrant pain in adductor tendinopathy, osteitis pubis or pubic symphysis instability	C/D
• Hip arthroscopy is a useful method for diagnosis and treatment of athletes with groin pain from intra-articular hip disorders	C/D
• Diagnostic nerve or injury site local anesthetic blocks may be useful	C/D

MRI, magnetic resonance imaging; NSAID, nonsteroidal anti-inflammatory drugs.

References

1 Fricker PA. Management of groin pain in athletes. *Br J Sports Med* 1997; **31**(2):97–101.
2 Fricker PA, Taunton JE, Amman W. Osteitis pubis in athletes: infection, inflammation or injury? *Sports Med* 1991; **12**:266–279.
3 O'Brien M, Delaney M. The anatomy of the hip and groin. *Sports Med Arthrosc Rev* 1997; **5**:252–267.
4 Skandalakis JE, Gray SW, Skandalakis LJ, *et al.* Surgical anatomy of the inguinal area. *World J Surg* 1989; **13**:490–498.
5 Tuite DJ, Finnegan PJ, Saliaris AP, *et al.* Anatomy of the proximal musculotendinous junction of the adductor longus muscle. *Knee Surg Sports Traumatol Arthrosc* 1998; **6**:134–137.

6 Akita K, Niga S, Yamato Y, *et al.* Anatomic basis of chronic groin pain with special reference to sports hernia. *Surg Radiol Anat* 1999; **21**:1–5.
7 Prather H. Pelvis and sacral dysfunction in sports and exercise. *Phys Med Rehab Clin North Am* 2000; **11**(4):805–836.
8 Ekberg O, Persson NH, Abrahamsson P, *et al.* Longstanding groin pain in athletes. A multidisciplinary approach. *Sports Med* 1988; **6**:56–61.
9 Lovell G. The diagnosis of chronic groin pain in athletes: a review of 189 cases. *Aust J Sci Med Sport* 1995; **27**:76–79.
10 Derman WE. A clinical approach to chronic groin pain in the adult athlete. *Int Sportmed J* 2000; **1**(1) March.
11 Holmich P, Holmich LR, Bjerg AM. Clinical examination of athletes with groin pain: an intraobserver and interobserver reliability study. *Br J Sports Med* 2004; **38**:446–451.
12 Verrall GM, Slavotinek JP, Barnes PG, *et al.* Description of pain provocation tests used for the diagnosis of sports-related chronic groin pain: relationship of tests to defined clinical (pain and tenderness) and MRI (pubic bone marrow oedema) criteria. *Scand J Med Sci Sports* 2005; **15**:36–42.
13 Croft PR, Nahit ES, Macfarlane GJ, *et al.* Interobserver reliability in measuring flexion, internal rotation, and external rotation of the hip using a plurimeter. *Ann Rheum Dis* 1996; **55**:320–323.
14 Byrd JW, Jones KS. Diagnostic accuracy of clinical assessment, magnetic resonance imaging, magnetic resonance arthrography, and intra-articular injection in hip arthroscopy patients. *Am J Sports Med* 2004; **32**:1668–1674.
15 Van den Berg JC, De Valois JC, Go PMNYH, *et al.* Detection of groin hernia with physical examination, ultrasound, and MRI compared with laparoscopic findings. *Investig Radiol* 1999; **34**:739–743.
16 Holmich P. Adductor-related groin pain in athletes. *Sports Med Arthrosc Rev* 1997; **5**:285–291.
17 Miller C, Major N, Toth A. Pelvic stress injuries in the athlete. *Sports Med* 2003; **33**:1003–1012.
18 Verrall GM, Slavotnik JP, Fon GT. Incidence of pubic bone marrow oedema in Australian Rules football players: relation to groin pain. *Br J Sports Med* 2001; **35**:28–33.
19 Williams JGP. Limitation of hip joint movement as a factor in traumatic osteitis pubis. *Br J Sports Med* 1978; **12**:129–133.
20 Verrall GM, Hamilton IA, Slavotnik JP, *et al.* Hip joint range of motion reduction in sports-related chronic groin injury diagnosed as pubic bone stress injury. *J Sci Med Sport* 2005; **8**:77–84.
21 Harris NH, Murray RO. Lesions of the symphysis in athletes. *Br Med J* 1974; **4**:211–214.
22 Coventry MB, Mitchell WC. Osteitis pubis. observations based on a study of 45 patients. *J Am Med Assoc* 1961; **178**:898–905.
23 Besjakov J, von Scheele C, Ekberg O, *et al.* Grading scale of radiographic findings in the pubic bone and symphysis in athletes. *Acta Radiol* 2003; **44**:79–83.
24 Chamberlain EW. The symphysis pubis in the roentgen examination of the sacro-iliac joint. *Am J R* 1930; **24**:621–625.
25 Walheim G, Olerud S, Ribbe T. Mobility of the pubic symphysis: measurements by an electromechanical method. *Acta Orthop Scand* 1984; **55**:203–208.
26 Ghebontni L, Roger B, Christel P, *et al.* Pubalgie du sportif: interêt de l'IRM dans le démembrement des lésions. *J Traumatol Sport* 1996; **13**:86–93.
27 Verrall GM, Oakeshott RD, Henry LW, *et al.* Bone biopsy of the parasymphyseal region of athletes with osteitis pubis diagnosed by MRI demonstrates new woven bone formation. *Aust J Sci Med Sport* 2003; **6**:S95.
28 Jurzel RB, Au AH, Rooholamini SA, *et al.* Magnetic resonance imaging of peripartum rupture of the symphysis pubis. *Obstet Gynecol* 1996; **87**:826–829.
29 Mandelbaum B, Mora SA. Osteitis pubis. *Oper Tech Sports Med* 2005; **13**:62–67.
30 De Paulis F, Cacchio A, Michelini O, *et al.* R Sports injuries in the pelvis and hip: diagnostic imaging. *Eur J Radiol* 1998; **27**:S49–S59.
31 Malycha P, Lovell G. Inguinal surgery in athletes with chronic groin pain: the "sportsman's" hernia. *Aust N Z J Surg* 1992; **62**:123–125.
32 Taylor DC, Meyers WC, Moylan JA, *et al.* Abdominal musculature abnormalities as a cause of groin pain in athletes: inguinal hernias and pubalgia. *Am J Sports Med* 1991; **19**:239–242.
33 Albers SL, Spritzer CE, Garrett WE, *et al.* MR findings in athletes with pubalgia. *Skelet Radiol* 2001; **30**:270–271.

34 Hackney RG. The sports hernia: a cause of chronic groin pain. *Br J Sports Med* 1993; **27**:58–62.
35 Orchard JW, Read JW, Neophyton J, *et al.* Groin pain associated with ultrasound finding of inguinal canal posterior wall deficiency in Australian Rules footballers. *Br J Sports Med* 1998; **32**:134–139.
36 Gullmo A. Herniography. *World J Surg* 1989; **13**:560–568.
37 Ekberg O, Kesek P, Besjakov J. Herniography and magnetic resonance imaging in athletes with chronic groin pain. *Sports Med Arthrosc Rev* 1997; **5**:274–279.
38 Leander P, Ekberg O, Sjöberg S, *et al.* MR imaging following herniography in patients with unclear groin pain. *Eur Radiol* 2000; **10**:1691–1696.
39 Robinson P, Barron DA, Parsons W, *et al.* Adductor related groin pain in athletes: correlation of MR imaging with clinical findings. *Skeletal Radiology* 2004; **33**:451–457.
40 Karlsson J, Sward L, Kalebo P, *et al.* Chronic groin injuries in athletes: recommendations for treatment and rehabilitation. *Sports Med* 1994; **17**:141–148.
41 Renstrom PAFH. Groin injuries: a true challenge in orthopaedic sports medicine. *Sports Med Arthrosc Rev* 1997; **5**:247–251.
42 Noakes TD, Smith JA, Lindenberg GM, *et al.* Pelvic stress fractures in long distance runners. *Am J Sports Med* 1985; **13**:120–123.
43 Karpos PA, Spindler KP, Pierce MA, *et al.* Osteomyelitis of the pubic symphysis in athletes: a case report and literature review. *Med Sci Sports Exerc* 1995; **27**:473–478.
44 Combs JA. Bacterial osteitis pubis in a weight lifter without invasive trauma. *Med Sci Sports Exerc* 1998; **30**:1561–1563.
45 McCrory P, Bell S. Nerve entrapment syndromes as a cause of pain in the hip, groin and buttock. *Sports Med* 1999; **27**:261–274.
46 Ziprin P, Williams P, Foster ME. External oblique aponeurosis nerve entrapment as a cause of groin pain in the athlete. *Br J Surg* 1999; **86**:566–568.
47 Bradshaw C, McCrory P, Bell S, *et al.* Obturator nerve entrapment. A cause of groin pain in athletes. *Am J Sports Med* 1997; **25**:402–408.
48 Macnab I. *Backache*. Baltimore: Williams and Wilkins, 1979: 91.
49 Bogduk N, Twomey LT. *Clinical Anatomy of the Lumbar Spine*, 2nd ed. Melbourne: Churchill Livingstone, 1991: 154.
50 Peterson L, Renström P. *Sports Injuries: Their Prevention and Treatment.* North Ryde, NSW: Methuen Australia, 1986: 265.
51 Johnston CAM, Wiley JP, Lindsay DM, *et al.* Iliospoas bursitis and tendinitis. *Sports Med* 1998; **25**:271–283.
52 Roos HP. Hip pain in sport. *Sports Med Arthrosc Rev* 1997;**5**:292–300.
53 Karlsson J, Jerre R. The use of radiography, magnetic resonance, and ultrasound in the diagnosis of hip, pelvis and groin injuries. *Sports Med Arthrosc Rev* 1997; **5**:268–273.
54 Reid DC. *Sports Injury Assessment and Rehabilitation.* New York: Churchill Livingstone, 1992: 626–627.
55 Boyd KT, Peirce NS, Batt ME. Common hip injuries in sport. *Sports Med* 1997; **24**:273–288.
56 McCarthy J, Barsoum W, Puri L, *et al.* The role of hip arthroscopy in the elite athlete. *Clin Orthop Rel Res* 2003; **406**:71–74.
57 Narvani AA, Tsiridis E, Kendall S, *et al.* A preliminary report on prevalence of acetabular labrum tears in sports patients with groin pain. *Knee Surg Sports Traumatol* 2003; **11**:403–408.
58 Mitchell B, McCrory P, Brukner P, *et al.* Hip joint pathology: clinical presentation and correlation between magnetic resonance arthrography, ultrasound and arthroscopic findings in 25 cases. *Clin J Sports Med* 2003; **13**:152–156.
59 Saw T, Villar R. Footballer's hip: a report of six cases. *J Bone Joint Surg Br* 2004; **86**:655–658.
60 Narvani AA, Tsiridis C, Tai CC, *et al.* Acetabular labrum and its tears. *Br J Sports Med* 2003; **37**:207–211.
61 Kelly BT, Williams RJ, Philippon MJ. Hip arthroscopy: current indications, treatment options, and management issues. *Am J Sports Med* 2003; **31**:1020–1037.
62 Dienst M. Hip arthroscopy: technique and anatomy. *J Oper Tech Sports Med* 2005; **13**:13–23.
63 Byrd JW. Hip arthroscopy in athletes. *J Oper Tech Sports Med* 2005; **13**:24–36.
64 Safran M. Evaluation of the hip: history, physical examination, and imaging. *J Oper Tech Sports Med* 2005; **13**:2–12.

65 Kiuru MJ, Pihlajamaki HK, Ahovuo JA. Fatigue stress injuries of the pelvic bones and proximal femur: evaluation with MR imaging. *Eur Radiol* 2003; **13**:605–611.
66 Wen DY, Propeck T, Singh A. Femoral neck stress injury with negative bone scan. *J Am Board Fam Pract* 2003; **16**:170–174.
67 Keene JS, Lash EG. Negative bone scan in a femoral neck stress fracture: a case report. *Am J Sports Med* 1992; **20**:234–236.
68 Sterling JC, Webb RF, Myers MC, *et al.* False negative bone scan in a female runner. *Med Sci Sports Exerc* 1993; **25**:179–185.
69 Bal BS, Sandow T. Bilateral femoral neck fractures with negative bone scans. *Orthopaedics* 1996; **19**:974–976.
70 Hackett GS. *Ligament and Tendon Relaxation Treated by Prolotherapy*, 3rd ed. Springfield, IL: Thomas, 1958: 27–28.
71 Rodriguez C, Miguel A, Lima H, *et al.* Osteitis pubis syndrome in the professional soccer athlete: a case report. *J Athl Train* 2001; **36**:437–440.
72 Holmich P, Uhrskou P, Ulnits L, *et al.* Effectiveness of active physical training as treatment for long-standing adductor-related groin pain in athletes: randomised trial. *Lancet* 1999; **353**:439–443.
73 Holmich P. Exercise rehabilitation for chronic groin pain in athletes. *Int Sportmed J* 2000; **1**:1–5.
74 Hogan A. A rehabilitation model for pubic symphysis injuries. In: Sports Medicine Australia, eds. *Australian Conference of Science and Medicine in Sport (Abstracts)*. Adelaide: Sports Medicine Australia, 1998: 143.
75 Hogan A, Lovell G. Pubic stress tests and rehabilitation of osteitis pubis: key reassessment criteria. In: Reilly T, ed. *Science and Football IV: Proceedings of the Sports Medicine Annual Conference (SA Branch)*. London: Routledge, 2002: 207–211.
76 Cowan S, Schache AG, Brukner P, *et al.* Delayed onset of transversus abdominis in long-standing groin pain. *Med Sci Sports Exerc* 2004; **36**:2040–2045.
77 McKim KR, Taunton JE. The effectiveness of compression shorts in the treatment of athletes with osteitis pubis. *NZ J Sports Med* 2001; **29**:70–73.
78 Holt MA, Keene JS, Graf BK, *et al.* Treatment of osteitis pubis in athletes: results of corticosteroid injections. *Am J Sports Med* 1995; **23**:601–606.
79 O'Connell MJ, Powell T, McCaffrey NM, *et al.* Symphyseal cleft injection in the diagnosis and treatment of osteitis pubis in athletes. *AJR Am J Roentgenol* 2002; **179**:955–959.
80 Topol GA, Reeves KD, Hassanein KM. Efficacy of dextrose prolotherapy in elite male kicking-sport athletes with chronic groin pain. *Arch Phys Med Rehabil* 2005; **86**:697–702.
81 Maksymowych WP, Aaron SL, Russell AS. Treatment of refractory symphysitis pubis with intravenous pamidronate. *J Rheumatol* 2001; **28**:2754–2757.
82 Stewart GW, Brunet ME, Manning MR, *et al.* Treatment of stress fractures in athletes with intravenous pamidronate. *Clin J Sports Med* 2005; **15**:92–94.
83 Williams PR, Thomas DP, Downes EM. Osteitis pubis and instability of the pubic symphysis: when operative measures fail. *Am J Sports Med* 2000; **28**:50–55.
84 Grace JN, Sim FH, Shives TC, *et al.* Wedge resection of the symphysis pubis for the treatment of osteitis pubis. *J Bone Joint Surg Am* 1989; **71**:358–364.
85 Moore RS Jr, Stover MD, Matta JM. Late posterior instability of the pelvis after resection of the symphysis pubis for the treatment of osteitis pubis: a report of two cases. *J Bone Joint Surg Am* 1998; **80**:1043–1048.
86 Mulhall KJ, McKenna J, Walsh A, *et al.* Osteitis pubis in professional soccer players: a report of outcome with symphyseal curettage in cases refractory to conservative management. *Clin J Sports Med* 2002; **12**:179–181.
87 Paajanen H, Heikkinen J, Hermunen H, Airo I. Successful treatment of osteitis pubis by using totally extraperitoneal endoscopic technique. *Int J Sports Med* 2005; **26**:303–306.
88 Hemingway AE, Herrington L, Blower AL. Changes in muscle strength and pain in response to surgical repair of posterior abdominal wall disruption followed by rehabilitation. *Br J Sports Med* 2003; **37**:54–58.
89 Fredberg U, Kissmeyer-Nielsen P. The sportsman's hernia: fact or fiction? *Scand J Med Sci Sports* 1996; **6**:201–204.
90 Polglase A, Frydman GM, Farmer KC. Inguinal surgery for debilitating chronic groin pain in athletes. *Med J Aust* 1991; **155**:674–677.

91 Ekstrand J, Ringborg S. Surgery versus conservative treatment in soccer players with chronic groin pain: a prospective randomised study in soccer players. *Eur J Sports Traumatol Rel Res* 2001; **23**:141–145.
92 Ingolby CJH. Laparoscopic and conventional repair of groin disruption in sportsmen. *Br J Surg* 1997; **84**:213–215.
93 Azurin DJ, Go LS, Schuricht A, *et al.* Endoscopic preperitoneal herniorrhaphy in professional athletes with groin pain. *J Laparoendosc Adv Surg Tech A* 1997; **7**:7–12.
94 Kluin J, den Hoad PT, van Linschoten R, *et al.* Endoscopic evaluation and treatment of groin pain in the athlete. *Am J Sports Med* 2004; **32**:944–949.
95 Martens MA, Hansen L, Mulier J. Adductor tendinitis and musculus rectus abdominis tendopathy. *Am J Sports Med* 1987; **15**:353–356.
96 Meyers WC, Foley DP, Garrett WE, *et al.* Management of severe lower abdominal or inguinal pain in high-performance athletes. *Am J Sports Med* 2000; **28**:2–8.
97 Biedert RM, Warnke K, Meyer S. Symphysis syndrome in athletes. *Clin J Sports Med* 2003; **13**:278–284.
98 Crichton KJ, Fricker PA, Purdam C, *et al.* Injuries to the pelvis and lower limb. In: Bloomfield J, Fricker PA, Fitch KD, editors. *Science and Medicine in Sport*, 2nd ed. Carlton, Victoria: Blackwell Science, 1995: 434.
99 Dahan R. Rehabilitation of muscle–tendon injuries to the hip, pelvis and groin areas. *Sports Med Arthrosc Rev* 1997; **5**:326–333.
100 Nicholas SJ, Tyler TF Adductor muscle strains in sport. *Sports Med* 2002; **32**:339–344.
101 Holmich P. Adductor-related groin pain in athletes. *Sports Med Arthrosc Rev* 1997; **5**:285–291.
102 Akermark C, Johansson C. Tenotomy of the adductor longus tendon in the treatment of chronic groin pain in athletes. *Am J Sports Med* 1992; **20**:640–643.
103 Pavlov M, Nelson TL, Warren RF, *et al.* Stress fractures of the pubic ramus. *J Bone Joint Surg Am* 1982; **64**:1020–1025.
104 Rolf C. Pelvis and groin fractures: a cause of groin pain in athletes. *Sports Med Arthrosc Rev* 1997; **5**:301–304.
105 Lynch SA, Renstrom PAFH. Groin injuries in sport: treatment strategies. *Sports Med* 1999; **28**:137–144.
106 Starling JR, Harms BA. Diagnosis and treatment of genitofemoral and ilioinguinal neuralgia. *World J Surg* 1989; **13**:586–591.
107 Jacobsen T, Allen WC. Surgical treatment of snapping iliopsoas tendon. *Am J Sports Med* 1990; **18**:470.
108 Busconi B, McCarthy J. Hip and pelvic injuries in the skeletally immature athlete. *Sports Med Arthrosc Rev* 1996; **4**:132–158.
109 Merrifield HH, Cowan RF. Groin strains in ice hockey. *J Sports Med* 1973; **1**:41–42.
110 Tyler TF, Nicholas SJ, Campbell RJ, *et al.* The association of hip strength and flexibility with the incidence of adductor muscle strains in professional ice hockey players. *Am J Sports Med* 2001; **29**:124–128.
111 Emery CA, Meeuwissee WH. Risk factor s for groin injuries in hockey. *Med Sci Sports Exerc* 2001; **33**:1423–1433.
112 Arnason A, Sigurdsson SB, Gudmundsson A, *et al.* Risk factors for injuries in soccer. *Am J Sports Med* 2004; **32**:S5–16S.
113 Ekstrand J, Gillquist J. The avoidability of soccer injuries. *Int J Sports Med* 1983; **4**:124–128.
114 O'Connor DM. Groin injuries in professional rugby league players: a prospective study. *J Sports Sci* 2004; **22**:629–636.

SECTION 6
Injuries to the lower leg

CHAPTER 26

How evidence-based is our clinical examination of the ankle?

C. Niek van Dijk

Introduction

Supination injuries of the ankle ligament are among the most common injuries. They account for about 25% of all injuries in the musculoskeletal system. The most commonly injured part of the lateral ligament complex is the anterior talofibular ligament. In cases of multiligament rupture, in addition to the anterior talofibular ligament the calcaneofibular ligament is ruptured concomitantly. The calcaneofibular ligament, apart from stabilizing the ankle joint, is a primary stabilizer of the subtalar joint as well. Theoretically, a subtalar instability is present in this situation. Although ruptures of the ankle ligaments are very common, treatment selection remains controversial. In a recent systematic review of the available literature, it was found that treatment for an acute lateral ligament rupture that was too short in duration or did not include sufficient support for the ankle joint and tended to result in more residual symptoms. It was concluded that a no-treatment strategy for acute ruptures of the lateral ankle ligament leads to more residual symptoms.[1] After a supination trauma, it is therefore important to distinguish a simple distortion from an acute grade II or III lateral ankle ligament rupture, since adequate treatment is associated with a better prognosis. Because of the suspected poor reliability of physical diagnosis of ligament ruptures after inversion trauma of the ankle, stress radiography, arthrography, magnetic resonance imaging (MRI), and sonography are often performed simultaneously.[2] However, these methods are expensive, and their reliability is also debated.

Comparison of physical diagnostic features in one trial

The accuracy of physical examination has been determined in a series of 160 patients in which physical examinations within 48 hours of the injury were compared with examinations 5 days after the injury.[3,4] All of the patients had arthrography, but the outcome was not disclosed to the patient or the investigator until after the second delayed physical examination. The specificity and sensitivity of the delayed physical examination for the presence or absence or a lateral ankle ligament rupture were 84% and 96%, respectively. It is therefore concluded that a precise clinical diagnosis is possible. The most important features in the physical examination are swelling, hematoma discoloration, pain on palpation, and the anterior drawer test. Physical examination is unreliable in the acute situation because of the pain; the anterior drawer test cannot be adequately performed. Moreover, there is diffuse pain on palpation, and it is often difficult to judge whether the cause of the swelling is edema or hematoma. A few days after trauma, the swelling and pain have diminished, and it becomes obvious whether the cause of the swelling was edema or hematoma. The pain on palpation has become more localized, and the anterior drawer test can now be performed. The site of pain on palpation is important. If there is no pain on palpation of the anterior talofibular ligament (ATFL), there is no acute lateral ligament rupture. Pain on palpation of the ATFL in itself cannot distinguish between a rupture or a distortion. Pain on palpation in combination with hematoma discoloration, however, has a 90% chance of identifying acute lateral ligament rupture. A positive anterior drawer test has a sensitivity of 86% and a specificity of 75%. It is sometimes possible to detect the occurrence of a skin dimple when performing the anterior drawer test. If a skin dimple does occur during the anterior drawer test, there is a high correlation with a rupture of the lateral ligaments (positive predictive value 94%). However, a skin dimple occurs in only 50% of patients with a lateral ankle ligament rupture.[5] A positive anterior drawer test in combination with pain on palpation of the ATFL and hematoma discoloration has a sensitivity of 96% and a specificity of 84%. It has been demonstrated that the interobserver variation for the delayed physical examination is good, with an average kappa of 0.7.[4]

Meta-analysis of instability in the ankle joint

Materials and methods

A systematic literature search was performed for trials of various diagnostic modalities in acute ankle sprains. Only trials that used operative treatment or arthrography as the "gold standard" to verify the accuracy of a test were used. The search was performed using MEDLINE, EMBASE, and cross-bibliographic checks of the literature from 1966 to 2000.

Outcome measure

The diagnostic odds ratio was used as the outcome measure.

Data and analysis

Data were plotted using receiver operating characteristics (ROC) and were analyzed using Meta Tests software.

Results

A total of 41 studies were selected, of which 23 were excluded because surgery or arthrography were not used as the gold standard, because of unclear or poor randomization design, or because insufficient data were available to calculate the sensitivity and/or specificity.[6] With regard to delayed physical examination, the sensitivity and specificity of the anterior drawer test (ADT) are 85% and 79%, respectively.[7] For hematoma discoloration, the sensitivity is 88%, with a specificity of 78%. Pain on palpation just anterior to the lateral malleolus has a sensitivity of 98%, with a specificity of 7%. Combining the findings at the delayed physical examination (pain on palpation, hematoma discoloration, and ADT) leads to a sensitivity of 96% and a specificity of 84%.

Subtalar instability

In cases of multiligament rupture, the calcaneofibular ligament is ruptured concomitantly with the ATFL. Theoretically, subtalar instability is present in this situation. Apart from this combined problem, subtalar instability can also be an isolated problem.

In the acute phase, the combined ligament rupture resembles an isolated ATFL rupture, with swelling, hematoma discoloration, pain on palpation, and positive ADT. Chronic subtalar instability presents late, with symptoms of persistent instability. The clinical examination includes local pain over the tarsal sinus and increased inversion to the hindfoot, as well as increased external rotation or medial translation of the calcaneus—only described by very experienced examiners.

Several methods of imaging subtalar instability have been described, such as stress tomography, subtalar arthrography, Broden stress view, computed tomography, and more recently MRI and diagnostic subtalar arthroscopy. Arthrography and arthroscopy are invasive procedures with accompanying risks and complications. Stress radiography is still in favor, as subtalar instability is a dynamic problem. However, a gold standard has not been established in the recent literature.

Acute multiligament lesions are treated in the same way as ATFL lesions. There is no evidence to support primary surgery. As in other hindfoot injuries, many patients improve with conservative measures. Proprioceptive training and peroneal strengthening have shown better results than casting or taping and range of movement exercises.[8]

There is insufficient evidence in the literature on the clinical and radiographic diagnosis of subtalar instability, but since the treatment and final results resemble those for isolated ATFL rupture, diagnosis in the acute situation can be limited to diagnosis of ATFL.

Discussion

Until the 1960s, physical examination was used to distinguish between a distortion or a lateral ankle ligament rupture. Physical examination was thought to provide an unreliable outcome,[9–15] and this led to the development of stress radiographs. Stress radiographs have shown poor reliability, with a sensitivity of 50% and a specificity of 96%. In the 1970s, surgery became the treatment of choice. Since stress radiographs were found to be unreliable, arthrography of the ankle was introduced.[16–18] Arthrography is an invasive examination and therefore not without risks. Potential complications include bacterial arthritis, allergic reactions, and chemical arthritis.

With regard to therapy, functional treatment was found to be cost-effective in the 1980s. This led to the development of new noninvasive investigations such as ultrasonography and MRI. Most recently, a delayed physical examination has been introduced. Delaying the physical examination until 4–5 days after injury has been found to be the most reliable diagnostic strategy, with a sensitivity of 96% and a specificity of 84%.[7] The interobserver variation with this strategy has proved to be good, and the approach has also been found to be cost-effective.[19]

Once a diagnosis has been made, it is generally agreed that nonsurgical therapy with early functional rehabilitation is the treatment of choice.[2] A meta-analysis showed that surgical treatment is superior to functional treatment.[1] There are reasons to question the selection of surgery as a treatment of choice. Surgical treatment is associated with an increased risk of complications and is also associated with higher costs. Because of the high prevalence of ankle injuries, surgical treatment may be carried out by surgeons who are still in training in many cases, which may affect the outcome. Finally, when conservative treatment fails, secondary operative reconstruction of the elongated ligaments can be performed with similarly good results, even years after the initial injury.[20] Functional treatment therefore remains the treatment of choice.

Applying an inelastic tape bandage is only effective when it is done at the moment that the swelling has diminished. This type of treatment is inexpensive and not burdensome to the patient. The same is true of the delayed physical examination. Before the decision is made to apply an inelastic bandage or a lace-up support, a delayed physical examination must be carried out in order to reach a diagnosis and decide whether the treatment is really necessary.

Does performing an anterior drawer test 4–5 days after the injury disturb wound healing? Cell lysis, granulation, and phagocyte activity take up to 6 days to occur after an injury, and fibroblasts start to grow into the wound at 5 days. Subsequently, collagen grows along a fibrin mesh. After 10 days, the defect is filled with vascular inflammatory tissue.[21,22] Carrying out an anterior drawer test 4–5 days after the trauma will therefore not disturb wound healing.

The delayed physical examination is a diagnostic modality with a high degree of sensitivity and specificity. This approach has been confirmed to be the strategy of choice.[23,24]

Key message

- For detection of an acute lateral ankle ligament rupture, a delayed physical examination (4–5 days after trauma) is the strategy of choice.

Sample examination questions

Multiple-choice questions (answers on page 602)

1 The diagnosis of acute lateral ankle ligament rupture is based on:
   A The result of the physical examination
   B The result of the physical examination plus stress radiography
   C The result of the physical examination plus arthrography
   D The result of the physical examination plus ultrasonography
   E Stress radiography, arthrography, or echography

2 The outcome of physical examination for detection of an acute lateral ankle ligament rupture is based on:
   A Inspection
   B Palpation
   C Manual anterior drawer test
   D A + B + C
   E The talar tilt test

3 The best available treatment for an acute lateral ankle ligament rupture is
   A Supervised neglect (= no treatment)
   B Elastic support
   C Inelastic tape bandage
   D Brace
   E Operative treatment

Case study 26.1

David, an ambitious 26-year-old semiprofessional football player, was recently involved in an accident in which he sustained a significant supination trauma to the right ankle.

On investigation (on the day of the trauma), there is massive swelling of the ankle. Stability testing is not possible due to pain and swelling. There is pain on palpation in a large area around and on the lateral malleolus. He is unable to bear weight.

How would you proceed?

1 Radiography to exclude fracture (Ottawa ankle rules).
2 Temporary treatment with rest, ice, compression, and elevation (RICE).
3 New physical examination 4–5 days after the trauma to look for location of the palpation pain; to carry out an anterior drawer test; and to look for signs of hematoma discoloration.

Summarizing the evidence

Comparison	Results	Level of evidence*
Delayed physical examination versus arthrography	3 RCTs, all of moderate size, showed no difference in outcome	A1
Physical examination < 48 h versus arthrography	5 RCTs, 2 large, pooled in favor of arthrography	A4

* A1: evidence from large randomized controlled trials (RCTs) or systematic reviews (including meta-analysis).†
A2: evidence from at least one high-quality cohort.
A3: evidence from at least one moderate-sized RCT or systematic review.†
A4: evidence from at least one RCT.
B: evidence from at least one high-quality study of nonrandomized cohorts.
C: expert opinions.
† Arbitrarily, the following cut-off points have been used; large study size: ≥ 100 patients per intervention group; moderate study size ≥ 50 patients per intervention group.

References

1 Pijnenburg ACM, Dijk van CN, Bossuyt PMM, Marti RK. Treatment for lateral ankle ligament ruptures: a meta-analysis. *J Bone Joint Surg (Am)*, 2000; **82**:761–773.
2 Kannus P, Renström P. Treatment for acute tears of the lateral ligaments of the ankle. *J Bone Joint Surg* 1991; **73**:305–312.
3 Dijk van CN, Lim LSL, Bossuyt PMM, Marti RK. Physical examination is sufficient for the diagnosis of sprained ankles. *J Bone Joint Surg* 1996; **78**:958–962.
4 Dijk van CN. *On Diagnostic Strategies in Patients with severe ankle sprain* [thesis]. Amsterdam: University of Amsterdam, 1994.
5 Dijk van CN, Lim LSL, Bossuyt PMM, Marti RK. Diagnosis of sprained ankles. *J Bone Joint Surg* 1997; **79**:1039–1040.
6 Pijnenburg ACM. Acute Ankle Injuries. Diagnostic and Therapeutic Strategies on Evidence-based Grounds, chapter 4 Diagnostic modalities in ankle sprains; a systemic literature review. Thesis Amsterdam: University of Amsterdam 2006 ISBN 90-920346-X.
7 Van Dijk CN. [CBO-guideline for diagnosis and treatment of the acute ankle injury. National organization for quality assurance in hospitals; in Dutch.] *Ned Tijdschr Geneeskd* 1999; **143**:2097–2101.

8 Keefe DT, Haddad SL. Subtalar instability: etiology, diagnosis, and management. *Foot Ankle Clin* 2002; 7:577–609.
9 Percy EC, Hill RO, Callaghan JE. The "sprained" ankle. *J Trauma* 1969; **9**:972–985.
10 Sanders HW. [Importance of radiological methods for the diagnosis of (lateral) ligament lesions of the ankle; in Dutch.] *Ned Tijdschr Geneeskd* 1976; **120**:2035–2039.
11 Volkov MV, Mironova ZS, Badmin IA. Injuries to ligaments of the talocrural joint in ballet-dancers and their management [abstract in English]. *Orthop Traumatol (Moskous)* 1973; **9**:1–6.
12 Broström L, Liljedahl SO, Lindvall N. Sprained ankles, 2: arthrographic diagnosis of recent ligament ruptures. *Acta Chir Scand* 1965; **129**:485–499.
13 Broström L. Sprained ankles, 3: clinical observations in recent ligament ruptures. *Acta Chir Scand* 1965; **130**:560–569.
14 Rechfeld H. Ruptures of ligaments in the ankle and foot. *Reconstr Surg Traumat* 1976; **15**:70–80.
15 Lindstrand A. Clinical diagnosis of lateral ankle sprains. In: Chapchal G, ed. *Injuries of the Ligaments and Their Repair: Hand, Knee, Foot. 7th International Symposium on Topical Problems in Orthopedic Surgery, Lucerne (Switzerland), 1976.* Stuttgart: Thieme, 1977:178–180.
16 Ahuovuo J, Kaartinen E, Slätis P. Diagnostic value of stress radiography in lesions of ligament injuries and classification of ankle injuries. *Radiology* 1977; **125**:63–68.
17 Johannsen A. Radiological diagnosis of lateral ligament lesion of the ankle: a comparison between talar tilt and anterior drawer sign. *Acta Orthop Scand* 1978; **49**:295–301.
18 Moppes FI van, Hoogenband CR van den. *Diagnostic and therapeutic aspects of inversion trauma of the ankle joint* [thesis]. Maastricht: Croezen, 1982.
19 Dijk van CN, Mol BWJ, Marti RK, Lim LL, Bossuyt PMM. Diagnosis of ligament rupture of the ankle joint: physical examination, arthrography, stress radiography and sonography compared in 160 patients after inversion trauma. *Acta Orthop Scand* 1996; **67**:566–570.
20 Krips R, Van Dijk CN, Halasi T, *et al.* Anatomical reconstruction versus tenodesis for the treatment of chronic anterolateral instability of the ankle joint: a 2–10 year follow-up. *Knee Surg Sports Traumatol Arthrosc* 2000; **8**:173–179.
21 Jack EA. Experimental rupture of the medial collateral ligament of the knee. *J Bone Joint Surg Br* 1950; **32**:396–402.
22 Frank C, Woo SL, Amiel D, *et al.* Medial collateral ligament healing: a multidisciplinary assessment in rabbits. *Am J Sports Med* 1983; **11**:379–389.
23 Klenerman L. The management of sprained ankle. *J Bone Joint Surg Br* 1998; **80**:11–12.
24 Chan KM, Karlsson J. ISAKOS-FIMS World Consensus Conference on Ankle Instability. 2005 International Society of Arthroscopy, Knee Surgery and Orthopaedic sports Medicine (ISAKOS) International Federation of Sports Medicine (FIMS).

CHAPTER 27

Can we prevent ankle sprains?

Roald Bahr

Introduction

Ankle injuries are the most common injuries encountered, with an incidence of one per 100,000 inhabitants per day, accounting for about 20% of all sports injuries. Ankle sprains occur with a high frequency in sports characterized by running and jumping. In other words, they are common in most sports, in contact as well as in noncontact sports, and in team sports as well as in individual sports. Most ankle injuries are moderate ligament sprains. With proper functional treatment, the patient can return to work or sport within a few weeks or even a few days, and most injuries heal without sequelae. However, some ankle sprains cause prolonged disability in the form of persisting pain or instability.

The most important risk factor for ankle injuries is a history of a previous sprain. Sensorimotor control is reduced in athletes with persistent instability complaints after injury,[1–4] and even in the immediate recovery period after an acute injury.[5] This may account for the several-fold increased risk of injury in athletes with previous ankle problems.

The high rate of ankle sprains in and outside sports calls for preventive measures, and the first attempts to prevent ankle injuries were published by Quigley *et al.*[6] in 1946 and Thorndike[7] in 1956. The objective of the present chapter is to examine the evidence that ankle sprains in sport can be prevented.

Methods

This review was written using information from articles on the prevention of ankle injuries identified through the MEDLINE database (1966–September 2001) using "ankle injuries" and "prevention" as keywords. The search identified 185 studies that were considered for inclusion in the present review. The same search was repeated in 2005, covering the period October 2001–August 2005, and this revealed an additional 71 studies. A study was included if it met criteria modified from Verhagen *et al.*[8] as follows:

- The study contained research questions regarding the prevention of lateral ankle ligament injuries.
- The study was a randomized clinical trial (RCT), a clinical trial, or a cohort study.
- The results of the study contained incidence rates of lateral ankle ligament injuries as a study outcome.

Reference lists of included studies were also searched for relevant original research studies. Five formal review papers[8–13] on ankle sprain prevention published from 1997 to 2001 and an additional two reviews[14,15] from 2001 to 2005 were identified in the two literature searches (Table 27.1).[8–13,15–33] Original research studies identified from these review papers were also included in the current review.

Table 27.1 Ankle injury prevention studies. The table shows all papers included in the present review, and whether they were identified in the previous or current search or from review papers published in 1999–2001. Evaluation scores from previous reviews are shown where available

First author, ref.	Year	Study design	Search 1966–2001	Search 2001–2005	Evaluation scores in previous review papers						
					Verhagen[8] (max. 14)	Handoll[16] (max. 22)	Quinn[9] (max. 33)	Thacker[10] (max. 100)	Hume[11]	Robbins[12]	Callaghan[13]
Olsen[33]	2005	RCT (of teams)		X							
Stasinopoulos[32]	2004	RCT		X							
Verhagen[15]	2004	Prospective controlled		X							
Schumacher[31]	2000	Retrospective cohort	X								
Holme[30]†	1999	RCT	X			6					
Amoroso[29]	1998	RCT	X		10	12	15*				
Bahr[28]	1997	Prospective cohort	X		9			32			
Sharpe[27]	1997	Retrospective cohort							X		
Wester[26]	1996	RCT	X			5					
Sitler[25]	1994	RCT	X		13	12	24	60	X		X
Surve[24]	1994	RCT	X		9	7	17	39	X	X	X
Barrett[23]	1993	RCT	X		13	8	19	68			
Rovere[22]	1988	Retrospective cohort	X		9			48	X	X	X
Tropp[21]	1985	RCT (of teams)	X		9	5	16	31	X	X	X
Ekstrand[20]	1983	RCT (of teams)				6		45	X		
Cameron[19]	1973	Prospective cohort						11			
Garrick[18]	1973	RCT	X		10			23	X	X	X
Simon[17]	1969	RCT				3		40			

* Referred to in abstract form as Ryan. 1994.[34]

† Also published in Danish as Barkler. 2001.[35]

Previous reviews

The conclusions and recommendations of reviews published 1997 to 2001 will be presented briefly before examining the available original research studies. Notably, the reviews have reached similar conclusions—although nearly all have some reservations regarding the methodology of the research available.

Callaghan in 1997 reviewed the role of taping and bracing in the treatment and prevention of ankle sprains.[13] He describes six studies on injury prevention in the section on taping and bracing for acute ankle sprain, concluding that both taping and braces have been shown to prevent ankle sprains in basketball and soccer players, though the study design of the studies reported should be considered before applying tape or recommending a brace for the prevention of ankle sprains. He also reviewed the effect of orthoses on performance, concluding that they do not lead to any negative effects in performance tests.

Hume and Gerrard in 1998 also reviewed the effect of external ankle support on ankle injury rates based on eight studies, and pointed out several limitations in these studies (small study size, self-selection, inadequate controls).[11] They concluded that the studies reviewed failed to provide unequivocal evidence of the effectiveness of external ankle support. However, they also state that several studies, even given the limitations mentioned, do seem to indicate that taping or bracing reduces the ankle injury rate, particularly for athletes with previous injuries. They also recommend that external ankle support during both practice and training should be encouraged where there is a clear history of recurrent ankle injury in a sports player, in combination with an ankle proprioception training program.

Robbins and Waked in 1998 briefly touched on the preventive effect of taping and rigid/semirigid devices, in a paper focusing on the importance of incorrect foot position caused by footwear.[12] They conclude that the studies are unconvincing, because all of them were small-scale, retrospective, without adequate controls, often sponsored by manufacturers, and they also utilize self-reporting of injuries or diagnoses made by coaches. Nevertheless, they state that the reports suggest that both taping and semirigid devices effectively prevent first ankle sprains and are perhaps more effective still in preventing re-injury.

Thacker *et al.* in 1999 reviewed the evidence on the effectiveness of any kind of prevention program for ankle sprains—not just including taping or bracing.[10] They identified seven randomized controlled trials and three cohort studies that compared methods to prevent ankle sprains using shoes and taping, bracing, or specialized training. This was the first review to develop a rigorous scoring instrument for ankle injury prevention studies, and the quality scores of the papers ranged from 11 to 68 out of a maximum of 100. In other words, the study quality was low to medium. They recommend that athletes with a sprained ankle complete supervised rehabilitation before returning to practice or competition, and those athletes suffering from a moderate or severe sprain should wear an appropriate orthosis for at least 6 months.

Verhagen *et al.* in 2000 conducted a formal literature search on any method of preventing ankle ligament injuries and also included a design and methodology evaluation in their paper.[8] The eight studies included were given methodology scores between 65% and 93% of the maximum attainable score. In other words, it appears that their methodology score resulted in more favorable results than Thacker *et al.* They conclude that the use of either tape or braces reduces the incidence of ankle sprains, and that the use of tape and braces results in less severe ankle sprains. Also, they found that braces seem to be more effective in preventing ankle sprains than tape. They were unable to determine which athletes benefit more from the use of external ankle support—those with or those without previous ankle sprains. Also, the role of shoe type is unclear. They also conclude that proprioceptive training reduces the incidence of ankle sprains in athletes with recurrent ankle sprains to the same level as subjects without any history of ankle sprains.

Finally, Quinn *et al.* completed a formal Cochrane review on interventions for preventing ankle ligament injuries in 1996, which was amended in 1997[9] and again in 2001.[16] They identified five randomized trials with data for 3682 participants using external ankle support (semirigid orthoses, Aircast brace or high top shoes) or ankle disk training. The methodology scores given to the studies included ranged between 45% and 73% of the maximum attainable score.[9] They found a significant reduction in the number of ankle sprains in people allocated external ankle support (odds ratio 0.51; 95% confidence interval, 0.38 to 0.67).[16] The interventions resulted in a large reduction in risk for those with a previous history of ankle sprains (OR 0.31; 95% CI, 0.20 to 0.53), but a non-significant result for those who did not have a prior history of ankle sprains (OR 0.73; 96% CI, 0.52 to 1.03). They also found that the treatment effect differed significantly between the two subgroups ($P < 0.01$)—i.e., that there is evidence that external ankle support provides a greater support for those with a previous ankle sprain than for subjects with no previous ankle sprain. They did not find any difference in the severity of ankle sprains or any change in the incidence of other leg injuries. Finally, they concluded that the protective effect of high-top shoes remains to be established and that there was limited evidence for reduction in ankle sprain risk for those with previous ankle sprains who did ankle disk training exercises.

In summary, although there is general agreement that most studies suffer from methodology and design limitations, most reviewers conclude that external ankle support provides protection for ankle ligament injuries—at least among those who have suffered a previous ankle sprain. However, there is no consensus on whether balance training on an ankle disk reduces the risk of future ankle sprains—whether the athlete has previously been injured or not. This disagreement stems from a lack of high-quality studies on balance training.

Original research papers

This section is summarized in Table 27.2.[15,17–33]

In a randomized trial, Simon[17] compared the effect of taping with cloth strapping to prevent ankle sprains in a group of 148 college football players over two spring seasons. The players were divided alphabetically into two groups, half wearing tape and half with their ankles wrapped with cloth wrapping ("Louisiana wrapping"). The treatment was reversed for the second season. There were four ankle injuries in both groups. Although this is a small study and no difference was observed between the groups, since there was no control group we do not know whether the injury rate was lower than what would be expected without treatment.

In 1973, Garrick and Requa[18] performed the first randomized clinical trial to examine the effect of ankle taping on the frequency of sprains. They also classified the shoe types used, although the shoe type (high-top or low-top) was self-selected. A total of 2562 player exposures in an intramural college basketball program were studied over two seasons, and the teams were randomly assigned to taping (mostly inelastic taping with stirrups and

Table 27.2 Characteristics and outcomes of ankle injury prevention studies

First author, ref.	Year	Study design	n	Setting	Duration of study	Intervention	Outcome
Olsen[33]	2005	RCT (of teams)	1837 players aged 15–17 (1586 female, 251 male)	Youth team handball, Norway	One season (8 months)	A structured warm-up program to improve running, cutting, and landing technique, as well as neuromuscular control, balance, and strength	Decreased incidence in knee or ankle sprains in intervention group
Stasinopoulos[32]	2004	RCT	52 female athletes with previous ankle sprains	Amateur volleyball, Greece	One season	Three groups: Balance training vs. technical training vs. external ankle support	No statistical comparisons presented, study too small to conclude
Verhagen[15]	2004	Prospective controlled (RCT of regions)	1127 athletes	Amateur volleyball, Netherlands	One season	Balance-board training program	Decreased incidence in training group
Schumacher[31]	2000	Retrospective cohort	13,782 parachute jumps	Army parachute jumping training, USA	38 months	Outside-the-boot brace	Decreased incidence in braced group
Holme[30]	1999	RCT	92 recreational athletes with acute ankle sprains	Hospital emergency room, Denmark	12-month follow-up	Supervised training program, including balance-board training	Decreased incidence in training group
Amoroso[29]	1998	RCT	3674 parachute jumps; 745 men	Army parachute jumping training course, USA	Unknown	Outside-the-boot brace	Decreased incidence in braced group

Continued

Table 27.2 *(Continued)*

First author, ref.	Year	Study design	n	Setting	Duration of study	Intervention	Outcome
Bahr[28]	1997	Prospective cohort	819 athlete seasons (420 men, 394 women)	Elite amateur club volleyball, Norway	Three years	Three-part prevention program: injury awareness session, balance-board training, and technical training	Decreased incidence after introduction of prevention program
Sharpe[27]	1997	Retrospective cohort	38 female players with 56 previously injured ankles	College soccer, USA	Five years	Canvas-laced brace, tape, combination or no treatment	Decreased incidence with prophylactic bracing
Wester[26]	1996	RCT	48 recreational athletes with acute ankle sprains	Hospital emergency room, Denmark	230-day follow-up (mean)	12 weeks balance-board training program	Decreased incidence in training group
Sitler[25]	1994	RCT	1601 male military cadets (177 with history of ankle sprain, 1424 without)	Intramural college basketball at West Point, USA	Two years	Semirigid orthosis	Decreased incidence in orthosis group
Surve[24]	1994	RCT	504 male soccer players (258 with history of ankle sprain, 246 without)	Four divisions, from highest to lowest level in Western Province, South Africa	One season	Semirigid orthosis	Decreased incidence of recurrent sprains in orthosis group

Barrett[23]	1993	RCT	569 college students (91.7% male)	Intramural college basketball, USA	One season (2 months)	Low- and high-top shoes	No effect of shoe type
Rovere[22]	1988	Retrospective cohort	297 male football players	One college team, USA	Six seasons	Tape and laced orthosis	Laced orthoses more effective than tape; additional effect of low-top shoes
Tropp[21]	1985	RCT (of teams)	439 male soccer players	Soccer teams in the 6th division, Sweden	One season	Soft orthosis and balance-board training	Decreased incidence of recurrent sprains in both groups
Ekstrand[17]	1983	RCT (of teams)	180 male soccer players	Soccer teams in the 4th division, Sweden	6 months out of two seasons	Seven-part prevention program—including prophylactic taping	Decreased incidence of ankle sprains in intervention group
Cameron[19]	1973	Prospective cohort	2839 male football players	High-school football, USA	One season	Four different shoe types: Cleats, heel plates, soccer shoes, swivel shoes	Decreased incidence with swivel shoes
Garrick[18]	1973	RCT	2562 player exposures, gender unknown (all male?)	Intramural college basketball, USA	Two season	Tape (randomized) combined with high/low-top shoes (self-selected)	Decreased incidence in taped group—additional effect of high-top shoes
Simon[17]	1969	RCT	148 football players	College football, USA	Two spring practice seasons	Taping vs. cloth strapping	No difference between groups

RCT, randomized controlled trial.

horseshoe strips finished with a figure-of-eight lock; a few used an elastic taping material) or control. The results showed that the lowest injury rate was observed in the taped groups (high-top shoes: 6.5 injuries per 1000 player exposures; low top shoes 17.6) in comparison with the untaped control group (high-top shoes: 30.4 injuries per 1000 player exposures; low-top shoes: 33.4). Among players with a history of previous sprains, the injury rate was 16.4 per 1000 player exposures in the taped groups (high-top shoes: 8.3; low-top shoes: 19.9), in comparison with 55.2 in the untaped control group (high-top shoes: 28.8, low-top shoes: 63.6). From this study, it therefore appears that taping reduces the risk of ankle sprains, and that there is an additional protective effect of high-top shoes. Moreover, it appears that the protective effect is even more pronounced among players with a history of previous sprains.

Cameron prospectively followed 2839 male high-school players over one season to compare the effect of wearing specially designed shoes with swivel plates for football with shoes with cleats, heel plates, or soccer shoes.[19] He found a 2.7-fold decrease in the rate of ankle sprains in athletes wearing the swivel shoes (3.0% with injury) compared with those wearing cleats (8.5%), heel plates (7.7%), or soccer shoes (5.6%).

Ekstrand *et al.* conducted a randomized controlled trial examining the effects of an injury prevention program in sports.[20] Twelve male fourth-division teams (180 players) were followed for the first 6 months of the 1980 and 1981 seasons. Between these two observation periods, the teams were allocated at random to two groups of six teams. One group was given a prophylactic program, and the other served as control. The program was based on previous studies of injury mechanisms in soccer and consisted of:

- Correction of training
- Provision of optimum equipment
- Prophylactic ankle taping of players with previous injury and/or clinical instability (43 of 90 players, 52 ankles)
- Controlled rehabilitation
- Exclusion of players with grave knee instability
- Information about the importance of disciplined play and the increased risk of injury at training camps
- Correction and supervision by doctors and physiotherapists

The six control teams had a mean of 2.6 injuries per month during the first 6 months of 1981, an incidence equal to the mean for all 12 teams in the division during the same period in 1980. After the introduction of the prophylactic program, the six test teams reduced the incidence to 0.6 injuries per month in 1981, which was 75% less than in the control group ($P < 0.001$). Of interest here is that the incidence of sprains to the ankle was reduced significantly ($P < 0.05$). The authors concluded that the prevention program, which included prophylactic ankle taping of players with ankle problems, significantly reduces soccer injuries. The main difficulty when interpreting the study in the context of ankle injury prevention is that it is difficult to determine which of the seven program components contributed most to the result.

Tropp *et al.* compared two different methods—ankle orthoses and ankle disk training—for the prevention of ankle sprains in a prospective study in which players were randomized to treatment groups by team.[21] Ten teams (n = 171) served as controls, whereas in seven teams (n = 124; 60 used the orthosis and 64 did not) were offered ankle orthoses and players on eight teams with a history of previous ankle sprains were assigned to ankle disk training (n = 65). The results were analyzed separately for players with and without a history of previous ankle sprains. Among players with previous ankle problems, 19 of 75 players (25%) in the control group sustained a sprain during the study period; the corresponding figure for the orthosis group and ankle disk groups were one of 45 (2%, $P < 0.01$) and three of 65 (5%, $P < 0.01$), respectively. Among players without any history of previous ankle problems, the authors found no difference in the frequency of ankle sprains. They also observed that in the ankle disk group, the frequency of injury was 5% both among players with a history of problems who all did ankle disk training ($n = 65$) and among players without previous problems who did not train. In other words, this study suggested that ankle disk training and orthosis use was equally effective in preventing ankle sprains, whereas there was no preventive effect among players with previously healthy ankles. Their results also suggest that ankle disk training can normalize the risk of injury among players with a history of previous ankle sprains.

Rovere *et al.* examined the effectiveness of taping or wearing a laced ankle stabilizer in a retrospective cohort study covering one college football team for six seasons.[22] For 18 months, the players all had taped ankles, and for the remaining 4.5 years the players chose their ankle support. Over the entire period, the players chose high-top or low-top shoes as preferred. The 297 players sustained 224 ankle injuries and 24 re-injuries. They found that a player wearing the ankle stabilizers had half the risk of injury of a player wearing tape (95% CI, 0.42 to 0.85; $P = 0.003$). They also found that low-top shoes were relatively more effective than high-top shoes in preventing injury. However, this was a retrospective study in which players self-selected their shoe type and whether to use a stabilizer or tape. When interpreting the results, it is important to keep in mind that players at greater risk—for example, because of playing position or previous injury status—may have selected the equipment they perceived as giving them the greatest protective effect. Although the group comparisons were stratified by position, a selection bias may still exist to inflate the injury risk for any group. In fact, nearly all the re-injuries occurred in the tape group.

Barrett *et al.* used a prospective randomized design to evaluate the effect of shoe type on ankle sprain risk.[23] Out of a predominantly male population of 622 college intramural basketball players, 569 players completed the study requirements, and of these, 43.3% had a history of ankle sprains. The randomization procedure was stratified by previous history of ankle sprains, and the players were randomized to wear a new pair of either high-top ($n = 208$), high-top with inflatable air chambers ($n = 203$), or low-top basketball shoes ($n = 158$) during all games for a complete season. The authors found that there was no significant difference in injury rates between the groups wearing high-top shoes ($n = 7$; 4.8 injuries per 1000 playing hours), high-top shoes with inflatable air chambers ($n = 4$; 2.7 injuries per 1000 playing hours), or low-top basketball shoes ($n = 4$; 4.1 injuries per 1000 playing hours). It should be noted that the total number of injuries, and consequently the statistical power of the study, was low. Thus, this study can not be taken as final evidence that there is no preventive effect of high-top shoes.

Surve *et al.* undertook a randomized clinical study to evaluate the effect of a semirigid ankle stabilizer on the incidence of ankle sprains during one playing season.[24] Senior male soccer players, who represented all the soccer teams from four divisions, were asked to participate in the study, and they were randomly assigned to a control group (no treatment) or an intervention group who wore a semirigid Aircast Sport Stirrup orthosis during soccer practice and games. The randomization was stratified according to previous injury status, and this resulted in four groups with similar size: two control groups (131 with a history of previous ankle sprain and 129 with no history) and two intervention groups (127 with a history of previous ankle sprain and 117 with no history). The results showed that the incidence of ankle sprains was reduced among players with a previous history of ankle sprains ($P < 0.001$). The incidence was 0.46 per 1000 playing hours among those who wore a brace and 1.16 per 1000 playing hours among those who did not. However, among players with no previous history of ankle sprains, there was no difference in the incidence of ankle injuries between those who wore orthoses (0.97 per 1000 playing hours) and those who did not (0.92 per 1000 playing hours). Thus, the authors conclude that a semirigid orthosis significantly reduced the incidence of recurrent ankle sprains in soccer players with a previous history of ankle sprains. They recommend the use of orthoses for players with a previous ankle sprain, in conjunction with a comprehensive rehabilitation program to decrease the risk of recurrent ankle injuries.

Sitler *et al.* designed a randomized clinical trial to determine the efficacy of a semirigid ankle stabilizer in reducing the frequency and severity of acute ankle injuries in basketball.[25] Participants in the study were 1601 United States Military Academy cadets with no preparticipation, clinical, functional, or radiographic evidence of ankle instability. The subjects were randomly assigned to a control group (812 subjects, 90 of these with previous injury) or an intervention group (789 subjects, 87 previously injured) who wore a semirigid Aircast Sports Stirrup orthosis during basketball practice and games. The authors found that the injury rate was 5.2 injuries per 1000 athlete exposures (n = 35) in the control group and 1.6 per 1000 athlete exposures in the intervention group (n = 11). Thus, the relative risk of sustaining an ankle injury was approximately three times greater for control subjects as for ankle stabilizer subjects ($P < 0.01$). However, it should be noted that this reduction was only evident from contact injuries; there was no effect on non-contact injuries. The corresponding results were 4.8 (control) versus 1.7 (intervention) injuries per 1000 athlete exposures among athletes with no previous injury and 8.0 (control) versus 1.4 (intervention) injuries per 1000 athlete exposures among athletes with a history of previous ankle sprain. In the interpretation of the results, this study should be given particular weight, since the prestudy status of the subjects, playing conditions (shoe type worn, floor type), diagnostic methods, and compliance were carefully controlled and reported. However, the number of participants and exposures was too small to allow for a statistical evaluation of the effect in subgroups of healthy and previously injured subjects, although it appears that the protective effect may have been similar in both groups. The authors conclude that the use of ankle stabilizers significantly reduced the rate of ankle injuries, but that injury severity was not statistically reduced. They also conclude that wearing the ankle stabilizer did not affect the frequency of knee injuries.

Wester *et al.* examined the effect of a training program on a wobble board on residual symptoms and re-injuries following an ankle sprain.[26] The subjects were 61 recreational athletes who reported to the hospital emergency room with an acute ankle sprain from sports participation, but had no previous ankle problems. The patients were randomized to a control group or a training group. The training group was provided with a wobble board and instructed to follow a daily program with progressively difficult balance exercises for 12 weeks. Thirteen patients withdrew before the final follow-up. Of the remaining 24 patients in the training group, six had recurrent sprains (25%) and none had subjective instability of the ankle. Among the 24 patients in the control group there were 13 with recurrent sprains (54%, $P < 0.05$) and six felt instability of the ankle (25%, $P < 0.01$). The authors conclude that training on a wobble board early after a primary ankle sprain is effective in reducing residual symptoms.

Sharpe *et al.* retrospectively examined the medical records of female varsity soccer players at a third-division college to determine the effect of bracing and taping.[27] From a review of medical records for the team over five seasons, they identified 38 players with 56 previously injured ankles, and whether the injured players had used no external ankle support (n = 17), tape (n = 12), bracing with a Swede-O canvas lace-up brace (n = 19), or both taping and bracing (n = 8). The ankle sprain recurrence frequency was 35% for the untreated ankles, 25% for the taped ankles, 25% for the taped and braced ankles, and 0% for the untreated ankles. On the basis of this, the authors suggest that ankle bracing is effective in reducing the incidence of ankle sprains in female soccer players with a previous history of ankle sprains. However, the results must be interpreted with caution, since it is a small study with retrospective data collection, and the treatment received was—at least in part—self-selected and not randomly assigned.

Bahr *et al.* conducted a prospective cohort study to examine the effects of a three-part injury prevention program on the incidence of ankle sprains among approximately 270 senior elite volleyball players over three seasons.[28] The program consisted mainly of an injury awareness session, technical training (with emphasis on proper take-off and landing technique for blocking and attacking), and a balance-board training program (for players with previous ankle sprains). Baseline data were collected during the first season, the program was introduced during the second season, and the effects of the prevention program were evaluated during the third season. The authors found that the incidence of ankle injuries was reduced from 0.9 ± 0.1 per 1000 player hours during the first season (48 injuries) to 0.5 ± 0.1 during the third season (24 injuries), with a risk ratio of 0.53 ($P < 0.01$). It is not possible to establish with certainty how the main elements of the prevention program, technical training and balance-board training, as well as increased awareness of typical injury mechanisms, each contributed to the overall results. However, the risk of re-injury seemed to be reduced for previously injured ankles, and this may be taken as an indication that the balance-board training program had some effect. Also, there was a reduction in the number of injuries due to landing on the foot of an opponent, which indicates that the special technical training program and increased awareness about the main mechanisms of injury may have contributed as well. The authors conclude that further studies are needed to identify the effects of each program component. Also, since this was an intervention study using historical baseline data, the results must be interpreted with caution. It is possible that factors other than those introduced as a prevention program changed during the three study years and therefore contributed to the results observed.

Amoroso *et al.* conducted a randomized trial involving 777 parachuters during the final week of an army airborne training course.[29,34] Of this group, 745 completed all study requirements. The subjects were randomly assigned to one of two groups—either wearing an Aircast outside-the-boot brace or no brace (369 brace wearers and 376 non-brace wearers). Each subject made five parachute jumps, for a total of 3674 jumps. The authors found that the incidence of inversion ankle sprains was 1.9% in non-brace wearers and 0.3% in brace wearers (risk ratio 6.9; $P = 0.04$). There appeared to be no effect on other injuries. The authors concluded that inversion ankle sprains during parachute training could be significantly reduced by using an outside-the-boot ankle brace, with no increase in risk for other injuries. However, although about half of the subjects reported having had a previous ankle sprain upon entry, no results are provided regarding the effect in previously healthy versus previously injured ankles. Thus, it is not possible to evaluate whether the protective effect was limited to those with previous sprains or not.

Holme *et al.* examined the effect of an early rehabilitation program, which included balance training, on ankle function.[30,35] The subjects were 92 recreational athletes who reported to the hospital emergency room with an acute ankle sprain from sports participation, but had no prior complaints of ankle joint instability. All subjects were given the same standardized information regarding early ankle mobilization, including strength (standing on heels/toes, one-foot hopping), mobility (circular movements), and balance exercises (standing on one foot with eyes open and with eyes closed, and standing on a balance board). After 5 days, the subjects were matched for age, sex, and level of sports activity and randomized to a control group (n = 46) or a training group (n = 46). The training group was offered supervised group physical therapy for 1 hour twice weekly. The training program included comprehensive balance exercises on both legs, figure-of-eight running, standing on a balance board, on the inside or outside of the foot, with eyes open and closed. The authors found that 6 weeks after the acute injury, the subjects displayed a side-to-side reduction in ankle strength and postural control, but that these factors were normalized 4 months after the injury in both groups. It should be noted that there was a considerable loss to follow-up—17 patients in the training group did not complete the entire study (37%). However, although the training program had no measurable effect on strength or postural control, there were significantly fewer re-injuries in the training group (two of 29, 7%) than in the control group (11 of 38, 29%) during the first 12-month period after the original injury. Although there is a considerable loss to follow-up in both studies, this study[30] and that by Wester *et al.*[26] indicate that early balance training after a primary ankle sprain provides protection from recurrent injuries.

Schumacher *et al.* presented results from a cohort study that evolved as a natural experiment by the introduction of mandatory use of an outside-the-boot ankle brace developed by the U.S. Army for parachute jumping.[31] Results from parachute jumps before (n = 7857) and after (n = 5928) were compared by retrospective review of medical records. The results show that there were 4.45 injuries per 1000 jumps before the braces were introduced, and that the injury rate was reduced to 1.52 injuries per 1000 jumps after braces were made mandatory ($P = 0.002$). In other words, the results of this study corroborate the conclusions of the randomized trial by Amoroso *et al.*[29] that inversion ankle sprains during parachute training can be significantly reduced by using an outside-the-boot ankle brace.

Stasinopoulos[32] conducted a study in volleyball that aimed to compare the effects of the three components included in the program previously tested by Bahr *et al.*[28]—technical training, balance training, and external support. The objective was to investigate which of these three interventions is the most effective in preventing ankle sprain in female volleyball players. Participants were 52 players who suffered ankle sprains during the 1998–1999 season. They were divided randomly into three preventive groups: group 1 (n = 18) followed the technical training program; group 2 (n = 17) followed the balance training program; group 3 (n = 17) used the Sport Stirrup orthosis. The players followed their respective programs for the whole of the 1999–2000 season, and data were collected at the end of the season. A total of 11 ankle sprains were observed during the intervention season —two in group 1, three in group 2, and six in group 3. The author concluded that the three preventive strategies were all effective in preventing further ankle sprain, and that technical training was slightly more so than the other two methods. However, it is difficult to see how this conclusion can be justified by the results, since there was no control group and the number of participants and cases is too small for meaningful statistical comparisons.

Verhagen and co-workers wanted to test whether a proprioceptive balance-board program is effective for prevention of ankle sprains in volleyball players.[15] They did a prospective controlled intervention study during the 2001–2002 season in which they included 116 male and female volleyball teams from the second and third volleyball divisions in the Netherlands. Teams were randomized by four geographical regions to an intervention group (66 teams, 641 players) and control group (50 teams, 486 players). Intervention teams followed a prescribed balance-board training program, control teams followed their normal training routine, and coaches recorded exposure on a weekly basis for each player. Injuries were also registered by the players within 1 week after onset. The authors found that there were significantly fewer ankle sprains in the intervention group in comparison with the control group (risk difference 0.4 per 1000 playing hours; 95% CI, 0.1 to 0.7). However, it should be noted that a significant reduction in ankle sprain risk was found only for players with a history of ankle sprains. The authors therefore concluded that the use of a proprioceptive balance-board program is effective for prevention of ankle sprain recurrences.

Since there was a lack of research on youth and adolescents participating in sports, Olsen *et al.*[33] investigated the effect of a structured warm-up program designed to reduce the incidence of knee and ankle injuries in this age group. Theirs was a cluster-randomized controlled trial with 120 Norwegian team handball clubs (1837 players, aged 15–17 years), which were randomized to an intervention (61 clubs, 958 players) or control group (59 clubs, 879 players) for one league season (8 months). The intervention group used a structured warm-up program to improve running, cutting, and landing technique, as well as neuromuscular control, balance, and strength. The study was designed to examine the effect of the intervention on the rate of acute injuries to the knee or ankle combined, and the authors found that the relative risk in the intervention group was 0.53 in comparison with the control group (95% CI, 0.35 to 0.81; 81 acute knee or ankle injuries in the control group and 48 in the intervention group). Although the study was not powered to examine the effect on ankle sprains alone, the authors reported 28 acute ankle injuries in the intervention group and 40 in the control group (relative risk 0.63; 95% CI, 0.36 to 1.09; $P = 0.097$). Thus, although the authors concluded that a structured program of warm-up exercises can prevent knee and ankle injuries in young athletes, and that such preventive training should therefore be an integral part of youth sports programs, the specific effect of the program on ankle sprains alone has not yet been conclusively proven.

Directions for future research

Although there is convincing evidence that external ankle support provides protection from future injury, some questions remain that need to be addressed in large scale randomized trials. First, very little evidence exists on ankle taping; most of the quality research to date on the effect of external ankle support has been done on orthoses, principally one particular brand. Furthermore, it is not entirely clear whether prophylactic bracing benefits all athletes, regardless of previous injury status. Many studies do not report their results separately for subjects with or without previous problems, and in those that do, conflicting results have been seen among athletes who do not have a history of ankle sprains. Also, the studies in which pre-injury status has been taken into account have generally used players, rather than ankles, as the unit of analysis. This makes the interpretation of the results difficult. Needless to say, subjects have a left and a right ankle, and it is not clear how players who have one ankle with a previous injury and one with no prior injury have been classified. It is recommended that in future studies, randomization procedures should be stratified according to the previous injury status of the players, and that the results should be reported using ankles, not players, as the unit of analysis.

The evidence for balance training as a preventive measure is convincing, but in the same way as for bracing, it appears that the effect may be limited to athletes with a history of previous injury. Further larger-scale studies are necessary to examine this question further, taking previous injury history into account. There is also a need to conduct appropriately sized randomized clinical studies to examine the effects of high-top shoes alone or in combination with taping or bracing.

Since it is conceivable that the protective effects of bracing and taping or balance training may depend on the injury mechanism involved, this should be reported in future studies. For instance, although balance training may help an athlete avoid noncontact injuries (for example, a volleyball player tripping over when running to retrieve a ball on defense), they may not protect against contact injury (for example, a volleyball player landing on the foot of an opponent or a soccer player being tackled by an opponent). The injury mechanisms for ankle injuries in many sports (for example, soccer) have not been examined in detail, and this information may help suggest new ways to prevent injury.

Finally, it is important to keep in mind that nearly all the evidence on ankle injury prevention has been collected using adult, almost exclusively male, athletic study populations. This means that the conclusions reached do not necessarily apply to women, adolescents and children, older individuals, or non-sport settings. Consequently, there is a need to conduct studies in these and other settings, as well.

Conclusion

External ankle support (Fig. 27.1) can prevent ankle sprains—at least in athletes with previous ankle problems. It also appears likely that a balance training program can improve sensorimotor control,[36,37] and that such a program (Fig. 27.2) reduces the risk of re-injury to the same level as that in healthy ankles.[15,21,30]

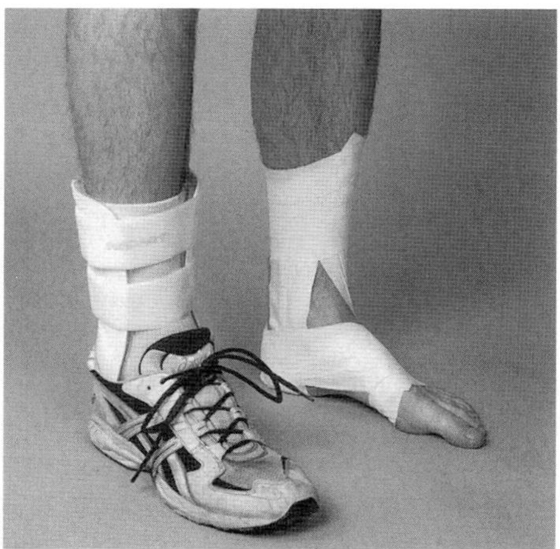

Figure 27.1 An ankle brace (right ankle) or tape (left ankle) should be worn during sporting and other high-risk activities at least until completion of a supervised rehabilitation program, including 6–10 weeks of balance-training exercise.

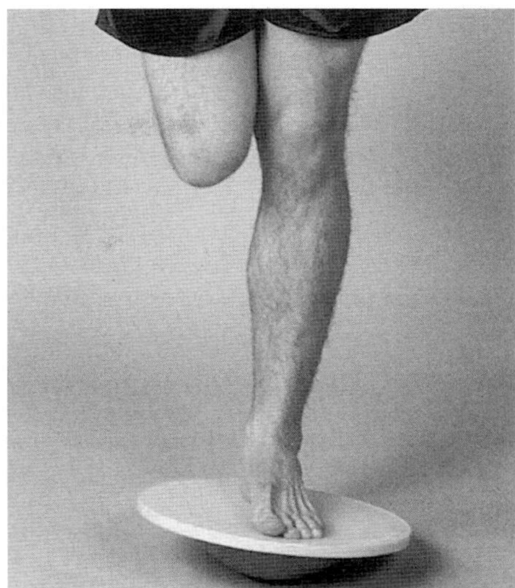

Figure 27.2 Balance-board training is performed with the player standing on one leg on a balance board. The objective is to control balance using an ankle strategy—i.e., without using hands, hips, or knees to adjust body position, but to correct balance using the ankle only, as much as possible. Thus, arms are held across the chest and the opposite leg is held still at 90° knee flexion.

How balance training and orthoses work is uncertain, but they may simply enhance sensorimotor control of the ankle joint. This view is corroborated by the fact that their effect mainly seems to be limited to players with previous injury,[21,24,25] in whom postural control, position sense, and postural reflexes appear to be reduced,[1,3,4,30,38–41] and that orthoses do not seem to restrict inversion enough to substantiate their prophylactic effect.[8,42,43] If the protective effect of orthoses were mechanical, one would expect an effect in healthy ankles as well. However, it may also be that the mechanism by which orthoses work is simply by guiding the foot.[44–46] In other words, the external ankle support may help ensure that the athlete lands with the foot in the proper position.

Bracing is generally seen as being more comfortable than tape, as well as being more cost-effective with long-term use.[8,10,42] However, in some sports in which foot control is essential, such as soccer, some players may resist using braces and prefer tape. Most studies indicate that appropriately applied tape or orthoses do not adversely affect performance.[10]

Thus, athletes with a sprained ankle should complete supervised rehabilitation, including a 6–10-week program of balance training exercise, before returning to practice or competition. An appropriate orthosis should be worn at least until the completion of rehabilitation.

Summary

- External ankle support prevents ankle injuries—at least in athletes with previous injury.
- It is not clear whether high-top shoes reduces the risk of ankle sprains.
- Balance training improves sensorimotor control in athletes with previous injury, and prevents ankle sprains in this population.
- Athletes with a sprained ankle should complete supervised rehabilitation, including a 6–10-week program of balance training exercise, before returning to practice or competition and an appropriate orthosis should be worn at least until completion of rehabilitation.

Key messages

- The preventive effects of bracing have been clearly documented, although the evidence is more convincing for players with previous ankle injury than for healthy athletes.
- Although there are some indications that braces seem to be more effective in preventing ankle sprains than tape, this has not been clearly documented. It should be noted that all of the quality research to date on the effect of external ankle support has been done on orthoses, very little evidence exists on ankle taping.
- The efficacy of wearing high-top shoes is unclear.
- Balance training reduces the risk of ankle sprains in athletes with previous injury.

Sample examination questions

Multiple-choice questions (answers on page 602)

1 Which is the most important risk factor for an ankle sprain?
   A A history of a previous sprain
   B Gender
   C Generalized joint laxity
   D Short Achilles tendon
   E Rear foot valgus

2 Which statement correctly reflects currently available evidence for the effectiveness of balance training in preventing ankle sprains?
   A There is no evidence to support the effectiveness of balance training to prevent ankle sprains
   B There is evidence to show that balance training reduces the risk of ankle sprains in athletes with a history of previous injury
   C The preventive effects of balance training have been clearly documented, both for athletes with no prior ankle sprain and athletes with a history of previous ankle injury
   D Current evidence suggests that there is no effect of balance training in preventing ankle sprains

3 Which statement correctly reflects currently available evidence for the effectiveness of external ankle support (taping or bracing) in preventing ankle sprains?
   A There is insufficient evidence to support or refute the effectiveness of taping and bracing to prevent ankle sprains
   B The preventive effects of taping or bracing have been clearly documented, although the evidence is more convincing for players with previous ankle injury than for healthy athletes
   C The preventive effects of taping or bracing have been clearly documented, both for athletes with no prior ankle sprain and athletes with a history of previous ankle injury
   D Current evidence suggests that there is no effect of taping and bracing in preventing ankle sprains

Essay questions

1 When reading a paper on the effectiveness of external ankle support or balance training for preventing ankle sprains, we should try to take the methodological quality of the study into account. What are important aspects of the design of a randomized clinical trial for the prevention of ankle sprains?

2 As yet, only a few studies have examined the effectiveness of balance training to prevent ankle injuries. What are the most important results of these studies?
3 Many questions regarding the effectiveness of ankle injury prevention programs remain unanswered, and further research is needed. In your opinion, what are the most important research questions, and which studies should be given a high priority on the research agenda?

Summarizing the evidence

Comparison/treatment strategies	Results	Level of evidence*
External ankle support	5 RCTs, one of moderate size†, all in favor of external ankle support	A1
Balance training	1 moderate-size RCT, 2 small size RCTs, in favor of balance training	A2
Shoe type (low-top vs. high-top)	1 small size RCT, two cohort studies, conflicting results	A4

* A1: evidence from large randomized controlled trials (RCTs) or systematic review (including meta-analysis).†
A2: evidence from at least one high-quality cohort.
A3: evidence from at least one moderate-sized RCT or systematic review.
A4: evidence from at least one RCT.
B: evidence from at least one high-quality study of nonrandomized cohorts.
C: expert opinions.
† Arbitrarily, the following cut-off points have been used: large study size, total number of injuries ≥ 100 per intervention group; moderate study size, total number of injuries ≥ 50 per intervention group.

References

1 Tropp H, Odenrick P, Gillquist J. Stabilometry recordings in functional and mechanical instability of the ankle joint. *Int J Sports Med* 1985; **6**:180–182.
2 Konradsen L, Ravn JB. Ankle instability caused by prolonged peroneal reaction time. *Acta Orthop Scand* 1990; **61**:388–390.
3 Karlsson J, Peterson L, Andreasson G, Högfors C. The unstable ankle: a combined EMG and biomechanical modeling study. *Int J Sport Biomech* 1992; **8**:129–144.
4 Konradsen L, Ravn JB. Prolonged peroneal reaction time in ankle instability. *Int J Sports Med* 1991; **12**:290–292.
5 Konradsen L, Olesen S, Hansen HM. Ankle sensorimotor control and eversion strength after acute ankle inversion injuries. *Am J Sports Med* 1998; **26**:72–77.
6 Quigley TB, Cox J, Murphy MH. Protective device for the ankle. *JAMA* 1946; **123**:924.
7 Thorndike AJ. *Athletic injuries: Prevention, Diagnosis and Treatment.* Philadelphia: Lea and Febiger, 1956.
8 Verhagen EA, van Mechelen W, de Vente W. The effect of preventive measures on the incidence of ankle sprains. *Clin J Sport Med* 2000; **10**:291–296.
9 Quinn K, Parker P, de Bie R, Rowe B, Handoll H. Interventions for preventing ankle ligament injuries. *Cochrane Database Syst Rev* 2000; (2):CD000018.

10 Thacker SB, Stroup DF, Branche CM. The prevention of ankle sprains in sports: a systematic review of the literature. *Am J Sports Med* 1999; **27**:753–760.

11 Hume PA, Gerrard DF. Effectiveness of external ankle support: bracing and taping in rugby union. *Sports Med* 1998; **25**:285–312.

12 Robbins S, Waked E. Factors associated with ankle injuries: preventive measures. *Sports Med* 1998; **25**:63–72.

13 Callaghan MJ. Role of ankle taping and bracing in the athlete. *Br J Sports Med* 1997; **31**:102–108.

14 Osborne MD, Rizzo TD Jr. Prevention and treatment of ankle sprain in athletes. *Sports Med* 2003; **33**:1145–1150.

15 Verhagen E, van der Beek A, Twisk J. The effect of a proprioceptive balance board training program for the prevention of ankle sprains: a prospective controlled trial. *Am J Sports Med* 2004; **32**:1385–1393.

16 Handoll HH, Rowe BH, Quinn KM, de Bie R. Interventions for preventing ankle ligament injuries. *Cochrane Database Syst Rev* 2001; (**3**):CD000018.

17 Simon JE. Study of the comparative effectiveness of ankle taping and ankle wrapping on the prevention of ankle injuries. *J Natl Athl Trainers Assoc* 1969; **4**:6–7.

18 Garrick JG, Requa RK. Role of external support in the prevention of ankle sprains. *Med Sci Sports* 1973; **5**:200–203.

19 Cameron BM. The swivel football shoe: a controlled study. *J Sports Med* 1973; 1:16–27.

20 Ekstrand J, Gillquist J, Liljedahl SO. Prevention of soccer injuries: supervision by doctor and physiotherapist. *Am J Sports Med* 1983; **11**:116–120.

21 Tropp H, Askling C, Gillquist J. Prevention of ankle sprains. *Am J Sports Med* 1985; **13**:259–262.

22 Rovere GD, Clarke TJ, Yates CS, Burley K. Retrospective comparison of taping and ankle stabilizers in preventing ankle injuries. *Am J Sports Med* 1988; **16**:228–233.

23 Barrett JR, Tanji JL, Drake C, Fuller D, Kawasaki RI, Fenton RM. High- versus low-top shoes for the prevention of ankle sprains in basketball players: a prospective randomized study. *Am J Sports Med* 1993; **21**:582–585.

24 Surve I, Schwellnus MP, Noakes T, Lombard C. A fivefold reduction in the incidence of recurrent ankle sprains in soccer players using the Sport-Stirrup orthosis. *Am J Sports Med* 1994; **22**:601–606.

25 Sitler M, Ryan J, Wheeler B. The efficacy of a semirigid ankle stabilizer to reduce acute ankle injuries in basketball: a randomized clinical study at West Point. *Am J Sports Med* 1994; **22**:454–461.

26 Wester JU, Jespersen SM, Nielsen KD, Neumann L. Wobble board training after partial sprains of the lateral ligaments of the ankle: a prospective randomized study. *J Orthop Sports Phys Ther* 1996; **23**:332–336.

27 Sharpe SR, Knapik JJ, Jones B. Ankle braces effectively reduce recurrence of ankle sprains in female soccer players. *J Athletic Train* 1997; **32**:21–24.

28 Bahr R, Bahr IA, Lian Ø. A twofold reduction in the incidence of acute ankle sprains in volleyball after the introduction of an injury prevention program: a prospective cohort study. *Scand J Med Sci Sports* 1997; **7**:172–177.

29 Amoroso PJ, Ryan JB, Bickley B. Braced for impact: reducing military paratroopers' ankle sprains using outside-the-boot braces. *J Trauma Inj Inf Crit Care* 1998; **45**:575–580.

30 Holme E, Magnusson SP, Becher K. The effect of supervised rehabilitation on strength, postural sway, position sense and re-injury risk after acute ankle ligament sprain. *Scand J Med Sci Sports* 1999; **9**:104–109.

31 Schumacher JT Jr, Creedon JF, Pope RW. The effectiveness of the parachutist ankle brace in reducing ankle injuries in an airborne ranger battalion. *Mil Med* 2000; **165**:944–948.

32 Stasinopoulos D. Comparison of three preventive methods in order to reduce the incidence of ankle inversion sprains among female volleyball players. *Br J Sports Med* 2004; **38**:182–185.

33 Olsen OE, Myklebust G, Engebretsen L, Holme I, Bahr R. Exercises to prevent lower limb injuries in youth sports: cluster randomised controlled trial. *BMJ* 2005; **330**:449.

34 Ryan JB, Amoroso PJ, Jones BH. Impact of an outside-the-boot ankle brace on sprains associated with military airborne training [abstract]. *Orthop Trans* 1994; **18**:557.

35 Barkler EH, Magnusson SP, Becher K. [The effect of supervised rehabilitation on ankle joint function and the risk of recurrence after acute ankle distortion; in Danish.] *Ugeskr Laeger* 2001; **163**:3223–3226.

36 Gauffin H, Tropp H, Odenrick P. Effect of ankle disk training on postural control in patients with functional instability of the ankle joint. *Int J Sports Med* 1988; **9**:141–144.

37 Sheth P, Yu B, Laskowski ER, An KN. Ankle disk training influences reaction times of selected muscles in a simulated ankle sprain. *Am J Sports Med* 1997; **25**:538–543.

38 Karlsson J, Bergsten T, Peterson L, Zachrisson BE. Radiographic evaluation of ankle joint stability. *Clin J Sport Med* 1991; **1**:166–175.

39 Freeman MAR, Wyke B. Articular reflexes at the ankle joint: an electromyographic study of normal and abnormal influences of ankle-joint mechanoreceptors upon reflex activity in the leg muscles. *J Bone Joint Surg (Br)* 1967; **54**:990–1001.

40 Michelson JD, Hutchins C. Mechanoreceptors in human ankle ligaments. *J Bone Joint Surg (Br)* 1995; **77**:219–224.

41 Fridén T, Zätterström R, Lindstrand A, Moritz U. A stabilometric technique for evaluation of lower limb instabilities. *Am J Sports Med* 1989; **17**:118–122.

42 Verhagen EA, van Mechelen W, van der Beek AJ. The effect of tape, braces and shoes on ankle range of motion. *Sports Med* 2001; **31**:667–677.

43 Cordova ML, Ingersoll CD, LeBlanc MJ. Influence of ankle support on joint range of motion before and after exercise: a meta-analysis. *J Orthop Sports Phys Ther* 2000; **30**:170–177.

44 Wright IC, Neptune RR, van den Bogert AJ, Nigg BM. The influence of foot positioning on ankle sprains. *J Biomech* 2000; **33**:513–519.

45 Eils E, Rosenbaum D. The main function of ankle braces is to control the joint position before landing. *Foot Ankle Int* 2003; **24**:263–268.

46 Konradsen L. Factors contributing to chronic ankle instability: kinesthesia and joint position sense. *J Athl Train* 2002; **37**:381–385.

CHAPTER 28

How should you treat a stress fracture?

Kim Bennell and Peter Brukner

Introduction

Stress fractures are overuse injuries of bone commonly seen in physically active individuals such as athletes[1,2] and military recruits.[3,4] They can occur in any bone, but are most frequently seen in the lower limb, particularly in the region of the tibia.[5]

Stress fractures are partial or complete fractures of bone that develop when bone does not successfully adapt to the repeated application of load. During physical activity, microdamage that develops is normally repaired by the remodeling process. However, if microdamage accumulates, symptoms of excessive bone strain may result.[6–8] Bone's ability to resist damage depends on a number of factors, including its structural and material properties and the activity of muscles in attenuating loads.

Stress fracture represents one end of the continuum of bone's response to repetitive loading, but a patient may present with symptoms of bone strain anywhere along this continuum. Current imaging techniques show a range of appearances depending on this time course. Early changes in bone, commonly termed "stress reactions," are visualized by scintigraphy and magnetic resonance imaging,[9] but not by conventional radiographs, which only show evidence of a stress fracture at a later stage.[10]

Search methods and results

A computer search was conducted up to April 2005 using the Cochrane Library, MEDLINE, Current Contents and CINAHL to identify relevant articles using the search terms: stress fracture, fatigue fracture, treatment, and prevention (Table 28.1). The bibliographies of relevant papers were also searched, and other studies relevant to the area were included. The management of osteoporotic fractures in the elderly was excluded. Few randomized controlled trials (RCTs) were found that evaluated an intervention to prevent or treat stress fractures. A Cochrane review of the area up until 2000, using a comprehensive search strategy to identify RCTs or quasi-experimental trials, found nine studies reporting the outcomes of strategies to prevent stress fractures and three studies reporting the efficacy of treatment programs for stress reactions or stress fractures.[11] Assessment of these studies by the authors revealed that the methodological quality was generally poor. Since then, four additional studies have been identified. The prevention studies have all been performed in military recruits, and the types of interventions include shock-absorbing insoles (n = 4),[12–15] orthotic inserts (n = 2),[16,17] basketball shoes (n = 1),[18] training modifications (n = 2),[19,20] calcium supplements (n = 1),[21] and prophylactic risedronate (n = 1).[22] The treatments evaluated include pneumatic air braces (n = 3),[23–25] low-energy laser (n = 1)[26]

Table 28.1 Results of search strategy—number of journal articles identified

Terms	MEDLINE*	CINAHL†
Stress fracture	984	108
Stress fracture and treatment	264	13
Stress fracture and prevention	38	3
Fatigue fracture	155	2
Fatigue fracture and treatment	36	1
Fatigue fracture and prevention	3	0

* Limited to humans and English-language publications.
† Limited to research in English-language publications.

and low-intensity pulsed ultrasound (n = 1).[27] These studies are summarized in Table 28.2, and the findings have been incorporated in detail into the later sections. Given the small number of clinical trials, lower levels of evidence have also been included in this review in order to make recommendations about how to treat stress fractures in clinical practice.

Diagnosis

Patients with stress fractures usually complain of localized pain and tenderness over the fracture site. There will often be a history of a recent change in training, or taking up a new activity. Stress fracture is primarily diagnosed clinically. Clinical suspicion may be confirmed by radiography. The radiographic appearance of a stress fracture is often quite subtle, with the most frequent finding being a periosteal reaction. However, radiographs may fail to show a stress fracture until after it has been present for some time, and some fractures are notoriously difficult to detect using plain radiography. Thus, further investigation is often indicated in the patient in whom stress fracture is suspected but the radiographic findings are normal.

A more sensitive examination is the radioisotopic bone scan (scintigraphy), which can demonstrate the location of an overuse bony lesion. A localized area of increased uptake, or "hot spot," indicates a stress fracture. Until the 1990s, a triple-phase bone scan was considered perfectly sensitive, so a negative bone scan essentially ruled out a stress fracture.[28] In recent years, a few authors have reported finding stress fractures with magnetic resonance imaging (MRI) when the bone scans have been negative.[29] The clinical implication of these cases is that a negative bone scan only represents a 99% probability that there is no stress fracture, rather than a 100% probability. Thus, a bone scan remains a very valuable investigation. The bone scan, however, is a nonspecific investigation, and other bony abnormalities such as tumors and osteomyelitis may therefore cause similar pictures. It may also be difficult to localize the site of the area of increased uptake precisely, especially in an area such as the foot, where numerous small bones are in close proximity.

In most cases of stress fracture, a radioisotopic bone scan is sufficient to confirm the diagnosis, and no further investigations are required. However, in a few sites that are known to present problems with treatment, such as the tarsal navicular, further information regarding the site and extent of the fracture is required. In these cases, a computed-tomographic (CT) scan or MRI may be performed to show the exact site and extent of the fracture.

Table 28.2 Summary of controlled trials investigating prevention or treatment strategies for stress fractures

First author, ref.	Design	Strategy	SF definition	Intervention	Group	Results
Andrish (1974)[12]	RCT	P	Radiography	Foam rubber heel pad	M	No effect
Scully (1982)[20]	QE	P	NS	Training modification	M	Reduction in fractures
Milgrom (1985)[14]	RCT	P	BS	Orthotic inserts	M	Reduction in fractures
Giladi (1985)[19]	QE	P	BS	Training modification	M	No effect
Smith (1985)[13]	QE	P	NS	Shock-absorbing insole	M	No effect
Gardner (1988)[16]	QE	P	Radiography	Polymer insole	M	No effect
Schwellnus (1990)[15]	RCT	P	Radiography	Shock-absorbing insole	M	No effect
Milgrom (1992)[18]	RCT	P	BS	Basketball boot	M	Reduced foot fractures
Schwellnus (1992)[21]	QE	P	Radiography	Calcium supplements	M	No effect
Mundermann (2001)[17]	QE	P	SR	Orthotic inserts	M	Reduced foot fractures
Milgrom (2004)[22]	RCT	P	BS, Radiography	Risedronate	M	No effect
Nissen (1994)[26]	RCT	T	Clinical	Low power laser	M	No effect
Slayter (1995)[23]	RCT	T	BS	Pneumatic leg brace	M	Reduced duty return time
Swenson (1997)[24]	RCT	T	Radiography	Pneumatic leg brace	A	Reduced sport return time
Allen (2004)[25]	RCT	T	BS	Pneumatic leg brace	M	No effect
Rue (2004)[27]	RCT	T	Radiography	Pulsed ultrasound	M	No effect

A, athletes; BS, bone scan; M, military; NS, not stated; P, prevention; QE, quasi-experimental; RCT, randomized, controlled trial; SF, stress fracture; SR, stress reaction; T, treatment.

Table 28.3 Factors influencing the length of time to return to sport following a stress fracture

- Duration of symptoms
- Stage of continuum of bone strain
- Site of stress fracture
- Level of competition

MRI is being increasingly advocated as the investigation of choice for stress fractures. While MRI does not image fractures as clearly as do CT scans, it is of comparable sensitivity to radioisotopic bone scans in assessing bony damage. The typical MRI appearance of a stress fracture shows periosteal and marrow edema plus or minus the actual fracture line.[9]

Treatment

The actual time from diagnosis of a stress fracture to full return to sport or physical activity depends on a number of factors, including the site of the fracture, the length of the symptoms, and the severity of the lesion (stage in the spectrum of bone strain) (Table 28.3). Most stress fractures with a relatively brief history of symptoms will heal without complication or delay and permit a return to sport within the 4–8-week range. However, there is a group of stress fractures that require additional treatment and special consideration. These are listed separately later in this chapter.

While there are many subtleties involved in the treatment of stress fractures, the primary treatment is modified activity. During the phase of modified activity, a number of important issues are attended to including modification of risk factors, maintenance of muscular strength and fitness, pain management, investigation of bone health, and prescription of orthotic devices. We divide the treatment of stress fractures into two phases: phase 1 is the early treatment using modified activity, and phase 2 is the period from the reintroduction of physical activity to full return to sport. The evidence to support the treatment options will be discussed.

Phase 1

Pain management

Pain is seldom severe, but can be a problem even with normal walking. Mild analgesics can be used, as well as physical therapy modalities (e.g., ice, interferential, electrical stimulation). In some cases in which activities of daily living (ADLs) are painful, it may be necessary for the patient with a stress fracture to be non–weight-bearing or partially weight-bearing on crutches for a period of up to 7–10 days. In the majority of cases this is not necessary, and merely avoiding the aggravating activity will be sufficient.

Potential pharmaceutical therapies

Given the pathology of stress fractures, pharmacological agents that accelerate repair and remodeling may assist with healing. According to a review by Burr,[30] one potential agent is intermittently administered parathyroid hormone (PTH). This agent is known to accelerate intracortical bone turnover without any long-term negative effects on bone mass or short-term or long-term negative effects on bone strength. Furthermore, because intermittently administered PTH stimulates the apposition of periosteal bone, this could have beneficial effects on bone strength even after the withdrawal of treatment and lead to a reduced risk for future fracture. However, controlled trials need to be conducted in an animal stress fracture model and then in humans before this drug therapy can be recommended for the treatment of stress fractures.

Practitioners often suggest nonsteroidal anti-inflammatory drugs (NSAIDs) to assist with initial pain reduction and healing of stress fractures. Because they inhibit cyclooxygenases, NSAIDs will help control inflammatory processes that may accompany injury or overload. However, prostaglandins are essential for normal bone turnover and fracture healing and the treatment could thus slow or prevent repair of the stress fracture. This area has been well reviewed by Wheeler and Batt.[31] Since there is no conclusive evidence to date, it would be prudent to limit the use of NSAIDs in patients with stress fractures.

Electrotherapy modalities

Low-energy laser

There has only been one study investigating the application of low-powered laser treatment in the healing of stress fractures.[26] This RCT was performed in army recruits who presented with a diagnosis of "shin splints." The treatment consisted of laser therapy at 40 mW in 60 s/cm of tender tibial edge, and a placebo group was included. The results do not support the use of this modality for reducing symptoms of tibial periostitis/stress reaction, as there was no difference in the number of recruits fit for duty after 2 weeks when the active and placebo groups were compared.

Electrical stimulation

Various methods of electrical stimulation have all been shown to have a positive effect on healing of nonunion of traumatic fractures. These include pulsed electromagnetic fields,[24,32–36] direct electric current,[37–40] and capacitively coupled electric field.[38,41–43] There have been no studies of the efficacy of this treatment on the healing of stress fractures and only one nonblinded, uncontrolled study of its effect on the time to return to sport in stress fractures in athletes.

Benazzo *et al.*[44] reported the results of a study on the treatment of stress fractures in athletes by capacitive coupling, a bone healing stimulation method promoting bone formation by application of alternating current in the form of a sinusoidal wave. Twenty-two of 25 stress fractures were healed, and two more showed improvement. The majority of these fractures were stress fractures of the navicular and fifth metatarsal, which are prone to delayed union or nonunion. Further controlled studies are required to determine the efficacy of this treatment in the management of both the acute stress fracture and in cases of nonuniting stress fractures.

Low-intensity pulsed ultrasound

A growing body of evidence provides support for the application of low-intensity pulsed ultrasound (US) during fracture repair. In animals, US has been found to facilitate endochondral bone formation,[45] increase bone mineral return, and enhance mechanical strength return at the fracture site.[46] In humans, the most convincing evidence for the use of US during acute fracture repair is provided by three well-designed RCTs,[47–49] in which US accelerated the rate of fresh tibial, radial, and scaphoid fracture repair by a factor of

1.4–1.6 (or 30–38%). In addition, ultrasound has been shown to reduce the incidence of delayed unions[50] and to facilitate healing in fractures displaying delayed union and nonunion.[51–54]

The results of a case study[55] and a case series of athletes with stress fractures treated with low-intensity pulsed US appeared promising.[56] However, a recent randomized, double-blind, placebo-controlled trial failed to find an effect of US on healing time in 46 tibial stress fractures treated for 20 minutes daily with a commercially available US system.[27] This lack of effect may be due to the relatively small sample size. At this stage, US would not be recommended for routine treatment of stress fractures, but might be an option for stress fractures at sites prone to delayed union or nonunion or in elite athletes. Research is needed to further assess the effects of pulsed US on stress fracture healing, including different dosages and different sites.

Muscle strengthening

Skeletal muscle plays an important role in stress fracture development. At some regions, bone load is increased by muscular force, while at other sites load is reduced as muscles absorb energy.[57] In endurance sports, it is possible that even low levels of muscular fatigue can affect the total impact load to bone, particularly in the lower extremity. Following fatiguing exercise, bone strain, particularly strain rate, has been shown to increase.[58,59] Some studies have shown that reduced muscle strength[60] and smaller muscle size[61–63] predispose to stress fractures in athletes and military recruits. Biomechanical analyses of how muscular forces act on bone to cause stress fractures have only been done for the rib, fibula, tibia, and metatarsals. The role of muscular forces in the development of other stress fractures is generally speculative.[64]

While there are no studies that have evaluated the role of muscle strengthening in the treatment of stress fractures, it is logical to include a specific strengthening program because of the important role of muscles in shock absorption and to help counteract the effects of detraining. In the clinical setting, decrements in muscular strength and endurance may be undetectable whether testing manually or using a machine such as an isokinetic dynamometer. Thus, all athletes with stress fractures of the lower extremity should receive a specific program of muscular strengthening exercises in muscle groups surrounding the joints above and below the fracture line. Attention should be paid to developing muscle endurance. Muscle strengthening programs are usually prescribed for a period of 6–12 weeks and can begin immediately after diagnosis of the stress fracture. However, it is important that the exercises do not cause pain at the stress fracture site.

Maintaining fitness

Maintenance of fitness during periods of forced inactivity due to injury is a major concern to coaches and athletes. Inactivity has marked detrimental effects on the cardiovascular system, as well as on the metabolic and morphological characteristics of skeletal muscle. Reductions in various parameters of fitness have been reported after relatively brief periods of inactivity. Decrements in maximal stroke volume, cardiac output, and maximal oxygen uptake of approximately 25% have been reported after 20 days of bedrest.[65] Other studies have shown a decline of 14–16% in maximal oxygen uptake with cessation of training for 6 weeks.[66,67]

The effect of rest on performance varies from one athlete to another and depends on the particular sport. It should be emphasized to the athlete that during phase 1, the rehabilitation program is designed to allow the damaged bone time to heal and gradually develop or regain full strength while maintaining the person's fitness in ways that avoid overloading the bone.

Nonloading activities that maintain fitness are those that use as many large muscle groups as possible without overloading the bone. The recruitment of many large muscles results in high oxygen uptake, and in substituting a nonloading activity for the athlete's sport, the goal is to place an equal or greater demand on the cardiopulmonary system to supply large quantities of oxygen to the working muscles. The most common methods of maintaining fitness are cycling, swimming, water running, rowing, and StairMaster. For muscular strength, upper and lower body weight programs can usually be prescribed without risk. These work-outs should as much as possible mimic the athlete's normal training program in both duration and intensity.

Deep water running (DWR), involving immersion up to the neck using a vest as a flotation device, is particularly attractive to runners because it closely simulates their sport. Training studies comparing DWR and land running have reported no significant differences in maximal oxygen uptake,[68–70] anaerobic threshold, running economy,[70] leg strength,[68] and 2-mile performance[69] after 4–8 weeks of land versus DWR training. Avellini *et al.*[71] reported similar improvements in land maximal oxygen uptake after a 12-week DWR program in comparison with a land cycling ergometer program.

The effectiveness of DWR is dependent on the simulation of land-based running style and workouts in the water. However, DWR is not identical to land running, and some important differences must be taken into account when setting a DWR program. The viscosity friction of the water environment and the non–weight-bearing nature of DWR make this form of running mechanically different from land running. Stride frequency in DWR has been reported to be 60–65% that of land values.[72] While heart rate can be used to monitor exercise intensity in DWR sessions, it is important to note that water immersion results in a cephalad shift in blood volume, resulting in an increase in stroke volume[73] and a decline in maximal heart rate[72–74] during water immersion exercise. The effect of water immersion on heart rate has been reported to be a reduction of approximately 10–13 beats per minute when exercising at high workloads, but similar to land values at lower intensities of exercise.[75]

It is possible to maintain fitness even in elite athletes. Frangolias *et al.*[76] reported the case of an elite middle distance runner who sustained a Jones fracture of the right foot that required a lengthy (10–12-week) period of non–weight-bearing cast immobilization. Limited activity was allowed during the first 3 weeks after injury, due to discomfort. A more structured program consisting of a 6-day training and 1-day rest schedule was initiated in week 4 (Table 28.4). Treadmill $\mathrm{Vo}_{2\max}$ and ventilatory threshold showed small decreases but progressive improvement when measured at 23 and 30 weeks post-injury in comparison with pre-injury levels. The 10-km race performance at 31 weeks post-injury was 6 seconds faster than the pre-injury time.

Alternate activities have been shown to maintain $\mathrm{Vo}_{2\max}$ and muscular strength, but specific metabolic and neuromuscular adaptations that affect skill are not easily duplicated. For this reason, isolated skill-related activities are resumed as early as possible in phase 1. It is possible in most cases for the athlete to maintain specific sports skills. In ball sports, these can involve activities either seated or standing still. This active rest approach also greatly assists the athlete psychologically.

Table 28.4 Weekly water running training regimen

Day	Training regimen
1	Interval training, simulated mile repeats: 4 × 5 min to 6 × 5 min with 1 min rest; HR 175–180 bpm
2	Low-intensity run: 30–45 min; HR 130–150 bpm
3	Interval training, hard intervals: 6 × 3 min with 1 min rest; HR 175–180 bpm
4	Low-intensity run, as for day 2
5	Interval training, short: 5–15 × 2 min or 5–15 × 1 min, with 30-s rest; HR 175–180 bpm
6	Long steady-state run: 40–90 min; HR 145–165 bpm
7	Rest day (or low-intensity run performed)

Source: adapted and reproduced with permission from Frangolias *et al.*[76]
HR, heart rate; bpm, beats per minute.

Modification of risk factors

As with any overuse injury, it is not sufficient to merely treat the stress fracture itself. Stress fractures represent the result of incremental overload. Subtle adjustments to modifiable factors that contribute to the total load are an essential component of the management of an athlete with a stress fracture. A thorough history and clinical examination will assist in identifying the factors that may have contributed to the injury and those that can be modified to reduce the risk of injury recurring (Table 28.5). The fact that stress fractures have a high rate of recurrence is an indication that this part of the management program is often neglected.[1,77] However, it should be pointed out that there have been few clinical trials to evaluate the effectiveness of risk factor modification in reducing stress fracture development or recurrence. Instead, most of the studies are cohort studies in which the relationship of the risk factor to stress fracture is evaluated in either a prospective or retrospective manner. The following section briefly reviews the evidence to support the role of modifiable risk factors for stress fractures.

Training

While training errors have been anecdotally linked to stress fracture development, there is little research to identify the contribution of each training component (type, volume, intensity, frequency and rate of change) especially in athletes. There are only two RCTs that have evaluated the effect of training modifications on stress fracture development,[19,20] and these are in the military setting. It appears that reducing high-impact activities such as running and jumping decreases stress fracture incidence, whereas reducing marching distance has no effect.[11] Other studies have shown that training interventions such as the inclusion of rest periods,[20,78] elimination of running and marching on concrete,[79,80] and pre-entry physical conditioning[81,82] may also reduce stress fracture risk in the military. In female recruits, reducing marching speed and allowing individual step lengths, running on softer surfaces, and replacing longer runs with interval running significantly reduced pelvic stress fracture incidence.[83]

In athletes, Brunet *et al.*[84] surveyed 1505 runners and found that increasing mileage correlated with an increase in stress fractures in women, but not men. In a study of ballet dancers, a dancer who trained for more than 5 hours per day had an estimated risk for stress fracture that was 16 times greater than a dancer who trained for less than 5 hours

Table 28.5 Risk factor assessment in a patient presenting with a stress fracture

Risk factor	Variables
Training	• Type • Volume • Intensity • Surface • Changes in training
Footwear	• Type • Age of shoe • Use of insoles
Lower limb alignment	• Foot type • Tibial torsion • Knee varus/valgus • Femoral anteversion • Leg length
Muscle length and joint range	• Flexibility of calf, hamstrings, hip flexors • Range of ankle dorsiflexion, hip internal/external rotation
Menstrual status	• Current and past menstrual patterns • Use of the oral contraceptive pill • Sex hormonal levels if irregular
Bone density—dual-energy X-ray absorptiometry (DXA)	• If amenorrheic or multiple stress fracture history
Dietary intake	• Calcium • Energy • Other nutrients influencing absorption of calcium or bone health—e.g., protein, fiber • Presence of eating disorder

per day.[85] These studies support a role for training volume as a risk factor for stress fracture in athletes.

In the clinical setting, it is imperative to obtain a detailed training history to try and identify any training parameters that may have contributed to that individual's stress fracture. In particular, questions should be directed at establishing volume, intensity, degree of rest periods, type of training and any recent changes in these parameters. Furthermore, athletes should be encouraged to keep an accurate training log book. This will allow the athlete to monitor his or her training and to gauge the appropriateness of training changes. Coaches should ensure that training regimens for athletes are individualized. What may be appropriate for most members of a team may be excessive for some.

Footwear and insoles

A Cochrane review identified six RCTs or quasi-experimental trials that evaluated the effect of insoles or other footwear modifications on prevention of stress fractures.[12–16,18] All were conducted in the military setting. The authors of the review concluded that "the use of insoles inside boots in military recruits during their initial training appears to reduce the number of stress fractures and/or stress reactions of bone by over 50%."[11] Another study published since then also found that various types of orthotic insert were associated with fewer foot stress fractures.[17] Whether the results can be generalized to the sporting population, who often wear different footwear and perform different training, is not clear. This is emphasized by a laboratory experiment study that found that semirigid orthoses lowered tibial bone strain when worn in boots while walking, but increased strains during running.[86]

Another important contributing factor to stress fracture development may be inadequate training shoes. These shoes may be inappropriate for the particular foot type of the individual, may have generally inadequate support/shock absorption, or may be worn out. In a randomized trial, training in basketball shoes compared with normal military boots was associated with a significant reduction in the incidence of stress fractures in the foot, but not in overall stress fractures.[18] Mechanical durometry tests confirmed that the basketball shoes had superior shock attenuation than the military boots, and *in vivo* tests showed significantly lower tibial accelerometry when recruits wore the basketball shoes.[87] The potential effect of footwear is further highlighted by an increase in second metatarsal stress fractures in Swedish military recruits, which accompanied the introduction of a new boot with a more flexible outer sole.[88] The new boot was shown to increase dorsal metatarsal tension.

Biomechanical abnormalities

Intrinsic biomechanical abnormalities are also thought to be contributing factors to the development of overuse injuries in general and stress fractures in particular. While associations between stress fractures and various factors influencing skeletal alignment have been sought in military populations, there are few data pertaining to athletes.

The structure of the foot will partly determine how much force is absorbed by the bones in the foot and how much force is transferred to proximal bones such as the tibia during ground contact. The high-arched (pes cavus) foot is more rigid and less able to absorb shock, resulting in more force passing to the tibia and femur. The low-arched (pes planus) foot is more flexible, allowing stress to be absorbed by the musculoskeletal structures of the foot. It is also often associated with prolonged pronation or hyperpronation, which can induce a great amount of torsion on the tibia and may exacerbate muscle fatigue as the muscles have to work harder to control the excessive motion, especially at toe-off. Theoretically, either foot type could predispose to a stress fracture. Several studies have indicated that the risk of stress fracture is greater for male recruits with high foot arches than for those with low arches,[89–91] although not all have corroborated these findings.[92] Most of the athlete studies are case series that do not allow comparison of injured and uninjured athletes. While pes planus may be the most common foot type in athletes presenting to sports clinics with stress fractures,[93,94] pes planus may be equally as common in athletes who remain uninjured. A high foot arch and greater forefoot varus was more likely in athletes with recurrent stress fractures than in athletes without stress fractures.[95] It is also possible that a relationship between foot type and stress fracture may vary depending on the site of stress fracture.[5,90] Therefore, studies may fail to find an association between certain foot types and stress fractures because they have not analyzed the data separately by stress fracture site.

There is evidence from cohort studies to show that a leg length discrepancy increases the likelihood of stress fractures in both military[96] and athletic[62,84,95] populations, but the injury does not seem to occur on either the shorter or longer leg preferentially. Other alignment features include the presence of genu varum, valgum or recurvatum, Q angle, and tibial torsion. Of these, only an increased Q angle has been found in association with stress fractures,[97] although this is not a universal finding.[92,98]

The literature suggests that foot type may play a role in stress fracture development, but the exact relationship probably depends upon the anatomical location of the injured region and the activities undertaken by the individual. However, a leg length discrepancy does appear to be a risk factor in both military and civilian populations, and thus a heel raise should be provided to the patient if necessary. The failure to find an association between other biomechanical features and stress fractures in cohort studies does not necessarily rule out their importance. A thorough biomechanical assessment is an essential part of both treatment and prevention of stress fractures. Until the contribution of biomechanical abnormalities to stress fracture risk is clarified through scientific research, correction of such abnormalities should be attempted, if possible.

Muscle flexibility and joint range of motion

The role of flexibility is difficult to evaluate, as flexibility encompasses a number of characteristics, including active joint mobility, ligamentous laxity, and muscle length. Numerous variables have been assessed in relation to stress fractures, including range of rearfoot inversion/eversion, ankle dorsiflexion/plantarflexion, knee flexion/extension, and hip rotation/extension, together with length of the calf, hamstring, quadriceps, hip adductors, and hip flexor muscles.[62,92,98–102] Of these, only increased range of hip external rotation[100,101,103] and decreased range of ankle dorsiflexion[99] have been associated with stress fracture development, and even these findings have been inconsistent.

The difficulty in assessing the role of muscle and joint flexibility in stress fractures may relate to a number of factors, including the relatively imprecise methods of measurement, the heterogeneity of these variables, and the fact that both increased and decreased flexibility may be contributory. Until better evidence is available to the contrary, it is worth prescribing stretches if muscle flexibility and joint range are found to be restricted in the athlete who presents with a stress fracture.

Menstrual status

Women with stress fractures should be questioned about their current and past menstrual status. There is sufficient evidence from cross-sectional and cohort studies to show that menstrual disturbances increase the risk of stress fracture[62,85,98,104–115] and lead to premature bone loss, particularly at trabecular sites.[116–120] Lower bone density in women may be associated with a greater risk of stress fractures, although results from studies are mixed.[62,110–114,121–123] It may be that low bone density plays a greater role in predisposing to stress fractures at cancellous bone sites rather than cortical sites.[124]

The management of the amenorrheic female athlete with a stress fracture is controversial, and we would suggest treating each case individually. It is now thought that the primary cause of bone loss in athletic amenorrhea is not a lack of estrogen, but rather low energy availability due to dietary restriction and/or excessive exercise.[125,126] Low energy availability has been found to uncouple bone turnover and suppress bone formation.[127] This has implications for treatment and may explain why improvements in bone density with the oral contraceptive pill are not as great[128,129] as those demonstrated with hormone replacement therapies in postmenopausal women.[130] It may also explain why prospective cohort studies in athletes[62] and military recruits[98] have failed to support a protective effect of oral contraceptive pill use on stress fracture development.

On the basis of the research to date, it would seem that treatment of the amenorrheic athlete should focus on reducing the energy imbalance, either by reducing the amount and intensity of her activity and/or increasing her daily energy intake.

The role of bone density measurement in these patients is still unclear. Bone density measurements compare the patient's bone density to the "average," but it is known that bone density is increased in those involved in weight-bearing exercise,[131] and there are no normative databases for athletes. We find bone density measurement useful in the amenorrheic athlete, both to provide a baseline measurement prior to treatment and as a potential additional factor in convincing the athlete to commence treatment.

Dietary intake

Dietary surveys of various sporting groups often reveal inadequate intakes of macronutrients and micronutrients, which are important for skeletal health.[132,133] Furthermore, athletes report a greater frequency of disordered eating patterns than the general population, especially those in sports emphasizing leanness and/or those competing at higher levels.[134] As discussed, low caloric intake has been hypothesized as one of the mechanisms for menstrual disturbances in sportswomen.[126] Disordered eating, amenorrhea, and osteopenia often occur simultaneously in athletic females, a syndrome that has been referred to as the "female athlete triad."[135] This syndrome appears to be encountered less frequently in female military personnel.[136]

There is currently little evidence to support low calcium intake as a risk factor for stress fractures in athletic[62,85,110,111,113,137,138] or military[121] populations. In the only controlled trial, calcium supplementation of 500 mg daily had no significant effect on stress fracture incidence in male military recruits.[21] Conversely, abnormal and restrictive eating behaviors and low energy intake do seem to increase the likelihood of fracture in women.[61,62,111,114,138,139]

Healthy eating habits should be promoted in all individuals. If one is concerned about dietary intake in those presenting with a stress fracture, food records as well as biochemical and anthropometric indices should be used to assess dietary adequacy and nutritional status. Appropriate nutritional counseling should be provided if necessary.

Bracing

The use of a pneumatic air brace may assist with stress fracture healing in the leg and reduce the time taken to return to sport. Swenson and colleagues[24] propose that the pneumatic leg brace shifts a portion of the weight-bearing load from the tibia to the soft tissue, which results in less impact loading with walking, hopping, and running. They also suggest that the brace facilitates healing at the fracture site by acting to compress the soft tissue, thereby increasing the intravascular hydrostatic pressure and resulting in a shifting of the fluid and electrolytes from the capillary space to the interstitial space. This theoretically enhances the piezoelectric effect and enhances osteoblastic bone formation.

Two case series reported excellent results with the use of a pneumatic leg brace. Dickson and Kichline[140] found that all athletes were able to return immediately to their sports without disabling symptoms. Whitelaw *et al.*[141] reported that resumption of activity occurred after an average of 3.7 weeks, with return to full, unrestricted activity occurring after an average of 5.3 weeks. Recently, it was reported that four patients with delayed union of anterior mid-tibial stress fractures all avoided the need for surgery with the use of the leg brace together with modified rest.[142] However, being case series, none of these three studies had a control group.

Two RCTs, one in military recruits[23] and one in athletes,[24] showed a significant reduction in the time to recommencing training after diagnosis of stress fracture with the use of a pneumatic leg brace (weighted mean difference –42.6 days; 95% CI, –55.8 to –29.4 days.[11] Swenson *et al.*[24] found that the median time from the initiation of treatment to the completion of a standard functional progression program was 21 days in the brace group (n = 8) in comparison with 77 days in the traditional group (n = 10). However, a more recent study with similar numbers of military recruits with tibial stress fractures (n = 20 completing) failed to find an effect of the brace on time to pain free hop and run.[25] While results are conflicting, there is some evidence to suggest that a pneumatic brace accelerates the return to activity[11] after fibular or tibial stress fractures.

Phase II

When normal, day-to-day ambulation is pain-free, resumption of the impact loading activities begins. The rate of resumption of activity is individual and should be modified according to symptoms and physical findings. The time to return to sport is variable, depending on a number of factors such as the site of stress fracture, the person's age, competitive level, and time to diagnosis.[143] Table 28.6 shows the percentage of stress fractures healed at various times in a case series of 368 stress fractures in athletes.[144] It is apparent that at some sites, such as the femoral neck, sesamoids, and middle third of the tibia, recovery generally takes longer than 2 months. However, at other sites, such as the fibula and metatarsals, recovery takes less than 2 months.

There are no studies that have compared different return-to-sport programs. However, since healing bone is weaker, a progressive increase in load is needed so that the bone will

Table 28.6 Percentage of stress fractures healed at different times in a case series of 368 stress fractures in athletes

Stress fracture site	**Healing period**		
	2–4 weeks (%)	**1–2 months (%)**	**> 2 months (%)**
Tibia			
Proximal third	0	43	57
Middle third	0	48	52
Distal third	0	53	47
Fibula	7	75	18
Metatarsals	20	57	23
Sesamoids	0	0	100
Femur			
Shaft	7	7	86
Neck	0	0	100
Pelvis	0	29	71
Olecranon	0	0	100

Source: adapted with permission from Hulkko and Orava.[144]

Table 28.7 Progression of activities based on their degree of tibial bone loading

- Cycling
- Walking, leg press, StairMaster
- Treadmill running
- Straight line outdoor running
- Sprinting, running on curved track
- Zig-zag running, up/down hills, jumping
- Zig-zag hopping, rebounding

adapt with increases in strength. Some studies have evaluated the degree of tibial bone loading during various activities, using strain gauges cemented onto the tibia of a small number of healthy volunteers.[145–148] The results provide some insight into a possible progression of activities during rehabilitation after tibial stress fractures (Table 28.7).

For lower limb stress fractures in which running is the aggravating activity, we recommend a program that involves initial brisk walking, increasing by 5–10 minutes per day up to a length of 45 minutes. Resumption of activity should not be accompanied by pain, but it is not uncommon to have some discomfort at the site of the stress fracture. If bony pain occurs, then activity should cease for 1–2 days. If the individual is pain-free with normal ambulation, the activity is resumed at the volume and pace below the level at which the pain occurred. The patient should be clinically reassessed at 2-weekly intervals to assess the progress of the training program and any symptoms related to the stress fracture.

Once 45 minutes of continuous brisk walking is achieved without pain, slow jogging can begin for a period of 5 minutes within the 45-minute walk. Treadmill running provides less tibial strain than running outdoors. Assuming that this increase in activity does not reproduce the patient's symptoms, the amount of jogging can be increased by 5 minutes per session on a daily or every-other-day basis to a total of 45 minutes at slow jogging pace. This period of time is necessary to load the bone slowly and to be sure that adequate healing has occurred. Once the 45-minute goal is achieved, the pace can be increased—initially half-pace and then gradually increasing to full-pace striding. Once full sprinting is achieved pain-free, functional activities such as hopping, skipping, jumping, twisting, and turning can be introduced gradually (Table 28.7). It is important that this process is a graduated one, and it is important to err on the side of caution rather than try to return too quickly. A typical program for an individual with an uncomplicated lower limb stress fracture resuming activity after a period of initial rest and activities of daily living is shown in Table 28.8.

This pattern of reintroduction of activity can be followed for other sports. For example, with aerobics classes, reintroduction of aerobic floor exercises should begin at 2 minutes per session with the remaining 18 minutes of "cardio" being spent on the exercise bike. This ratio is gradually increased until the patient is back to full-time floor exercise.

It is not infrequent for the patient to experience pain at some point during the reintroduction of activity. This by no means is an indication of a return of the stress fracture. In each instance, the activity should be discontinued, followed by several days of modified rest, and then training should resume at a level lower than at which the pain occurred. If the clinician places the patient on an accelerated program for the reintroduction of activity, monitoring periods should be adjusted accordingly, and in some cases, should be weekly. Progress should be monitored clinically by the presence or absence of symptoms

Table 28.8 Activity program following uncomplicated lower limb stress fracture following a period of rest and activities of daily living

			a period of rest and activities of daily living				
	Day 1 (min)	**Day 2 (min)**	**Day 3 (min)**	**Day 4 (min)**	**Day 5 (min)**	**Day 6 (min)**	**Day 7 (min)**
Week 1	Walk 5	Walk 20	Walk 25	Walk 30	Walk 35	Walk 40	Walk 45
Week 2	Walk 20 Jog 5 Walk 15	Walk 15 Jog 15 Walk 15	Walk 15 Jog 20 Walk 15	Walk 10 Jog 25 Walk 10	Walk 5 Jog 30 Walk 10	Walk 5 Jog 35 Walk 5	Jog 45
Week 3	Jog 45 Stride 10	Jog 45 Stride 10	Jog 45 Stride 15	Jog 45 Stride 15	Jog 45 Sprint 0	Jog 45 Sprint 10	Jog 45 Sprint 15
Week 4	Add functional activities			Gradually increase all week			
Week 5				*Resume full training*			

and local signs. It is not necessary to monitor progress by radiography, scintigraphy, CT, or MRI, since radiological healing often lags behind clinical healing.

When training resumes, it is important to allow adequate recovery time after hard sessions or hard weeks of training. This can be accommodated by developing microcycles and macrocycles. Alternating hard and easy training sessions is a microcycle adjustment, but graduating the volume of work or alternating harder and easier sessions can also be done weekly or monthly. During periods of increases in training, it is worth introducing these on a stepwise basis. For example, introduce the increase, then stay at this level for a few weeks until bone becomes adapted. In view of the history of stress fracture, it is advisable that some form of cross-training—e.g., swimming and cycling for a runner—be introduced to reduce the stress on the previously injured area and reduce the likelihood of a recurrence. Given the role of muscles in helping to absorb bone load, interventions to assist in muscle recovery may be implemented such as massage, icing, etc.

Recently, it was hypothesized that short-term suppression of bone turnover using bisphosphonates might prevent the initial loss of bone during the remodeling response to high bone strains and potentially prevent stress fractures. This was evaluated in a randomized, double-blind, placebo-controlled study using risedronate or placebo given as 30 mg daily for 10 weeks, then once a week for the next 12 weeks, in 324 military recruits.[22] However, the results showed no statistically significant differences in the total, tibial, femoral, or metatarsal stress fracture incidence between the groups. Thus, risedronate does not appear to be a viable option for lowering stress fracture risk in active, healthy populations.

Surgery

Surgery is virtually never required in the management of the routine stress fracture. However, in the case of a displaced stress fracture (e.g., neck of the femur) or established nonunion (e.g., anterior cortex of the tibia, navicular, sesamoids), surgery may be required.

Table 28.9 Stress fractures that require specific treatment and potential treatments

Stress fracture site	Potential treatment
Neck of femur	Superior: internal fixation Inferior: non–weight-bearing rest
Pars interarticularis	Bracing depending on stage
Patella	Non–weight-bearing cast in extension
Anterior cortex, mid-shaft tibia	Prolonged immobilization or surgery
Medial malleolus	Undisplaced: pneumatic leg brace 6 weeks Displaced: Surgery
Talus	Non–weight-bearing rest or surgery
Navicular	Non–weight-bearing cast immobilization 6 weeks
5th metatarsal	6 weeks cast immobilization or surgical fixation
2nd metatarsal (base)	4–6 weeks cast immobilization
Sesamoid	Non–weight-bearing cast immobilization 6 weeks

Stress fractures requiring specific treatment

While the majority of stress fractures will heal without complications in a relatively short time frame with relative rest, there are a number of stress fractures that have a tendency to develop complications such as delayed union or nonunion, which require specific additional treatment such as cast immobilization or surgery. These are described in Table 28.9. While it is beyond the scope of this chapter to cover the treatment of these in detail, readers are referred to other reviews in this area.[149–151]

Conclusion

The treatment of stress fractures can therefore be divided into two phases. The initial phase involves pain management, modification (or cessation) of the aggravating activity, muscle strengthening, and maintenance of aerobic fitness. An important component of this phase is the identification and subsequent modification of risk factors, which may be training errors, biomechanical problems, hormonal abnormalities, and diet. The use of braces has been shown to reduce the time to return to full activity in some lower limb stress fractures. Similarly, the use of electrical stimulation and ultrasound may be helpful. When the athlete is pain-free, gradual resumption of the aggravating activity should commence, but this must be done in a graduated manner as long as the athlete remains pain-free. While modified rest is the basis of treatment for most stress fractures, there is a group of fractures that require specific treatment because of their site or their tendency to delayed union or nonunion. These include stress fractures of the neck of the femur, anterior cortex of the tibia, navicular, fifth metatarsal, and sesamoid bones. A summary of the evidence to date is provided in the table at the end of the chapter. It is apparent that further research is needed in order to provide better-quality evidence for the prevention and treatment of stress fractures (Box 28.1).

Key messages

- Athletes should be pain-free during recovery and return to sport.
- Nonsteroidal anti-inflammatory medication should be avoided.

Box 28.1 Summary of how to treat a stress fracture

Treatment	Strategies
• Decide on overall management approach	• Consider site of stress fracture —If problematic, may require special treatment • Decide on stage of continuum of bone strain —Use of appropriate diagnostic procedures
• Relieve pain and any swelling	• Gait aids if necessary • Ice • Electrotherapy modalities
• Accelerate repair and remodeling	• Potential therapies not yet proven —Drug regimens—e.g., intermittent PTH —Low-intensity pulsed ultrasound —Electrical stimulation • Avoid use of NSAIDs
• Modified rest	• Maintain fitness —Deep water running —Low-impact activities (e.g., cycling, stepper) • Muscle strengthening —Major muscle groups
• Modification of risk factors	• Training • Footwear and insoles • Biomechanical abnormalities • Muscle flexibility and joint range • Menstrual status • Dietary intake
• Facilitate return to sport	• Use of a pneumatic air brace for leg fractures • Progressive loading regimen • Monitor symptoms

NSAID, nonsteroidal anti-inflammatory drug; PTH, parathyroid hormone.

- A pneumatic leg brace for tibial stress fractures may speed the return to sport.
- Risk factors must be identified and corrected.
- Aerobic fitness can be maintained with non–weight-bearing activities.
- Certain high-risk stress fractures need specific treatment.
- Healing should be monitored clinically.

Sample examination questions

Multiple-choice questions (answers on page 602)

1 Which of the following has been shown to be a risk factor for the development of a stress fracture in females?
  A Low calcium intake
  B Eating disorders
  C Menstrual disturbances

D Excessive subtalar pronation
E Leg length discrepancy

2 There is evidence that the following techniques have a positive effect on the healing of certain stress fractures:
A Pneumatic leg brace
B Electrical stimulation
C Nonsteroidal anti-inflammatory medication
D Low-intensity pulsed ultrasound
E Corticosteroid injection

3 Which of the following stress fractures requires specific treatment other than rest and gradual resumption of activity?
A Navicular
B Shaft of femur
C First rib
D Anterior cortex of tibia
E Medial malleolus

Essay questions

1 Discuss the role of risk factors in the development of stress fractures.
2 What are the principles involved in the rehabilitation of an uncomplicated stress fracture?
3 Draw up an activity program for the return to sport after an uncomplicated lower limb stress fracture.

Case study 28.1

A 20-year-old female distance runner presents with a 3-week history of increasing pain over the distal tibia. She is preparing for her first marathon and has recently increased her mileage significantly. She is a vegetarian and has had only one menstrual period in the past 12 months. A bone scan reveals a focal area of increased uptake in the tibia. How should this patient be managed?

Summarizing the evidence

	Results	**Level of evidence***
Treatment strategies		
Low-intensity pulsed ultrasound	1 RCT in military—no effect	A4
Low-energy laser	1 RCT in military—no effect	A4
Electrical stimulation	1 case series in athletes	D
Pneumatic air cast	3 RCTs, 2 in military and 1 in athletes—positive effect in 2, no effect in 1	A4
Modified rest	No formal trials	C
Progressive bone loading exercise	No formal trials	C
NSAIDs	No formal trials	–
Prevention strategies		
Training modifications	2 quasi-randomized trials in military—positive effect with reduced high-impact activity, no effect with reduced marching distance	B

Continued

Summarizing the evidence (*Continued*)

	Results	Level of evidence*
Shoe insoles/orthotics	3 RCTs and 3 quasi-randomized trials in military—positive effect in pooled data	A3
Basketball shoes	1 RCT in military—positive effect for foot stress fractures	A4
Calcium supplements	1 quasi-randomized trial in military—no effect	B
Bisphosphonates—risedronate	1 RCT in military–no effect	A4
Oral contraceptive pill	No formal trials	–
Lower limb muscle strengthening	No formal trials	C
Correction of biomechanical features, range of motion	No formal trials	C

NSAID, nonsteroidal anti-inflammatory drug; RCT, randomized controlled trial.
* Grade A1: evidence from large RCTs or systematic review (including meta-analysis).†
Grade A2: evidence from at least one high-quality cohort.
Grade A3: evidence from at least one moderate-sized RCT (≥ 50 patients per intervention group) or systematic review.†
Grade A4: evidence from at least one RCT.
Grade B: evidence from at least one high-quality study of nonrandomized cohorts.
Grade C: expert opinions.
Grade D: case series.

References

1 Bennell KL, Malcolm SA, Thomas SA, Wark JD, Burkner PD. The incidence and distribution of stress fractures in competitive track and field athletes. *Am J Sports Med* 1996; **24**:211–217.

2 Johnson AW, Weiss CB, Wheeler DL. Stress fractures of the femoral shaft in athletes—more common than expected: a new clinical test. *Am J Sports Med* 1994; **22**:248–256.

3 Kaufman KR, Brodine S, Shaffer R. Military training-related injuries: surveillance, research, and prevention. *Am J Prev Med* 2000; **18**:S54–63.

4 Pope RP, Herbert R, Kirwan JD, Graham BJ. Predicting attrition in basic military training. *Mil Med* 1999; **164**:710–714.

5 Matheson GO, Clement DB, McKenzie DC, *et al.* Stress fractures in athletes: a study of 320 cases. *Am J Sports Med* 1987; **15**:46–58.

6 Burr DB, Milgrom C, Boyd RD, *et al.* Experimental stress fractures of the tibia. *J Bone Joint Surg* 1990; **72**:370–375.

7 Schaffler MB, Radin EL, Burr DB. Mechanical and morphological effects of strain rate on fatigue of compact bone. *Bone* 1989; **10**:207–214.

8 Schaffler MB, Radin EL, Burr DB. Long-term fatigue behavior of compact bone at low strain magnitude and rate. *Bone* 1990; **11**:321–326.

9 Aoki Y, Yasuda K, Tohyama H, Ito H, Minami A. Magnetic resonance imaging in stress fractures and shin splints. *Clin Orthop* 2004; **421**:260–267.

10 Zwas ST, Elkanovitch R, Frank G. Interpretation and classification of bone scintigraphic findings in stress fractures. *J Nucl Med* 1987; **28**:452–457.

11 Gillespie WJ, Grant I. Interventions for preventing and treating stress fractures and stress reactions of bone of the lower limbs in young adults. *Cochrane Database Syst Rev* 2000; (**2**):CD000450.

12 Andrish JT, Bergfeld JA, Walheim J. A prospective study of the management of shin splints. *J Bone Joint Surg Am* 1974; **56**:1697–1700.

13 Smith W, Walter J, Bailey M. Effect of insoles in coastguard basic training footwear. *J Am Podiatr Assoc* 1985; **45**:644–647.

14 Milgrom C, Giladi M, Kashtan H, *et al.* A prospective study of the effect of a shock-absorbing orthotic device on the incidence of stress fractures in military recruits. *Foot Ankle* 1985; **6**:101–104.

15 Schwellnus MP, Jordaan G, Noakes TD. Prevention of common overuse injuries by the use of shock absorbing insoles. *Am J Sports Med* 1990; **18**:636–641.

16 Gardner LI, Dziados JE, Jones BH, *et al.* Prevention of lower extremity stress fractures: a controlled trial of a shock absorbent insole. *Am J Public Health* 1988; **78**:1563–1567.

17 Mundermann A, Stefanyshyn DJ, Nigg BM. Relationship between footwear comfort of shoe inserts and anthropometric and sensory factors. *Med Sci Sports Exerc* 2001; **33**:1939–1945.

18 Milgrom C, Finestone A, Shlamkovitch N, *et al.* Prevention of overuse injuries of the foot by improved shoe shock attenuation: a randomized, prospective study. *Clin Orthop* 1992; **281**:189–192.

19 Giladi M, Milgrom C, Danon Y, Aharonson A. The correlation between cumulative march training and stress fractures in soldiers. *Mil Med* 1985; **150**:600–601.

20 Scully TJ, Besterman G. Stress fracture: a preventable training injury. *Mil Med* 1982; **147**:285–287.

21 Schwellnus MP, Jordaan G. Does calcium supplementation prevent bone stress injuries? A clinical trial. *Int J Sport Nutr* 1992; **2**:165–174.

22 Milgrom C, Finestone A, Novack V, *et al.* The effect of prophylactic treatment with risedronate on stress fracture incidence among infantry recruits. *Bone* 2004; **35**:418–424.

23 Slayter M. *Lower Limb Training Injuries in an Army Recruit Population* [thesis]. Newcastle: University of Newcastle, 1995.

24 Swenson EJ, DeHaven KE, Sebastianelli WJ, *et al.* The effect of a pneumatic leg brace on return to play in athletes with tibial stress fractures. *Am J Sports Med* 1997; **25**:322–328.

25 Allen CS, Flynn TW, Kardouni JR, *et al.* The use of a pneumatic leg brace in soldiers with tibial stress fractures: a randomized clinical trial. *Mil Med* 2004; **169**:880–884.

26 Nissen LR, Astvad K, Madsen L. [Low-energy laser therapy in medial tibial stress syndrome; in Danish.] *Ugeskr Laeger* 1994; **156**:7329–7331.

27 Rue JP, Armstrong DW, Frassica FJ, Deafenbaugh M, Wilckens JH. The effect of pulsed ultrasound in the treatment of tibial stress fractures. *Orthopedics* 2004; **27**:1192–1195.

28 Matheson GO, Clement DB, McKenzie DC, *et al.* Scintigraphic uptake of 99m Tc at non-painful sites in athletes with stress fractures. *Sports Med* 1987; **4**:65–75.

29 Keene JS, Lash EG. Negative bone scan in a femoral neck stress fracture. *Am J Sports Med* 1992; **20**:234–236.

30 Burr D. Pharmaceutical treatments that may prevent or delay the onset of stress fractures. In: Burr DB, Milgrom C, eds. *Musculoskeletal Fatigue and Stress Fractures.* Boca Raton: CRC Press, 2001: 259–270.

31 Wheeler P, Batt ME. Do non-steroidal anti-inflammatory drugs adversely affect stress fracture healing? A short review. *Br J Sports Med* 2005; **39**:65–69.

32 Bassett CAL, Mitchell SN, Gaston SR. Treatment of ununited tibial diaphyseal fractures with pulsing electromagnetic fields. *J Bone Joint Surg Am* 1981; **63**:511–523.

33 Barker AT, Dixon RA, Sharrard WJ, Sutcliffe ML. Pulsed magnetic field therapy for tibial non-union: interim results of a double-blind trial. *Lancet* 1984; **i**:994–996.

34 O'Connor BT. Pulsed magnetic field therapy for tibial non-union. *Lancet* 1984; **ii**:171–172.

35 De Haas WG, Beaupre A, Cameron H, English E. The Canadian experience with pulsed magnetic fields in the treatment of ununited tibial stress fractures. *Clin Orthop* 1986; **208**:55–58.

36 Sharrard WJW. A double-blind trial of pulsed electromagnetic fields for delayed union of tibial fractures. *J Bone Joint Surg Br* 1990; **72**:347–355.

37 Brighton CT, Black J, Friedenberg ZB, *et al.* A multicenter study of the treatment of non-union with constant direct current. *J Bone Joint Surg Am* 1981; **63**:2–13.

38 Brighton CT, Shaman P, Heppenstall RB, *et al.* Tibial nonunion treated with direct current, capacitive coupling, or bone graft. *Clin Orthop* 1995; **321**:223–234.

39 Esterhai JL, Brighton CT, Heppenstall RB, Alavi A, Desai AG. Detection of synovial pseudarthrosis by 99mTc scintigraphy: application to treatment of traumatic non-union with constant direct current. *Clin Orthop* 1981; **161**:15–23.

40 Parnell EJ, Simons RB. The effect of electrical stimulation in the treatment of non-union of the tibia. *J Bone Joint Surg Br* 1991; **73**:S178.

41 Brighton CT, Pollack SR. Treatment of nonunion of the tibia with a capacitively coupled electric field. *J Trauma* 1984; **24**:153–155.

42 Brighton CT, Pollack SR. Treatment of recalcitrant non-union with a capacitively coupled electric field: a preliminary report. *J Bone Joint Surg Am* 1985; **67**:577–585.

43 Scott G, King JB, A prospective, double blind trial of electrical capacitive coupling in the treatment of non-union of long bones. *J Bone Joint Surg Am* 1994; 76-A:820–826.

44 Benazzo F, Mosconi M, Beccarisi G, Galli U. Use of capacitive coupled electric fields in stress fractures in athletes. *Clin Orthop* 1995; **310**:145–149.

45 Duarte LR. The stimulation of bone growth by ultrasound. *Arch Orthop Trauma Surg* 1983; **101**:153–159.

46 Pilla AA, Mont MA, Nasser PR, Khan A, *et al.* Non-invasive low-intensity pulsed ultrasound accelerates bone healing in the rabbit. *J Orthop Trauma* 1990; **4**:246–253.

47 Heckman JD, Ryaby JP, McCabe J, Frey JJ, Kilcoyne RF. Acceleration of tibial fracture-healing by non-invasive, low-intensity pulsed ultrasound. *J Bone Joint Surg Am* 1994; **76**:26–34.

48 Kristiansen TK, Ryaby JP, McCabe J, Frey JJ, Roe LR. Accelerated healing of distal radius fractures with the use of specific, low-intensity ultrasound. *J Bone Joint Surg Am* 1997; **79**:961–973.

49 Mayr E, Rutzki M, Hauser H, Ruter A. Low intensity ultrasound accelerates healing of scaphoid fractures. [Paper presented at the American Academy of Orthopaedic Surgeons 67th Annual Meeting, Orlando, Florida, 2000.]

50 Cook SD, Ryaby JP, McCabe J, *et al.* Acceleration of tibia and distal radius fracture healing in patients who smoke. *Clin Orthop* 1997; **337**:198–207.

51 Frankel VH. Results of prescription use of pulse ultrasound therapy in fracture management. In: Szabó Z, Lewis JE, Fantini GA, Savalgi RS, eds. *Surgical Technology International VII.* San Francisco: Universal Medical Press, 1998: 389–393.

52 Frankel VH, Koval KJ, Kummer FJ. Ultrasound treatment of tibial nonunions. [Paper presented at the American Academy of Orthopaedic Surgeons 66th Annual Meeting, Anaheim, California, 1999.]

53 Fujioka H, Tsunoda M, Noda M, Matsui N, Mizuno K. Treatment of ununited fracture of the hook of hamate by low-intensity pulsed ultrasound: a case report. *J Hand Surg Am* 2000; **25**:77–79.

54 Mayr E, Frankel V, Ruter A. Ultrasound: an alternative healing method for nonunions? *Arch Orthop Trauma Surg* 2000; **120**:1–8.

55 Jensen JE. Stress fracture in the world class athlete: a case study. *Med Sci Sports Exerc* 1998; **30**:783–787.

56 Brand JCJ, Brindle T, Nyland J, Caborn DN, Johnson DL. Does pulsed low intensity ultrasound allow early return to normal activities when treating stress fractures? A review of one tarsal and eight tibial stress fractures. *Iowa Orthop J* 1999; **19**:26–30.

57 Scott SH, Winter DA. Internal forces at chronic running injury sites. *Med Sci Sports Exerc* 1990; **22**:357–369.

58 Yoshikawa T, Mori S, Santiesteban AJ, *et al.* The effects of muscle fatigue on bone strain. *J Exp Biol* 1994; **188**:217–233.

59 Fyhrie DP, Milgrom C, Hoshaw SJ, *et al.* Effect of fatiguing exercise on longitudinal bone strain as related to stress fracture in humans. *Ann Biomed Eng* 1998; **26**:660–665.

60 Hoffman JR, Chapnik L, Shamis A, Givon U, Davidson B. The effect of leg strength on the incidence of lower extremity overuse injuries during military training. *Mil Med* 1999; **164**:153–156.

61 Armstrong DW 3rd, Rue JP, Wilckens JH, Frassica FJ. Stress fracture injury in young military men and women. *Bone* 2004; **35**:806–816.

62 Bennell KL, Malcolm SA, Thomas SA, *et al.* Risk factors for stress fractures in track and field athletes: a 12 month prospective study. *Am J Sports Med* 1996; **24**:810–818.

63 Milgrom C. The Israeli elite infantry recruit: a model for understanding the biomechanics of stress fractures. *J R Coll Surg Edinb* 1989; **34**:S18–S22.

64 Donahue SW. The role of muscular force and fatigue in stress fractures. In: Burr DB, Milgrom C, eds. *Musculoskeletal Fatigue and Stress Fractures*, Boca Raton, FL: CRC Press, 2001: 131–150.

65 Saltin B, Blomqvist G, Mitchell JH, *et al.* Response to exercise after bed rest and after training. *Circulation* 1968; **38**(5 Suppl):VII/1–78.

66 Pedersen PK, Jorgensen K. Maximal oxygen uptake in young women with training, inactivity and retraining. *Med Sci Sports Exerc* 1978; **10**:223–237.

67 Coyle EF, Martin WH, Sinacore DR. Time course of loss of adaptations after stopping prolonged intense endurance training. *J Appl Physiol* 1984; **57**:1857–1864.

68 Hertler L, Provost-Craig M, Sestili D. Water running and the maintenance of maximum oxygen consumption and leg strength in runners [abstract]. *Med Sci Sports Exerc* 1992; **24**:S23.

69 Eyestone ED, Fellingham G, George J, *et al.* Effect of water running and cycling on maximum oxygen consumption and 2 mile run performance. *Am J Sports Med* 1993; **21**:41–44.
70 Wilber RL, Moffatt RJ, Scott BE, *et al.* Influence of water-run training on running performance [abstract] *Med Sci Sports Exerc* 1994; **26**:S4.
71 Avellini BA, Shapiro Y, Pandolf KB. Cardiorespiratory physical training in water and on land. *Eur J Appl Physiol* 1983; **50**:255–263.
72 Frangolias DD, Rhodes EC. Maximal and ventilatory threshold responses to treadmill and water immersion running. *Med Sci Sports Exerc* 1995; **27**:1007–1013.
73 Christie JL, Shelddahl LM, Tristani FE, *et al.* Cardiovascular regulation during head-out water immersion exercise. *J Appl Physiol* 1990; **69**:657–664.
74 Butts NK, Tucker M, Greening C. Physiological responses to maximal treadmill and deep water running in men and women. *Am J Sports Med* 1991; **19**:612–614.
75 Frangolias DD, Rhodes EC, Belcastro AN, *et al.* Comparison of metabolic responses of prolonged work at Tvent during treadmill and water immersion running [abstract]. *Med Sci Sports Exerc* 1994; **26**:S10.
76 Frangolias DD, Taunton JE, Rhodes EC, *et al.* Maintenance of aerobic capacity during recovery from right Jones' fracture (case report). *Clin J Sport Med* 1997; **7**:54–58.
77 Milgrom C, Giladi M, Chisin R, Dizian R. The long-term followup of soldiers with stress fractures. *Am J Sports Med* 1985; **13**:398–400.
78 Worthen BM, Yanklowitz BAD. The pathophysiology and treatment of stress fractures in military personnel. *J Am Podiatr Med Assoc* 1978; **68**:317–325.
79 Reinker KA, Ozburne S. A comparison of male and female orthopaedic pathology in basic training. *Mil Med* 1979; **144**:532–536.
80 Greaney RB, Gerber RH, Laughlin RL, *et al.* Distribution and natural history of stress fractures in U.S. marine recruits. *Radiology* 1983; **146**:339–346.
81 Milgrom C, Simkin A, Eldad A, Nyska M, Finestone A. Using bone's adaptation ability to lower the incidence of stress fractures. *Am J Sports Med* 2000; **28**:245–251.
82 Shaffer RA, Brodine SK, Almeida SA, Williams KM, Ronaghy S. Use of simple measures of physical activity to predict stress fractures in young men undergoing a rigorous physical training program. *Am J Epidemiol* 1999; **149**:236–242.
83 Pope RP. Prevention of pelvic stress fractures in female army recruits. *Mil Med* 1999; **164**:370–373.
84 Brunet ME, Cook SD, Brinker MR, Dickinson JA. A survey of running injuries in 1505 competitive and recreational runners. *J Sports Med Phys Fit* 1990; **30**:307–315.
85 Kadel NJ, Teitz CC, Kronmal RA. Stress fractures in ballet dancers. *Am J Sports Med* 1992; **20**:445–449.
86 Ekenman I, Milgrom C, Finestone A, *et al.* The role of biomechanical shoe orthoses in tibial stress fracture prevention. *Am J Sports Med* 2002; **30**:866–870.
87 Finestone AS. Prevention of stress fractures by modifying shoe wear. In: In: Burr DB, Milgrom C, eds. *Musculoskeletal Fatigue and Stress Fractures.* Boca Raton: CRC Press, 2001: 233–245.
88 Arndt A, Westblad P, Ekenman I, Lundberg A. A comparison of external plantar loading and in vivo local metatarsal deformation wearing two different military boots. *Gait Posture* 2003; **18**:20–26.
89 Giladi M, Milgrom C, Stein M, *et al.* The low arch, a protective factor in stress fractures: a prospective study of 295 military recruits. *Orthop Rev* 1985; **14**:709–712.
90 Simkin A, Leichter I, Giladi M, Stein M, Milgrom C. Combined effect of foot arch structure and an orthotic device on stress fractures. *Foot Ankle* 1989; **10**:25–29.
91 Brosh T, Arcan M, Toward early detection of the tendency to stress fractures. *Clin Biomech* 1994; **9**:111–116.
92 Montgomery LC, Nelson FRT, Norton JP, Deuster FA. Orthopedic history and examination in the etiology of overuse injuries. *Med Sci Sports Exerc* 1989; **21**:237–243.
93 Taunton JE, Clement DB, Webber D. Lower extremity stress fractures in athletes. *Phys Sportsmed* 1981; **9**:77–86.
94 Sullivan D, Warren RF, Pavlov H, Kelman G. Stress fractures in 51 runners. *Clin Orthop* 1984; **187**:188–192.
95 Korpelainen R, Orava S, Karpakka J, Siira P, Hulkko A. Risk factors for recurrent stress fractures in athletes. *Am J Sports Med* 2001; **29**:304–310.
96 Friberg O. Leg length asymmetry in stress fractures: a clinical and radiological study. *J Sports Med* 1982; **22**:485–488.

97 Cowan DN, Jones BH, Frykman PN, *et al.* Lower limb morphology and risk of overuse injury among male infantry trainees. *Med Sci Sports Exerc* 1996; **28**:945–952.

98 Winfield AC, Bracker M, Moore J, Johnson CW. Risk factors associated with stress reactions in female marines. *Mil Med* 1997; **162**:698–702.

99 Hughes LY. Biomechanical analysis of the foot and ankle for predisposition to developing stress fractures. *J Orthop Sports Phys Ther* 1985; **7**:96–101.

100 Giladi M, Milgrom C, Stein M, *et al.* External rotation of the hip: a predictor of risk for stress fractures. *Clin Orthop Rel Res* 1987; **216**:131–134.

101 Milgrom C, Finestone A, Shlamkovitch N, *et al.* Youth is a risk factor for stress fracture: a study of 783 infantry recruits. *J Bone Joint Surg Br* 1994; **76**:20–22.

102 Ekenman I, Tsai-Fellander L, Westblad P, Turan I, Rolf C. A study of intrinsic factors in patients with stress fractures of the tibia. *Foot Ankle Int* 1996; **17**:477–482.

103 Giladi M, Milgrom C, Simkin A, Danon Y. Stress fractures: identifiable risk factors. *Am J Sports Med* 1991; **19**:647–652.

104 Lindberg JS, Fears WB, Hunt MM, *et al.* Exercise-induced amenorrhea and bone density. *Ann Intern Med* 1984; **101**:647–648.

105 Marcus R, Cann C, Madvig P, *et al.* Menstrual function and bone mass in elite women distance runners. *Ann Intern Med* 1985; **102**:158–163.

106 Lloyd T, Triantafyllou SJ, Baker ER, *et al.* Women athletes with menstrual irregularity have increased musculoskeletal injuries. *Med Sci Sports Exerc* 1986; **18**:374–379.

107 Warren MP, Brooks-Gunn J, Hamilton LH, Warren LF, Hamilton WG. Scoliosis and fractures in young ballet dancers. *N Engl J Med* 1986; **314**:1348–1353.

108 Nelson ME, Clark N, Otradovec C, Evans WJ. Elite women runners: association between menstrual status, weight history and stress fractures. *Med Sci Sports Exerc* 1987; **19**:S13.

109 Barrow GW, Saha S. Menstrual irregularity and stress fractures in collegiate female distance runners. *Am J Sports Med* 1988; **16**:209–216.

110 Carbon R, Sambrook PN, Deakin V, *et al.* Bone density of elite female athletes with stress fractures. *Med J Aust* 1990; **153**:373–376.

111 Frusztajer NT, Dhuper S, Warren MP, Brooks-Gunn J, Fox RP. Nutrition and the incidence of stress fractures in ballet dancers. *Am J Clin Nutr* 1990; **51**:779–783.

112 Myburgh KH, Hutchins J, Fataar AB, Hough SF, Noakes TD. Low bone density is an etiologic factor for stress fractures in athletes. *Ann Intern Med* 1990; **113**:754–759.

113 Grimston SK, Engsberg JR, Kloiber R, Hanley DA. Bone mass, external loads, and stress fractures in female runners. *Int J Sport Biomech* 1991; **7**:293–302.

114 Bennell KL, Malcolm SA, Thomas SA, *et al.* Risk factors for stress fractures in female track-and-field athletes: a retrospective analysis. *Clin J Sports Med* 1995; **5**:229–235.

115 Tomten SE. Prevalence of menstrual dysfunction in Norwegian long-distance runners participating in the Oslo marathon games. *Scand J Med Sci Sport* 1996; **6**:164–171.

116 Hetland ML, Haarbo J, Christiansen C, Larsen T. Running induces menstrual disturbances but bone mass is unaffected, except in amenorrheic women. *Am J Med* 1993; **95**:53–60.

117 Jonnavithula S, Warren MP, Fox RP, Lazaro MI. Bone density is compromised in amenorrheic women despite return of menses: a 2-year study. *Obstet Gynecol* 1993; **81**:669–674.

118 Myburgh KH, Bachrach LK, Lewis B, Kent K, Marcus R. Low bone mineral density at axial and appendicular sites in amenorrheic athletes. *Med Sci Sports Exerc* 1993; **25**:1197–1202.

119 Robinson TL, Snow-Harter C, Taaffe DR, *et al.* Gymnasts exhibit higher bone mass than runners despite similar prevalence of amenorrhea and oligomenorrhea. *J Bone Miner Res* 1995; **10**:26–35.

120 Gremion G, Rizzoli R, Slosman D, Theintz G, Bonjour JP. Oligo-amenorrheic long-distance runners may lose more bone in spine than in femur. *Med Sci Sports Exerc* 2001; **33**:15–21.

121 Cline AD, Jansen GR, Melby CL. Stress fractures in female army recruits: implications of bone density, calcium intake, and exercise. *J Am Coll Nutr* 1998; **17**:128–135.

122 Lauder TD, Dixit S, Pezzin LE, *et al.* The relation between stress fractures and bone mineral density: evidence from active-duty army women. *Arch Phys Med Rehabil* 2000; **81**:73–79.

123 Girrbach RT, Flynn TW, Browder DA, *et al.* Flexural wave propagation velocity and bone mineral density in females with and without tibial bone stress injuries. *J Orthop Sports Phys Ther* 2001; **31**:54–62.

124 Marx RG, Saint-Phard D, Callahan LR, Chu J, Hannafin JA. Stress fracture sites related to underlying bone health in athletic females. *Clin J Sport Med* 2001; **11**:73–76.

125 Kaufman BA, Warren MP, Dominguez JE, *et al.* Bone density and amenorrhea in ballet dancers are related to a decreased resting metabolic rate and lower leptin levels. *J Clin Endocrinol Metab* 2002; **87**:2777–2783.

126 Zanker CL, Swaine IL. Relation between bone turnover, oestradiol, and energy balance in women distance runners. *Br J Sports Med* 1998; **32**:167–171.

127 Ihle R, Loucks AB. Dose–response relationships between energy availability and bone turnover in young exercising women. *J Bone Miner Res* 2004; **19**:1231–1240.

128 Lavienja AJ, Braam LM, Knapen MHJ, *et al.* Factors influencing bone loss in female endurance athletes. *Am J Sports Med* 2003; **31**:889–895.

129 Hergenroeder AC, Smith EOB, Shypailo R, *et al.* Bone mineral changes in young women with hypothalamic amenorrhea treated with oral contraceptives, medroxyprogesterone, or placebo over 12 months. *Am J Obstet Gynecol* 1997; **176**:1017–1025.

130 Prince RL, Smith M, Dick IM, *et al.* Prevention of postmenopausal osteoporosis: a comparative study of exercise, calcium supplementation, and hormone-replacement therapy. *N Engl J Med* 1991; **325**:1189–1195.

131 Wallace BA, Cumming RG. Systematic review of randomized trials of the effect of exercise on bone mass in pre- and postmenopausal women. *Calcif Tissue Int* 2000; **67**:10–18.

132 Ronsen O, Sundgot-Borgen J, Maehlum S. Supplement use and nutritional habits in Norwegian elite athletes. *Scand J Med Sci Sports* 1999; **9**:28–35.

133 Ziegler PJ, Nelson JA, Jonnalagadda SS. Nutritional and physiological status of US national figure skaters. *Int J Sport Nutr* 1999; **9**:345–360.

134 Picard CL. The level of competition as a factor for the development of eating disorders in female collegiate athletes. *J Youth Adolesc* 1999; **28**:583–594.

135 Otis CL, Drinkwater B, Johnson M, Loucks A, Wilmore J. American College of Sports Medicine position stand: the female athlete triad. *Med Sci Sports Exerc* 1997; **29**:i–ix.

136 Lauder TD, Williams MV, Campbell CS, *et al.* The female athlete triad: prevalence in military women. *Mil Med* 1999; **164**:630–635.

137 Warren MP, Brooks-Gunn J, Fox RP, *et al.* Lack of bone accretion and amenorrhea: evidence for a relative osteopenia in weight bearing bones. *J Clin Endocrinol Metab* 1991; **72**:847–853.

138 Warren MP, Brooks-Gunn J, Fox RP, *et al.* Osteopenia in exercise-associated amenorrhea using ballet dancers as a model: a longitudinal study. *J Clin Endocrinol Metab* 2002; **87**:3162–3168.

139 Nattiv A, Puffer JC, Green GA. Lifestyles and health risks of collegiate athletes: a multi-center study. *Clin J Sport Med* 1997; **7**:262–272.

140 Dickson TB, Kichline PD. Functional management of stress fractures in female athletes using a pneumatic leg brace. *Am J Sports Med* 1987; **15**:86–89.

141 Whitelaw GP, Wetzler MJ, Levy AS, Segal D, Bissonnette K. A pneumatic leg brace for the treatment of tibial stress fractures. *Clin Orthop Rel Res* 1991; **270**:302–305.

142 Batt ME, Kemp S, Kerslake R. Delayed union stress fractures of the anterior tibia: conservative management. *Br J Sports Med* 2001; **35**:74–77.

143 Benazzo F, Barnabei G, Ferrario A, Castelli C, Fischetto G. Stress fractures in track and field athletes. *J Sports Traumatol Rel Res* 1992; **14**:51–65.

144 Hulkko A, Orava S. Stress fractures in athletes. *Int J Sports Med* 1987; **8**:221–226.

145 Milgrom C, Finestone A, Segev S, *et al.* Are overground or treadmill runners more likely to sustain tibial stress fracture? *Br J Sports Med* 2003; **37**:160–163.

146 Kawamoto R, Ishige Y, Watarai K, Fukashiro S. Influence of curve sharpness on torsional loading of the tibia in running. *J Appl Biomech* 2002; **18**:218–230.

147 Milgrom C, Finestone A, Levi Y, *et al.* Do high impact exercises produce higher tibial strains than running? *Br J Sports Med* 2000; **34**:195–199.

148 Milgrom C, Finestone A, Simkin A, *et al.* In vivo strain measurements to evaluate the strengthening potential of exercises on the tibial bone. *J Bone Joint Surg Br* 2000; **82**:591–594.

149 Egol KA, Frankel VH. Problematic stress fracture. In: Burr DB, Milgrom C, eds. *Musculoskeletal Fatigue and Stress Fractures.* Boca Raton: CRC Press, 2001: 305–319.

150 Brukner P, Bennell K, Matheson G. *Stress Fractures.* Melbourne: Blackwell Science, 1999.

151 Brukner PD, Bennell KL. Stress fractures. *Crit Rev Phys Rehabil Med* 1997; **9**:151–190.

CHAPTER 29

What is the best treatment of subcutaneous rupture of the Achilles tendon?

Deiary Kader, David J. Deehan, and Nicola Maffulli

Introduction

The Achilles tendon is the thickest and strongest tendon in the human body, yet it is the most frequently ruptured. Over the past few decades, subcutaneous rupture of the Achilles tendon has become increasingly common.[1,2] Despite the extensive research interest in the management of acute Achilles tendon rupture (ATR), there is still no agreed management protocol, and the choice of management regimen still lies largely with the preference of the surgeon and/or of the patient.[3–5] The managements modalities for an acutely ruptured Achilles tendon can be broadly classified into nonoperative (cast immobilization or functional bracing) and operative (open or percutaneous). In the past three decades, open repair has been the method of choice in athletes, young people, and patients with chronic ruptures. Prior to this, conservative management was favored due to the low reported complication rates. More recent studies on conservative management of acute ATR have utilized mobile splints, which allow early mobilization.[6–8] These studies have reported promising outcomes, often equivalent to operative repair studies, making conservative management a valid option.

In general, most surgeons would opt for operative management in physically active patients. Controversy remains over which operative technique gives the best outcomes. Some authorities have reported an overall higher complication rate using open repair,[9–12] noting predominantly skin healing problems, while others show few complications[13–15] and a low repeat rupture rate.[16–18] Percutaneous repair[19] may minimize the skin healing problems associated with operative repair, and has the advantage of being easily performed under local anesthetic. However, the original attempts produced a relatively high rate of sural nerve injury[20,21] and higher re-rupture rates in comparison with open methods of repair.[22] Percutaneously repaired Achilles tendons are also less thick than those repaired by open procedures,[23] and some patients may prefer the better cosmesis that this may afford.[24] More recent techniques minimize the risk of sural nerve injury, and have a remarkably low risk of re-rupture.[25]

Many methods for operative repair of an ATR have been described (Table 29.1), with some recent articles reporting the use of prosthetic materials such as Marlex mesh, Dacron weave, and lactic acid polymers.[26–28] External fixation[29–31] has yielded impressive results, although the technique is seldom used in the West.

Table 29.1 Summary of the management and outcome of Achilles tendon rupture

Type of management	Period of publication	Publications (n)	Patients (n)	Average age of patients (y)	Period of immobilization (weeks)	Mean follow-up mean (months)	Skin complications	General complications	Re-rupture rate
Conservative and immobilization	1966–1979	7	152	42.7	8.4	18.5	1 (0.7%)	18 minor (11.8%) 0 major	25 (16.4%)
	1980–1989	7	172	38.8	8.9	33.5	0 (0%)	7 minor (4.1%) 2 major (1.2%)	19 (11.4%)
	1990–2000	9	254	40.8	9.6	39.7	2 (0.8%)	19 minor (7.5%) 2 major (0.8%)	18 (6·3%)
	2001–2005	1	140	41	8	33	0 (0%)	3 minor (2.1%)	8 (5.7%)
Total		24	718	40.8	9	31.2	3 (0.4%)	47 minor (6.5%) 4 major (0.6%)	70 (9.7%)
Percutaneous repair and immobilization	1966–1979	1	18	43.1	8	26.5	2 (11.1%)	0	0
	1980–1989	2	21	36.7	7	10.5	2 (9.5%)	2 minor (9.5%) 0 major	0
	1990–2000	10	208	41.0	7.8	28.8	8 (3.8%)	19 minor (9.1%) 2 major (1%)	9 (4.3%)
Total		13	247	40.8	7.7	25.8	12 (4.9%)	21 minor (8.5%) 2 major (0.8%)	9 (3.6%)
Open repair and immobilization	1966–1979	23	774	41.1	6.7	55.4	127 minor (16.4%) 34 major (4.4%)	63 minor (8.1%) 7 major (0.9%)	14 (1.8%)
	1980–1989	27	1036	39.9	7	30.5	151 minor (14.6%) 17 major (1.6%)	137 minor (13.2%) 5 major (0.5%)	20 (1.9%)
	1990–2000	37	1908	40.0	6.7	43.9	179 minor (9.24%) 35 major (1.8%)	101 minor (5.3%) 17 major (0.9%)	48 (2.5%)
	2001–2005	3	689	40	Variable	Variable	12 minor 14 major	11 minor 12 major	25 (3.6%)
Total		90	4407	40.2	6.8	42.6	469 minor (10.6%) 100 major (2.3%)	312 minor (7%) 41 major (0.9%)	107 (2.4%)

Continued

Table 29.1 *(Continued)*

Type of management	Period of publication	Publications (n)	Patients (n)	Average age of patients (y)	Period of immobilization (weeks)	Mean follow-up mean (months)	Skin complications	General complications	Re-rupture rate
Conservative management and early mobilization	1966–1979	–	–	–	–	–	–	–	–
	1980–1989	–	–	–	–	–	–	–	–
	1990–2000	3	67	40	2	22.3	0	11 minor	1
Total		3	67	40	2	22.3	0 (0%)	11 minor (16.4%)	1 (1.5%)
Percutaneous repair and early mobilization	1966–1979	–	–	–	–	–	–	–	–
	1980–1989	–	–	–	–	–	–	–	–
	1990–2000	4	122	38.8	N/A	9.8	8 minor (6.6%) 4 major (3.3%)	18 minor (14.8%) 1 major (0.8%)	8 (6.6%)
	2001–2005	1	66	42	N/A	12	None	None	1
Total		5	188	40.4	N/A	10.9	8 minor (4.2%) 4 major (2.1%)	18 minor (9.6%) 1 major (0.5%)	9 (4.8%)
Open repair and early mobilization	1966–1979	–	–	–	–	–	–	–	–
	1980–1989	1	6	39	N/A	12	0	0	0
	1990–2000	11	277	37.9	N/A	20.5	14 minor (5.0%) 1 major (0.4%)	15 minor (5.4%) 1 major (0.4%)	4 (1.4%)
Total		12	283	37.9	N/A	20.3	14 minor (4.9%) 1 major (0.4%)	15 minor (5.3%) 1 major (0.4%)	4 (1.4%)
External fixation	1966–1979	–	–	–	–	–			
	1980–1989	2	41	42	7.5	17.6	3 minor	3 minor	0
	1990–2000	1	314	?	?	120	?	?	?
		3	355				2 (4.9%)	3 (7.3%)	0 (0%)

Table 29.2 Keywords used to search the MEDLINE database

Keywords for main MEDLINE literature search • Achilles tendon • Incidence • Postoperative complications • Rupture • Tendon • Tendon injuries
Subheadings used for MEDLINE literature search • Abnormalities • Anatomy & histology • Injuries • Grafting • Physiopathology • Pathology • Physiology • Surgery • Transplantation

In this chapter, we update our quantitative review of the published literature on the management of ATR originally published in the previous edition of this volume.

Methods

A computerized literature search of the entire MEDLINE database, covering the years 1966–2005, was conducted. Keywords used in the search are listed in Table 29.2. We retrieved all articles relevant to the subject. The search was not limited to articles in English, and articles were also considered if they were published in French, German, Italian, or Spanish. The authors' own personal collection of papers and any relevant personal correspondences were also included. To be included in this chapter, each article had to be published in a peer-reviewed journal and contain an exhaustive description of patients and methods. We excluded case reports and reviews of the literature. The conduct and validity of all clinical studies were carefully considered, and the outcomes of management protocols were carefully scrutinized. From a total of 218 publications, case reports, reviews of the literature, and articles that did not mention outcomes were excluded. This left a total of 140 publications, all of which included the outcomes of studies of Achilles tendon ruptures. We examined all the articles identified in this fashion, extracting and coding the information contained in each article.

Data extraction

From each article, we extracted the year of publication, the number of patients, the number of patients excluded, the average age, the type of management, follow-up, complications and their rate, and outcomes. The complications from each article were divided into three categories:

- Wound complications
- General complications
- Re-rupture rates

Table 29.3 Definitions of complications

Minor complications	Major complications
Wound	
Superficial infection	Deep infection
Wound hematoma	Chronic fistula
Delayed wound healing	
Adhesion of the scar	
Suture granuloma	
Skin necrosis	
General	
Pain	Deep vein thrombosis
Disturbances in sensibility	Pulmonary embolism
Suture rupture	Tendon lengthening
	Death

The raw data were converted into percentages of the number of cases per management group. Wound complications and general complications were also further subdivided into major and minor (Table 29.3).

Where available, we also extracted data from 92 of the 140 studies that mentioned patient satisfaction, and "good" or "excellent" results were taken as a percentage of the study group for each individual study and correlated with the methodology score for that particular article.

Statistics

Data were entered in a commercially available database and analyzed using the Statistical Package for the Social Sciences (SPSS), version 12. We utilized Spearman's correlation for the study, as we found that there was marked skew in the distribution of publications, with the bulk being published between 1990 and 2000. There was also a skew in the distribution of the complication rates and patient satisfaction, with a large majority of the studies having low complication rates and the majority of patients being satisfied with their management.

Results

The 140 studies contained information on 7686 patients. Many articles contained material on several types of management, and data comparing different management methods were therefore separated into:

- Conservative management and immobilization
- Conservative management and early mobilization
- Percutaneous repair and immobilization
- Percutaneous repair and early mobilization
- Open repair and immobilization
- Open repair and early mobilization
- External fixation

We identified 27 articles with 786 patients on conservative management, 18 articles with 435 patients on percutaneous repair, 102 articles with 4690 patients on open repair, and three articles with 355 patients on Achilles tendon repair with external fixation.

The vast majority of the studies were retrospective. There were only 13 randomized controlled trials—five comparing surgical versus nonsurgical treatment, six comparing postoperative immobilization, and two trials comparing percutaneous with open repair.

The average age of the patients through all categories of management (conservative and immobilization, percutaneous and immobilization, open and immobilization, conservative and early mobilization, percutaneous and early mobilization, open and early mobilization, and external fixation) remained remarkably constant (40.8, 40.6, 40.2, 40.0, 38.8, 37.7 and 42 years, respectively), ranging from 12 to 86 years of age.

Management methods

Conservative techniques

The patients managed conservatively generally underwent immobilization in a below-knee cast in gravity equinus position for 4 weeks, and were then placed in a more neutral position for a further 4 weeks.[11,12,32–38] Variations involved application of above-knee casts[39–41] and shorter[8,40] or longer[32,39,41,42] periods of immobilization. The average period of immobilization was 9 weeks, and the average follow-up period was 31.2 months for the conservatively immobilized group.

Three studies described management purely by functional bracing.[6–8] All reported good functional outcome and low re-rupture rates. The average time of immobilization in these studies was only 2 weeks, with an average follow-up of 22.3 months.

The number of skin complications reported from all conservative management methods was remarkably low, at three out of 718 (0.4%). All three reported complications were minor adhesions arising from direct trauma to the Achilles tendon prior to rupture. There were 58/785 (7.4%) minor general complications, 4/785 (0·5%) major complications, and 71/785 (9%) cases of re-rupture in the conservative group (Table 29.1).

Recently, Wallace *et al.*[43] assessed the results in 140 patients with a complete rupture of the Achilles tendon who had been treated nonoperatively with the use of cast and a removable orthosis. The authors reported excellent results in 56% of the patients; good, 30%; fair, 12%; and poor, 2%. The overall complication rate was 8%, with three complete and five partial tendon re-ruptures, two deep vein thromboses, and one temporary dropfoot. The authors concluded that the results of nonoperative orthotic management were better overall than the published results of operative repair of acute Achilles tendon rupture.[43]

Percutaneous techniques

Nine studies utilized the technique described by Ma and Griffith in 1977.[18–21,44–48] Variations of the technique were also described using both general and local anesthetic techniques.[49–52] Relatively high levels of sural nerve entrapment were noted in some studies utilizing the six percutaneous stab wounds technique[23,42,47,50] and the five percutaneous stab wounds technique,[49] accounting for up to 16.7% (8/48) of treated cases. However, Kosanovic *et al.*[48] presented a series of 36 patients using a six stab wounds percutaneous technique under local anesthesia, reporting no sural nerve complications, and a recent study of 16 patients by Atherton *et al.*[45] also reported similarly good results. Webb and Bannister[25] devised a three transverse incision approach to further minimize the complication of sural nerve injury. Thirteen studies described similar immobilization techniques to the conservatively managed groups, whereas four studies described early mobilization in a splint or removable cast.[49–52]

The average age of patients undergoing percutaneous repair was 40.8 years for the immobilized group and 40.4 years for the early mobilized group. The average period of immobilization in the percutaneous group was 7.7 weeks, with average follow-up periods of 25.8 months and 9.8 months for the immobilized and early mobilized groups, respectively. A total of 247 patients had percutaneous repair and immobilization, and 188 patients had percutaneous repair and early mobilization. The number of minor wound complications reported was 12/247 (4.9%). The general complication rate was 21/247 (8.5%) minor complications and 2/247 (0.8%) major complications, with 9/247 (3.6%) cases of re-rupture in the immobilized group. The early mobilized group sustained 8/188 (4.2%) minor and 4/188 (2.1%) major wound complications, 18/188 (9.5%) minor and 1/188 (0.5%) major general complications, and 9/188 (4.8%) cases of re-rupture.

Lim *et al.*,[53] in a prospective randomized controlled trial comparing open and percutaneous repair of closed Achilles tendon rupture, reported a higher rate of complications with open repair. There were seven cases of wound infection (21%) and two cases of re-rupture (6%) out of 33 in the open group, compared with three cases of wound puckering (9%), one re-rupture (3%), and one case of persistent paresthesia in the sural nerve territory (3%) out of 33 in the percutaneous group. The difference in infective wound complications between the two groups was statistically significant (Fisher's exact test, $P = 0.01$). The authors advocated percutaneous repair on the basis of the low rate of complications and improved cosmetic appearance.[53] Recently, Gorschewsky *et al.* reported their results with percutaneous repair of the Achilles tendon, using two Lengemann extension wires for coadaptation of the ruptured tendon and applying fibrin sealant to the rupture site, followed by early postoperative mobilization. Of 66 patients, only one (i.e., less than 2%) suffered a re-rupture due to trauma. There were no other complications reported.[54]

Open techniques

Many different open methods of repair have been described. The preferred method for early diagnosed ruptures has been simple end-to-end suture.[55] For neglected ruptures, allografts have been used.[14,56–58] More recently, however, synthetic materials have been utilized for augmentation, allowing early mobilization with promising results.[27,28,59] The use of augmentation for repair was not limited to delayed repair in neglected ATRs, and the identification of all neglected ATRs from the pool of studies was therefore not possible. This meant that data were often a combination of all open techniques. Our analysis revealed at least 41 different open techniques (Table 29.1). There were 3718 ATRs managed with open repair and immobilization, and 283 ATRs that were managed with open repair and early mobilization.

The average time of immobilization was 7 weeks in the open repair group, with a mean follow-up of 42.6 months and 20.3 months for the immobilized group and early mobilized group, respectively. A total of 469/4407 (10.6%) minor and 100/4407 (2.3%) major wound complications, 312/4407 (7%) minor and 41/4407 (0.9%) major general complications, and 107/4407 (2.4%) cases of re-rupture were noted in the immobilized group. A total of 14/283 (4.9%) minor and 1/283 (0.4%) major wound complications, 15/283 (5.4%) minor and 1/283 (0.4%) major general complications, and 4/283 (1.4%) re-ruptures were noted in the early mobilization group.

External fixation techniques

We identified three studies that used this technique.[29–31] The method of external fixation utilizes proximal and distal Kirschner wires with the foot in equinus for 7–8 weeks without postoperative plaster immobilization. Unfortunately, one of the articles[31] had very little information on the postoperative complications, and only mentioned a 95.55% excellent outcome rate from 314 ATRs. In the other two studies, 41 patients were managed with external fixation techniques. The average age of these patients was 42 years. In the 41 patients, three minor wound complications (7.3%) were noted, three minor general complications (7.3%), and no re-ruptures. The methodology scores for these two studies were 45[29] and 73,[30] respectively. The article by Tokmakov[31] had a methodology score of 35.

Randomized controlled trials

In this review, 13 randomized controlled trials were included. Six trials involving 313 patients compared cast immobilization versus functional brace (Table 29.4)[8,60–64] and five trials involving 663 patients comparing nonsurgical with surgical treatment (Table 29.5).[12,55,65–67] Two trials involving 94 patients compared percutaneous to open repair. A few other trials were excluded for various reasons, including inadequate methodology and insufficient reporting of outcomes.

Postoperative splinting in a functional brace (107/273 patients) was associated with a shorter in-patient stay, less time off work, a quicker return to sporting activities, and a lower complication rate (excluding re-rupture). Open operative treatment compared with nonoperative treatment (five trials, 568 patients) was associated with a lower risk of re-rupture. Results give a pooled incidence of 16/305 (5.2%) in the operatively treated group and 27/263 (10.2%) in the nonoperatively treated group, but a higher risk of other complications, including infection with an overall incidence of 25/305 (8%) in surgically managed patients and none in the nonsurgical group.

Percutaneous repair was associated with a shorter operating time and lower risk of infection. None of the 48 patients undergoing percutaneous repair had an infection, in comparison with nine of 46 in the open surgical group.

Review articles and the Cochrane database

In addition to the recent Cochrane review, a few quantitative reviews have been published on the management of Achilles tendon.

Wills *et al.*[56] reviewed 20 papers (1003 patients). They reported a re-rupture rate of 40/226 (17.7%) with conservative management, in comparison with 12/777 (1.5%) with operative management. They concluded that surgical management is superior for reducing the incidence of re-rupture, and that nonsurgical management is useful in high-risk patients.

Cetti[57] reviewed 66 papers (4597 patients). He reported a re-rupture rate of 69/514 (13.4%) with conservative management in comparison with 58/4083 (1.4%) re-ruptures with operative management. He concluded that surgical management leads to fewer re-ruptures and significantly better functional results.

Lo *et al.*[58] reviewed 19 papers (990 patients). They reported a re-rupture rate of 29/248 (11.7%) with conservative management in comparison with 21/742 (2·8%) with operative management. They again concluded that nonoperative management is preferable in patients with poor healing potential. Both forms of management can be offered to healthy active individuals.

Table 29.4 Randomized controlled trials comparing postoperative immobilization: functional brace versus cast immobilization

First author, ref.	Publication year	Patients (n)	Functional brace	Cast immobilization	Follow-up	Functional brace	Cast immobilization	Recommendation
Saleh[8]	1992	40	Below-knee cast in equinus 2 weeks and in semi-equinus 1 week, followed by early mobilization in a Sheffield splint for 6–8 weeks; weight-bearing allowed after 3 weeks)	Above-knee cast in equinus 4 weeks, below-knee cast in semi-equinus 4 weeks, below-knee cast in neutral 2 weeks; weight-bearing allowed after 8 weeks)	1 y	1/20 re-rupture No excessive lengthening Rapid recovery of dorsiflexion	1/20 re-rupture No excessive lengthening	Patients treated with the splint regained mobility significantly more quickly ($P < 0.001$) and preferred the splint to the plaster cast
Cetti[60]	1994	60	Postoperative functional brace allowing weight-bearing (dorsal splint plus stirrup in equinus for 6 weeks, heel-raise 2 weeks)	Cast immobilization (complete cast in equinus non-weight-bearing for 6 weeks, heel raise 2 weeks)	1 y	1/30 re-rupture Fewer minor complications Better recovery of normal ankle movement Fewer had calf atrophy Statistically significantly shorter sick leave Less elongation of the tendon	2/30 re-ruptures 1 infection	Postoperative mobile cast proved safe and convenient and preferable to management with the traditional rigid below-knee cast
Mortensen[61]	1999	71	Functional brace dorsal splint in equinus for 2 weeks, Don-Joy brace in 30° flexion 2 weeks, and Don-Joy brace in neutral, FWB 2 weeks	Complete cast in equinus for 6 weeks, neutral cast FWB 2 weeks	Median 16 mo	1/36 re-rupture 1 infection No patient had excessive lengthening of the tendon Return to work and sports activities sooner Strength of plantar flexion same	2/35 re-rupture	Early restricted motion appears to shorten the time needed for rehabilitation. There were no complications related to early motion in these patients. However, early unloaded exercises did not prevent muscle atrophy

Kerkhoffs[62]	2002	39	Cast in equinus for 1 week; semirigid "wrap" (for 6 weeks; partial weight-bearing for 4 weeks; full thereafter)	Cast immobilization (complete cast in neutral for 6–8 weeks; weight-bearing allowed when cast removed	5–8 y	0/16 re-rupture Shorter hospital stay Shorter period to return to pre-injury sports level	1/23 re-rupture	Functional management with a wrap is preferable to management with a walking cast with respect to hospitalization time and return to sports
Kangas[63]	2003	50	Functional brace (dorsal splint in neutral, allowing active plantar flexion, for 6 weeks)	Cast immobilization (complete cast in neutral for 6 weeks)[25] Weight-bearing at 3 weeks	60 weeks	1/25 re-rupture	2/25 re-rupture 1 infection	The calf muscle strength was better in the early motion group, whereas the other outcome results obtained in the two groups of patients were very similar. Therefore recommend early functional postoperative management
Maffulli[64] (two studies, quasi – RCT)	2003	53	Cast in equinus (for 2 weeks) followed by functional brace (dorsal splint in neutral, allowing active plantar flexion, for 4 weeks) Weight-bearing as soon as possible	Cast immobilization (complete cast in equinus for 2 weeks, mid-equinus for 2 weeks and neutral for 2 weeks) Weight at 2–4 weeks	16–26 mo	No re-rupture 2 superficial infections 1 hypertrophic scar 3 scar hypersensitivity	No re-rupture 2 superficial infections 6 scar hypersensitivity	Early weight-bearing with the ankle plantigrade is not detrimental to the outcome of repair after acute rupture of the Achilles tendon and shortens the time needed for rehabilitation. However, strength deficit and muscle atrophy are not prevented

FWB, full weight-bearing.

Table 29.5 Randomized controlled trials comparing surgical versus nonsurgical management

First author, ref.	Publication year	Patients (n)	Surgical	Nonsurgical	Follow-up	Outcome	Recommendation
Nistor[12]	1981	105	Bunnel repair below-knee plantar flexion at 2–3 weeks Total immobilization 6–9 weeks	4 weeks above knee in planter flexion and 4 weeks below knee	1–5 y	2 re-ruptures and two deep infections in patients who had operations, in comparison with five re-ruptures in the conservatively treated patients	Nonsurgical management
Cetti[55]	1993	111	Bunnel repair below-knee plantar flexion 6 weeks	4 weeks below knee in plantar flexion and 4 weeks neutral	1 y	In operative management group there were 3 re-ruptures and 2 deep infections in comparison with 7 re-ruptures, one second re-rupture, and one extreme residual lengthening of the tendon in the nonoperative group	Surgical management is preferable, but nonoperative management is an acceptable alternative
Schroeder[65]	1997	43	Single or double Kessler repair (13) and percutaneous repair (15)	A special boot immobilization for 8 weeks. Heel-raise reduced after 4 weeks (15)	6–12 mo	No re-rupture in any of the groups. Two wound infections in open surgical repair	
Moller[66]	2001	112	Modified Kessler repair Cast in plantar flexion for 6 weeks	4 weeks below knee in plantar flexion and 4 weeks neutral	2 y	Re-rupture rate in the nonoperative group was 20.8% compared with 1.7% in the operated group. No significant difference in patient outcomes when re-ruptures were excluded	Surgical management
Van der Linden (quasi-RCT)	2004	292	Surgical suture Plaster for 6 weeks	Splinting for 12 weeks		10 re-ruptures, 7 major wound problems, 11 minor wound complications, and 6 patients with complaints from the sural nerve after surgical repair; compared with 4 re-rupture and one pulmonary embolism 3 months after a re-rupture in the nonsurgical management group	Nonsurgical treatment is preferred. However, surgical treatment may be indicated in young athletes

Popovic and Lemaire[68] concluded that a satisfactory outcome may be achieved with either nonoperative or operative treatment of ATR, but surgical repair appears to provide better functional capacity, lower re-rupture rates, and slightly improved strength, but with a higher rate of minor complications.

Wong *et al.*[59] provided an extensive analysis of 125 articles published between 1965 and 2000 including 5370 patients. They concluded that open repair and early mobilization provide the best functional recovery and an acceptable complication rate. The general complication rates were highest in the percutaneous and early-mobilization groups. Re-rupture rates were highest in the immobilized conservative management groups (62 of 578, 10.7%), and lowest in groups with external fixation (0%).

Bhandari *et al.*[69] provided a review of only prospective randomized controlled trials of surgical methods versus nonoperative management of ATR from 1969 to 2000. They identified six publications and corrected for variance and heterogenicity between the study data. From the pooled analysis of results, they calculated a 68% reduction in the risk of re-rupture with surgery in comparison with conservative management, but they highlighted the bias from nonrandomized controlled trials promoting operative management.

Kocher *et al.*[70] conducted a similar review from 1966 to 2001. They excluded review articles and studies that did not involve cohorts with matching variables or randomized controlled trials. This identified 35 publications, 25 on operative repair and 10 on conservative management. The authors found a higher rate of rupture in conservatively managed ATRs (12.1% vs. 2.2%), whereas the mild moderate and major complication rate was higher in operative management groups (21.6% vs. 3.3%). Most of the operative complications are secondary to wound problems, and are usually mild to moderate.

Lynch[71] conducted a literature search to determine the method of choice in treating ATR. He identified five prospective randomized trials, six nonrandomized comparative studies, and 13 studies on surgical treatment only. He concluded that surgical management of ATR is the method of choice due to the lower incidence of re-rupture, while nonsurgical treatment may be acceptable for patients who refuse surgery or who are unfit for surgery. He also confirmed that early mobilization is associated with an improved functional outcome.

Khan *et al.*[72] performed a comprehensive review of the literature for the Cochrane Database in 2004. The authors reached the same conclusion as the previous review articles with regard to the low risk of re-rupture following open surgical treatment of ATR and the higher risk of other complications, including wound infection, which can be reduced by percutaneous surgery.

Outcome assessment

The vast majority of studies assessed the patients clinically, measuring calf circumference, gait, and the ability to stand on tiptoe. Many studies used other means of assessment, such as isokinetic or isometric dynamometry.[12,16,17,21,22,24,46,49,52,73–87] Dynamic fatigability tests, such as the heel-raise test, have been used to assess functional recovery following rupture.[7,75,87] Imaging has also been utilized to assess abnormalities in structural recovery in healing Achilles tendon ruptures. Ultrasonography (US) is a cheap and quick method of assessing Achilles tendons for abnormalities such as tendinopathies.[5] However, US does not provide information about the return in the tensile strength of ruptured Achilles tendons.[5] Computed tomography has been used to assess calf atrophy following ruptures, and studies have indicated that calf atrophy is more significant in patients who are managed conservatively. Magnetic resonance imaging has been used to objectively assess scar formation following the use of various open repair techniques, but only as a research tool.[27,88,89]

Subjective scoring

Few studies used formal subjective scoring to assess patient satisfaction and recovery following ATR. There were a number of subjective scoring scales to assess patient satisfaction, but like the repairs themselves, a single, simple, standardized method was not used repeatedly. Examples of scoring methods used include the Arner and Lindholm scale,[90–92] visual analogue scales,[49] Visick's scale,[93] Tegner's score,[40] the ankle–hindfoot scale,[73] the Percy and Connochie scale,[74,94] the modified Boyden score,[95] the Mandelbaum and Pavinini scale,[96] and the Holz scale.[97]

Discussion

This chapter has focused on the current state of knowledge on the treatment of isolated closed early rupture of the Achilles tendon. We have not dwelt upon delayed reconstruction or revision surgery for re-rupture. The key to correct management continues to be early and accurate diagnosis, allowing for an informed treatment plan subsequent to detailed discussion with the patient. Despite this being such a common and well-described injury, the management remains controversial. Furthermore, there is a paucity of well-designed controlled randomized trials of various treatment options. To compound this confusion, no single agreed outcome measure or scoring system has either been adopted universally or validated. There is as yet no "gold standard" management protocol.

In this chapter, we have deliberately included all studies describing the management of Achilles tendon rupture so that the whole spectrum of management techniques could be represented. Overselection of studies, we hoped, would allow for inclusion and scrutiny of more novel approaches to ATR management. We found a lack of consistency in the design and presentation of the various studies, especially when reporting outcomes. Enthusiastic advocates of outcome measurement for this condition, such as Leppilahti *et al.*,[95] have designed scoring methods to determine objective outcomes and prognostic factors for Achilles tendon rupture outcome. Standardization of reporting is aimed at making the interpretation of different studies easier. Despite this, even such injury-specific scoring systems may not be adopted easily, due to difficulty with key aspects such as isokinetic dynamometry, which may not be available to the wider orthopedic community.

By commencing our review in 1966 (with a span of 39 years), we have identified a clear trend towards reporting of outcome following surgical intervention, as opposed to conservative measures. Indeed, approximately 60% of the retrieved articles describe the outcome following open repair of Achilles tendon ruptures. This may reflect an increased enthusiasm for aggressive treatment, disappointment with the high rate of re-rupture subsequent to nonoperative measures, or a bias against assessment of conservative measures. This publication bias may further reflect the fact that open repair is the most popular method of management of a ruptured Achilles tendon, although no such information, to our knowledge, from a regional or national register currently exists. It may also be seen in the context of a trend towards more aggressive surgical intervention for acute injuries.[98]

The treating surgeon has to make two crucial decisions at the outset of management. These are either to treat nonoperatively or operate, and then whether to initiate a program

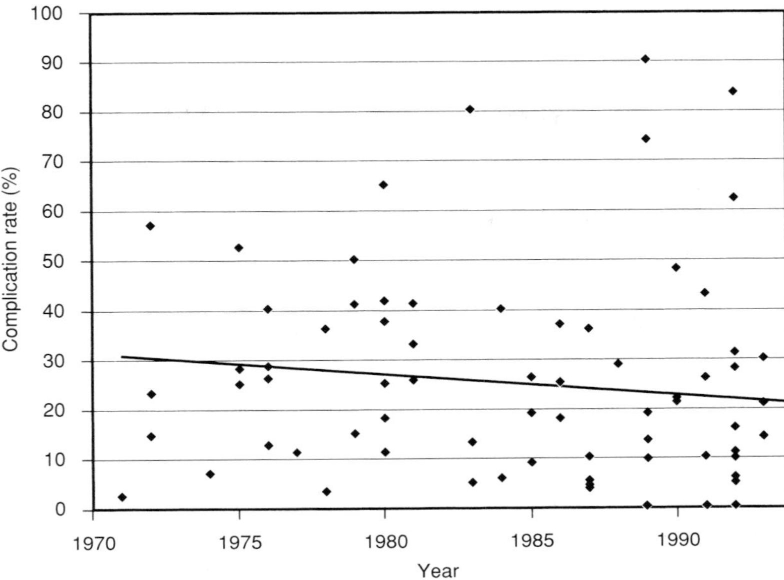

Figure 29.1 The complication rate over time.

of early rehabilitation with or without a functional brace. It is clear from the majority of the reviewed studies that surgical intervention is associated with a lower incidence of re-rupture. This is in general approximately half the rate reported for conservative management. The risk of re-rupture is equivalent with an open technique and a limited exposure technique. No consistent significant differences for re-rupture between these two surgical techniques were found. Indeed, the existence of more than one surgical technique may underscore the fact that no one procedure is without risk or universally accepted. Whether this is a reflection of the orthopedic psyche or the precarious local vascular supply to the adjacent soft tissues is unclear. Despite a concerted effort to achieve minimal soft-tissue dissection and scrutiny of the outcome, the reported rate of complications remains depressingly high for surgical treatment. The risk is often used to justify a nonoperative route, but with the attendant higher risk of re-rupture and requirement for later, technically challenging, surgery.

We have paid particular attention to the way in which complication rates may have changed with time. In comparison with other review articles, there did not seem to be a clear difference in the overall reported complication rates. However, upon analysis of individual studies published in specific years, a trend towards a decreasing number of complications has emerged (Fig. 29.1). This would imply that the results of management of ATR are improving. Certainly, a focus on minimizing skin healing complications, better surgical soft-tissue handling, and stronger emphasis on early mobilization may underlie such a trend; however, the true impact of early mobilization on the reduction in local complications remains unclear and requires closer study.

We do accept that the overall complication rate in the present study may be artificially high, as it was not possible to account for the fact that wound, general, and re-rupture complications may have occurred in the same patient. The overall complication rate was calculated at 664/5046 patients (22.4%). This is lower than the report by Lo *et al.*[58] (256/990, 25.9%), but greater than that reported by Wills *et al.*[56] (209/1003, 20.8%), Cetti[57] (576/4597, 12.5%) and Popovic and Lemaire[68] (664/5046, 13.1%) (Table 29.5).

There is a general perception that conservative measures should be reserved for the older age group and that the younger patient with ATR should have surgical treatment as a primary management modality in the absence of clear contraindications. However, we failed to identify any differences in the mean age of treated patients, despite reports that conservative management was reserved predominantly for older patients. An explanation for the relatively young age of the affected patients probably lies in the fact that the vast majority of ruptures are associated with sport. In a prospective study by Cetti *et al.*,[55] it was found that 82.9% (92/111) of the patients were active in sport prior to rupture of their Achilles tendons.

There appear to have been several new key developments over the last three decades that have allowed for the evolution in the management of ATR. Functional bracing, used in both conservative and operative procedures, appears to have produced a trend towards a decrease in the number of re-ruptures. In particular, contributions by McComis *et al.*[7] and Eames *et al.*[6] in the sphere of conservative management and early mobilization have favorably influenced the overall re-rupture rate for such treatment (63/645, 9.8% vs. 62/578, 10.8%). Future widespread use of functional bracing in ATR studies may consolidate the benefits of early mobilization.

We found that the rate of wound complications was by far greatest in the open repair and immobilized group of patients (569/4407, 12.9%). With the open repair and early-mobilization group, the percutaneous repair and immobilization group, and the externally fixated group, the rates of wound complications were approximately half of that found in the previous study group (15/283, 5.4%; 12/247, 4.9%; and 2/41, 4.9%, respectively). The patients managed with percutaneous repair and early mobilization also demonstrated a slightly higher rate of wound complications (12/188, 6.4%). Sural nerve injury is still a matter of the utmost concern for the operating surgeon. Iatrogenic injury may occur as a result of unrecognized division, compression due to either local scar formation or hematoma, or suture entrapment. This results in a permanently altered or absent sensation over the lateral aspect of the foot. In terms of general complications, the highest rates were found in the percutaneous and early mobilization groups (19/188, 10.1%), largely due to the high number of sural nerve injuries, and in the early-mobilized conservative group (11/67, 16.4%). Buchgraber and Passler[49] reported this complication in eight of 48 patients who underwent the procedure. However, Atherton *et al.*[45] and Kosanovic *et al.*[48] avoided this complication altogether in 16 and 36 patients, respectively. Expertise by a given surgeon in the use of this technique may explain these discrepancies. For the other management groups, the general complication rate remained relatively low, affecting less than 10% of the study population.

External fixation of 355 ATRs resulted in no reported re-ruptures. Conservatively managed patients with functional bracing had a re-rupture rate of only 1.5% (one of 67). Open repair and functional bracing led to similar rates of re-rupture (4/283, 1.4%), and the highest rates of re-rupture were found in the conservative management and immobilized group (62/578, 10.8%). The high re-rupture rate in the conservatively managed group has been noted in many other studies, which may be a reason for its decline in popularity over the years. External fixation is a very seldom mentioned and rarely used means of managing ATR, yet in our analysis it has the lowest reported re-rupture rate, which is a major outcome measure when assessing the success of ATR management. Meticulous maintenance and follow-up of external fixation in other orthopedic domains have probably affected the uptake of this method as a routine management option for ATR.[99]

Overall, the best outcomes with regard to minimization of complication rates were found in those patients managed with open repair and early mobilization (35/283, 12.4%). Complication rates using external fixation (excluding the study by Tokmakov[31]) were also relatively low at 14.6% (5/41). Patients who underwent percutaneous repair with early mobilization sustained higher complication rates (40/188, 21.27%) but had a better functional outcome than those immobilized for longer periods of time, whilst those patients who had undergone conservative management with whatever mobilization regime had a complication rate of about 17%. The highest complication rate was in the open repair and immobilization group (1029/4407, 23.3%). Unfortunately, as a consequence of the large number of different surgical techniques reported for repair of the ruptured Achilles tendon and the paucity of controlled studies and large number of extraneous variables, we have found it very difficult to advocate a particular surgical method. The evidence would tend to favor the use of simple end-to-end suturing (Kessler, Bunnel, and Masson), which accounts for 1394/4001 (34.8%) of all open techniques used. Other open repair techniques usually use end-to-end techniques with additional peripheral reinforcement. The Ma and Griffith[19] repair and Delponte technique[51] are the most commonly used percutaneous methods, accounting for 91/269 (33.8%) and 92/269 (34.2%) of percutaneous repairs. The popularity of these techniques probably bears witness to their simplicity.

In general, it seems that the simpler surgical principles are favored. It is essential that the treating surgeon should have a thorough knowledge of the risks and potential benefits of each modality of management. Crucially, we believe that it is imperative that a balanced opinion be offered with regard to the risks of re-rupture, nerve injury, skin complications, and the immobilization period required for each potential mode of intervention.

Conclusions

Operative management is the most common management modality reported following spontaneous rupture of the Achilles tendon in relatively young patients. Open repair and early mobilization is probably the method of choice, offering a relatively low complication rate and reliable early functional recovery. Promising results have also been demonstrated in patients managed conservatively and mobilized early, and this option may well be acceptable in those patients who are unfit for surgery. It should be noted, however, that the articles detailing the results of conservative management and early mobilization mostly do not deal with highly athletic patients, and that the good results achieved with this management modality are therefore probably biased. Despite the excellent results achieved in the patients managed by external fixation, this method is seldom used, and it is difficult to envisage that it will be widely adopted, especially when others are technically easier to perform and require less intensive follow-up.[100]

The management of uncomplicated subcutaneous tears of the Achilles tendon should probably be individualized in accordance with the concerns, occupation, sports participation, and health of the patient. If optimal performance is required in athletes and patients with high levels of physical activity, operative management is probably the modality of choice. Percutaneous repair should be considered in patients who do not wish to undergo formal open operative repair, possibly for cosmetic reasons, or perhaps because they view an open operative repair as a more invasive procedure. Conservative management should probably be reserved for older patients who are unlikely to achieve any major benefit from an operative procedure, or for those patients who view surgery as an unnecessary risk; if available, functional bracing should be used. We stress, however, that the lack of randomized controlled trials, and the inevitable publication bias in the studies published, means these recommendations are based on only on partial, possibly biased, evidence. Ultimately, the management regime should be tailored to the individual and to local expertise. However, the literature emphasizes keeping these regimes simple, and hence reproducible.

Summary

- Achilles tendon ruptures are common, and their incidence is rising.
- There are few randomized controlled trials studying different modalities of management.
- Operative management is the most common management modality reported following spontaneous rupture of the Achilles tendon in relatively young patients.

Key messages

- Management of uncomplicated subcutaneous tears of the Achilles tendon should be individualized according to the concerns, occupation, sports participation, and health of the patient.
- If optimal performance is required in athletes and patients with high levels of physical activity, operative management is probably the management of choice, with the present techniques offering a low complication rate and reliable early functional recovery.
- Percutaneous repair should be considered in patients who do not wish to undergo formal open operative repair, possibly for cosmetic reasons, or perhaps because they view an open operative repair as a more invasive procedure.
- Conservative management should probably be reserved for older patients who are unlikely to achieve any major benefit from an operative procedure, or for those patients who view surgery as an unnecessary risk; and, if available, functional bracing should be used.

Sample examination questions

Multiple-choice questions (answers on page 602)

1 With regard to subcutaneous tears of the Achilles tendon:
  A The management of subcutaneous tears of the Achilles tendon is well codified
  B Subcutaneous tears of the Achilles tendon are rare
  C In general, most surgeons would opt for operative management in physically active patients
  D The choice of operative technique is unclear
  E High-quality randomized controlled trials are available to guide physicians in evidence-based choices

2 With regard to percutaneous repair of subcutaneous tears of the Achilles tendon:
  A The technique minimizes skin healing problems associated with operative repair
  B The technique can be performed under local anesthetic
  C Using the original techniques, the sural nerve is rarely injured
  D Re-rupture rates are lower than following conservative management, but higher than following open methods of repair
  E Most complications experienced with this method of repair are minor

3 With regard to operative management of subcutaneous tears of the Achilles tendon:
   A Operative management is the most common management modality reported following spontaneous rupture of the Achilles tendon in young patients
   B Open repair and early mobilization results in a low rate of functional recovery
   C The rate of complications reported in recent studies is high
   D Highly athletic patients are best treated with operative methods
   E When using open repair techniques, there is a clear advantage in using a core suture and strong peripheral reinforcement with nonabsorbable materials

Essay questions

1 Conservative management of Achilles tendon ruptures: an option in selected patients?
2 Discuss the risks and benefits of open repair of Achilles tendon ruptures.
3 A 72-year-old smoker with chronic obstructive airways disease on long-term oral corticosteroids has ruptured his right Achilles tendon. He would like to know what the options for management are. Write short notes about what you would tell him.

Case study 29.1

A 32-year-old fit male doctor, playing five-a-side soccer, sprinted towards the ball and experienced a sudden acute and excruciating pain distal to his left calf. The patient can put weight on the affected limb, but cannot push off with his left foot. A gap is palpable 4 cm proximal to the insertion of the Achilles tendon, and the calf squeeze test shows no motion at the left ankle. The patient goes to the local gymnasium two or three times per week, and plays with his children at the weekend. He wants “everything to be sorted out in the best possible way.”

Summarizing the evidence

Comparison/management strategies	Results	Level of evidence*
Surgery vs. conservative management	Eight quantitative reviews of the literature, collecting a variety of data from RCTs and prospective and retrospective studies	A1

* A1: evidence from large randomized controlled trials (RCTs) or systematic review (including meta-analysis).†
A2: evidence from at least one high-quality cohort.
A3: evidence from at least one moderate-sized RCT or systematic review.†
A4: evidence from at least one RCT.
B: evidence from at least one high-quality study of nonrandomized cohorts.
C: expert opinions.
† Arbitrarily, the following cut-off points have been used; large study size: total number of injuries ≥ 100 per intervention group; moderate study size: total number of injuries ≥ 50 per intervention group.

Further reading

1 Leppilahti J, Puranen J, Orava S. Incidence of Achilles tendon rupture. *Acta Orthop Scand* 1996; 67:277–279.
2 Moller A, Astron M, Westlin N. Increasing incidence of Achilles tendon rupture. *Acta Orthop Scand* 1996; 67:479–481.

3 Maffulli N. Ultrasound of the Achilles tendon after surgical repair: morphology and function. *Br J Radiol* 1995; **68**:1372–1373.

4 Nyyssonen T, Luthje P. Achilles tendon ruptures in South-East Finland between 1986–1996, with special reference to epidemiology, complications of surgery and hospital costs. *Ann Chir Gynaecol* 2000; **89**:53–57.

5 Leppilahti J, Orava S. Total Achilles tendon rupture: a review. *Sports Med* 1998; **25**:79–100.

6 Eames MH, Eames NW, McCarthy KR, Wallace RG. An audit of the combined non-operative and orthotic management of ruptured tendo Achillis. *Injury* 1997; **28**:289–292.

7 McComis GP, Nawoczenski DA, DeHaven KE. Functional bracing for rupture of the Achilles tendon: clinical results and analysis of ground-reaction forces and temporal data. *J Bone Joint Surg Am* 1997; **79**:1799–1808.

8 Saleh M, Marshall PD, Senior R, MacFarlane A. The Sheffield splint for controlled early mobilisation after rupture of the calcaneal tendon: a prospective, randomised comparison with plaster treatment. *J Bone Joint Surg Br* 1992; **74**:206–209.

9 Bomler J, Sturup J. Achilles tendon rupture: an 8-year follow up. *Acta Orthop Belg* 1989; **55**:307–310.

10 Gillespie HS, George EA. Results of surgical repair of spontaneous rupture of the Achilles tendon. *J Trauma Inj Infect Crit Care* 1969; **9**:247–249.

11 Jacobs D, Martens M, Van Audekercke R, Mulier JC, Mulier F. Comparison of conservative and operative treatment of Achilles tendon rupture. *Am J Sports Med* 1978; **6**:107–111.

12 Nistor L. Surgical and non-surgical treatment of Achilles tendon rupture: a prospective randomized study. *J Bone Joint Surg Am* 1981; **63**:394–399.

13 Cetti R, Christensen SE. Surgical treatment under local anesthesia of Achilles tendon rupture. *Clin Orthop Rel Res* 1983; **173**:204–208.

14 Goldman S, Linscheid RL, Bickel WH. Disruptions of the tendo Achillis: analysis of 33 cases. *Mayo Clin Proc* 1969; **44**:28–35.

15 Hooker CH. Rupture of the tendo Achillis. *J Bone Joint Surg Br* 4 1963; **45**:360–363.

16 Beskin JL, Sanders RA, Hunter SC, Hughston JC. Surgical repair of Achilles tendon ruptures. *Am J Sports Med* 1987; **15**:1–8.

17 Inglis AE, Sculco TP. Surgical repair of ruptures of the tendo Achillis. *Clin Orthop Rel Res* 1981; **156**:160–169.

18 Zell RA, Santoro VM. Augmented repair of acute Achilles tendon ruptures. *Foot Ankle Int* 2000; **21**:469–474.

19 Ma GW, Griffith TG. Percutaneous repair of acute closed ruptured Achilles tendon: a new technique. *Clin Orthop Rel Res* 1977; **128**:247–255.

20 Rowley DI, Scotland TR. Rupture of the Achilles tendon treated by a simple operative procedure. *Injury* 1982; **14**:252–254.

21 Steele GJ, Harter RA, Ting AJ. Comparison of functional ability following percutaneous and open surgical repairs of acutely ruptured Achilles tendons. *J Sports Rehabil* 1993; **2**:115–127.

22 Bradley JP, Tibone JE. Percutaneous and open surgical repairs of Achilles tendon ruptures: a comparative study. *Am J Sports Med* 1990; **18**:188–195.

23 Sutherland A, Maffulli N. A modified technique of percutaneous repair of ruptured Achilles tendon. *Oper Orthop Traumatol* 1999; 7:288–295.

24 Boyden EM, Kitaoka HB, Cahalan TD, An KN. Late versus early repair of Achilles tendon rupture: clinical and biomechanical evaluation. *Clin Orthop Rel Res* 1995; **317**:150–158.

25 Webb JM, Bannister GC. Percutaneous repair of the ruptured tendo Achillis. *J Bone Joint Surg Br* 1999; **81**:877–880.

26 Cottalorda J, Kelberine F, Curvale G, Groulier P. Surgical treatment of ruptures of the Achilles tendon in athletes: 31 cases operated on with an average follow up of 4 years. *J Chir* 1992; **129**:436–440.

27 Liem MD, Zegel HG, Balduini FC, *et al.* Repair of Achilles tendon ruptures with a polylactic acid implant: assessment with MR imaging. *AJR Am J Roentgenol* 1991; **156**:769–773.

28 Ozaki J, Fujiki J, Sugimoto K, Tamai S, Masuhara K. Reconstruction of neglected Achilles tendon rupture with Marlex mesh. *Clin Orthop Rel Res* 1989; **238**:204–208.

29 Casteleyn PP, Opdecam P, De Clercq D. Surgical treatment of Achilles tendon ruptures, combined with an external fixation system. *Acta Orthop Belg* 1980; **46**:310–313.

30 Nada A. Rupture of the calcaneal tendon: treatment by external fixation. *J Bone Joint Surg Br* 1985; **67**:449–453.

31 Tokmakov P. Treatment of ruptures of Achilles' tendons by an external fixator. *Folia Med (Plovdiv)* 1995; **37** (4A Suppl):92.
32 Christensen IB. Rupture of the Achilles tendon: analysis of 57 cases. *Acta Chir Scand* 1943; **106**:50–60.
33 Coombs RRH. Prospective trial of conservative and surgical treatment of Achilles tendon rupture. *J Bone Joint Surg Br* 1981; **63**:288.
34 Edna T. Non-operative treatment of Achilles tendon ruptures. *Acta Orthop Scand* 1980; **51**:991–993.
35 Gillies H, Chalmers J. The management of fresh ruptures of the tendo Achilles. *J Bone Joint Surg* 1970; **52**:337–343.
36 Lea RB, Smith L. Non-surgical treatment of tendon Achilles rupture. *J Bone Joint Surg Am* 1972; **54**:1398–1407.
37 Lildholdt T, Munch-Jorgensen T. Conservative treatment of Achilles tendon rupture: a follow-up study of 14 cases. *Acta Orthop Scand* 1976; **47**:454–458.
38 Perrson A, Wredmark T. The treatment of total rupture of the Achilles tendon by plaster immobilisation. *Int Orthop* 1979; **3**:149–152.
39 Arlettaz Y, Chevalley F, Gremion G, Levyraz PF. Les ruptures fraîches du tendon d'Achilles. A propos de 14 cas traités conservativement. *Swiss Surg* 1998; **4**:75–81.
40 Fruengaard S, Helmig P, Riis J, Stovring JO. Conservative treatment for acute rupture of the Achilles tendon. *Int Orthop* 1992; **16**:33–35.
41 Keller J, Rasmussen TB. Closed treatment of Achilles tendon rupture. *Acta Orthop Scand* 1984; **55**:548–550.
42 Stein SR, Luekens CA. Closed treatment of Achilles tendon ruptures. *Orthop Clin North Am* 1976; **7**:241–246.
43 Wallace RG, Traynor IE, Kernohan WG, Eames MH. Combined conservative and orthotic management of acute ruptures of the Achilles tendon. *J Bone Joint Surg Am* 2004; **86**:1198–1202.
44 Aracil J, Pina A, Lozano JA, Torro V, Escriba I. Percutaneous suture of Achilles ruptures. *Foot Ankle* 1992; **13**:350–351.
45 Atherton WG, Dangas S, Henry APJ. Advantages of semi-closed over open method of repair of ruptured Achilles tendon. *Foot Ankle* 2000; **6**:27–30.
46 FitzGibbons RE, Hefferon J, Hill J. Percutaneous Achilles tendon repair. *Am J Sports Med* 1993; **21**:724–727.
47 Klein W, Land DM, Saleh M. Percutaneous repair of rupture of the Achilles tendon. *J Bone Joint Surg Br* 1990; **72**:1087.
48 Kosanovic M, Cretnik A, Batista M. Subcutaneous suturing of the ruptured Achilles tendon under local anaesthesia. *Arch Orthop Trauma Surg* 1994; **113**:177–179.
49 Buchgraber A, Passler HH. Percutaneous repair of Achilles tendon rupture: immobilisation versus functional postoperative treatment. *Clin Orthop Rel Res* 1997; **341**:113–122.
50 Buisson P, Batisse J, Porter L, Fabre A, Guillemot E. Traitement des ruptures du tendon d'Achille selon la technique de tenorraphie percutanée. *J Traumatol Sport* 1996; **13**:204–211.
51 Delponte P, Potier L, de Poulpiquet P, Buisson P. Treatment of subcutaneous ruptures of Achilles tendon with a percutaneous tenorrhaphy. *J Orthop Surg* 1992; **6**:404–407.
52 Merti P, Jarde O, Tranvan F, Doutrrellot P, Vives P. Tenorraphie percutanée pour rupture du tendon d'Achille. Etude de 29 cas. *Rev Chir Orthop* 1999; **85**:277–285.
53 Lim J, Dalal R, Waseem M. Percutaneous vs. open repair of the ruptured Achilles tendon: a prospective randomized controlled study. *Foot Ankle Int* 2001; **22**:559–568.
54 Gorschewsky O, Pitzl M, Putz A, Klakow A, Neumann W. Percutaneous repair of acute Achilles tendon rupture. *Foot Ankle Int* 2004; **25**:219–224.
55 Cetti R, Christensen SE, Ejsted R, Jensen NM, Jorgensen U. Operative versus nonoperative treatment of Achilles tendon rupture: a prospective randomized study and review of the literature. *Am J Sports Med* 1993; **21**:791–799.
56 Wills CA, Washburn S, Caiozzo V, Prietto CA. Achilles tendon rupture: a review of the literature comparing surgical versus nonsurgical treatment. *Clin Orthop Rel Res* 1986; **207**:160–163.
57 Cetti R. Rupture of the Achilles tendon: operative vs. nonoperative options. *Foot Ankle Clin* 1997; **2**:501–519.
58 Lo IKY, Kirkley A, Nonmeiler B, Kumbhare DA. Operative versus nonoperative treatment of acute Achilles tendon ruptures: a quantitative review. *Clin J Sports Med* 1997; **7**:207–211.

59 Wong J, Barrass V, Maffulli N. Quantitative review of operative and nonoperative management of Achilles tendon ruptures. *Am J Sports Med* 2002; **30**:565–574.
60 Cetti R, Henriksen LO, Jacobsen KS. A new treatment of ruptured Achilles tendons: a prospective randomized study. *Clin Orthop Rel Res* 1994; **308**:155–165.
61 Mortensen HM, Skov O, Jensen PE. Early motion of the ankle after operative treatment of a rupture of the Achilles tendon: a prospective, randomized clinical and radiographic study. *J Bone Joint Surg Am* 1999; **81**:983–990.
62 Kerkhoffs GM, Struijs PA, Raaymakers EL, Marti RK. Functional treatment after surgical repair of acute Achilles tendon rupture: wrap vs. walking cast. *Arch Orthop Trauma Surg* 2002; **122**:102–105.
63 Kangas J, Pajala A, Siira P, Hamalainen M, Leppilahti J. Early functional treatment versus early immobilization in tension of the musculotendinous unit after Achilles rupture repair: a prospective, randomized, clinical study. *J Trauma Inj Infect Crit Care* 2003; **54**:1171–1180.
64 Maffulli N, Tallon C, Wong J, Lim KP, Bleakney R. Early weightbearing and ankle mobilization after open repair of acute midsubstance tears of the Achilles tendon. *Am J Sports Med* 2003; **31**:692–700.
65 Schroeder D, Lehmann M, Steinbrueck K. Treatment of acute Achilles tendon ruptures: open vs. percutaneous repair vs. conservative treatment. A prospective randomized study. *Orthop Trans* 1997; **21**:1228.
66 Moller M, Movin T, Granhed H, *et al.* Acute rupture of tendon Achillis: a prospective randomised study of comparison between surgical and non-surgical treatment. *J Bone Joint Surg Br* 2001; **83**:843–848.
67 Van der Linden-van der Zwaag HM, Nelissen RG, Sintenie JB. Results of surgical versus non-surgical treatment of Achilles tendon rupture. *Int Orthop* 2004; **28**:370–373.
68 Popovic N, Lemaire R. Diagnosis and treatment of acute ruptures of the Achilles tendon: current concepts review. *Acta Orthop Belg* 1999; **65**:458–471.
69 Bhandari M, Guyatt GH, Siddiqui F, *et al.* Treatment of acute Achilles tendon ruptures: a systematic overview and metaanalysis. *Clin Orthop Rel Res* 2002; **400**:190–200.
70 Kocher MS, Bishop J, Marshall R, Briggs KK, Hawkins RJ. Operative versus nonoperative management of acute Achilles tendon rupture: expected-value decision analysis. *Am J Sports Med* 2002; **30**:783–790.
71 Lynch RM. Achilles tendon rupture: surgical versus non-surgical treatment. *Accid Emerg Nurs* 2004; **12**:149–158.
72 Khan RJ, Fick D, Brammar TJ, Crawford J, Parker MJ. Interventions for treating acute Achilles tendon ruptures. *Cochrane Database Syst Rev* 2004; (3):CD003674.
73 Fernandez-Fairen M, Gimeno C. Augmented repair of Achilles tendon ruptures. *Am J Sports Med* 1997; **25**:177–181.
74 Gerdes MH, Brown TD, Bell AL, *et al.* A flap augmentation technique for Achilles tendon repair: postoperative and functional outcome. *Clin Orthop Rel Res* 1992; **220**:241–246.
75 Haggmark T, Liedberg H, Eriksson E, Wredmark T. Calf muscle atrophy and muscle function after non-operative versus operative treatment of Achilles tendon ruptures. *Orthopedics* 1986; **9**:160–164.
76 Kissel CG, Blacklidge DK, Crowley DL. Repair of neglected Achilles tendon ruptures: procedure and functional results. *J Foot Ankle Surg* 1994; **33**:46–52.
77 Kruger-Franke M, Siebert CH, Scherzer S. Surgical treatment of ruptures of the Achilles tendon: a review of long-term results. *Br J Sports Med* 1995; **29**:121–125.
78 Leppilahti J, Siira P, Vanharanta H, Orava S. Isokinetic evaluation of calf muscle performance after Achilles rupture repair. *Int J Sports Med* 1996; **17**:619–623.
79 Mandelbaum BR, Myerson MS, Forster R. Achilles tendon ruptures: a new method of repair, early range of motion, and functional rehabilitation. *Am J Sports Med* 1995; **23**:392–395.
80 Quigley TB, Scheller AD. Surgical repair of the ruptured Achilles tendon: analysis of 40 patients treated by the same surgeon. *Am J Sports Med* 1980; **8**:244–250.
81 Respizzi S, Ribas MM. Valutazione isocinetica delle riconstruzioni del tendine d'Achille. *J Sports Traumatol Rel Res* 1991; **13**:35–43.
82 Richter J, Pommer A, Hahn M, David A, Muhr G. Möglichkeiten und Grenzen der funktionell konservativen Therapie akuter Achillessehnenrupturen. *Chirurg* 1997; **68**:517–524.
83 Roberts C, Rosenblum S, Uhl R, Fetto J. Surgical treatment of Achilles tendon rupture. *Orthop Rev* 1989; **18**:513–519.
84 Shields CL, Kerlan RK, Jobe FW, Carter VS, Lombardo SJ. The Cybex II evaluation of surgically repaired Achilles tendon ruptures. *Am J Sports Med* 1978; **6**:396–372.

85 Speck M, Klaue K. Early full weightbearing and functional treatment after surgical repair of acute Achilles tendon rupture. *Am J Sports Med* 1998; **26**:789–793.

86 Soldatis JJ, Goodfellow DB, Wilber JH. End-to-end operative repair of Achilles tendon rupture. *Am J Sports Med* 1997; **25**:90–95.

87 Moberg A, Nordgran B, Solveborn. Surgically repaired Achilles tendon ruptures with postoperative mobile ankle cast: a 12-month follow-up study with an isokinetic and a dynamic function test. *Scand J Med Sci Sports* 1992; **2**:231–233.

88 Aoki M, Ogiwara N. Early active motion and weightbearing after cross stitch Achilles tendon repair. *Am J Sports Med* 1998; **26**:794–800.

89 Karjalainen PT, Aronen HJ, Pihlajamaki HK, *et al.* Magnetic resonance imaging during healing of Achilles tendon ruptures. *Am J Sports Med* 1997; **25**:164–171.

90 Anderson E, Hvass I. Suture of Achilles tendon rupture under local anesthesia. *Acta Orthop Scand* 1986; **57**:235–236.

91 Arner O, Lindholm A. Subcutaneous rupture of the Achilles tendon: a study of 92 cases. *Acta Chir Scand* Suppl 1959; **239**:7–51.

92 Solveborn S, Moberg A. Immediate free ankle motion after surgical repair of acute Achilles tendon ruptures. *Am J Sports Med* 1994; **22**:607–610.

93 Crollo RMPH, van Leeuwen DM, van Ramshorst B, van der Werken C. Acute rupture of the tendo calcaneus. *Acta Orthop Belg* 1987; **53**:492–494.

94 Percy EC, Conochie LB. The surgical treatment of ruptured tendo Achillis. *Am J Sports Med* 1978; **6**:132–136.

95 Leppilahti J, Forsman K, Puranen J, Orava S. Outcome and prognostic factors of Achilles rupture repair using a new scoring method. *Clin Orthop Rel Res* 1998; **346**:152–161.

96 Maniscalco P, Bertone C, Bonci E, Donelli L, Pagliantini L. Titanium anchors for the repair of distal Achilles tendon ruptures: preliminary report of a new surgical technique. *J Foot Ankle Surg* 1998; **37**:96–100.

97 Winter E, Weise K, Weller S, Ambacher T. Surgical repair of Achilles tendon rupture; Comparison of surgical with conservative treatment. *Acta Orthop Trauma Surg* 1998; **117**:364–367.

98 Sarmiento A. Thoughts of the future of orthopedics: I am concerned. *J Orthop Sci* 2000; **5**:425–430.

99 Coyte PC, Bronskill SE, Hirji ZZ, *et al.* Economic evaluation of 2 treatments for pediatric femoral shaft fractures. *Clin Orthop Rel Res* 1997; **336**:205–215.

100 Porter D, Mannarino F, Snead D, Gabel S, Ostrowski M. Primary repair without augmentation for early neglected Achilles tendon ruptures in the recreational athlete. *Foot Ankle Int* 1997; **18**:557–564.

101 Lynn TA. Repair of the torn Achilles tendon, using the plantaris tendon as a reinforcing membrane. *J Bone Joint Surg Am* 1966; **48**:268–272.

102 Perez-Teuffer AR. Traumatic rupture of the Achilles tendon: reconstruction by transplant and graft using the lateral peroneus brevis. *Orthop Clin North Am* 1974; **5**:89–93.

103 Wapner KL, Hecht PJ, Mills RH. Reconstruction of neglected Achilles tendon injury. *Orthop Clin North Am* 1995; **26**:249–263.

104 Saw Y, Baltzopoulos V, Lim A, *et al.* Early mobilisation after operative repair of ruptured Achilles tendon. *Injury* 1993; **24**:479–488.

105 Sutherland A, Maffulli N. Naht der rupturienten Achillessehne. *Oper Orthop Traumatol* 1998; **10**:50–58.

106 Volpe A, Girotto Riga B, Giunchi F, Melaotte PL. La riparazione del tendine d'Achile con utilizzo di PDS band: indicazioni, tecnica, risultati. *Ital J Orthop Traumatol* 1995; **21**:157–166.

107 Carter TR, Fowler PJ, Blokker C. Functional postoperative treatment of Achilles tendon repair. *Am J Sports Med* 1992; **20**:459–462.

108 Kakiuchi M. A combined open and percutaneous technique for repair of tendo Achillis: comparison of open repair. *J Bone Joint Surg Br* 1995; **77**:60–63.

109 Keller J, Bak B. The use of anesthesia for surgical treatment of Achilles tendon rupture. *Orthopedics* 1989; **12**:431–433.

110 Merkel M, Neumann HW, Merk H. A new score for the comparison of results after operative treatment of ruptures of the Achilles tendon. *Chirurg* 1996; **67**:1141–1146.

111 Sejberg D, Hansen LB, Dalsgaard S. Achilles tendon ruptures operated on under local anesthesia: retrospective study of 81 nonhospitalized patients. *Acta Orthop Scand* 1990; **61**:549–550.

112 Carden DG, Noble J, Chalmers J, Lunn P, Ellis J. Rupture of the calcaneal tendon: the early and late management. *J Bone Joint Surg Br* 1987; **69**:416–420.
113 Jessing P, Hansen E. Surgical treatment of the 102 tendo Achillis rupture: suture or tenontoplasty? *Acta Chir Scand* 1975; **141**:170–177.
114 Kasinathan ST. Open injuries of tendon Achillis. *J West Pac Orthop Assoc* 1980; **17**:96–99.
115 Kellam JF, Hunter GA, McElwain JP. Review of the operative treatment of Achilles tendon rupture. *Clin Orthop* 1985; **210**:80–83.
116 Kiviluoto O, Santavirta S, Klosser O, Sandelin J, Hakkinen S. Surgical repair of the Achilles tendon. *Arch Orthop Trauma Surg* 1985; **104**:327–329.
117 Kouvalchouk JF, Monteau M. Bilan du traitement chirgical des ruptures du tendon d'Achille. *Rev Chir Orthop* 1976; **62**:253–266.
118 Kvist-Kristensen J, Thastrup-Andersen P. Rupture of the Achilles tendon: a series and review of literature. *J Trauma* 1972; **12**:794–798.
119 Lawerence GL, Cave EF, O'Connor H. Injury to the Achilles tendon, experience in a Massachusetts General Hospital, 1900–1954. *Am J Surg* 1955; **89**:795–802.
120 Lennox DW, Wang GJ, McCue FC, Stamp WG. The operative treatment of Achilles tendon injuries. *Clin Orthop Rel Res* 1980; **148**:152–155.
121 Rantanen J, Hurme T, Pannanen M. Immobilisation in neutral versus equinus position after Achilles tendon repair. *Acta Orthop Scand* 1993; **64**:333–335.
122 Tobin WJ. Repair of the neglected rupture and severed Achilles tendon. *Am Surg* 1953; **19**:514–522.
123 Turco VJ, Spinella AJ. Achilles tendon ruptures: peroneus brevis transfer. *Foot Ankle* 1987; **7**:253–259.
124 Mann RA, Holmes GB, Seale KS, Collins DN. Chronic rupture of the Achilles tendon: a new technique of repair. *J Bone Joint Surg Am* 1991; **73**:214–219.
125 Abraham E, Pankovich AM. Neglected rupture of the Achilles flap: treatment by V–Y tendinous flap. *J Bone Joint Surg Am* 1975; **57**:253–256.
126 Barnes MJ, Hardy AE. Delayed construction of the calcaneal tendon. *J Bone Joint Surg Br* 1986; **68**:121–124.
127 Lindholm A. A new method of operation in subcutaneous rupture of the Achilles tendon. *Acta Chir Scand* 1959; **117**:261–270.
128 Lieberman JR, Lozman J, Czajka J, Dougherty J. Repair of Achilles tendon ruptures with Dacron vascular graft. *Clin Orthop* 1988; **234**:204–208.
129 Choksey A, Soonawalla D, Murray J. Repair of neglected Achilles tendon ruptures with Marlex mesh. *Injury* 1996; **27**:215–217.
130 Howard CB, Winston I, Bell W, Mackie I, Jenkins DHR. Late repair of the calcaneal tendon with carbon fibre. *J Bone Joint Surg Br* 1984; **66**:206–208.
131 Parson JR, Weiss AB, Schenk RS, Alexander H, Pavlisko F. Long-term follow-up of Achilles tendon repair with an absorbable polymer carbon fibre composite. *Foot Ankle* 1989; **9**:179–184.
132 Aldam CH. Repair of calcaneal tendon ruptures. *J Bone Joint Surg Br* 1989; **71**:486–488.
133 DiStefano VJ, Nixon JE. Achilles tendon rupture: pathogenesis, diagnosis and treatment by a modified pullout wire technique. *J Trauma* 1972; **12**:671–677.
134 Motta P, Errichiello C, Pontini I. Achilles tendon rupture: a new technique for easy surgical repair and immediate movement of the ankle and foot. *Am J Sports Med* 1997; **25**:172–176.
135 Marti RK, van der Werken C, Schutte PR, Bast TJ. Operative repair of ruptured Achilles tendon and functional after-treatment, 1: acute repair. *Neth J Surg* 1983; **35**:61–64.
136 Massari L, Cinotti A, Mannella P, Traina GC. Clinical and ultrasound follow-up of 62 patients submitted to the surgical treatment of subcutaneous rupture of the Achilles tendon. *Chir Organi Mov* 1994; **79**:213–218.
137 Ralston EL, Schmidt ER. Repair of the ruptured Achilles tendon. *J Trauma* 1971; **11**:15–21.
138 Mohammed A, Rahamatalla A, Wynne-Jones CH. Tissue expansion in late repair of tendo Achillis rupture. *J Bone Joint Surg Br* 1995; **77**:64–66.
139 Fahlstrom M, Bjornstig U, Lorentzon R. Acute Achilles tendon ruptures in badminton players. *Am J Sports Med* 1998; **26**:467–470.
140 Rubin BD, Wilson HJ. Surgical repair of the interrupted Achilles tendon. *J Trauma* 1980; **20**:248–249.
141 Farizon F, Pages A, Azoulai JJ, Larison R, Bousquet G. Traitement chirurgical des ruptures du tendon d'Achille. A propos de 42 cas traités selon la technique Bosworth. *Rev Chir Orthop* 1997; **83**:65–69.

142 Helgeland J, Odland P, Hove LM. Akillesseneruptur: operative eller ikke-operativ behandling. *Tidsskr Nor Loegeforen* 1997; **117**:1763–1766.

143 Postacchini F, Puddu G. Subcutaneous rupture of the Achilles tendon. *Int Surg* 1976; **61**:14–18.

144 Soodan VM, Bhagat OP, Gulati DS, Kachroo BB. Surgical repair of neglected tendo Achillis tear. *Indian J Orthop* 1986; **20**:174–176.

145 Traina GC, Vitale G. Risultati a distanza el trattamento delle lesioni sottocutanee del tendine di Achille. *Clin Orthop Univ* 1975; **62**:315–323.

146 Wagdy-Mahmoud S, Megahed AA, El-Sheshtawy OE. Repair of the calcaneal tendon: an improved technique. *J Bone Joint Surg Br* 1992; **74**:114–117.

147 Van der Werken C, Marti RK. Operative repair of ruptured Achilles tendon and functional after-treatment, 2: delayed rupture. *Neth J Surg* 1983; **35**:65–68.

148 Wredmark T, Carlstedt CA. Tendon elongation and muscle function after repair of Achilles tendon rupture. *Scand J Med Sci Sports* 1992; **2**:139–142.

149 Stein SR, Luekens CA. Methods and rationale for closed treatment of Achilles tendon ruptures. *Am J Sports Med* 1976; **4**:162–169.

150 Clark CR. The prospective, randomized, double-blind clinical trial in orthopaedic surgery. *J Bone Joint Surg Am* 1997; **79**:1119–1120.

151 Mortensen NH, Saether J, Steinke MS, Staehr H, Mikkelsen SS. Separation of tendon ends after Achilles tendon repair: a prospective, randomized, multicenter study. *Orthopedics* 1992; **15**:899–903.

152 Levi N. The incidence of Achilles tendon rupture in Copenhagen. *Injury* 1997; **28**:311–313.

153 Cretnik A, Frank A. Incidence and outcome of rupture of the Achilles tendon. *Wien Klin Wochenschr* 2004; **116** (Suppl 2):33–38.

154 Bruggeman NB, Turner NS, Dahm DL, *et al.* Wound complications after open Achilles tendon repair: an analysis of risk factors. *Clin Orthop Rel Res* 2004; **427**:63–66.

155 Haji A, Sahai A, Symes A, Vyas JK. Percutaneous versus open tendo Achillis repair. *Foot Ankle Int* 2004; 25:215–218.

156 Rettig AC, Liotta FJ, Klootwyk TE, Porter DA, Mieling P. Potential risk of rerupture in primary Achilles tendon repair in athletes younger than 30 years of age. *Am J Sports Med* 2005; **33**:119–123.

157 Rajasekar K, Gholve P, Faraj AA, Kosygan KP. A subjective outcome analysis of tendo-Achilles rupture. *J Foot Ankle Surg* 2005; **44**:32–36.

158 Menegaldo LL, de Toledo FA, Weber HI. Moment arms and musculotendon lengths estimation for a three-dimensional lower-limb model. *J Biomech* 2004; **37**:1447–1453.

159 Weber M, Niemann M, Lanz R, Muller T. Nonoperative treatment of acute rupture of the Achilles tendon: results of a new protocol and comparison with operative treatment. *Am J Sports Med* 2003; **31**:685–691.

160 Coutts A, MacGregor A, Gibson J, Maffulli N. Clinical and functional results of open operative repair for Achilles tendon rupture in a non-specialist surgical unit. *J R Coll Surg Edinb* 2002; **47**:753–762.

161 Majewski M, Widmer KH, Steinbruck K. Achilles tendon ruptures: 25 years' experience in sport-orthopedic treatment. *Sportverletz Sportschaden* 2002; **16**:167–173.

162 Pajala A, Kangas J, Ohtonen P, Leppilahti J. Rerupture and deep infection following treatment of total Achilles tendon rupture. *J Bone Joint Surg Am* 2002; **84**:2016–2021.

163 Moller M, Movin T, Granhed H, *et al.* Acute rupture of tendon Achillis: a prospective randomised study of comparison between surgical and non-surgical treatment. *J Bone Joint Surg Br* 2001; **83**:843–848.

CHAPTER 30
How to manage plantar fasciitis

Gerald Ryan

Introduction

Plantar fasciitis is the most common cause of dorsal heel pain. Despite this frequency, medical providers are often misinformed regarding the etiology and treatment of this disorder. This misunderstanding can lead to inappropriate and often ineffective treatment plans. Even with appropriate intervention, plantar fasciitis may prove resistant to a variety of treatments and can be a source of frustration for the provider and patient. This chapter will review the available medical information regarding the pathophysiology, evaluation, and treatment plans for this common condition.

Internet search strategies

MEDLINE, SportDiscus, and Best Evidence were searched using the terms "plantar fasciitis," "heel pain," and "heel pain syndrome." In addition, the same categories were combined with the various treatment modalities, including orthotics, heel cups and pads, night splints, casting, surgery, and extracorporeal shock-wave therapy. Few prospective randomized trials were identified. Weight was then given to case–control and large retrospective studies in the evaluation of the various treatment modalities.

Anatomy

The plantar fascia consists of a medial, central (intermediate), and lateral segment. Anatomy texts often refer to the plantar fascia as the plantar aponeurosis.[1] Magnetic resonance imaging (MRI) studies performed on patients with heel pain indicate that only the central (intermediate) portion of the fascia is abnormal in these patients.[2] The plantar aponeurosis originates on the inferomedial surface of the calcaneus, deep to the fat pad of the heel. The fascia then fans out anteriorly and inserts onto the dorsal surface of the proximal phalanges.[3] This anatomical configuration forms the longitudinal arch of the foot. The medial calcaneal nerve, a branch of the posterior tibial nerve, innervates the origin of the plantar aponeurosis. The first branch of the lateral plantar nerve passes beneath the calcaneal tuberosity, innervating the abductor digiti quinti as well as supplying sensory branches to the plantar fascia. A collection of fat globules is contained within a honeycombed matrix between the calcaneus and the skin of the heel. In addition, the skin of the heel is the thickest skin of the body. This combination of a specialized heel pad and thickened skin functions as a shock absorber for the heel and mitigates the effects of impact and friction on the heel during heel strike.[4] The thickness of the fat pad decreases with age, transmitting greater forces to the calcaneus with heel strike as the fat pad thins.

Windlass effect

The insertion of the distal fascia onto the proximal phalanges produces a windlass effect first described by Hicks.[5] Dorsiflexion of the toes pulls the plantar fascia around the metatarsal heads, much like the windlass of a sailboat. This anatomical arrangement increases traction and strain on the plantar fascia and shortens the fascia between its origin at the calcaneus and the metatarsal heads. The shortening of the fascia raises the longitudinal arch and supinates the foot. In contrast, plantar flexion of the toes lengthens the aponeurosis between the calcaneus and the metatarsal heads, causing the arch to fall and the foot to pronate.[6] The windlass mechanism provides passive variation of the flexibility of the forefoot. Plantar flexion of the toes pronates the foot and increases the flexibility of the forefoot during the heel strike phase of gait. Dorsiflexion of the toes during the push-off phase raises the arch and supinates the foot, increasing the rigidity of the foot and improving the efficiency of push-off. These changes in the flexibility are achieved without an active muscular component, increasing the efficiency of the gait and improving endurance. The windlass mechanism has been confirmed in cadaver studies.

Etiology

The term "fasciitis" is a misnomer. Histopathological studies of the plantar fascia in patients with heel pain reveal disorganization of the collagen fibers, an increase in the amount of mucoid ground substance, and an increase in number of fibroblasts, with minimal inflammation of the fascia. These changes are similar to those found in overuse injuries of the Achilles and patellar tendon and the rotator cuff mechanism, and more accurately describe a tendinosis of these structures. Tendinosis is a degenerative condition due to chronic damage resulting from overuse, and is not an inflammatory reaction.[7] Thickening of the plantar fascia has been confirmed by MRI and ultrasound studies. The plantar fascia in asymptomatic patients is 2–4 mm thick. The plantar fascia of symptomatic patients is 6–10 mm thick.[5,8] Due to the apparent lack of an inflammatory component in the typical patient with heel pain, it has been suggested that a more appropriate term would be "heel pain syndrome" rather than plantar fasciitis.

Microtears in the collagen fibers of the plantar fascia are thought to be the etiology of these histopathological changes. Heel impact does not appear to cause the pathological changes found in patients with heel pain syndrome. Gait studies performed on patients with heel pain revealed no difference between the force of heel strike in the affected and unaffected heel.[9] Radiographs of many patients with heel pain reveal a calcification of the plantar aponeurosis at its origin on the calcaneus. This radiological finding is commonly referred to as a heel spur. Heel spurs serve as markers for chronic heel pain, but are not the cause of the pain. Radiographs of asymptomatic patients often reveal heel spurs,[10] and the presence of a heel spur does not alter the response to therapy.[11]

Diagnosis

The diagnosis of painful heel syndrome is made by history and physical examination. Ancillary studies may be necessary to exclude other similar conditions, but are not necessary in most patients with plantar fasciitis.

History

The symptom most suggestive of painful heel syndrome is a sharp heel pain when the patient first attempts to bear weight on the heel after sleeping or being recumbent for several hours. The pain is frequently severe enough to prevent the individual from putting his or her full weight on the heel for several minutes. Gradually, the pain subsides as the patient ambulates. The pain may recur during the day when the patient attempts to walk after sitting for a prolonged period of time. The etiology of this pain is conjectured to be either edema of the aponeurosis from microtears of the fascia or a disruption of the tendon matrix that is laid down as the body attempts to repair these microtears. Most individuals will also experience a dull, aching pain of the medial heel throughout the day. The intensity of this pain is most often dependent on the amount of time the individual stands on his or her feet during the day, and/or on the patient's weight. The heel pain may radiate distally towards the metatarsal heads. Pain radiating to the Achilles tendon or more proximally is unusual. The medial heel is most commonly involved, but in severe cases the patient may describe pain of the entire dorsal heel.

Most patients do not recall a history of trauma or change in their usual routine prior to the onset of the heel pain. Injury to the plantar aponeurosis is rarely associated with trauma. An important exception to this rule is young male runners. Runners will often report an increase in either the intensity of training or a significant increase in average mileage prior to the onset of the heel pain. There is little evidence that either a change in running shoes or the condition of the shoes increases the risk of plantar fasciitis. For most patients, an increase in body mass and daily activity are the likely causes of their symptoms.

Physical examination

Essentially, all patients with plantar fasciitis will have pain on palpation of the medial calcaneus at the origin of the plantar aponeurosis. Failure to elicit pain while palpating the medial calcaneus should prompt a search for an alternative cause of the patient's symptoms. Dorsiflexion of the great toe increases plantar fascia tension and may also cause medial calcaneus pain. This finding is very specific for plantar fasciitis, but unlike direct palpation of the calcaneus, is not found in the majority of patients.

Although not critical in the diagnosis of painful heel syndrome, the forefoot should be evaluated for any abnormalities. Individuals with either a high, rigid arch (pes cavus) or a flattened arch (pes planus) and excessive forefoot pronation (forefoot valgus) have an increased incidence of plantar fasciitis. It may be helpful when evaluating runners to ask the patient to bring in a well-worn pair of running shoes. Examination of the wear pattern on the soles of running shoes can be very helpful in the identification of an abnormal gait. The abnormal gait may increase the strain on the plantar aponeurosis and increase the likelihood of an overuse injury.

The posterior heel should be carefully examined for other potential causes of heel pain. The insertion of the Achilles tendon, the calcaneal bursa, and the posterior point of the heel should be firmly palpated in an attempt to discover additional areas of pain. The Achilles tendon is evaluated for the presence of a bump or thickening of the calcaneal bursa. The medial and lateral calcaneus should be percussed along the path of the medial calcaneal and lateral plantar nerves in an attempt to elicit a Tinel's sign, indicating nerve entrapment. Pain on palpation of the metatarsal heads suggests metatarsalgia or metatarsal fracture. Careful note should be made of any warmth or erythema of the skin, an unusual finding in plantar fasciitis. The dorsal surface of the heel is examined for signs of trauma or ecchymosis, and the skin is evaluated for the presence of calluses or plantar warts.

In the absence of a history of trauma, radiographs are not necessary to diagnose plantar fasciitis. A history of trauma, however, should prompt the examiner to rule out a fracture or other bony abnormality. Radiographs are not indicated initially to evaluate the calcaneus for the presence or absence of a heel spur, as the presence of a heel spur adds little to the initial evaluation and management of plantar fasciitis.[11,12] More extensive studies, such as MRI, ultrasound, or bone scan should be reserved for patients with recalcitrant pain and atypical presentations. Radiographs are indicated, however, for the initial evaluation of pediatric and elderly patients presenting with heel pain, due to the low incidence of plantar fasciitis in these populations. A prospective study of a thousand consecutive visits to a pediatric practice revealed only eight visits for heel pain, all due to Sever's disease, an apophysitis of the calcaneus.[13] Radiographs of the heel are usually adequate in making this diagnosis, but a bone scan or MRI are indicated if radiographs are normal and the examination is highly suggestive of Sever's disease. Plantar fasciitis is also rarely a cause of heel pain in the elderly. The most likely reason for this low incidence is the decreased activity level of the geriatric population. Radiographs should be obtained in all elderly patients to rule out bony metastases to the heel, or fracture.

Differential diagnosis

A careful physical examination should allow the diagnosis of plantar fasciitis to be made in most patients. An alternative diagnosis should be considered in patients with an atypical history and pain on palpation of areas other than the medial calcaneus, as well as patients who fail to respond to therapy (Table 30.1).

Musculoskeletal

Bony abnormalities should always be considered in children and the elderly. In addition, a history of trauma or sudden onset of pain warrants a search for an alternative diagnosis. Fractures resulting from seemingly minor trauma necessitate a search for underlying abnormalities such as Paget's disease, osteoporosis, or metastatic disease.

Table 30.1 Differential diagnosis

Musculoskeletal
- Calcaneal apophysitis
- Fractures
- Metastatic disease
- Contusion
- Achilles tendinitis and bursitis

Neurological
- Posterior tibial nerve (tarsal tunnel syndrome)
- Medial branch of the posterior tibial nerve
- Lateral plantar nerve

Systemic disease
- Reiter's syndrome
- Ankylosing spondylitis
- Lupus

Pain due to Achilles tendinitis or bursitis rarely involves the dorsal aspect of the heel and can usually be distinguished on physical examination from plantar fasciitis. Runners may have both Achilles tendinitis and plantar fasciitis, as both injuries are frequently the result of excessive mileage. Fortunately, the treatments for both these conditions are similar, and most patients will respond even if it is difficult to determine which injury is the primary cause of a runner's symptoms.

Neuralgia

Injury or entrapment of either the posterior tibial nerve or the lateral calcaneal nerve can produce heel pain. Unlike plantar fasciitis, neuropathic pain is often worse at bedtime or awakens the patient from sleep. Patients may report hypoesthesia or hyperesthesia of the distal foot. Patients with neuralgia as the source of their heel pain do not typically have pain with palpation at the insertion of the medial plantar aponeurosis, nor does dorsiflexion of the great toe exacerbate symptoms. Nerve conduction studies may be of value in patients with tarsal tunnel syndrome, but are not helpful in the evaluation of patients with suspected neuralgia due to an abnormality of the branch of the lateral calcaneal nerve innervating the abductor digiti minimi.

Systemic disease

Heel pain may be due to a systemic inflammatory illness. Reiter's syndrome (arthritis, urethritis, and conjunctivitis), ankylosing spondylitis, systemic lupus erythematosus, and other connective-tissue illnesses may present as heel pain. Clinicians should be on the alert for an underlying illness if the physical examination reveals any evidence of erythema, warmth, or effusion of the heel suggesting an inflammatory process. Radiographs are of limited use in differentiating plantar fasciitis from an inflammatory illness, but bone scans and MRI are useful if the diagnosis is in doubt. The concurrent onset of heel pain and other connective-tissue abnormalities should always prompt an investigation for an underlying illness. If an underlying illness is discovered, treatment of the underlying illness should be initiated and therapy of plantar fasciitis should be reserved for those who do not respond to treatment of the underlying illness.

Treatment

Although plantar fasciitis is surpassed only by ankle sprains as the cause of lower extremity pain in runners,[14] the treatment of the condition has not been extensively evaluated. Two recent systematic reviews yielded a limited number of prospective randomized controlled trials of frequently utilized treatments for plantar fasciitis.[15,16] In addition, available studies would suggest that 80–85% of patients presenting with plantar fasciitis will experience improvement of symptoms within the first 6 months, regardless of the treatment utilized.[17–19] Keeping these limitations in mind, commonly utilized treatments will be ranked according to the quality of the available evidence. Recommendations will be made on the basis of the strength of this information.

Rest

No randomized trials were found addressing this intervention. Two retrospective studies surveyed patients and asked them to rank their satisfaction with the interventions they had received. Rest was ranked third behind casting and injection amongst the 11 interventions evaluated in one study, and as the most effective in the other. A combined total of 514 patients were surveyed in the two studies.[18,19]

Recommendation. Rest is likely to be helpful, but has little support in the literature. Most patients will experience a significant decrease in pain within the first 6 months, regardless of the initial intervention chosen.

Heel cord stretching

Although heel cord stretching is included in virtually all treatment plans for plantar fasciitis, only one study was found that looked at stretching as an isolated treatment. Seventy-two percent of patients assigned to stretching alone reported improvement of symptoms, in comparison with 88% of patients who used prefabricated splints and stretching.[20] The trial did not include an observational group to serve as a control, so the effectiveness of the stretching program could not be assessed. In patients with pain that had persisted for more than 10 months, DiGiovanni *et al.* reported improved resolution of pain using a stretching program of dorsiflexion of the forefoot and toes, in comparison with heel cord stretching.[21]

Recommendation. Heel cord stretching is likely to be helpful, but has little support in the literature.

Heel pads and orthotics

A review of the available information on the efficacy of heel pads and orthotics in the treatment of plantar fasciitis reveals conflicting information. Lynch *et al.* found that only 30% of the patients they studied rated symptom improvement as fair to excellent with the use of heel cups, while 70% of the patients treated with custom-molded orthotics reported a similar level of improvement.[17] In contrast, Pfeffer *et al.* found that the use of prefabricated heel cups was significantly more effective in relieving symptoms than were custom-molded orthotics.[20] It should be noted that the study by Pfeffer *et al.* was funded primarily by the makers of prefabricated heel pads. The surveys by Gill *et al.*[18] and Wolgin *et al.*[19] both found that patients ranked arch supports as highly effective interventions. The survey by Gill *et al.* ranked the use of a heel cup as the least effective intervention.[18]

Biomechanical studies do not support the use of heel cups in the treatment of plantar fasciitis. Heel force impact studies reveal that the heel strike forces in patients with plantar fasciitis are the same in painful and asymptomatic[22] heels. An earlier study on impact forces revealed similar findings, and heel pads were found to be effective only in those individuals with localized heel pain from contusions, but not in patients with plantar fasciitis.[23] In contrast to these findings, custom-molded orthotics have been shown to reduce the tension of the plantar aponeurosis, although preformed orthotics did not produce a similar reduction in tension.[24] As stated previously, excessive tension at the origin of the plantar aponeurosis is thought to be the cause of plantar fasciitis. Reducing plantar fascia tension would be expected to reduce pain and aid healing. No similar biomechanical model exists for the action of heel pads.

Recommendation. Heel pads were found to be effective in a single study, but were ineffective in the remainder of the investigations. Heel pads are not recommended for the treatment of plantar fasciitis, but may benefit patients with heel pain due to a contusion.

Orthotics. Although studies do not universally support the use of orthotics, the weight of the evidence favors a benefit from orthotics. Custom-molded orthotics are likely to be more effective than preformed orthotics, but the high cost of custom orthotics limits their use in the initial treatment of plantar fasciitis. Orthotics are recommended in the initial treatment of plantar fasciitis.

Taping

Various methods of taping are employed, but all methods run the length of the longitudinal arch. The tape decreases the amount the arch flattens during the stance phase, decreasing the tension of the plantar fascia during the stance phase. Due to the inconvenience of frequently reapplying the tape, taping is typically used to provide immediate relief until the patient is able to obtain orthotics or modified footwear. Despite the frequent use of taping in the acute care of plantar fasciitis, no studies were found evaluating the effectiveness of taping.

Recommendation. Taping has not been adequately evaluated, and no recommendation can be made regarding its use in the treatment of plantar fasciitis.

Night splints

Tension night splints have been utilized to maintain the foot in maximum dorsiflexion while the patient sleeps. This form of therapy is purported to allow the fascia tissue to begin to heal with the plantar aponeurosis in full extension and reduce the tension at the origin of the fascia at the calcaneus. Biomechanical models have not confirmed this mechanism of action. Preformed and custom-molded splints have been utilized.

The use of tension night splints was first evaluated by Wapner and Sharkey.[25] Fourteen patients who had had symptomatic plantar fasciitis for more than 1 year who had not responded to multiple interventions were splinted in 5° of dorsiflexion overnight. Eleven of the patients had complete relief of their symptoms within 4 months. Subsequent studies revealed similar improvements.[26,27] A more recent prospective study compared the use of nonsteroidal anti-inflammatory drugs, shoe modifications, and stretching with a program utilizing these same interventions and night splints.[28] A total of 116 patients were followed for 12 weeks. There was no difference in the outcomes between the two groups. The discrepancies in these studies are likely due to the different populations investigated. Studies that demonstrated the efficacy of night splints enrolled patients who had failed to respond to other modes of therapy for extended periods of time. The study that did not demonstrate a treatment advantage with the use of night splints utilized the splints as an initial treatment modality. As described earlier, up to 85% of patients will experience significant relief of symptoms regardless of the initial therapy chosen. In addition, due to the small size of this study, it would be very difficult to demonstrate a treatment advantage from any intervention used for the initial treatment of plantar fasciitis.

Recommendation. Tension night splints are likely effective in the treatment of recalcitrant plantar fasciitis.

Casting

Patients with severe heel pain are frequently fitted with a short leg walking cast. A retrospective study of 411 patients with plantar fasciitis listed casting as the most effective therapy among the multiple therapies employed.[18] Only one small prospective study was found addressing the use of casting for the treatment of plantar fasciitis. Thirty-two patients with prolonged heel pain in whom multiple other modes of therapy had failed were treated with a short leg walking cast. Only 24 patients completed the study, and 86% of these patients reported significant improvement following treatment with the cast.[29] The study is limited, however, by the high drop-out rate (eight of 32 patients) and the lack of a control group. The efficacy of casting is limited, as prolonged use of a cast may induce atrophy of the lower leg musculature.

Recommendation. Casting may be helpful in the treatment of recalcitrant plantar fasciitis, but no quality studies have been done to document its effectiveness.

Steroid therapy

Corticosteroids are often used to treat plantar fasciitis. Separate prospective randomized controlled trials (RCT) have demonstrated an initial treatment effect for the use of iontophoresis[30] and percutaneous injection[17,31] to infiltrate the plantar fascia with corticosteroids. These studies also found the benefits to be transient. No significant difference in pain relief was discernible between the control patients and those treated with steroids after the first month. All of the RCTs of corticosteroid injections involved small numbers of patients.

Steroid injections may carry a significant risk of precipitating rupture of the plantar fascia. Acevedo and Beskin reviewed the records of 765 patients treated for plantar fasciitis.[32] Fifty-one patients experienced a rupture of the plantar fascia. Forty-four of these patients received a steroid injection prior to the rupture. The authors performed corticosteroid injections in 122 patients, and 12 of these patients later ruptured their plantar fascia. Ultrasound has been utilized to guide the placement of the corticosteroid, but there is no evidence that this technique enhances the outcome or decreases long-term complications. If corticosteroid injections are used, the proper method of injection is a medial approach at the point of greatest pain on the medial calcaneus. The injection should not be administered by puncturing the heel pad, as this approach results in greater discomfort to the patient. No studies were found that demonstrated a risk from the application of corticosteroids with iontophoresis.

Recommendation. Although corticosteroids are frequently utilized in the initial treatment of plantar fasciitis, the benefits of the treatment appear to be short-lived. In addition, corticosteroid injections have the potential to precipitate rupture of the plantar fascia. In view of the limited evidence of lasting relief of symptoms and the potential for significant harm, corticosteroid injections are not recommended in the initial treatment of plantar fasciitis. The value of steroid injections in the treatment of recalcitrant plantar fasciitis is uncertain and also carries the risk of patient harm. Although iontophoresis has not been shown to increase the risk of plantar aponeurosis rupture, the limited benefit provided by the treatment does not justify the cost of this treatment.

Extracorporeal shock-wave therapy (ESWT)

Extracorporeal shock-wave therapy is advocated in the treatment of plantar fasciitis. Enthusiasm for this mode of therapy is centered in Germany, Switzerland, and Austria. The same countries are home to the manufacturers of the ESWT apparatus. Two small RCTs and one moderate-sized RCT have been published, but all have significant shortfalls.

Earlier studies by Rompe *et al.* have unusual patient selection criteria.[33,34] A later study by Speed *et al.* was a small study with a high drop-out rate in the placebo group (five of 15).[35] An intention-to-treat analysis would not have shown any treatment advantage. Due to concerns regarding the cost of the procedure and limited evidence supporting the use of ESWT, the health ministries in Germany, Austria, and Switzerland have suspended reimbursement for ESWT pending further investigations of its effectiveness.[36]

Subsequent studies have done little to resolve the controversy over ESWT. Rompe *et al.* performed a prospective RCT including 45 runners with chronic heel pain and found a significant decrease in pain at 6 months and 1 year in patients treated with three applications of 2100 impulses of low-energy shock waves.[37] Theodore *et al.* also reported a treatment advantage for ESWT.[38] Careful review of this study reveals some concerns, however. The initial improvement of pain at 3 months was modest, with 56% of patients who received ESWT reporting success at 3 months in comparison with 46% of patients receiving a sham therapy; in addition, no long-term results were available, as the investigators allowed patients to cross over to the active treatment arm after the 3-month follow-up. Improvement in the symptoms of tennis elbow and plantar fasciitis was also reported by Mehra *et al.* using three treatments with ESWT with a mobile lithotripter.[39] In contrast, several studies have failed to show benefit from ESWT. Three RCTs with a combined total of 301 patients failed to show a treatment advantage with ESWT.[40–42]

Recommendation. The use of ESWT remains controversial in the treatment of chronic plantar fasciitis. Studies supporting its use are in large part supported by a single investigator (Rompe), and several studies done by others have shown no benefit. There is no evidence of harm from the therapy. A Cochrane review of ESWT concluded that "There is conflicting evidence for the effectiveness of low-energy extracorporeal shock-wave therapy in reducing night pain, resting pain, and pressure pain in the short term (6 and 12 weeks) and therefore its effectiveness remains controversial."[43] At this time, there is insufficient evidence to recommend for or against the use of ESWT. The cost of this as yet unproven therapy should be borne in mind when treatment is being chosen.

Radiofrequency therapy

A single study was found utilizing radiofrequency therapy in the treatment of plantar fasciitis. Sollitto and Plotkin utilized a fluoroscopy-guided radiofrequency probe to cauterize the plantar fascia at its insertion on the medial calcaneus. Ninety-two percent of the 39 patients treated experienced complete relief of their pain.[44] These results, however, must be viewed with some caution. Most of the patients had less than 6 months of pain prior to the procedure, and many had only experienced pain for 2–3 months. Most of these patients would be expected to have improved with other less invasive measures. In addition, there was no control group in the study.

Recommendation. Due to the invasive nature of this therapy and the limited evidence supporting its use, radiofrequency lesioning of the plantar fascia cannot be recommended at present for the treatment of plantar fasciitis.

Surgery

Patients should not be considered for surgery unless conservative measures have been unsuccessful for 12 months. A waiting period of 6 months is frequently recommended, but a significant number of patients will experience resolution of symptoms between 6 and 12 months.[19] Plantar fasciotomy is often combined with a neurolysis of the nerve to the abductor digiti quinti.[45] Endoscopic and open fasciotomy appear to have similar results, although this has only been studied in retrospective patient surveys.[46] Initial relief of recalcitrant heel pain after surgery is reported to be 70–90% in several studies.[45–49] Long-term results are not as encouraging. Fasciotomy results in a flattening of the longitudinal arch and a shifting of peak forces of ambulation from the heel to the midfoot.[48] This shift results in an increase in midfoot and forefoot problems following surgery. Davies *et al.* found that despite initial satisfaction with the surgical results, 48% of 43 patients who underwent fasciotomy were unhappy with the results.[47] Although patients surveyed by Fishco *et al.* as well as Sammarco and Helfrey reported a higher level of satisfaction postoperatively, one-third of these patients reported persistent midfoot and forefoot pain.[45,49] MRI analysis of patients with persistent pain revealed recurrent plantar fasciitis, pathology related to arch instability, and structural failure from overload as the most common abnormalities in patients with persistent or recurrent pain following plantar fasciotomy.[50]

Recommendation. Surgical intervention should be reserved for patients with heel pain resistant to all other more conservative measures. A significant number of patients with plantar fasciitis may experience relief of symptoms as late as 1 year following presentation, without invasive interventions. Due to the likelihood of resolution of symptoms, significant pain should be persistent for a minimum of 6 months, and more typically 1 year, before conservative therapies are considered to have failed. Although surgery is likely to provide short-term relief to the great majority of patients, long-term results are not as encouraging. Before surgery is carried out, patients should be made aware of the potential for subsequent forefoot problems resulting from the lysis of the plantar aponeurosis.

Conclusions

Heel pain due to plantar fasciitis frequently prompts patients to seek medical treatment (Figure 30.1). The diagnosis can in most cases be made after a careful examination. Atypical history or physical findings, as well as heel pain in very young or very old patients, should prompt an evaluation for other causes of heel pain. Radiographs are of little value for most patients. Once the diagnosis has been established, a conservative treatment plan of rest, stretching, and orthotics will provide relief for the majority of patients, although the evidence supporting these measures is limited. Although heel cups are frequently utilized in the initial treatment of plantar fasciitis, the majority of current studies do not support their use. For patients with persistent symptoms, a trial of night splints or casting is appropriate. Due to the limited long-term relief of symptoms and the risk of fascia rupture, steroid injections should be reserved for patients with symptoms persisting more than 3–6 months. Surgery should be considered only if patients remain symptomatic for more than 12 months, and patients should be warned of the increased risk of midfoot and forefoot problems following surgery. The use of ESWT is controversial and should likely be reserved for patients who have not responded to other less costly therapies. Radiofrequency lesioning should be considered investigational at present and cannot be recommended as a routine treatment for plantar fasciitis.

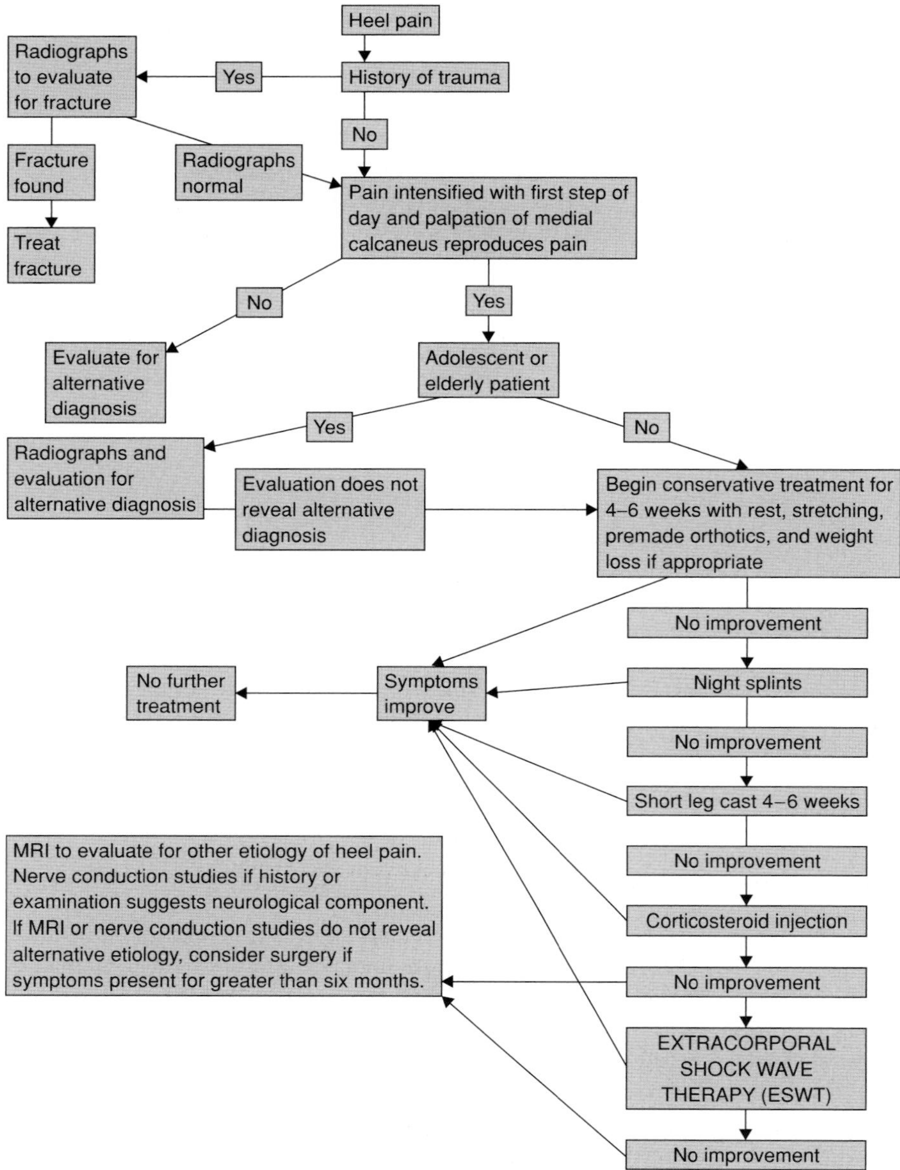

Figure 30.1 The approach to the patient with heel pain.

Summary

- Plantar fasciitis is an overuse injury, not associated with trauma.
- Symptoms are due to microtears at the tendon insertion, due to tendon strain during the take-off phase of walking, not the impact phase.
- The condition is unusual in adolescents and elderly patients—alternative causes of heel pain should be sought in these populations.

- The diagnosis is made clinically. Radiographs are of limited use outside of adolescent and elderly populations.
- Most patients (85%) will improve regardless the form of therapy, if any.
- There is limited evidence for most forms of treatment.

Key messages

- Give rest and stretching an adequate trial before more aggressive therapies.
- Corticosteroid injections provide only short-term relief and involve a risk of tendon rupture.
- There is limited evidence of efficacy for orthotics, heel pads, and night splints.
- Extracorporeal shock-wave therapy remains a controversial form of treatment due to conflicting reports in the literature.
- Surgery should be considered only as a last resort.
- There is no support in the literature for other forms of treatment.

Sample examination questions

Multiple-choice questions (answers on page 602)

1 Plantar fasciitis is an uncommon cause of heel pain in which of the following patients?
   A Ten-year-old athlete
   B Twenty-year-old long distance runner
   C Thirty-year-old obese female
   D Forty-year-old factory worker

2 Which of the following therapies increases the potential for rupture of the plantar fascia?
   A Stretching of the plantar fascia
   B Night splints
   C Corticosteroid injections
   D Casting

3 Surgery for relief of heel pain due to plantar fasciitis should only be considered if the patient has not responded to conservative therapy for a minimum of:
   A Six weeks
   B Three months
   C Six months
   D One year

Essay questions

1 Describe the pathophysiological mechanism for plantar fasciitis.
2 Explain why the pain of plantar fasciitis is greatest on the medial calcaneus.
3 Describe the role of radiographs in the evaluation of plantar fasciitis.

Case study 30.1

A 10-year-old child presents with his parents to your office with a 3-week history of heel pain. The child is active in soccer, but does not report any recent injury. The pain improves after several days of rest, but recurs with resumption of activities. What is the most likely cause of the child's pain, and what studies should be considered?

Case study 30.2

A patient with a long history of plantar fasciitis presents to your office. The patient reports several heel injections in the past. On each occasion, the pain was relieved for a short period of time, but recurred. Following the most recent injection, the pain did not recur but now the patient is experiencing midfoot pain with prolonged walking. What is most likely to have occurred and how should the patient be treated?

Case study 30.3

A patient presents with a 6-week history of heel pain on walking first thing in the morning. Your examination reveals pain to palpation of the medial side of the lower calcaneus. You make the diagnosis of plantar fasciitis. What would be a logical sequence of treatments to alleviate the patient's symptoms?

Summarizing the evidence

Intervention	Results	Level of evidence*
Rest	Although most patients are likely to respond to simple rest, no RCTs exist verifying its effectiveness in comparison with more active forms of therapy	C
Stretching	Recommended in most treatment guidelines, but no RCTs to confirm effectiveness over simple rest	C
Orthotics	Two small RCTs showed trend toward benefit of orthotics over stretching for initial treatment. Most evidence supporting use based on retrospective surveys	A4
Heel cups	One RCT showed improvement over stretching. alone. Large retrospective survey revealed little benefit	A4
Night splints	Three small RCTs showed significant improvement in recalcitrant plantar fasciitis with the use of night splints. One moderate-sized RCT for initial treatment of plantar fasciitis did not show improvement when adding the use of night splints to stretching, anti-inflammatories, and shoe recommendations. The lack of efficacy of night splints for the initial treatment of plantar fasciitis is not surprising, as 80–85% of patients with acute plantar fasciitis will experience symptom improvement regardless of the initial form of treatment	A3
Casting	No RCT, but cohort studies reveal benefit for recalcitrant plantar fasciitis	B

Summarizing the evidence (*Continued*)

Intervention	Results	Level of evidence*
Corticosteroid injections	One small RCT showed initial benefit for steroid injection and one small RCT showed initial benefit for iontophoresis, but benefit was transient in both groups. Large retrospective study of patients who received corticosteroid injections revealed significant risk for plantar fascia rupture following injection	A4
Surgery	No RCTs, cohort studies of patients with recalcitrant plantar fasciitis support improved outcomes following surgery. Surgery may increase long-term risk of later midfoot and forefoot problems	B
Extracorporeal shock-wave therapy	RCTs have shown both no benefit and benefit from therapy. Studies showing benefit have primarily been reported by a single investigator. Benefit of therapy has not been demonstrated by other investigators	A3
Radiofrequency lesioning	No RCTs and no high-quality cohort studies. Not recommended at present for treatment of plantar fasciitis	C

* A1: evidence from large randomized controlled trials (RCTs) or systematic reviews (including meta-analysis).†
A2: evidence from at least one high-quality cohort.
A3: evidence from at least one moderate-sized RCT or systematic review.
A4: evidence from at least one RCT.
B: evidence from at least one high-quality study of nonrandomized cohorts.
C: expert opinion.
† Arbitrarily, the following cut-off points were used: large study size: ≥ 100 patients per intervention group; moderate study size: ≥ 50 patients per intervention group.

References

1 Netter FH. In: *Atlas of Human Anatomy*. Summit, New Jersey: Ciba-Geigy, 1995: Plate 500.
2 Kier R. Magnetic resonance imaging studies of plantar fasciitis and other causes of heel pain. *MRI Clin North Am* 1994; 2:97–107.
3 Gray's Anatomy – The Anatomical Basis of Clinical Practice 39th Edition Editor in Chief Susan Standring. 2005 Elsevier Churchhill Livingstone, Philadelphia; 1509–1531.
4 Jahss MH, Kummer F, Michelson JD. Investigations into the fat pads of the sole of the foot: heel pressure studies. *Foot Ankle* 1992; 13:227–232.
5 Hicks J. The mechanics of the foot, II: the plantar aponeurosis and the arch. *J Anat* 1954; **88**:25.
6 Fuller EA. The windlass mechanism of the foot: a mechanical model to explain pathology. *J Am Podiatr Med Assoc* 2000; **90**:35–46.
7 Khan KM, Cook JL, Bonar F, Harcourt P, Astrom M. Histopathology of common tendinopathies: update and implications for clinical management. *Sports Med* 1999; 27:393–408.

8 Gibbon WW, Long G. Ultrasound of the plantar aponeurosis (fascia). *Skelet Radiol* 1999; **28**:21–26.
9 Liddle D, Rome K, Howe T. Vertical ground reaction forces in patients with unilateral plantar heel pain: a pilot study. *Gait Posture* 2000; **11**:62–66.
10 Berkowitz JF, Kier R, Rudicil S. Plantar fasciitis: MR imaging. *Radiology* 1991; **179**:665–667.
11 Schepsis AA, Leach RE, Gorzyca J, Plantar fasciitis: etiology, treatment, surgical results and review of the literature. *Clin Orthop* 1991; **266**:185–196.
12 Rubin G, Witten M. Plantar calcaneal spurs. *Am J Orthop* 1963; **5**:38–41.
13 De Inocencio J. Musculoskeletal pain in primary pediatric care: analysis of 1000 consecutive general pediatric clinic visits. *Pediatrics* 1998; **102**:E63.
14 Brody D. Running injuries. In: Nicholas JA, Hershman EB, eds. *The Lower Extremity and Spine in Sports Medicine*. St. Louis, Mosby: 1986: 1564–1566.
15 Atkins D, Crawford F, Edwards J, Lambert M. A systematic review of treatments for the painful heel. *Rheumatology* 1999; **38**:968–973.
16 Crawford F. Plantar heel pain (including plantar fasciitis). *Clin Evid* 2001; (**6**):823–831.
17 Lynch DM, Goforth WP, Martin JE, *et al.* Conservative treatment of plantar fasciitis: a prospective study. *J Am Podiatr Med Assoc* 1998; **88**:375–380.
18 Gill LH, Kiebzak GM. Outcome of nonsurgical treatment of plantar fasciitis. *Foot Ankle Int* 1996; **17**:527–532.
19 Wolgin M, Cook C, Graham C, Mauldin D. Conservative treatment of heel pain: long-term follow-up. *Foot Ankle Int* 1994; **15**:97–102.
20 Pfeffer G, Bacchetti P, Deland J, *et al.* Comparison of custom and prefabricated orthoses in the initial treatment of proximal plantar fasciitis. *Foot Ankle Int* 1999; **4**:214–221.
21 DiGiovanni BF, Nawoczenski DA, Lintal ME, *et al.* Tissue-specific plantar fascia-stretching exercise enhances outcomes in patients with chronic heel pain. *J Bone Joint Surg Am* 2003; **85**:1270–1277.
22 Liddle D, Rome K, Howe T. Vertical ground reaction forces in patients with unilateral plantar heel pain: a pilot study. *Gait Posture* 2000; **11**:62–66.
23 Katoh Y, Chao EY, Morrey BF, Laughman RK. Objective technique for evaluating painful heel syndrome and its treatment. *Foot Ankle* 1983; **3**:227–237.
24 Kogler GF, Solomonidis SE, Paul JP. Biomechanics of longitudinal arch support mechanisms in foot orthoses and their effect on plantar aponeurosis strain. *Clin Biomech* 1996; **11**:243–252.
25 Wapner KL, Sharkey PF. The use of night splints for treatment of recalcitrant plantar fasciitis. *Foot Ankle* 1991; **12**:135–137.
26 Batt ME, Tanji JL, Skattum N. Plantar fasciitis: a prospective randomized clinical trial of the tension night splint. *Clin J Sport Med* 1996; **6**:158–162.
27 Powell M, Post WR, Keener PT, Wearden S. Effective treatment of chronic plantar fasciitis with dorsiflexion night splints: a crossover prospective randomized outcome study. *Foot Ankle Int* 1998; **19**:10–18.
28 Probe RA, Baca M, Adams R, Preece C. Night splint treatment for plantar fasciitis: a prospective randomized study. *Clin Orthop* 1999; **368**:190–195.
29 Tisdel CL, Harper MC. Chronic heel pain: treatment with a short leg walking cast. *Foot Ankle Int* 1996; **17**:41–42.
30 Gudeman SD, Eisele SA, Heidt RS, Colosimo AJ, Stroupe AL. Treatment of plantar fasciitis by iontophoresis of 0.4% dexamethasone. *Am J Sports Med* 1997; **25**:312–316.
31 Crawford F, Atkins D, Young P, Edwards J. Steroid injection for heel pain: evidence of short-term effectiveness. A randomized controlled trial. *Rheumatology* 1999; **38**:974–977.
32 Acevedo JI, Beskin JL. Complications of plantar rupture associated with corticosteroid injection. *Foot Ankle Int* 1998; **19**:91–97.
33 Rompe JD, Hopf C, Nafe B, *et al.* Low energy extracorporeal shock wave therapy for painful heel: a prospective single-blind study. *Arch Orthop Surg* 1996; **115**:75–79.
34 Rompe JD, Kullmer K, Riehle HM, *et al.* Effectiveness of low energy extracorporeal shock waves for chronic plantar fasciitis. *Foot Ankle Surg* 1996; **2**:215–221.
35 Speed CA, Nicholls DW, Burnet SP, Richards CA, Hazelman BL. Extracorporeal shock wave therapy in plantar fasciitis: a pilot double blind, randomised placebo controlled study. *Rheumatology* 2000; **39** (Suppl 123):230.
36 Wild C, Khene M, Wanke S. Extracorporeal shock wave therapy in orthopedics: assessment of an emerging health technology. *Int J Technol Assess Health Care* 2000; **16**:199–209.

37 Rompe JD, Decking J, Schoellner C, Neff B. Shock wave application for chronic fasciitis in running athletes: a prospective randomized, placebo-controlled trial. *Am J Sports Med* 2003; **31**:268–275.
38 Theodore GH, Buch M, Amendola A, *et al.* Extracorporeal shock wave therapy for the treatment of plantar fasciitis. *Foot Ankle Int* 2004; **25**:290–297.
39 Mehra A, Zaman T, Jenkin AI. The use of a mobile lithotripter in the treatment of tennis elbow and plantar fasciitis. *Surgeon* 2003; **1**: 290–292.
40 Hammer DS, Adam F, Kreutz A, Kohn D, Seil R. Extracorporeal shock wave therapy (ESWT) in patients with chronic proximal plantar fasciitis: a 2-year follow-up. *Foot Ankle Int* 2003; **24**:823–828.
41 Speed CA, Nichols D, Wies J, *et al.* Extracorporeal shock wave therapy for plantar fasciitis: a double blind randomised controlled trial. *J Orthop Res* 2003; **21**:937–940.
42 Buchbinder R, Ptasznik R, Gordon J, *et al.* Ultrasound-guided extracorporeal shock wave therapy for plantar fasciitis: a randomized controlled trial. *JAMA* 2002; **288**:1364–1372.
43 Crawford F, Thomson C. Interventions for treating plantar heel pain. *Cochrane Database Syst Rev* 2003; (3):CD000416.
44 Sollitto RJ, Plotkin EL. Early clinical results of the use of radiofrequency lesioning in the treatment of plantar fasciitis. *J Foot Ankle Surg* 1997; **36**:215–219.
45 Sammarco GJ, Helfrey RB. Surgical treatment of recalcitrant plantar fasciitis. *Foot Ankle Int* 1996; **17**:520–526.
46 Stone PA, Davies JL. Retrospective review of endoscopic plantar fasciotomy, 1994–1997. *J Am Podiatr Med Assoc* 1999; **89**:89–93.
47 Davies MS, Weiss GA, Saxby TS. Plantar fasciitis: how successful is surgical intervention? *Foot Ankle Int* 1999; **20**:803–807.
48 Daly PJ, Kitaoka HB, Chao EYS. Plantar fasciotomy for intractable plantar fasciitis: clinical results and biomechanical evaluation. *Foot Ankle* 1992; **13**:188–195.
49 Fishco WD, Goecker RM, Schwartz RI. The instep plantar fasciotomy for chronic plantar fasciitis: a retrospective review. *J Am Podiatr Med Assoc* 2000; **90**:66–69.
50 Yu JS, Spigos D, Tomczak. Foot pain after a plantar fasciotomy: an MR analysis to determine potential causes. *J Comput Assist Tomogr* 1999; **23**:707–712.

Multiple-choice question answers

Chapter 1
1 = C, 2 = A, 3 = A and B

Chapter 2
1 = B, 2 = B, 3 = D, 4 = B

Chapter 3
1 = E, 2 = C, 3 = B

Chapter 4
1 = C, 2 = E, 3 = D

Chapter 5
1 = A, 2 = D, 3 = C

Chapter 6
1 = A and B, 2 = all true, 3 = A, B and C, 4 = A, B and D

Chapter 7
1 = E, 2= B, 3 = D

Chapter 8
1 = all false, 2 = A, B, C, D and E, 3 = B, C and D

Chapter 9
1 = A and B, 2 = A and C, 3 = A, B and D

Chapter 10
1 = C, 2 = B and D, 3 = B, 4 = A and D

Chapter 11
1 = D, 2 = D, 3 = D

Chapter 13
1 = D, 2 = D, 3 = C

Chapter 14
1 = D, 2 = B, 3 = C, 4 = E, 5 = A

Chapter 15
1 = B, 2 = B and C, 3 = A, B and E

Chapter 16
1 = C, 2 = B, 3 = D

Chapter 17
1 = A, 2 = D, 3 = E

Chapter 18
1 = A, 2 = A, 3 = D

Chapter 19
1 = A, 2 = C, 3 = C

Chapter 20
1 = C, 2 = A, 3 = E

Chapter 21
1 = A and D, 2 = A, B and E, 3 = A, B and E

Chapter 22
1 = B, 2 = C, 3 = E, 4 = E

Chapter 23
1 = A and B, 2 = D and E, 3 = C

Chapter 24
1 = A, 2 = B, 3 = C

Chapter 25
1 = B, C and E, 2 = B and C, 3 = A, B and C

Chapter 26
1 = A, 2 = D, 3 = C

Chapter 27
1 = A, 2 = B, 3 = B

Chapter 28
1 = B, C and E, 2 = A, B and D, 3 = A, D and E

Chapter 29
1 = C and D, 2 = A, B, D and E, 3 =A and D

Chapter 30
1 = A, 2 = C, 3 = D

Index